CLINICAL DISORDERS
OF BONE AND MINERAL
METABOLISM

Copyright © 1989 by Henry Ford Hospital

ISBN: 0-913-113-21-2

All rights reserved.

No part of this book may be reproduced, stored in a retrieval system, or transmitted in any form or by any means, electronic, mechanical, photocopying, microfilming, recording, or otherwise, without written permission from the publisher.

Printed in the United States of America.

CLINICAL DISORDERS OF BONE AND MINERAL METABOLISM

Proceedings of the Laurence and Dorothy Fallis International Symposium

EDITORS

Michael Kleerekoper, M.D.
Henry Ford Hospital Bone & Joint Specialty Center
Detroit, MI

Stephen M. Krane, M.D.
Arthritis Unit
Massachusetts General Hospital
Boston, MA

Mary Ann Liebert, Inc. publishers New York • Basel

1651 Third Avenue, New York, NY 10128 • (212) 289-2300

Preface

This book contains a compilation of papers presented at the International Symposium on Clinical Disorders of Bone and Mineral Metabolism held at the Hyatt Regency Hotel, Dearborn, Michigan, U.S.A. from May 8–13, 1988. This was the third in the series of such symposia sponsored by Henry Ford Hospital in Detroit with previous symposia in 1972 and 1983. In part the symposium was made possible through the generous support of Mrs. Dorothy Fallis and the estate of her late husband, Dr. Laurence Fallis, a former chairman of the Department of Surgery at the hospital. The activities related to osteoporosis were cosponsored by the National Osteoporosis Foundation, an important new lay organization devoted to increasing public awareness of this disease and fostering research activity aimed at reducing morbidity and mortality from osteoporosis that remains the major metabolic bone disease in Western society.

The intent of the symposium was to update clinicians in this field on the many advances that have taken place in the five years since our last symposium. Particular emphasis was placed on those areas where new information from the basic science arena was maturing to the point where it was now relevant to clinical practice and understanding clinical medicine.

A major emphasis throughout the symposium was the free exchange of ideas amongst the registrants from the 26 countries who participated. We have included at the end of each paper an edited transcript of the discussion—edited only for ease of reading. These discussions add much useful information to the text.

Each section of the book, which follows the format of the presentations at the symposium, is preceded by an overview prepared by the moderator of the session, who was in great part responsible for the overall scientific content of the session and the selection of the presenters. We are greatly indebted to these colleagues for providing a very broad coverage of this rapidly advancing field of medicine.

The symposium opened with a tribute to the late Boy Frame, M.D.—for so many years the driving force behind the emerging clinical discipline of metabolic bone disease and disorders of mineral metabolism, not only in his home base at Henry Ford Hospital but on a truly international level. He was the prime mover in developing this series of International Symposia on Clinical Disorders of Bone and Mineral Metabolism and his influence was felt throughout the week. This published proceedings is dedicated to the memory of this dear friend and colleague to whom we all owe so much.

M. Kleerekoper
S.M. Krane

Contents

Preface
  M. Kleerekoper and S.M. Krane

I Boy Frame, M.D.—In Memoriam — 1

Tribute to Dr. Boy Frame
  J.T. Potts, Jr. — 3
Surface Specific Bone Remodeling in Health and Disease
  A.M. Parfitt — 7
Mechanical Usage, Bone Mass, Bone Fragility: A Brief Overview
  H.M. Frost — 15
Discussion — 41

II Bone Remodeling — 43

Overview
  A.M. Parfitt — 45
Biochemical Markers of Bone Remodeling
  R. Marcus — 49
Discussion — 57
Effects of Age, Sex, and Race on Bone Remodeling
  R.R. Recker and R.P. Heaney — 59
Discussion — 71
In Vivo Hormonal Effects on Trabecular Bone Remodeling, Osteoid Mineralization, and Skeletal Turnover
  F. Melsen, L. Mosekilde, E.F. Eriksen, P. Charles, and T. Steinicke — 73
Discussion — 87

III Allied Disciplines — 89

Overview
  S.M. Krane — 91
Application of Molecular Genetics to Osteopenic Bone Disease
  P. Tsipouras and D.W. Rowe — 95
Discussion — 102
Hematopoietic Growth Factors
  G.D. Roodman — 105
Discussion — 111

Bone Induction
   J.A. Glowacki   113
Discussion   116
Surgical Management of Patients with Skeletal Tumors
   M.H. McGuire   117
Discussion   126

IV   Clinical Case Presentations   127

Overview
   L.V. Avioli and H.G. Bone III   129

V   Spinal Osteoporosis   133

Overview
   C.H. Chesnut III   135
Osteoporosis: 1988 and Beyond
   W.A. Peck   141
Discussion   143
Further Characterization of the Heterogeneity of the Osteoporotic Syndromes
   L.J. Melton III and B.L. Riggs   145
Discussion   152
Appropriate Use of Bone Densitometry
   H.K. Genant, J.E. Block, P. Steiger, C.C. Glueer, B. Ettinger, and S.T. Harris   153
Discussion   162
Developing Strong Bones: The Teenage Female
   V. Matkovic and D. Dekanic   165
Discussion   171
Preserving Strong Bones: The Young Adult Female
   B.L. Drinkwater   173
Discussion   179
Optimizing Bone Mass in the Perimenopause: Calcium
   R.P. Heaney   181
Discussion   187
Optimizing Bone Mass in the Perimenopause: Estrogen
   C. Christiansen and B.J. Riis   189
Discussion   197
Optimizing Bone Mass in the Perimenopause: Calcitonin and Diphosphonates
   C.H. Chesnut III   199
Discussion   202
Use of Vitamin D Metabolites in Osteoporosis
   J.C. Gallagher   205
Discussion   209
Steroids and Osteoporosis: An Unsolvable Problem?
   L.G. Raisz   211
Discussion   218

VI Metabolic Bone Disease and the Hip   225

Overview
  R. Lindsay   227
Epidemiology of Hip Fractures and Falls
  S.R. Cummings and M.C. Nevitt   231
Noninvasive Measurement of Bone Loss in the Femoral Neck
  H.W. Wahner   237
Relationship Between the Iliac Crest Bone Biopsy and Other Skeletal Sites
  D.W. Dempster   247
Stochastic Models of Femoral Bone Loss and Hip Fracture Risk
  A. Horsman and L. Burkinshaw   253
Discussion   261
Femoral Fracture: The Role of Vitamin D
  M. Peacock and L. Hordon   265
Vitamin D Nutrition and Metabolism in Aging and Osteoporosis
  T.L. Clemens   273
Discussion   280
The Orthopaedist and Hip Fractures
  J.M. Lane, C.N. Cornell, M. Bansal, S.B. Schwartz, and R. Schneider   287
Medical Management of Osteoporosis of the Hip
  M.E. Kraenzlin, E.E. Schulz, C.R. Libanati, L.A. Tudtud-Hans,
  M.R. Mariano-Menez, and D.J. Baylink   293
Discussion   297

VII PTH-Related Disorders   303

Overview
  J.P. Bilezikian and T.J. Martin   305
Approaches to the Clonality of Human Tumors and Their Application to Parathyroid Adenomas
  A. Arnold and H.M. Kronenberg   311
Physiology and Pathophysiology of Ca^{++}-Regulated PTH Release
  E.M. Brown, C.J. Chen, and M.S. Leboff   317
Multiple Endocrine Neoplasia Type I: Role of a Circulating Growth Factor in Parathyroid Cell Hyperplasia
  M.L. Brandi, M.B. Zimering, S.J. Marx, D. DeGrange, P. Goldsmith, K. Sakaguchi,
  and G.D. Aurbach   323
Discussion   329
G Proteins as Signal Transducers
  M.A. Levine   333
Pseudohypoparathyroidism: Studies of the Pathogenesis of Parathyroid Hormone Resistance
  D. Goltzman, J.A. Mitchell, and G.N. Hendy   341
Discussion   347

Primary Hyperparathyroidism: The Surgically Cured Patient
    S. Ljunghall, C. Joborn, M. Palmér, J. Rastad, and G. Åkerström   353
Primary Hyperparathyroidism in the 1980s
    J.P. Bilezikian, S.J. Silverberg, and E. Shane   359
Discussion   362

VIII Metabolic Bone Disease in Children   367

Overview
    M.P. Whyte   369
Osteopetrosis with Renal Tubular Acidosis and Cerebral Calcification: The Carbonic
    Anhydrase II Deficiency Syndrome
    W.S. Sly   373
Discussion   381
Pediatric Forms of Hypophosphatasia
    M.P. Whyte   383
Discussion   392
Williams Syndrome
    R.W. Chesney   395
Discussion   403
The Molecular Basis of Clinical Heterogeneity in Osteogenesis Imperfecta
    P.H. Byers, D.H. Cohn, B.J. Starman, G.A. Wallis, and M.C. Willing   407
Discussion   414
Neonatal Disorders of Mineral Metabolism
    L.S. Hillman   415
Discussion   421
Vitamin D Resistant Hypophosphatemic Rickets (VDRR): Pathogenesis and Medical
    Treatment
    F.H. Glorieux   425
Discussion   429

IX Vitamin D in Health and Disease   433

Overview
    N.H. Bell   435
1,25-Dihydroxyvitamin D_3 Receptor Structure and Function
    M.R. Haussler   439
Hereditary Resistance to 1,25-Dihydroxyvitamin D: Pathophysiology, Diagnosis,
    and Treatment
    U.A. Liberman and S.J. Marx   447
The Role of Phosphorus in Modulating Vitamin D Metabolism in Health and Disease
    R.C. Morris, Jr., B.P. Halloran, and A.A. Portale   455
Discussion   464
Clinical Disorders of Phosphorus and Vitamin D Metabolism
    T. Nesbitt, G.A. Davidai, P.C. Brazy, and M.K. Drezner   469

Abnormal Vitamin D and Calcium Metabolism in Sarcoidosis and Related Diseases
  Y. Liel, J. Basile, and N.H. Bell 475
The Effects of Race and Body Habitus on the Vitamin D Endocrine System
  S. Epstein and N.H. Bell 481
Discussion 486

X Clinical Disorders of Bone and Mineral Metabolism 493

Overview
  G.R. Mundy 495
Pathophysiology of Hypercalcaemia
  J.A. Kanis, E. McCloskey, N. Hamdy, D. O'Doherty, and D. Bickerstaff 499
Discussion 508
Hypercalcemia—Solid Tumors
  T.J. Martin 509
Discussion 515
Mechanisms of Hypercalcemia in Hematologic Malignancies
  G.R. Mundy 517
Discussion 522
Paget's Disease of Bones: Assessment, Therapy, and Secondary Prevention
  O.L.M. Bijvoet, C.J.L.R. Vellenga, and H.I.J. Harinck 525
Renal Calculi: Update
  C.Y.C. Pak 543
Discussion 551
Current Problems in Renal Osteodystrophy
  B.F. Boyce, Z. Mocan, D.J. Halls, and B.J.R. Junor 553
Discussion 561
The Pathogenesis and Clinical Course of Multiple Endocrine Neoplasia, Type 2A
  R.F. Gagel 563
Discussion 570

XI Therapeutic Advances in Metabolic Bone Disease 573

Overview
  H. Heath III 575
Biphosphonate Treatment of Severe Hypercalcemia
  J.J. Body 581
Potential Use of Gallium Nitrate and WR-2721 in the Treatment of Hypercalcemia and Hyperparathyroidism
  J.-P. Bonjour, R. Rizzoli, and J. Caverzasio 589
Discussion 594
Therapy of Aluminum Related Bone Disease
  H.H. Malluche and M.-C. Faugere 597
Discussion 602
The Role of Sodium Fluoride in the Treatment of Osteoporosis
  B.L. Riggs, S.F. Hodgson, and R. Eastell 605
Discussion 611

New Methods of Administration of Estrogens 613
   R. Lindsay
Discussion 619
Parathyroid Peptide (hPTH 1-34) in the Treatment of Osteoporosis
   J. Reeve, U.M. Davies, M. Arlot, J.N. Bradbeer, J.R. Green, R. Hesp, C. Edouard,
   P. Hulme, R.D. Podbesek, D. Katz, J.M. Zanelli, and P.J. Meunier 621
Discussion 629

Author Index 631

Subject Index 633

I
Boy Frame, M.D.
In Memoriam

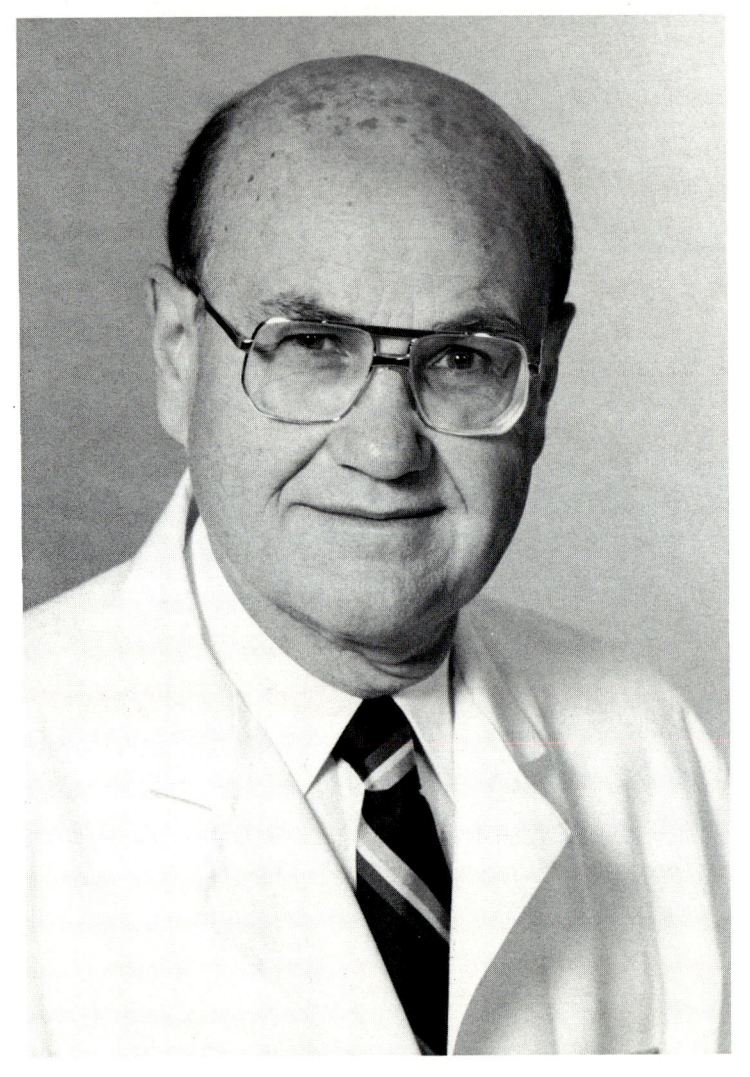

Boy Frame, M.D.
1923–1986

Tribute to Dr. Boy Frame

JOHN T. POTTS, JR.

*Harvard Medical School
and General Medical Services
Massachusetts General Hospital
Boston, MA*

I am deeply honored to be chosen to pay tribute to Dr. Boy Frame. Many of you here know him personally and have worked with him over a much longer period of time than I have. We began to work closely together when I served as his co-chairman for the previous symposium on calcium and bone metabolism, given here at the Henry Ford Hospital, a little over five years ago. From that time on I have had the pleasure of getting to know Boy well and have had the opportunity to learn first hand of his devotion to excellence, and his tireless energy.

I would like to speak about Boy Frame in terms of his remarkable professional accomplishments. He was an outstanding physician, a strong and original contributor in clinical investigation in calcium and bone metabolism, and a leader in medicine at the Henry Ford Hospital and in the American College of Physicians. As a person Boy was widely admired for his kindness and devotion to serving others. In order to capture something of the spirit of the personal qualities of Boy, particularly over earlier phases of his career when I did not know him so well, I will take the liberty of quoting from family, friends, and close colleagues who have paid tribute on earlier occasions to Boy Frame the man, as well as Boy Frame the professional.

A passion for education and learning, which marked him from an early period in his life, took him east from Iowa to Cheshire Academy, and then to Yale University. Yale held Boy's interest over an eight year period; after graduating as an undergraduate Boy continued in the Medical School, graduating as an MD cum laude in 1948 with an outstanding record of achievement, receiving awards for the best record in basic sciences and anatomy and the highest rank in his class. Boy then interned at the Massachusetts General Hospital in 1948-49, and then became an Assistant Resident for 1949-50. As an early sign of his interest in the educational and training philosophy of different institutions Boy then took an associate residency, 1950-51, back at the Yale Medical Center.

The Korean War then interrupted Boy's medical training. He served as a Captain in the US Air Force in Korea. One of Boy's colleagues, Dr. Raymond Mellinger, noted in his tribute to Boy that this period of serving in the military greatly impressed the then Captain Frame, and that his participation in the great military events of that time seemed to provide a stimulus to his life-long interest in history. Upon his discharge from the Air Force Boy next took an assistant residency in Neurology at the Neurological Institute and the Presbyterian Hospital in New York City 1954-55. He then returned to the Massachusetts General Hospital as a Senior Resident, 1955-56, during which period he also served as a Teaching Fellow at the Harvard Medical School. At this point Boy headed to the midwest and accepted his first staff and faculty position as Associate Physician in the Department of Internal Medicine at Henry Ford Hospital. This appointment signaled the beginning of Boy's remarkable career as a physician, clinical investigator, and medical leader. He served with great distinction in many phases of clinical and academic life at this institution over the next thirty years, until his death in August of 1986, at which point he was serving as the Chairman of the Department of Medicine and Clinical Professor of Medicine at the University of Michigan School of Medicine.

The remarkable qualities of Boy Frame, the physician, are well known to his hundreds of patients that he served with devotion, and to his many colleagues with whom he worked over the years at Henry Ford and elsewhere. He served as Physician in Charge of the Fifth Medical Divison and the Physician in Charge of the Bone and Mineral Divison at Henry Ford from 1961 onward. Dr. Fred Whitehouse of this institution who gave one of the tributes to Boy referred to him as Michigan's "internists' internist". This phrase is often applied but I think in Boy's case, from everything I know, it was truly an understatement. From his many colleagues here one learns of his enthusiasm on ward rounds, his skill in bedside teaching, and his emphasis on the importance of bedside teaching. His interest focused not only on the difficult and challenging problems in patient diagnosis and management, but also, typical of his warmth and broad perspective, on the sociological and psychological aspects of the care of his patients.

I remember my pleasure in talking with Boy about his clinical practice and his devotion to the educational efforts needed to keep internists at their best informed and sharpest. He repeatedly undertook the recertification examinations of the American Board of Internal Medicine and helped encourage others to do so. I enjoyed personally perusing his marvelous collections of textbooks, teaching reviews, and anatomical and radiological atlases.

His patients and his colleagues know better than those of us who did not work directly with him what an outstanding physician he was. All of us, however, can appreciate from the published record his outstanding contributions to clinical investigation in calcium and bone metabolism. Among his two hundred and thirty publications are many examples of descriptions or analyses of unusual clinical syndromes, particularly those involving the skeleton or mineral ion metabolism. Among the cases that interested him were migratory osteolysis, the association of spondylitis with hypoparathyroidism, osteomalacia induced by phenophthalein, mast cells and osteoporosis, pseudohypohyperparathyroidism (the puzzling association of osteitis fibrosa and hypoparathyroidism in patients with pseudohypoparathyroidism) unusual presentations of hypervitaminosis-A, cases of totally unexplained hypercalcemia, unusual variations of osteosclerosis combined with hyperostosis, and the bone disease seen in total parenteral nutrition. At the same time that Boy tackled with enthusiasm and a questioning mind these puzzling cases that he encountered in his busy clinical practice, and which he enthusiastically shared with colleagues in an attempt to understand the pathogenesis, he wrote in many highly useful classical reviews on syndromes of osteoporosis, osteomalacia, and diagnosis and management of patients with hyercalcemia.

In the proceedings of the conferences on calcium and bone metabolism from this institution published in 1973 and 1983 one finds many unusual case reports of puzzling syndromes that Boy encouraged his colleagues to present and discuss. What I always admired about Boy was that he would present the clinical problem as it was seen, challenging us to try to explain syndromes that had an annoying propensity for not fitting in with any of our comfortable schemes of classification or pathogenesis. This was typical of his deep zest for new knowledge and the challenging honesty of his clinical investigation. His great interest in the unusual aspects of metabolic bone disease led to his much deserved appointment to the Life Science Advisory Committee of NASA where he served with distinction.

A further and remarkable testament to Boy Frame's prodigious energy and personal effectiveness is evident when one considers his leadership role at the Henry Ford Hospital and in his beloved professional organization, the American College of Physicians. Despite and throughout his busy life as a general internist, specialist in clinical problems of calcium and bone metabolism, and clinical investigator, he served with great distinction at the Henry Ford Hospital and the College. At the hospital, as is evident from his curriculum vitae and from what I have learned from his colleagues, he made remarkable contributions in wide ranging areas of the hospital governance and issues of review and certification of professional standards and professional postgraduate education. The list of his hospital committee assignments is staggering. I was personally delighted when I learned that Boy had been named Chief of Medicine at Henry Ford Hospital in 1985, a recognition which he richly deserved and is a measure of the appreciation of his colleagues for his remarkable leadership role. Unfortunately, he did not have the opportunity to serve very long in a post to which he would have greatly added to his own and the institution's distinction, I am certain.

Boy did have the opportunity, however, to serve for many years in a variety of effective roles in the American College of Physicians. I know from my conversations with him and from many other colleagues around the country, how important this activity was to Boy and how effective he was in his several roles with the College in its professional and educational activities. He served as the Govenor for Michigan of the American College of Physicians from 1977 to 1982. He was made Chairman of the Board of Governors of the College in 1982 and then in 1983 a regent of The American College of Physicians. During this period of service, Boy made remarkable contributions to the vigor of the activities of the College, representing professional standards of physicians in Michigan and initiating a number of exciting postgraduate educational activities. Dr. Raymond Mellinger, in reflecting on Boy's service to the college stated, "no one in my recent memory has contributed more to the life of the Michigan chapter of the College, than did Boy Frame". Robert Moser stated, "the Michigan chapter became the prototype of what the ideal College chapter should be. He (Boy Frame) was like a bubbling fountain of new ideas. He exuded enthusiasm and optimism. His formula for the successful regional meeting became a College legend. It caught fire in a dozen states." Boy's remarkable contributions to the College were recognized by his colleagues posthumously by his election to the distinguished post of Mastership of the American College of Physicians.

I had the privilege of listening to an audiovisual tape of an interview that Dr. Marshall Goldberg held with Boy Frame after he became Chief of the Medical Service. Boy pointed out the enthusiasm that he had felt for the great medical educators in his past such as Dr. Peters at Yale and Drs. Walter Bauer, James Howard Means, and Chester Jones at the MGH. When he was asked why medicine had attracted him, he stated that he could not remember when it first occurred to him to enter medicine. Rather, he remembers only being sustained by two goals in his medical career: the intellectual challenge of medicine and the opportunity to help patients with disease.

Boy spoke warmly of the strength and critical help that Jane Frame provided for him throughout their personal life together and his professional career. He explained how Jane had helped him in editing many of his papers. He admitted that at times he was so busy that he forgot to relax, but that it was Jane who reminded him that it was time for them to play tennis. I remember well, incidentally, how formidable Jane and Boy were as a tennis doubles team when they quietly trounced my wife and me during an encounter on the court here at the time of last symposium. Boy was devoted to his children Richard, Abby and Robin and reveled in their successes in life and in work.

I recall, from the audiovisual interview, that Dr. Goldberg had great difficulty in getting Boy to list what he would like to be remembered by. Boy was very modest about any contributions that he had made and finally decided that if there was anything, it was the importance of strong and supportive interactions with patients and with young colleagues, most of all, stimulating young physicians to excel. When asked what advice he would give to young physicians starting their careers, he said the following. Set a goal and don't be diverted from achieving it. Maintain high standards and be broad as a clinician.

Boy Frame, indeed, epitomized in his own life these remarkable goals. His son, Dr. Richard Frame, in his moving tribute to Dr. Boy Frame, stated, "He had reached the pinnacle of his career and had done everything he wanted to do. There was really very little challenge left for him. In leaving this earth, I believe he transcended into a higher level of existence."

Dr. Boy Frame, we salute you. We hope that your example will inspire others; this is the greatest tribute that could be paid to you.

Surface Specific Bone Remodeling in Health and Disease

A.M. PARFITT

Bone and Mineral Research Laboratory
Henry Ford Hospital
Detroit, MI

INTRODUCTION:
   One of Harold Frost's early insights was that bone cells behave differently on different surfaces, even though exposed to the same concentrations of minerals and hormones (1). Frost first applied the term "envelope" to bone, but this term is often misused. It is the three-dimensional counterpart of a two-dimensional closed boundary, which divides space into two regions, an inside and an outside (2). A bone only has two envelopes, an outer and an inner. The outer, or periosteal envelope, includes the subchondral as well as the periosteal surface, and the inner or endosteal envelope includes cancellous, endocortical and intracortical (or Haversian) sub-divisions that are in continuity. All bone lies outside the endosteal envelope and all marrow and other soft tissues lie inside it. Throughout life the periosteal envelope gains bone, and the endosteal envelope loses bone, except for a brief period during the adolescent growth spurt. No more will be said about the periosteal envelope, but the differences between the three subdivisions of the endosteal envelope will be examined in detail.
   The distinction between cortical and cancellous bone tissue is generally familiar, but the distinction, long made by anatomists, between bones of the appendicular and axial skeleton (Table 1) has only recently been acknowledged

FEATURE	APPENDICULAR	AXIAL
Main bone tissue	Cortical	Cancellous
Main soft tissue	Muscle	Viscera
Main joint type	Synovial	Various
Cortices	Thick	Thin
With age, cancellous tissue	Contracts[a]	Expands[b]
Marrow	Fatty	Hematopoietic
Turnover	Low	High

TABLE 1. Subdivisions of the skeleton. a. Because of retreat of diaphyseal border towards metaphysis. b. Because of cancellization of inner region of cortex.

by clinical investigators. Anatomically the pelvis is classified as appendicular, but functionally it is more appropriate to classify it as axial. In general cortical bone has a higher turnover than cancellous bone, but the explanation for this resides mainly in their geometrical differences, particularly in the ratio of bone surface to bone volume. The generally lower turnover of the appendicular than the axial skeleton reflects its higher proportion of cortical bone, but is also influenced by the character of the bone marrow. Hematopoiesis normally disappears from the appendicular skeleton by age 25, but persists in the axial skeleton throughout life. It is the presence of hematopoietic marrow that makes the ilium reasonably representative of the axial skeleton. Because remodeling is more active adjacent to hematopoietic than to fatty marrow, the cancellous bone of the distal radius turns over more slowly than the cortical bone of the ilium (3). The cellularity of the marrow is not the only determinant of cancellous bone turnover in the appendicular skeleton, and other influences, most likely biomechanical, are also important.

Typical cortical bone tissue, with its pores of various sizes and typical cancellous bone tissue, with its much larger marrow spaces, are easy to recognize, but the demarcation between these two types of tissue is imprecise. Similarly, differentiation of the intracortical from the other two components of the endosteal envelope is usually straightforward, but distinction between the endocortical and cancellous sub-divisions is more difficult and subject to observer disagreement. We make the demarcation based on the sizes of the intracortical spaces, their distance from the endosteal envelope, and the diameters of the trabeculae as they merge with the cortex (4;Figure 1). The

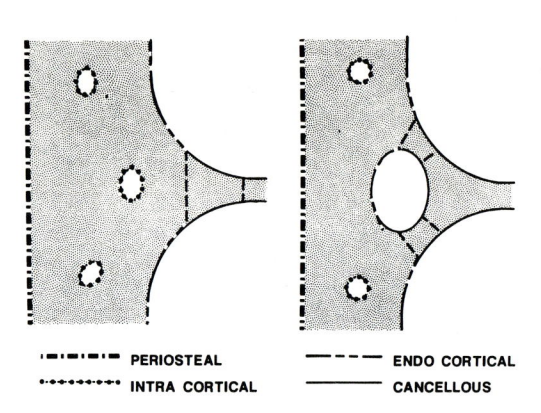

Figure 1. Demarcation between different subdivisions of the endosteal envelope. Since the subendocortical space enlarges with increasing age, a region of surface classified as intracortical in a young person (left) could be reclassified as either endocortical or cancellous in an older person (right).

complexity of the remodeling process in this region is such that the same element of surface can change from endocortical to intracortical, or from endocortical to cancellous even within a few months. There is much to be said for treating this as a separate region, termed the transitional zone (5). But in the studies reported, every region of surface present at the time of biopsy has been allocated to one of the three sub-divisions according to the observers best judgement; any errors in allocation would make it more difficult to detect systematic differences.

PRIMARY HYPERPARATHYROIDISM

18 post-menopausal women with primary hyperparathyroidism were compared with 27 healthy post-menopausal women of similar age. Bone formation rate per unit of bone surface, wall thickness and osteoclast extent were measured separately on the cancellous, endocortical and intracortical surfaces (6) and activation frequency was calculated as wall thickness divided by formation rate (7). An index of bone loss was also obtained for each surface. Since the increase in porosity was due more to an increase in the size rather than in the number of pores, mean pore radius indirectly calculated was used as the index of intracortical bone loss. Bone loss from the endocortical surface was estimated as mean cortical thickness, and loss from the cancellous surface estimated as one-half of mean trabecular thickness, since there was no difference between the groups in trabecular number.

The data were used to obtain an estimate of the change in mean resorption depth on each surface. The annual rate of loss was estimated by dividing the total loss by an estimated mean disease duration of 20 years. This is based on the mean age in the patients of about 60 years, and the epidemiologic observation that in the great majority of patients primary hyperparathyroidism is known to begin after the age of 40 (8). Dividing the annual loss by the probability of initiating remodeling gives an estimate of the average amount of bone lost by each complete cycle, which is the difference between the change in resorption depth and the change in wall-thickness. Rearranging this equation leads to an estimate of the change in resorption depth (Table 2). This is a minimum estimate; if the duration of the disease was less than

1. (BFR/BS)/W.Th = Activation frequency (Ac.f)
2. Total loss/duration = Annual loss
3. Annual loss/Ac.f = ΔR.De - ΔW.Th
4. ΔR.De = Annual loss/Ac.f + ΔW.Th

TABLE 2. Calculation of resorption depth (R.De) BFR/BS = Bone formation rate per unit of bone surface. W.Th = Wall thickness

20 years, as it likely was in many of the patients, the change in resorption depth required to produce the observed loss of bone would be greater than the estimate. The result represents an average resorption depth for all the previous teams of osteoclasts that have been active on the surface over the duration of the disease, and thus differs from the elegant reconstruction methods of Eriksen (9), which produce estimates of current resorption depth.

The hyperparathyroid patients showed an approximately two-fold increase in formation rate and activation frequency on each surface, no difference in wall thickness on any surface, and significant bone loss and increased osteoclast extent only on the endocortical surface (6). The calculated change in resorption depth was trivial on the cancellous and intracortical surfaces, but was substantial on the endocortical surface, amounting to about 40% of the mean value (Table 3). This indicates that the major cellular mechanism of

Surface	Total Loss (μm)	Annual loss[a] (μm)	Δ W.Th (μm)	Ac.f (/y)	Δ R.De (μm)
Cancellous	8	0.4	-0.34	0.91	+0.10
Cortical	8	0.4	-0.45	0.69	+0.13
Endocortical	414	20.7	-2.58	0.84	+22.1

TABLE 3. Remodeling imbalance in HPT   a. Mean disease duration of 20 y is assumed.

cortical bone loss from the axial skeleton is increased depth of resorption cavities on the endocortical surface, and as a more general conclusion, that adjacent bone surfaces in continuity may respond differently to the same humoral stimuli.

The inferred mechanism of cortical bone loss is probably also applicable to the appendicular skeleton. Garn's cross sectional data for metacarpal dimensions (10) suggest an average annual net loss from the endocortical surface of 20 μm between 30 and 80 years of age. Over the same period there is a reduction of approximately 15 μm in cancellous wall thickness (11); taking 10 μm as a generous estimate of the average reduction over this 50 year period, and making the unlikely assumption that the frequency of remodeling activation is 50% higher on the endocortical surface of the metacarpal than on the corresponding surface of the ilium, it is possible to explain only a small fraction of the observed loss without the assumption of a substantial increase in resorption cavity depth (12; Table 4). This concept has recently received

Observed total loss (30-80y)	=	1000 μm
Average annual loss	=	20 μm/y
Maximum net loss/cycle[a]	=	10 μm
Maximum activation frequency	=	0.5/y
Explained annual loss (=10 * 0.5)	=	5 μm/y

Table 4. Endocortical bone loss in the metacarpal a. Assuming constant resorption cavity depth.

direct confirmation in man by serial micro-radioscopy of the metacarpal (13), showing enlargement of sub-endocortical cavities and perforation of the thin shell of initially cortical bone overlying the cavity, leading ultimately to union with the marrow space. Although sub-endocortical cavities, whether demonstrated histologically or radiographically, appear to be separated from the marrow in a particular section or slice, in the third-dimension they communicate with, and undoubtedly arise from, a resorptive process initiated on the endocortical surface in contact with the marrow (14).

AGE-RELATED BONE LOSS AND VERTEBRAL FRACTURE PATHOGENESIS

The 27 healthy post-menopausal women of mean age 61 mentioned earlier, were compared with 24 healthy pre-menopausal women of mean age 37, and 78 women with at least one vertebral compression fracture of mean age 66 who met the entry criteria for a controlled clinical trial of sodium fluoride. The methods were the same as in the previous study with the addition of adjusted apposition rate, an index of the speed at which osteoblast teams work (15), and bone surface/bone volume and bone surface/tissue volume ratios (15). Since the endocortical surface is the inner border of the cortex and remodeling on the endocortical surface produces turnover of cortical bone, the endocortical and haversian components of the surface were added together as well as examined separately. Measurements on the endocortical and intra-cortical surfaces have been completed only on about 2/3 of the patients with osteoporosis.

In cancellous bone the bone surface/bone volume ratio does not change with age or menopause in normal subjects, but increases significantly in patients with compression fracture, as a reflection of the greater degree of trabecular thinning. In cortical bone the ratio, initially much smaller, increases with age or menopause in both groups, but to a greater extent in the osteoporotic patients. By contrast, the ratio of bone surface to tissue volume (including the soft tissues) in young healthy women is essentially identical in cancellous and cortical bone tissue, but after age or menopause the ratio decreases in cancellous bone but increases in cortical bone. The extent of surface available for remodeling per unit of bone tissue is significantly higher in cortical than in cancellous bone in post-menopausal women, a difference that is exaggerated in those with osteoporosis.

There was no significant fall in iliac cortical thickness after menopause, although the measurements were checked by both direct and indirect methods (15). A significant fall in iliac cortical thickness with age has been shown in autopsy studies (16), but the changes may be smaller in healthy free-living subjects, as recently reported for cancellous bone (17), because of the over-representation of ethanol abusers among subjects who have undergone sudden violent death. Cortical thickness was substantially reduced in the patients with osteoporosis, and the relative deficit was about 30% for both cortical thickness and cancellous bone volume. The likely mechanism was an increase in resorption activity depth on the endocortical surface, as in the rib (18). Cortical porosity also increased significantly after menopause, but to about the same extent in both normal and osteoporotic groups.

We confirmed that wall thickness fell significantly with age or menopause (11), but contrary to earlier reports (19) the magnitude of this change did not differ significantly between the normal and osteoporotic subjects. In both groups the fall in wall-thickness was confined to the cancellous surface, and no such fall was found on either the endocortical or haversian surfaces. Adjusted apposition rate fell significantly after menopause in both groups, and was significantly lower in the osteoporotic than in the normal subjects. But this change also was confined to the cancellous bone surface, and none of the differences for the endocortical or haversian surface were significant, either between pre- and post-menopause or between normal and osteoporotic subjects. Thus, the fall in osteoblast team work with age or menopause, both for amount and for rate and the further fall in rate in osteoporosis are surface specific.

Surface-based bone formation rate increased after menopause on all surfaces in normal subjects. Although statistically significant only on the cancellous surface, when the three surfaces were combined the difference became even more significant. In patients with fracture, the mean value was significantly lower on the cancellous surface than in healthy subjects of similar age, but just as high or even higher on the other surfaces, and on the endocortical surface formation wate was significantly higher than in the pre-menopausal normal subjects (20). The extent of osteoclast surface also increased after menopause on all surfaces, and the difference was more significant when the three surfaces were combined. In patients with fracture the extent of cancellous osteoclast surface was significantly lower than in post-menopausal normal subjects, but on the endocortical surface the post-menopausal increase was exaggerated.

By multiplying the surface-based bone formation rates by the appropriate ratio of surface to volume one obtains estimates of volume-based bone formation rates. When bone volume is used as the referent, the result of the calculation is an index of bone turnover. Although the probability of remodeling activation is the same on all subdivisions of the endocortical surface, because the ratio of surface to bone volume is higher in cancellous bone, the rate of turnover is also higher. In normal post-menopausal subjects this difference is exaggerated, but in patients with compression fracture the difference is reduced. When tissue volume, including the soft tissue, is used as the referent, the result of the calculation is a quantity that would be expected to have a greater influence on the various biochemical markers of bone remodeling (15). When the data are expressed in this way, bone formation is higher in cortical than in cancellous bone tissue, and this difference is exaggerated by normal menopause and exaggerated even further in patients with osteoporosis, in whom there is almost four times as much bone formed per unit of tissue volume in cortical bone tissue than in cancellous bone tissue.

We have confirmed once again our previous finding that in patients with vertebral compression fracture, cancellous bone formation rates are significantly lower than in healthy post-menopausal subjects without fracture (21-23). This observation appears to be in conflict with various biochemical indices of bone remodeling, which have suggested that formation rates are increased in patients with vertebral fracture. Several explanations have been suggested to account for this discrepancy (23), but the present data suggest that it is largely due to the different characteristics of remodeling on the cancellous and other bone surfaces. Those who favor the biochemical approach may regard this as a vindication of their methods, but I draw the entirely different conclusion that the biochemical methods fail completely to identify the abnormalities of bone remodeling that are most critical to the pathogenesis of vertebral fracture.

Osteopenia is a necessary but not a sufficient condition for the occurrence of fracture. Reduced axial bone mass in osteoporosis involves, both cortical and cancellous bone, and results from some combination of subnormal accumulation and excessive loss due to the systemic effects of menopause. Among the total population of women with untreated estrogen deficiency and disproportionate axial osteopenia who are thereby placed at risk, those who will sustain vertebral fracture are selected in part by two abnormalities of bone remodeling that are confined to the cancellous surface - reduced frequency of remodeling activation that leads to an increase in bone age and increased risk of microfracture, and an exaggeration of the age-related decline in osteoblast vigor that is likely to diminish the repair of microfracture (Figure 2). This must be the result of factors that are not only *local*, in the sense of intrinsic to bone rather than systemic, but additionally are *focal*, in the sense that they are confined only to one subdivision of the endosteal envelope.

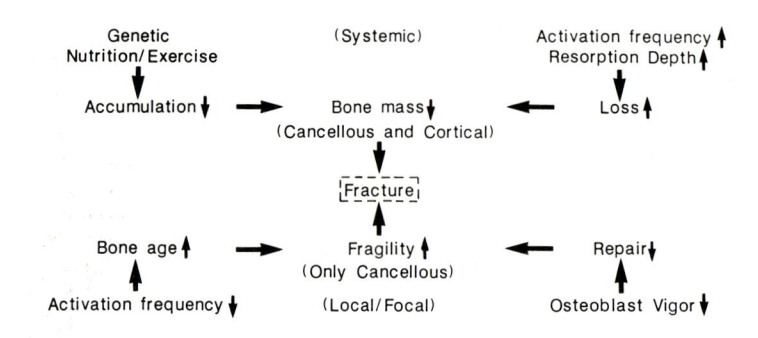

Figure 2. Pathogenesis of vertebral fracture. Preferential axial osteopenia involves both cancellous and cortical bone tissue and results mainly from systemic factors. Increased fragility affects only cancellous bone tissue and is the result of unidentified local and/or focal factors. Note that activation frequency may be increased and decreased at different times, each contributing in different ways to the final result.

CONCLUSIONS:

1. In both hyperparathyroidism and osteoporosis cortical thinning is probably the result of increased resorption depth on the endocortical surface.
2. In hyperparathyroidism there is preferential loss of cortical bone, whether axial or appendicular, but in osteoporosis there is preferential loss from the axial skeleton, whether cortical or cancellous.
3. The recruitment of new osteoclast and osteoblast teams increases with age or menopause on all surfaces, but the amount and rate of bone formed by osteoblast teams falls with age or menopause only on the cancellous surface.
4. In patients with vertebral fracture the increase in cell team recruitment is reversed on the cancellous surface and exaggerated on the endocortical surface, but the fall in osteoblast vigor with age or menopause is exaggerated on the cancellous but not on the other surfaces.
5. Bone formation per unit of tissue volume is higher in cortical than in cancellous bone, a difference that increases with age or menopause and even increases even further in patients with osteoporosis.
6. The discrepancy between biochemical and histologic approaches to the study of bone remodeling in osteoporosis is largely accounted for by differences in remodeling characteristics between different subdivisions of the endosteal envelope.
7. Current biochemical markers of bone remodeling give some indication of mechanisms and rates of bone loss, but are of no value in studying the pathogenesis of bone fragility.
8. Vertebral fracture pathogenesis reflects the interplay of systemic, local, and focal (or surface specific) factors, the latter accounting for defects in the recruitment and activity of osteoblast teams confined to the cancellous surface.

REFERENCES:

1. Frost HM. The Bone Dynamics in Osteoporosis and Osteomalacia. Charles C. Thomas, Springfield, Il. 1966.
2. Parfitt AM. Terminology and symbols in bone morphometry. In: Jaworski ZFG, ed. Proceedings of the First International Workshop on Bone Morphometry. Ottawa, Ottawa University Press, 1976:331-335.
3. Parfitt AM. The composition, structure and remodeling of bone: A basis for the interpretation of bone mineral measurements. In: Dequeker J,

Geusens P, Wahner HW, eds. Bone Mineral Measurements by Photon Absorptiometry: Methodological Problems. Leuven University Press, Leuven, Belgium, 1988.

4. Duncan H. Cortical porosis: A morphological evaluation. In: Jaworski ZFG, ed. Proceedings of the First International Workshop on Bone Morphometry. Ottawa, Ottawa University Press, 1979:331-335.

5. Keshawarz NM, Recker RB. Expansion of the medullary cavity at the expense of cortex in postmenopausal osteoporosis. Metab Bone Dis Rel Res 1984;5:223-228.

6. Parfitt AM, Kleerekoper M, Rao D. Stanciu J, Villanueva AR. Cellular mechanisms of cortical thinning in primary hyperparathyroidism (PHPT). J Bone Min Res 1987;2(Supp 1):384.

7. Parfitt AM. The physiologic and clinical significance of bone histomorphometric data. In: Recker R, ed. Bone Histomorphometry. Techniques and Interpretations. Boca Raton, CRC Press, 1983:143-223.

8. Heath H III, Hodgson SF, Kennedy MA. Primary hyperparathyroidism: Incidence, morbidity and potential impact in a community. N Engl J Med 302:189.

9. Eriksen EF. Normal and pathological remodeling of human trabecular bone: Three dimensional reconstruction of the remodeling sequence in normals and in metabolic bone disease. Endocrine Reviews 1986;4:379-408.

10. Garn SM. The earlier gain and the latter loss of cortical bone. Charles C. Thomas, Springfield, Il. 1970.

11. Lips P, Courpron P, Meunier PJ. Mean wall thickness of trabecular bone packets in the human iliac crest: changes with age. Calc Tiss Res 1978;26:13-17.

12. Parfitt AM. Age-related structural changes in trabecular and cortical bone: Cellular mechanism and biomechanical consequences. a) Differences between rapid and slow bone loss. b) Localized bone gain. Calc Tissue Int 1984;36:S123-S128.

13. Meema HE, Meema S. Longitudinal microradioscopic comparisons on endosteal and juxtaendosteal bone loss in premenopausal and postmenopausal women, and in those with end-stage renal disease. Bone 1988,8:343-350.

14. Duncan H, Hanson CA, Curtiss A. The different effects of soluble and crystalline hydrocortisone of bone. Calcif Tiss Res 1973;12:159-168.

15. Parfitt AM, Drezner MK, Glorieux FH, Kanis JA, Malluche H, Meunier PJ, Ott SM, Recker RR. Bone histomorphometry nomenclature, symbols and units. Report of the ASBMR Histomorphometry Nomenclature Committee. J Bone Min Res 1987;2:595-610.

16. Courpron P, Meunier P, Bressot C, Giroux JM. Amount of bone in iliac crest biopsy. Significance of the trabecular bone volume. Its values in normal and in pathological conditions. In: Meunier PJ, ed. Bone Histomorphometry, Second International Workshop, Armour Montagu, Paris, 1977.

17. Recker RR, Kimmel DB, Parfitt AM, Davies KM, Keshawarz N, Hinders S. Static and tetracycline-based bone histomorphometric data from 34 normal postmenopausal females. J Bone Min Res 1988;2:133-144.

18. Wu K, Frost HM. Bone resorption rates in physiological, senile and postmenopausal osteoporosis. J Lab Clin Med 1967;69:810-818.

19. Darby AJ, Meunier PJ. Mean wall thickness and formation periods of trabecular bone packets in idiopathic osteoporosis. Calcif Tissue Int 1981;33:199-204.

20. Brown JP, Delmas PD, Arlot M, Meunier PJ. Active bone turnover of the cortico-endosteal envelope in postmenopausal osteoporosis. J Clin Endo Metab 1987;5:954-959.

21. Parfitt AM, Mathews C, Rao D, Frame B, Kleerekoper M, Villanueva AR. Impaired osteoblast function in metabolic bone disease. In: DeLuca HF, Frost H, Jee W, Johnston C, Parfitt AM, eds. Osteoporosis: Recent Advances in Pathogenesis and Treatment. Baltimore, University Park Press, 1981:321-330.

22. Parfitt AM, Mathews CHE, Villanueva AR, Rao DS, Rogers M, Kleerekoper M,

Frame B. Microstructural and cellular basis of age related bone loss and osteoporosis. In: Frame B, Potts JT Jr, eds. Clinical Disorders of Bone and Mineral Metabolism. Amsterdam, Excerpta Medica, 1983:328-332.

23. Parfitt AM, Kleerekoper M. Diagnostic value of bone histomorphometry and comparison of histologic measurements and biochemical indices of bone remodeling. In: Christiansen C, Arnaud CD, Nordin BEC, Parfitt AM, Peck WA, Riggs BL, eds. Osteoporosis. Proc Copenhagen International Symposium on Osteoporosis, June 3-8, 1984. Aalborg Stiftsbogtrykkeri, pp. 111-120.

Mechanical Usage, Bone Mass, Bone Fragility: A Brief Overview

H.M. FROST

Southern Colorado Clinic
Pueblo, CO

I. Introduction.

After 1980 growing numbers of clinicians began to appreciate how mechanical usage effects on bone mass and architecture might relate to problems of metabolic bone disease, growth and development, orthopaedics, physical and sports medicine, rheumatology and skeletal pathology, among other things. Some formerly enigmatic pathogenetic mechanisms of those effects are now known, and in that regard this article summarizes how mechanical influences on three principal biologic activities of our skeletons can affect bone mass, architecture and fragility. Accumulated evidence has changed those once esoteric matters into ones of direct clinical usefulness. In the process it created new terminology and concepts that have weathered earlier controversies and confusion and begin to enter the human and veterinary clinical domains as useful and necessary enhancements of their expertise. This article assumes a familiarity with Dr. Parfitt's material in the article preceding it, and it will not discuss reactions of bone to infection, neoplasms or gross trauma. As background for what follows, fig (1) shows how our bone "bank" normally changes with age.

II. Three Principal Bone-Biologic Activities.

Three principal biologic activities of the skeleton determine, and completely so, how much bone our global bone bank contains and how it endures throughout life. They are named growth, modeling and remodeling. To preview what follows, at the organ and higher levels of organization and before maturity, growth and modeling normally control additions to but not losses from our bone bank, while throughout life BMU-based remodeling controls losses from but not additions to the bone bank. (36,38,40) We describe those activities next because what influences them can influence bone mass, and fragility and architecture too.

1) Growth. As described by Anderson and Kissane (5) and Jee (52), this increases size by increasing the numbers of cells and amounts of intercellular materials. Pure growth, meaning when not modified by other factors, can only produce unorganized masses of tissue, as in anaplastic malignancies. (38) Normally however longitudinal bone growth is oriented, partly by the anatomical relationships created during intrauterine life which make longitudinal bone growth happen at growth plates at the ends of most bones, as Bloom (9), Enlow

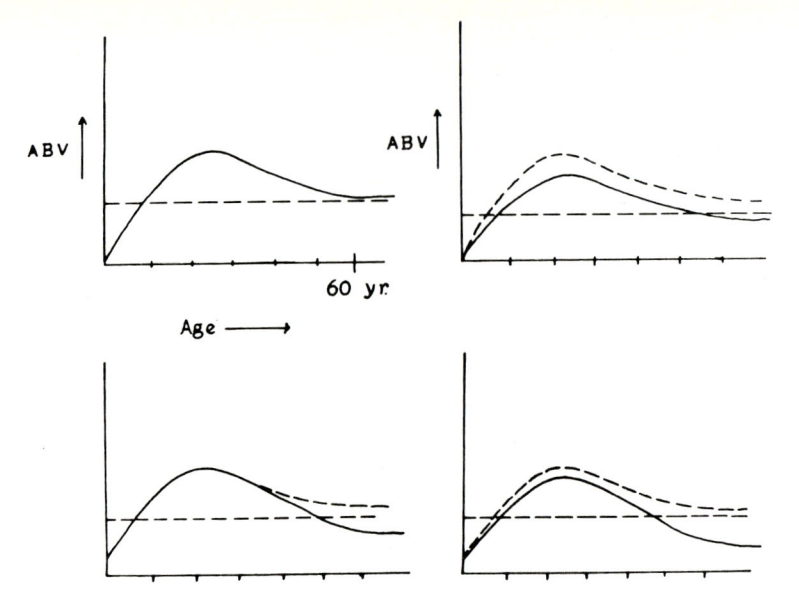

Figure (1). Bone mass and age. Graphs of changes in human bone mass (ABV) plotted against age in decades. Upper left: The norm, showing a peak between 20-30 years of age and subsequent age-related loss. (11,20,56,85,87,88) The accumulations to the left of the peak reflect new compact and spongy bone added by growth and modeling. The losses to the right of the peak reflect remodeling activity on trabecular and cortical-endosteal surfaces. The horizontal dashed line has been called the "fracture threshold" by some authors, below which clinical evidence of increased bone fragility tends to increase. This curve is shown in dashed line in the other 3 graphs. Upper right: Failure to accumulate a normal bone bank followed by a normal age-related adult loss can leave senior citizens with too little bone. So can pathological losses at the lower left, and combinations at the lower right. However the former assumption that insufficient bone is the sole cause of the pathologic bone fragility in osteoporoses is almost certainly wrong, as the text suggests later on (Reprinted by permission, H.M. Frost (1986) Intermediary Organization of the Skeleton, C.R.C. Press, Boca Raton).

(22) and Jee (52) describe, and that also make it add new spongiosa as primary spongiosa, and new length to bone cortices. Those bone bank additions stop at skeletal maturity, and growth alone cannot remove deposits already in the bank.

2) Modeling. Like modeling in clay, this means controlling architecture, which includes an organ's size and shape and the amount and distribution of structural tissue within it. (32,35) The modeling term, which was coined ca 1966 at one of the Sun Valley Bone Workshops, distinguishes certain activities and functions from an operationally different activity and function called remodeling which is described shortly. As general function, in part and at the organ level, various mechanical, nonmechanical, local and systemic influences cause modeling. In bone we recognize three kinds of modeling at present (analogous activities in chondral and fibrous tissues depend on different processes and game rules not discussed here). (13,38,42)

As shown in fig (2) and discussed by Jee (52) and Weinmann and Sicher, (96) two mechanisms provide macromodeling of cortical bone. Resorption drifts progressively remove bone from some cortical surfaces, while formation drifts progressively add bone on other surfaces in the form of circumferential and endosteal lamellae. (22) In whole bones, regular patterns of those drifts determine cortical bone shape, thickness and diameter during a child's growth, so they explain much of the naked-eye anatomy of bones. Minimodeling signifies similar drift processes at the magnifying-glass level that affect the size and orientation of trabecula in spongy bone. (19,41) Macromodeling, and to a lesser

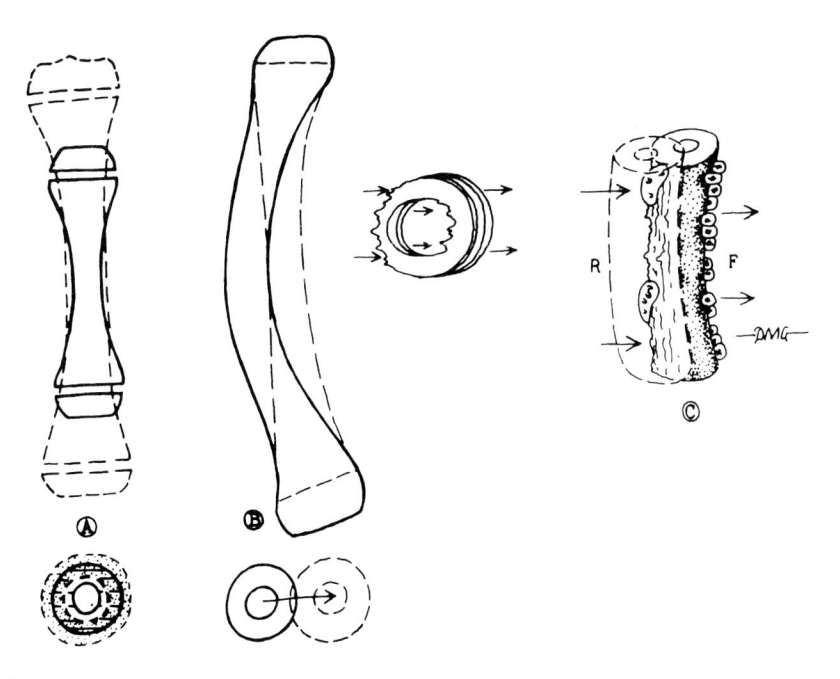

Figure (2). Macromodeling. As an infant's long bone in solid line at (A) grows in length at its growth plates, patterned resorption and formation drifts move its cortical surfaces transversely or sideways in tissue space as the dashed outline shows, to maintain the normal shape in the face of increasing size. Different patterns of the same two kinds of drifts can correct the postfracture deformity, in solid line at (B), towards the normal shape shown in dashed line (growth plate effects in such situations are ignored here). The insets to the right show the modeling drifts that cause corresponding motions in tissue space of the cortical-endosteal surfaces of the hollow bone (Reproduced by permission: H.M. Frost (1986) Osteogenesis imperfecta: The setpoint proposal. Clin. Orthop. Rel. Res. 216:280-277).

degree minimodeling, tend to become ineffective after general body growth stops. Their organ-level bone mass functions include adding to but not reducing deposits already in the global bone bank (clearly, at the tissue level a resorption drift does remove local bone).

Micromodeling, a cell-level process, (38) determines the microscopic grain of bone during its actual deposition, and in such a way that, as Ascenzi and Bonucci (7) and Evans (26) note, the overall orientation of its collagen fibers provides optimal support to the typical mechanical loads on it during its formation (see fig (3)). If later changes in a bone's mechanical loads require a different collagen fiber orientation, that occurs by removing and replacing that bone with new bone with a different grain. In part, different grains created by micromodeling give woven and lamellar bone different structural materials properties (and likewise scar and tendon, fibrocartilage and hyaline cartilage (52)). Macro- and minimodeling can affect bone mass and shape, but micromodeling only affects the mechanical quality and kind of whatever bone is present. The rest of this text concerns some effects of macro- and minimodeling, and not of micromodeling.

3) Remodeling. BMU-based remodeling described in the previous article by Dr. Parfitt occurs in discrete semimicroscopic packets or BMU, each in a sterotyped activation-resorption-formation or "ARF" sequence that normally consumes some 3-5 months per typical BMU. As in the 3rd row of drawings in fig (4), throughout our life span completed BMU typically leave a small excess of new bone on the periosteal envelope. They remove small deficits or "bites" (about .003 mm^3 bone per bite) from bone surfaces adjoining marrow, meaning trabecular and cortical-endosteal surfaces, and leave neither excesses nor

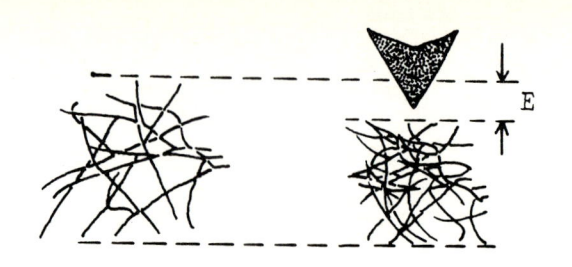

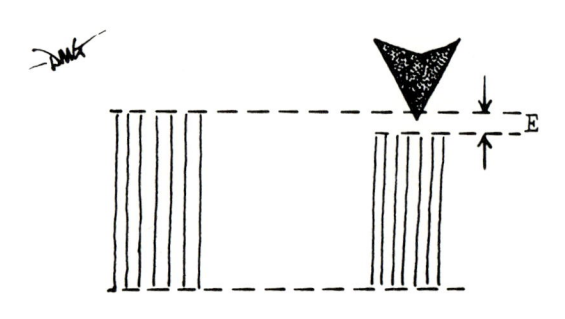

Figure (3). **Micromodeling.** Top: woven bone lacks long range order in the orientation of its collagen fibers, and thus also in its mineral crystals. As a result it shortens more (which is a compression strain, E) under a given load than lamellar bone at the bottom, because it is less stiff than lamellar bone. The collagen orientation of any small piece of bone is determined at the time osteoblasts lay down its organic matrix, and cannot change afterwards.

significant deficits on haversian surfaces (such increments and decrements have been signified by Δ B.BMU (33)). In humans that positive bone balance of periosteal BMU partly accounts for the adult's gradually expanding outside bone diameter first described by Sedlin (83) and confirmed by Garn, (43) Smith and Walker (85) and others, while the negative bone balance of BMU adjoining marrow causes the life-long enlargement of the marrow cavity of all mammals at the expense of spongiosa and cortical-endosteal bone, as originally described by Johnson. (55)

Four known functions of BMU-based remodeling concern this article. (i) It replaces the new primary spongiosa created by longitudinal growth beneath growth plates and made of mineralized cartilage and woven bone, with the secondary or permanent spongiosa made of lamellar bone. (22,38,52,71) (ii) It can turn bone over without necessarily changing its amount or architecture. (33) (iii) It controls most losses of bone adjoining marrow. (40) (iv) It repairs mechanical fatigue damage, of which more later. Two other roles, in homeostasis and fracture repair, lie outside this article's concerns. Fig (4) shows some BMU properties that concern us here, and Table (1) lists a few diseases and other conditions that involve BMU-based remodeling.

To recapitulate: Longitudinal growth adds new cortical length and spongiosa to the bone bank, while organ-level bone modeling adds new cortical bone to bone cross-sections. Both normally become ineffective after skeletal maturity, and height can reduce existing global bone bank deposits. Completed remodeling BMU have different bone balances on the four bone envelopes, and the latters' annual bone gains or losses due to remodeling add up how many increments or decrements of bone were left behind by all the BMU that were completed during the year, as in fig (4) bottom row (a typical adult completes some 6 million BMU per year in the whole skeleton). Increased recruitment of new BMU increases remodeling, meaning bone turnover, decreased activation does the opposite, and annual bone turnover by remodeling equals how much bone the typical completed BMU resorbed and replaced with new bone, *times* how many BMU

Table (1)

Some Clinical Affections that Involve the Pathophysiology of BMU-Based Remodeling*

Spontaneous fractures	March fractures
Pseudofractures	Bone pain
Osteoporoses, systemic	Osteomalacias
Osteoarthritis	Osteochondritis dissecans
Idiopathic aseptic necrosis	Osteogenesis imperfecta
Acute disuse osteoporosis	Migratory osteoporosis (algodystrophy)
Loosening of endoprostheses	Some biologic failures of bone healing
Mechanical incompetence	Biomechanical incompetence
Osteopetrosis	Posttraumatic osteodystrophy
Regional acceleratory phenomenon	Arthrokatadesis

---

*The text does not discuss some of these. Discussions do appear in the cited references.[1,37-39,55,71-77,96]

completed during the year. Accordingly both reversible and irreversible remodeling-dependent net gains/losses are directly proportional to changes in BMU activation, and in the separately controlled net gains or losses of bone in completed BMU. They do not, repeat not, depend on unilateral effects solely on osteoclasts or osteoblasts (although the older idea that they do or can dies hard). A belatedly appreciated purpose of remodeling activity consists of controlling global losses <u>but not gains</u> of bone adjoining marrow. (40)

Attention turns next to how mechanical usage affects those principal biologic activities and their bone mass effects. Both have novel features we only recognized after 1980, and that seemed illogical to many authorities when first described.

IV. Mechanical Usage Effects.

1). <u>Mechanical usage.</u> That usage means the mechanical muscle and body weight forces and motions on bones during daily activities. Carter, (13-15) Lanyon, (58) the author (41) and others (18,19) infer that the largest loads on a bone influence its bone mass more than smaller loads no matter how frequent. (34,38) As examples weight lifters, wrestlers and football guards tend to have more bone than marathon runners, who usually have more than healthy but sedentary people, who usually have more than chronically ill poeple. (3,20,40,56,63,69,87,98) From now on "vigor of mechanical" usage or simply MU, will refer to the typical largest loads on bones.

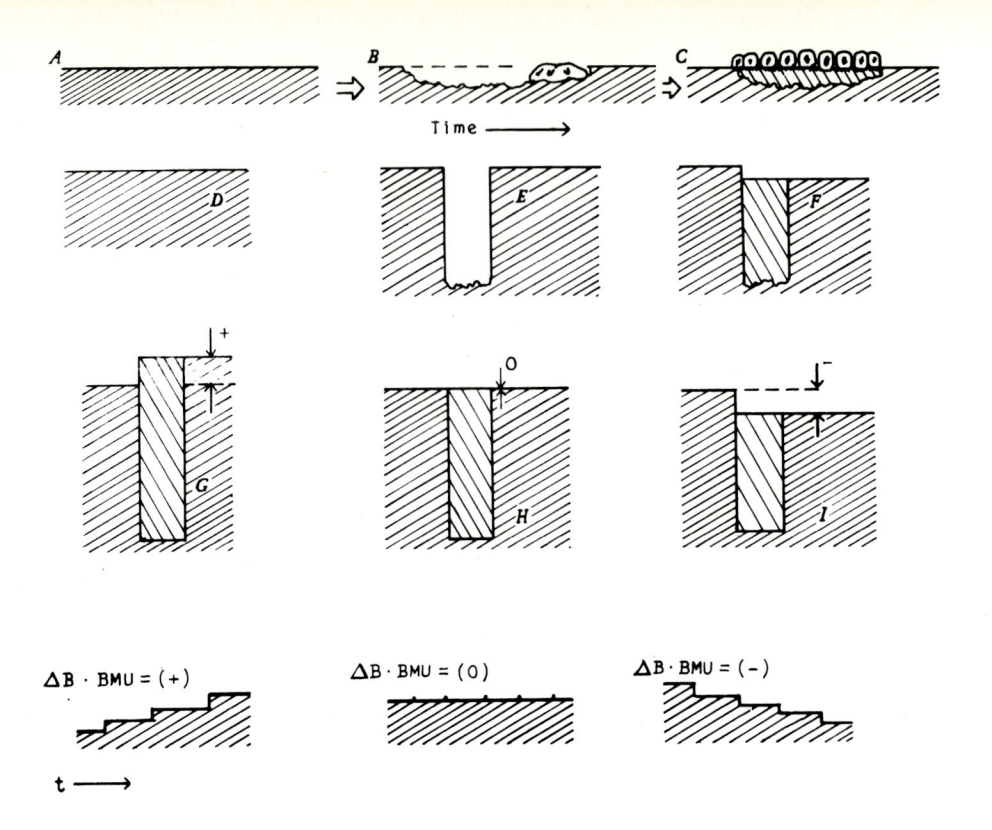

Figure (4). Some BMU physiology. Top row: On the quiescent bone surface at A, osteoclasts erode a resorption bay at B, and then osteoblasts fill the bay back up with bone at C. The multicellular entity causing that packet-style turnover is a BMU. Second row: A "BMU graph" (after the author) switches and idealizes the scales of those events to clarify how relative excesses of resorption or formation can affect bone balance.
Bottom row: These "stair graphs" (after Meunier) show the effects on local bone balance of a series of BMU with the Δ B.BMU values shown above: from left to right, a progressive gain, zero change, and progressive loss of bone. These two mechanisms, the Δ B.BMU and BMU activation, specifically and solely provide that part of the control of bone mass that depends on remodeling. It follows that their responses to mechanical and nonmechanical factors determine how such factors affect bone mass. Unilateral effects only on "bone resorption"-- or formation--which were conceived ca 1960 as the major determinants of bone mass effects, probably do not occur or occur rarely in life (See Section VI, 3), although many skeletal physiologists do not yet understand that.

2) Strain and stress. The mechanical loads put on a bone during daily activities cause physical strains and stresses in it. The strains may have the greater influence on how the principal biologic mechanisms respond to MU and, in the process, affect bone architecture and mass. (17,30)

The engineering definitions of strain and stress follow according to Cochran, (17) Currey, (19) Reilly and Burstein (78) and Popov (70) (see fig (5)).

A mechanical load or force on any structure always deforms it, e.g, makes it shorten, stretch, twist, bend, shear, or any combination. That deformation or strain stretches (e.g, deforms) the chemical bonds between the structure's molecules and those bonds resist deformation with an elastic force called a stress. When increasing strain increases a bone's internal stresses so they equal the applied load, increases in strain stop and the load and stress are in equilibrium. How much a given load strains a structure or material depends on

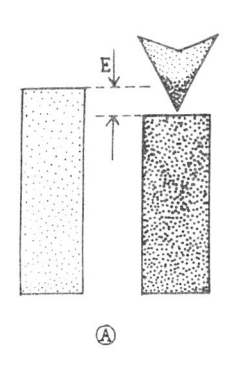

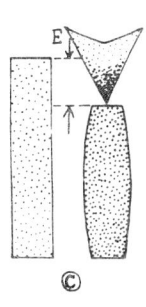

Figure (5) Strain. A vertical or compression load applied to the column above would make it shorten slightly. That compression strain would deform the chemical bonds holding its molecules together, and those bonds would resist that deformation with an elastic force called a stress. Thus: applied load strain → stress. Stiffness measures how much stress it takes to resist a given amount of strain. Below, the same load on a column of the same material and length but of smaller cross section area or thickness, would cause a larger strain. Strain can be expressed as microstrain, so a shortening of a bone from 100% to 99.9% of its original length equals 1000 microstrain in compression, while stretching it from 100% to 102.5% of its original length equals 25,000 microstrain in tension, which is usually enough to fracture a normal adult's lamellar bone.

its stiffness, which is not strength, and which can be expressed as Young's modulus of elasticity. Within the elastic limit of a material such as bone, the ratio of strain to stress tends to be constant, so doubling the load on a bone usually doubles both its strains and stresses. One can measure strain directly but stresses can only be inferred from other data.

3) Bone loads. Biomechanicians have learned that the largest or peak loads on most bones come from muscle forces rather than body weight. (17,19,72,73) The reason: body weight provides a resistance to muscle contraction, but to overcome that resistance most muscles must work against the additional resistance of such poor mechanical lever arms that their own forces on a bone, for example on the femur when walking up the stairs, can exceed twice the force of body weight. During strenuous sports they can briefly exceed even 10 times body weight.

Those preliminaries aside, the MU effects on bone mass in children and adults will be described next. Fig (1) earlier showed that bone mass normally increases during growth, peaks around age 30 and then begins a decline that continues for the rest of life, although at variable rates.

4) MU effects during growth. Increased vigor of MU somewhat increases longitudinal bone growth and its additions of new primary spongiosa and cortical length. (35,40) It also increases bone modeling, and therefore cortical

thickness and outside diameter. (38,40,98) At the same time it <u>retards</u> remodeling-dependent losses of already existing cortical-endosteal and trabecular bone. (40) The child's global bone bank increases because the growth and modeling additions exceed the remodeling losses. When growth and modeling stop in adults, the continuing bone losses of remodeling cause the so-called normal age-related loss of bone adjoining marrow.

Contrariwise, decreased MU and acute disuse retard additions to the bone bank by growth and modeling, and increase the losses due to remodeling of bone adjoining marrow. (49,51,92) Those effects can cause an osteopenia in children by slowing additions of new compacta and spongiosa, while removing normal or somewhat above normal amounts of bone adjoining marrow. Reducing but not stopping global gains relative to general body growth and age makes the bone bank's accumulations fall behind the norm, even though they still increase month after month. Examples: juvenile osteoporosis, osteogenesis imperfecta, Turner's syndrome. However the steady state effects of chronic complete disuse (e.g, lasting more than 2 years) on BMU-based remodeling (and on modeling too) still await definition by systematic studies.

5) <u>MU effects in adults.</u> Here longitudinal growth stops and modeling drifts become ineffective. That leaves BMU-based remodeling in control of most global bone mass effects of MU in adults. (32)

Increasingly vigorous MU tends to retard remodeling-dependent losses of bone adjoining marrow, and in the same three ways as for children. (<u>i</u>) It <u>depresses</u> recruitment of new BMU, which proportionally reduces net losses by taking fewer "bites" out of trabecular and cortical-endosteal bone as in fig (6) bottom left. (<u>ii</u>) It decreases the remodeling space as in fig (7), which Parfitt estimates normally occupies about 2-5% of the bone mass. (68) (<u>iii</u>) It can also reduce the net loss per completed BMU as in fig (6), 2nd row, left. Those effects tend to conserve but not to add bone adjoining marrow.

While few investigators studied how increased MU affects the principal biologic mechanisms, (69,98) many have studied the effects of disuse, including as examples Jaworski, (49-51) Uhthoff, (92,93) and Wronski (100) and colleagues. Greatly decreased MU or acute disuse increases loss of bone adjoining marrow in the same three ways as for children. (<u>i</u>) It derepresses and thus increases BMU recruitment as in fig (6) bottom right. (<u>ii</u>) It increases the reversible remodeling space as in fig (7b). (<u>iii</u>) It increases the net irreversible loss per completed BMU as in fig (6), 3rd row, left and middle. Those effects tend to enlarge the marrow cavity, thin the cortex and remove trabecular bone, so they can cause an osteopenia. Significantly, that same anatomical pattern of bone loss appears in most generalized adult-acquired osteoporoses and osteopenias that have nonmechanical causes. (40) Remember then: two kinds of remodeling effects can cause a bone loss: the initial and temporary remodeling space loss so named by Jaworski and shown in fig (7), and the more slowly accumulating and irreversible decrements or bites removed by completed BMU shown in fig (6). Furthermore, while remodeling space effects tend to occur on all bone envelopes, the irreversible losses tend to affect only spongiosa and cortical-endosteal bone.

Table (2) summarizes some of the above material.

6) <u>To recapitulate.</u> Global bone bank additions play a growth-modeling game before maturity, while net losses play a biologically separate but concurrent remodeling game throughout life. Modeling can adapt bone to gross <u>overloads</u> by adding cortical bone but primarily during growth, while BMU-based remodeling can adapt bone to gross <u>underloads</u> by removing bone adjoining marrow and throughout life. In essence (we will ignore some interesting nuances, of which there always seem to be some), BMU-based remodeling can turn bone over on all four envelopes, and can conserve or discard bone adjoining marrow, but without pharmacologic intervention and except on periosteal surfaces <u>it cannot</u>

Table (2)

Some General Physiologic (Not Pathologic) Mechanical Usage (MU) Effects on Bone Mass and Architecture

$\underline{\underline{MU}}$ ⟶ (MS$_1$) ⟶ <u>Longitudinal growth*</u> ⟶ creates new primary spongiosa + adds length to shaft
MU: I ⟶ I   MU: I ⟶ I
MU: D ⟶ D ($\propto$)   MU: D ⟶ D ($\propto$)

⟶ (MS$_2$) ⟶ <u>Cortical modeling*</u> ⟶ expands outside diameter + increases cortical cross section area
MU: I ⟶ I   MU: I ⟶ I
MU: D ⟶ D ($\propto$)   MU: D ⟶ D ($\propto$)

⟶ (MS$_3$) ⟶ <u>BMU-based remodeling</u> ⟶ replaces primary with permanent spongiosa*
MU: I ⟶ D
MU: D ⟶ I (?) (?)

⟶ turns over cortical and trabecular bone**
MU: I ⟶ D
MU: D ⟶ I ($\aleph$)

⟶ removes trabecular and cortical-endosteal bone**
MU: I ⟶ D
MU: D ⟶ I ($\aleph$)

<u>Code</u>: MU: mechanical usage. I: increased. D: decreased. <u>Exs</u>: MU: I ⟶ I means when MU increases the biologic activity increases too. MU: I ⟶ D means increased MU decreases the biologic activity.

$\propto$: biologic activity directly proportioned to change in MU.

$\aleph$: biologic activity inversely proportioned to change in MU. MS$_{1,2,3}$: putative mechanisms named mechanostats for convenience, that allow MU to control biologic activities. (*)Active mainly during general body growth. (**)Active throughout life. (?): This is the only feature of this table for which the direct evidence should be rated tenuous in 1988. The rest of its entries may be unfamiliar to some readers but they are not also dubious (See Current Concepts of Bone Fragility, Springer, 1986, and Intermediary Organization of the Skeleton, C.R.C. Press, 1986. This table was presented at the prestigious Bone Biology Workshop, Aug, 1987, which the University of Utah sponsored and Prof. W.S.S. Jee organized).

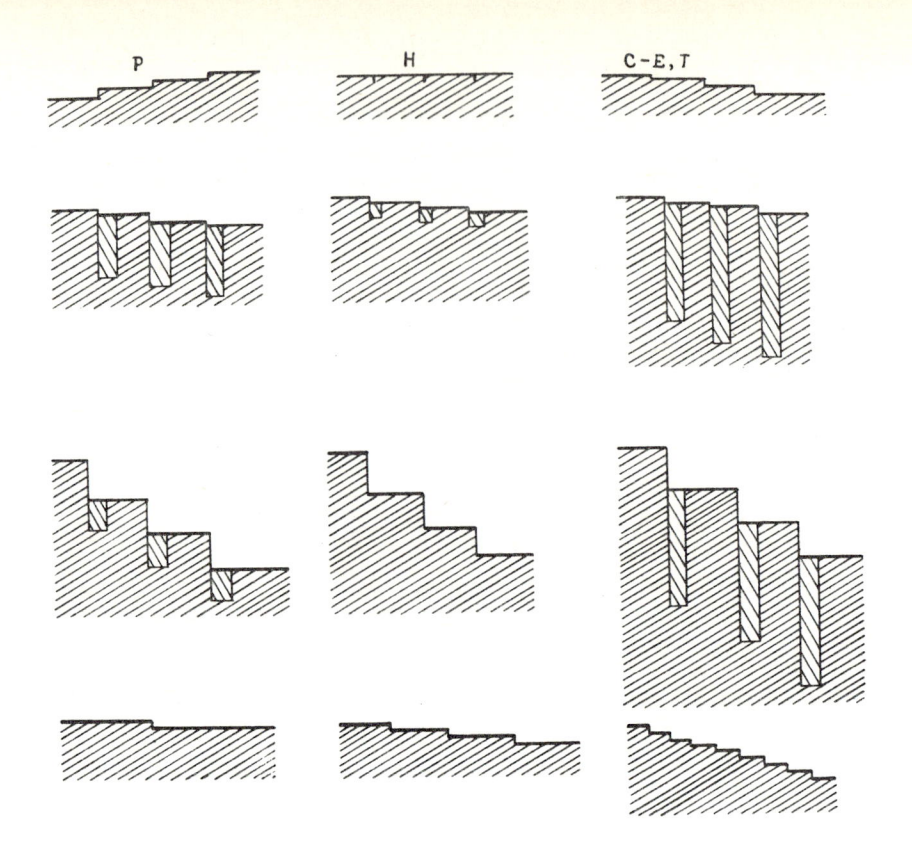

Figure (6). "Bite" and activation effects on bone mass. Top row: The envelope-specific bone balances described in the text and previous figure are shown: P = periosteal; H = haversian; C-E, T = cortical-endosteal and trabecular envelopes or bone surfaces.

Second and third rows: These illustrate how the same decrease or increase in the size of the decrement per typical completed BMU, or Δ B.BMU, can occur in the face of global increases or decreases in the accompanying total amount of bone turned over by completed BMU. The first two drawings in the 3rd row show what appears to happen during mechanical disuse.

Fourth row: Given the same sized decrement or "bite" per completed BMU on, say, a typical trabecular surface, then if the middle drawing shows the norm, the left one shows that depressing BMU activation takes fewer bites from the surface, which retards net irreversible bone loss. Increasing vigor of mechanical usage has that effect. The right drawing shows that increasing that activation increases the loss, and acute mechanical disuse has that effect. The time period represented by the horizontal axis of each graph could equal about 3 years for humans (Reprinted by permission H.M. Frost (1986) Intermediary Organization of the Skeleton C.R.C. Press, Boca Raton).

add significantly to existing global bone supplies (it might add bone locally in some circumstances). An osteopenic skeleton, meaning one with less bone than normal, can come from retarded accumulation during growth, or increased loss in childhood or adult life, or any combination. Mechanical usage has the predictable effects shown in Table (2) on the accumulations and losses provided by the principal biologic activities. Muscle size, strength and activity, rather than body weight, provide the major immediate causes of those effects.

Before concluding this section the reader should know that special modeling rules or laws can predict particular changes in a bone's longitudinal and cross sectional shape and size caused by mechanical factors. As evolutions of Wolff's Law, (97) and described in the cited references, (8,13,14,38,41) such rules

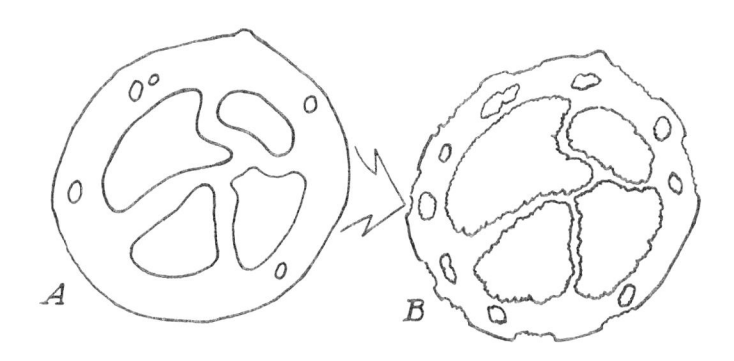

Figure (7). The remodeling space. In the bone cross section at (A), remodeling activity is normal on all 4 envelopes. An increase in BMU activation would pockmark all 4 envelopes with the holes produced during the ARF sequences of new remodeling BMU, as at (B). When BMU activation declined to normal, by the end of the subsequent remodeling period all those added holes would finally have refilled with bone, most of the interim temporary bone loss would become restored, and the situation would return to that shown at (A). Such remodeling space losses can temporarily remove over 20% of the compacta and 50% of the spongiosa. They occur often following fractures, and in migratory osteoporosis, inflammatory arthritides, high bone turnover states and during acute disuse situations.

belong in a separate subfield of skeletal science that touches on but lies apart from this text's focus on bone mass. It is not yet generally known that we do now have predictive, viable and testable modeling rules for bone, cartilage and fibrous tissues.

That background introduces the matters discussed in the next three sections of this text.

IV: The Mechanostat, the MES and Setpoints

During the 1950's a few people, including Snapper (86) and McLean and Urist, (61) speculated that some mechanism might control how mechanical factors affect bone mass. Several lines of evidence now show such mechanisms do exist. Collectively they could be called a "mechanostat." (40) What we know about them so far adds a fascinating new chapter to our understanding of skeletal biology. It includes the following matters.

First, and as Doyal et al (20) and Johnson (55) also noted, since ca 1850 many anatomists, anthropologists, paleontologists, pathologists and orthopaedists remarked that in healthy mammals the bone mass of most bones (but not all, e.g., the human calvarium) seems to fit the strength of the muscles they support. Large muscle groups act on large bones. That implies some natural mechanical criterion determines whether a growing bone is repeatedly and grossly overloaded or underloaded. Overloads would cause more bone to be added, and persistent underloads would cause removal of the excess bone. While plausible, the idea needs supporting quantitative evidence.

Second, firm supporting evidence has accumulated since 1974. Studies of in vivo bone strains in varied mammals and birds after 1970 that Beiwiener, (8) Currey, (19) Lanyon (58) and Rubin (79) have summarized, show the largest bone strains healthy subjects can cause by vigorous voluntary activity equal about 1/10 of the strain needed to fracture bone, which Evans (26), Currey (18) and Reilly and Burnstein (12,78) found equals about 25,000 microstrain (which corresponds to unit stresses of some 16,000 psi or 130 MPa; the legend to fig. 5 defines microstrain). In growing subjects, when strains repeatedly exceed that level then adaptive modeling begins to change bone mass and shape in ways that tend to lower subsequent peak strains back towards the 1/10 limit. (41) That "naturally acceptable strain limit" persists with little change between birth and maturity while the peak loads, on a femur for example, can increase well over 20 times. That proves that such a bone's architecture and mass fit its MU in a way that satisfies that criterion. Furthermore mechanically controlled bone modeling responds poorly to strains below that natural limit, no matter how often they occur. (38,41,46,59) It follows that a threshold range of strain must enable the bone modeling that reduces those strains. The search for and study of the transducing mechanism(s) that converts a bone's MU into signals that can control its modeling and remodeling activities forms a new biomechanics subfield that is not discussed here. (16,25,54,79)

The author named the threshold strain for modeling (which lies in the 1500-2500 microstrain region) the minimum effective strain; hence, MES. (34) In effect, MU that makes strains exceed that MES threshold turns mechanically controlled bone modeling ON, but lesser MU leaves it OFF. (38,47) The biologic system seems to respond more to some time-averaged history of repeated dynamic loads and strains than to single or constant ones, as the author and Epker originally proposed. (23,28,57) Like the author, some other authorities (13,18,42) suspect nature may "listen" to some three-dimensional effect of a bone's strains rather than to the simple longitudinal ones customarily considered as playing that role in the past. Nevertheless the longitudinal ones provide useful indices of the 3-D ones, and this text uses them as such.

Third, studies by Jaworski, (49,51) Uhthoff, (92) Lanyon, (58) Wronski, (100, 101) and colleagues, and among others, show that mechanically controlled BMU-based remodeling has a much smaller threshold strain range, probably in the 100-200 microstrain region, or about 1/100 of bone's fracture strain and the corresponding loads and stresses. (42) MU that causes smaller peak strains derepresses BMU activation, which increases remodeling as described earlier. That increases net losses of bone adjoining marrow. Contrariwise, MU that makes peak strains exceed that threshold but still remain within the physiologic range (which seems to span about 100-1500 microstrain) depresses activation and thus remodeling, which tends to conserve spongiosa and cortical-endosteal bone. As Cowin also suggested, (18) indirect MU effects such as changes in blood flow and hemodynamic pressure in bones may contribute to controlling the above responses, in addition to any direct influences of bone strains and stresses. Here too the biologic system seems to respond more to some history of repeated dynamic loads, than to single or constant ones. Fig (8) graphs the above activity and bone mass effects of mechanical usage.

Fourth, the above MES values should reveal the normal setpoints for the mechanostats that control modeling and remodeling responses to MU, (39) as shown in fig (8).

Fifth, the still scanty experimental data and the pertinent clinical observations suggest relatively few peak bone strain repititions per day, on the order of 10-30 load-deload cycles according to Lanyon (58) and Rubin, (79) might cause the above MU effects. That has a potential clinical use described later.

Attention turns now to another matter that many clinicians may find unfamiliar. Its role in medical as opposed to orthopaedic skeletal problems began to gain wide recognition only after 1985.

V: Microdamage Pathophysiology

Repeated mechanical loads or forces on structural materials such as bone can cause microscopic mechanical damage that weakens them, even though the individual loads remain well below the material's original breaking strength. Known to engineers as "fatigue damage," if not repaired (the usual cause in nonliving materials) it can accumulate until an ordinary load breaks the remaining undamaged material. (2,14,17,19,26,30,37) Several kinds of fatigue or "microdamage" occur in bone, (37,80,81,82) and in fibrous and chondral tissues

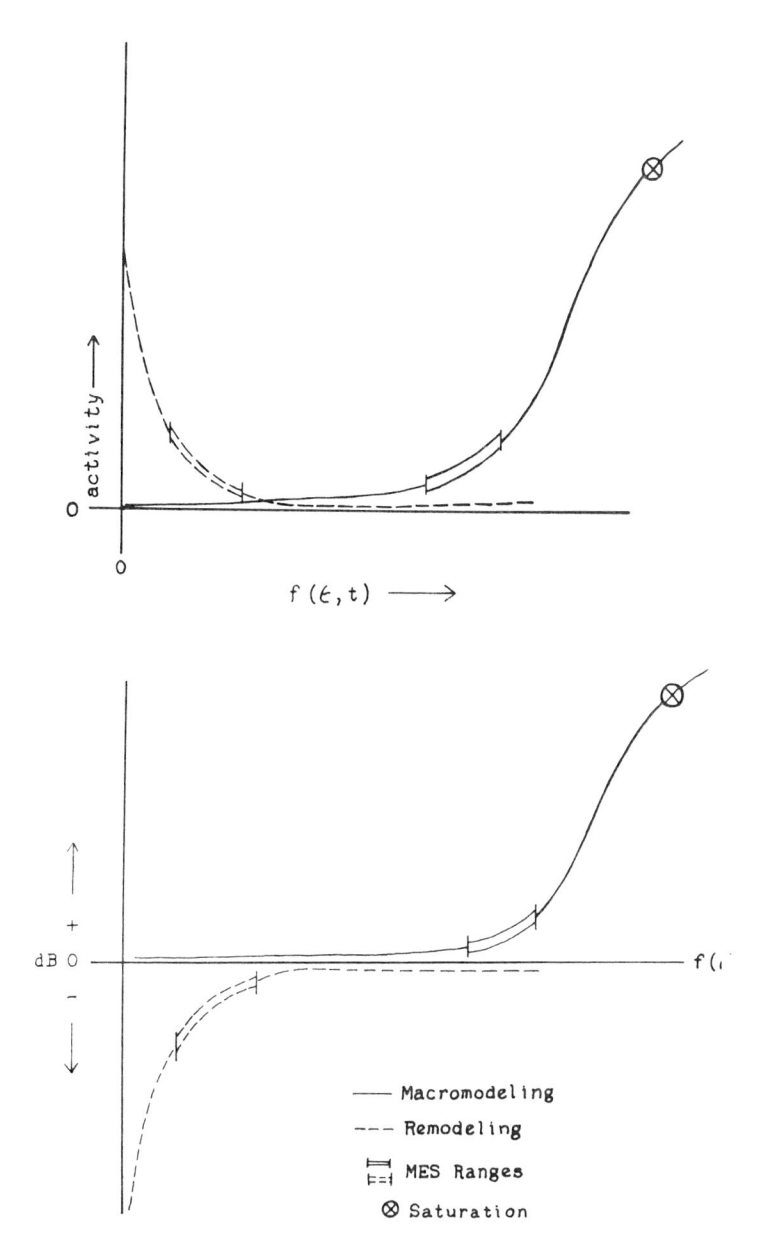

Figure (8). Activity and bone mass effects. Top: This graph plots how global macromodeling and BMU-based remodeling activities plotted on the vertical, appear to respond to increasing vigor of mechanical usage (f(E,t)) on the horizontal. In the plateau region between the two extremes relatively small activity changes accompany increases/decreases in mechanical usage, but large changes occur at the extremes. The peak bone strains at the left of the horizontal axis would approximate zero, equivalent to complete disuse. Peak strains at the right end of the axis would approximate 4000-5000 microstrain.
Bottom: These curves plot the global bone mass effects of the above activity changes, and show some fundamental differences in how modeling and remodeling respond to mechanical usage, including that increasing remodeling activity increases bone loss, while increasing modeling activity increases bone gains. The curves are approximate due to lack of systematic studies of these phenomena, and they ignore microdamage effects on remodeling (Reprinted by permission: H.M. Frost (1986) Intermediary Organization of the Skeleton, C.R.C. Press, Boca Raton).

too, but healthy bone can repair them so they do not accumulate, which can modify how they affect intact bones. Microdamage production and repair are discussed next.

1) <u>Microdamage production</u>. Microdamage increases under increased vigor of MU--meaning increased magnitudes of bone strains and stresses--and with increasing numbers of load-deload cycles, noting that each step a person takes causes one load-deload cycle in all the bones in that lower extremity. Also the larger strains caused by normal vigor of MU on a reduced bone mass cause much larger increases in new microdamage. That could contribute to the increased fragility and microfractures of trabecular bone associated with the loss of trabecular connectivity in many osteoporoses shown by Arnold (6) and Parfitt <u>et al</u> (67).

Therefore known causes of increased microdamage production include increased size and number of bone loads and loading cycles, and reduced bone mass in the presence of normal MU. While the quality of bone might also affect its susceptibility to microdamage, that matter needs more study. It was only recently proposed as a pertinent problem. (36) Any microdamage in a bone also makes it more fragile than normal, meaning it can fracture under a momentary force insufficient to fracture an identical bone with no microdamage. Since a bone's microdamage could vary from nil up to amounts that would let ordinary physical activity cause a fracture, the fragility due to microdamage should be able to vary correspondingly, that is, from nil to catastrophic. Larger and more frequent loads can occur in vigorous athletes and boot camp trainees and probably explain their stress fractures (see Section VII,2). Reduced bone mass occurs in osteoporoses, in many osteomalacias, and in osteopenias due to other causes.

2) <u>Microdamage repair</u>. Currey (19), the author (29,30,32) Martin and Burr, (60) Schaffler (81) and others (72,73) believe one function of remodeling BMU consists of replacing microdamaged bone with new bone so the microdamage does not accumulate. (38,60) It takes some 6 months for a BMU to repair one microdamage locus completely in that way. That repair differs from the grosser processes that heal complete fractures of bones.

That histologic repair of microdamage might slow down in at least four ways: by depressing or blocking recruitment of the new BMU that would repair it; by slowing down already recruited BMU (such slowdowns are shown by prolonged remodeling periods); by delaying full mineralization of the new bone (e.g., prolonging its "stiffness lag"); or by combinations. Histomorphometric studies show such abnormalities do occur in at least most osteomalacias and osteoporoses, (24,37) especially prolonged remodeling periods. Some drugs, including but not limited to corticosteroids, fluoride and Didronil, (27) can also cause those abnormalities.

This relation can encode the above ideas, where MDx means microdamage:

<u>new MDx</u> = <u>repair</u>:	<u>the system is stable</u>
<u>new MDx</u> < <u>repair</u>:	<u>fragility and risk of fracture decrease</u>
<u>new MDx</u> > <u>repair</u>:	<u>fragility and risk of fracture increase</u>

<u>Relation</u> (4)

We still do not know what causes the above abnormalities in metabolic bone diseases or even in some seemingly healthy people, nor how to correct them. Investigators only recently began to accept their clinical significance.

3) <u>Remodeling: a final common pathway</u>. Concentrating on how BMU-based remodeling responds to mechanics might suggest nothing else affects it, but other things can. They include in part sex, age, hormones, homeostatic challenge, disease, genetics, drugs, the envelope it occurs on, and "X": what we

Table (3)

Known* and Probable** Functions of BMU-based Remodeling

-Replaces mineralized cartilage at growth plates with woven bone*

-Replaces primary spongiosa with the permanent secondary spongiosa*

-Renews or turns over existing bone*

-Repairs microdamage**

-Replaces fracture callus with lamellar bone*

-Replaces woven bone with lamellar bone*

-Contributes to homeostasis and blood-bone interactions**

-Controls bone losses where bone adjoins marrow*

-Controls marrow cavity expansion in children and adults*

-Controls mean tissue age of bone*

do not know yet--but should. (38) Some of those factors could potentiate remodeling responses to mechanical factors, others could blunt them. Furthermore some evidence suggests the responses of BMU activation to MU effects, to microdamage, and to the above-mentioned nonmechanical influences, can be depressed or potentiated independently of each other. As one example, estrogen can reduce bone turnover (by depressing BMU activation) to less than 10% of its previous rate without impairing microdamage repair at all. (29,31,32,53,91,99) As another example, large doses of Didronil can suppress all remodeling including microdamage repair, yet humans and experimental animals--dogs--in which that was done showed no apparent abnormalities in calcium homeostasis. (27) Table (3) lists some known and probable functions provided by BMU-based remodeling. Its many functions probably tended to hide its strictly mechanical responses, and we may not know all of them yet.

4) _A role of bone macromodeling in microdamage physiology._ About 1983 two lines of evidence came together to suggest another clinically relevant property of bone. The studies that revealed the MES or the largest acceptable bone strains in life have been mentioned. As for the second, investigators such as Evans, (26) Carter (15) and Schaffler (81) found that normal bone has great resistance to fatigue below the modeling MES threshold of some 2000 microstrain, on the order of tens of millions of load-deload cycles. However above it, say at 4000 microstrain, which still equals only about 1/6 the fracture strain of normal bone, Carter found so much more new microdamage _in vitro_ that complete fatigue fractures could happen after only 5000-20,000 load-deload cycles. (15) Nunamaker (64) and Tschantz and Rutishauser (89) found similar phenomena _in vivo_. People normally put 20,000 load-deload cycles on their lower limb bones in less than 2 months.

Such evidence suggests two novel ideas. (i) A materials property threshold for microdamage in normal lamellar bone may make strains equal to or larger than 3000-4000 microstrain create more new microdamage than its repair mechanism can cope with. (35, 36) (ii) _Nature may fit bone mass and architecture to MU more to minimize fatigue damage than to provide great momentary strength._ (38) That modeling and remodeling do control bone mass and architecture suggests their functions include preventing bone strains from repeatedly exceeding the MES threshold for modeling, in turn to minimize fatigue damage and bone fragility (Carter voiced similar ideas in 1984). In at least one group of congenital diseases a genetic defect(s) seems specifically to blunt that purpose: osteogenesis imperfecta. (39)

VI: Three Bone-Biologic Nuances

One reason it took so long to perceive the biologic and MU phenomena described above amidst a wealth of pertinent evidence stems from our belated recognition of three ubiquitous properties of the living skeleton that confused us by mixing the pertinent evidence with their own features.

1) _The baseline properties._ (38,40,41) At birth our skeletons have architectures and anatomical relationships that arose _in utero_ as expressions of a predetermined genetic master blueprint, and independently of the postnatal MU influences that concern this text. At birth the skeleton also provides the principal growth, modeling and remodeling activities and how they respond to mechanics and other factors. The genes determine the inherent potentials and limits of those activities and local and circulating agents control them. A "natural experiment" shows those potentials: the growth, modeling and remodeling in bones in congenitally paralysed extremities, where the kinds of MU considered earlier do not occur.

Consequently the differences between bones in normal and paralysed limbs should reveal the influences of normal MU (and innervation) added to the baseline properties and potentials. The author's clinical observations suggest the baseline properties account for some 30-80% of the adult's bone mass and architecture, depending on the feature in question. (38) Ignoring possible direct effects of the innervation, both direct and indirect MU influences should account for the remainder. Thus normal MU would account for the _differences_ in bone curves, cross section areas, cortical thickness, lengths and bone mass in similar bones of similar age but in congenitally paralysed and normal limbs.

In general, and as Evans (26) and Gillespie (44) have observed, paralysed bones have shorter lengths and smaller outside diameters and cortical thickness, less spongy bone, reduced longitudinal curvatures and more circular cross sections. This relation can encode those observations, where f(B) signifies the baseline properties and f(MU) signifies the effects of mechanical usage after birth:

Bone mass = f(B) + f(MU)

Relation (5)

The details of such differences await systematic study; their importance in defining and quantitating MU effects was only pointed out in 1986. (38) One of their meanings: when _mechanically controlled_ growth, modeling and/or remodeling activities are in OFF states, (47) the baseline activities still can and do occur. (41) For that reason sudden disuse of a growing bone may turn its _mechanically controlled_ modeling OFF, but some inherent baseline modeling could still go on. Or, resumption of normal MU after acute disuse may depress _mechanically controlled_ remodeling, but remodeling responding to nonmechanical influences could and does go on. (47)

2) _Three tissue response modes._ Pathologists know that, like other tissues, living bone can respond in at least three ways or modes to the _intensity_ of a challenge as well as to its kind. They include the _trivial, physiologic_ and _pathologic._ (1,5,9,38,48,71,96) The trivial response mode means no significant response occurs, either because the stimulus is too small or the system is inherently unresponsive to it. Physiologic responses occur in healthy subjects from stimuli of normal kinds and intensity, and they include the MU responses described earlier. Pathologic responses to overly intense stimuli

(such as gross responses to gross overloads or trauma) or to abnormal kinds of stimuli, include two subsets. One extends physiologic responses into the pathologic range, such as increased tissue perfusion and bone turnover during infection or a regional acceleratory phenomenon, (38) or unusually retarded growth. The other includes reactions seen only in pathologic situations, such as woven bone formation on diaphyseal cortical surfaces, arrested growth, fracture callus, Paget's disease or inflammation. Many past interpretations of clinical and experimental evidence that failed to distinguish the above response modes assumed the game rules that governed evidence derived from one of them applied to the others. That can cause confusion when pundits try to explain to each other what caused such evidence.

This relation can encode the basic idea:

$$\begin{array}{c} \underline{\text{Pathologic mode}} \\ \uparrow \leftarrow \\ \underline{\text{physiologic mode}} \\ \uparrow \\ \underline{\text{trivial mode}} \leftarrow \end{array} \left\{ \begin{array}{l} \text{P-p threshold} \\ \text{t-p threshold} \\ \text{stimulus strength} \end{array} \right.$$

Relation (6)

This article concentrates on phenomena that happen in the trivial-physiologic domains.

3) <u>The transient-steady state distinction</u>. Short-term changes in global bone resorption or formation that happen hours to days after the onset of some challenge or treatment, whether mechanical or not, usually reflect corresponding changes in the activity of already existing osteoclasts or osteoblasts. (31,38,66) However, global long-term changes seen some two or more months after a challenge depend on the sluggish mechanisms that recruit those cells, and tend to become independent of the activity of individual osteoclasts or osteoblasts. (2,38,95) Several things create that novel property. First, Jaworski, (50) Owen (65) and others found that osteoclasts and osteoblasts have short functional lifetimes of about two weeks and months respectively, (9,52) so continuing modeling and remodeling activities require continual recruitment of new cells. Second, special mediator mechanisms provide that recruitment; they include precursor cells, "supporting cells" and capillaries that form essential parts of all modeling drifts and remodeling BMU. Third, the mediator mechanisms determine <u>how many</u> new 'clasts/'blasts are recruited, <u>if, when, where,</u> for <u>how long,</u> and <u>how active</u> each will be. (31,38) Fourth, the cumulative responses of those mediator mechanisms to the challenge account for any global changes in bone mass and architecture that happen over periods of months or longer. As one result a patient's typical osteoblast can function at only 1/2 of the normal rate, but the bone containing those 'blasts can be making twice as much new bone as normal (e.g, 4x more 'blasts than normal, each working 1/2 as fast as normal).

Because of the above arrangements, the initial responses of global resorption and formation to a challenge will not persist under continued treatment; they are <u>transients</u> for these two biologic systems. The final responses may take two or more months to become apparent but can persist under continued treatment; they are the systems' <u>steady state responses</u> which for clinical needs provide the more important ones. (38,66) Failure to distinguish transients from steady states has caused many misinterpretations of clinical and experimental evidence. This article focusses on the clinically more important steady state phenomena, of which equilibrium is only a special case, for a constant rate of loss or gain is also a steady state. The "lead time" a system needs to develop its steady state response to a challenge is called sigma by histomorphometrists, (75) and for BMU-based remodeling it equals the remodeling period described earlier and by Dr. Parfitt.

Attention turns next to how the above information might serve a few clinical needs.

VII: <u>Some Clinical Ways to Influence Bone Mass and Fragility</u>

1) <u>Influencing bone mass.</u> In 1988 these ways include those known on good evidence to work, and those that probably work but need more study before advising general clinical use.

<u>Proven means.</u> These include physical and pharmacologic ones. As for the former, at skeletal maturity the bone bank provides the material for an adult's age- and disease-related losses, so increasing that bank deposit during growth might minimize the development of osteopenias in adult life. Since physical activities that put large loads on bones tend to increase a child's bone bank deposits, it seems reasonable to foster them, and that could become an objective of physical education programs in our children's schools. Continued vigorous exercise in adult life helps to keep those deposits, so it seems reasonable to foster it in adults. One might implement it by lay education, and perhaps by special exercise programs for employees in business and industry, analogous to those going on for different reasons in Japan. In that regard we noted earlier that relatively few maximal loading events per day, perhaps only 10-30 of them, might retard mechanically controlled bone losses due to remodeling, and might enhance mechanically controlled additions of bone during growth. If so, then perhaps relatively simple and brief programs of daily exercise, lasting 10 minutes and devised for such purposes, could help the millions of children and adults in the developed nations who have chronic medical problems that make them incapable of sustained arduous exercise, such as 45 minutes of aerobics, swimming, tennis or jogging. While diet, race, drugs and other things might potentiate or reduce those effects, the systematic studies that could show that remain undone; their need and relevance were only recently recognized. This text does suggest some reasons for doing them and also more studies of <u>in vivo</u> strains and how they affect the bone mass responses of the principal biologic activities.

As for pharmacologic ways and to repeat, depressing (<u>not</u> arresting!) BMU activation retards remodeling-dependent losses of bone adjoining marrow in both children and adults. That explains some of the mechanical usage effects described earlier. As reported in 1966 and 1973, in adult women and men estrogen and perhaps some progesterones can also depress BMU activation. (29,32) Estrogen's proven ability to retard postmenopausal bone loss (76,77) probably depends on that effect more than on effects on existing osteoclasts. Recent experimental work by T. Jerome, R. Martin, C. Weaver and T. Wronski and colleagues vindicate those statements. Probably, and in spite of some recent minor controversy, supplemental dietary calcium ($\sim$1.5 gm/d) has a similar action, if by indirect means. (76,77) It is certainly safe.

<u>Potential means.</u> What causes the biologic BMU impairments that let microdamage accumulate in osteoporoses and osteomalacias remains obscure (24,36) but when we can correct those impairments by treatment that might let osteopenic bones function free of gross fatigue fractures without worrying too much about at least minor bone mass deficiencies, say masses equal to 85% or so of comparable norms. That suggests another way, so far unexplored, to modify the fragility of osteoporotic or otherwise osteopenic skeletons.

Three pharmacologic treatments can add bone to bone-deficient skeletons. They include fluoride, (10) low-dose parathyroid hormone (74,84) and the ADFR treatments. (4,33,45) Each has been used in several variations. However none of them is ready yet for genral clinical use. (8) Excepting the ADFR treatment, how the other two affect the modeling and remodeling processes and bone balance still needs study and definition. While other agents for achieving that goal will probably be discovered in the next decade or two, and some were discussed provocatively by W.B. High, W.S.S. Jee and M.R. Urist (94) at the 1987 Sun Valley Bone Biology Workshop, discussion of them is deferred here.

In healthy mammals the good fit between bone architecture and mass, and typical MU, shows living bone has a mechanism(s) or mechanostat that makes its biologic systems seek and maintain that fit. We already know its approximate setpoints for controlling the bone mass effects of modeling and remodeling. The mechanostat should have a mechanical side which converts mechanical usage of bone into signals cells can detect, and a biologic or cell-dependent side which detects and responds to those signals. (40) Or:

$$\underline{MU} \to \underline{bone} \to \underline{signals} \to \underline{detection} \to \underline{biologic\ response}$$
$$\xleftarrow{\text{mechanical}} \cdots \to | \xleftarrow{\text{biologic}} \cdots \to$$

Relation (7)

The author suggested recently that some circulating agents such as hormones and drugs might exert their bone mass and homeostatic effects by influencing how the biologic side of the mechanostat "perceives" a bone's true mechanical usage. (40) It could respond by conserving bone--and calcium-- if "deceived" into perceiving too vigorous mechanical usage, or by discarding bone and calcium if the contrary. Whether hypo- or hypercalcemia accompany those responses would then depend on how the agents affected the gut and kidney. If true, then bone added in response to pharmacologic treatment may not be retained after the treatment stops. Keeping it could require repeating the treatment periodically, and/or learning how to make the mechanostat "believe" the extra bone is needed by finding some treatment that lowers its setpoint, or both.

2) <u>Influencing microdamage physiology and bone fragility in orthopaedic, sports medicine and metabolic bone disease problems.</u> What follows offers salient points about matters too complex to explain in detail here.

Abrupt increases in the size and number of mechanical loads on bones occurs when people begin strenuous activities they were not accustomed to. Some examples: weight lifting, running, tennis, aerobics, wrestling, football, basketball and boot camp training. Abrupt but anatomically localized increases in loads can occur in the bone supporting the endo-prosthesis, such as a hip, knee, ankle, shoulder or other total joint replacement, and in bone supporting internal and external fixation devices.

Such situations would increase microdamage production in bone. Given healthy bone, then newly recruited remodeling BMU should repair the microdamage. However a time lag between beginning to repair a typical locus of microdamage, and its completion in a biomechanical sense, equals about 6 months in man (37) and it has two parts. In the first part, replacement of the damaged bone <u>tissue</u> takes about 3 months. In the second part achieving full <u>mineralization</u> and mechanical <u>stiffness</u> of the new bone takes another 3 months, and until it has finished the new bone cannot carry its due share of the loads on the whole bone, nor relieve the surrounding bone of its share while the repair process goes on.

Bone has a good safety factor for microdamage, for many people have few problems when they begin a new kind of strenuous activity. However during the above 6 month lag time, continuing the new activity continues to add more microdamage, and its amount in a bone will equal all the extra microdamage created during these 6 months. That 6 month period defines this system's transient phase, analogous to the remodeling period or sigma for BMU. After those 6 months the microdamage completely repaired during each month begins to equal what arises each month, so its amount tends to become constant. If that amount is not threatening the person should be unaware of it and could continue the activity free of subsequent problems. The time period after 6 months defines this system's steady state phase.

33

Clearly, if enough microdamage arose during the above 6 months lag time to leave too little undamaged bone to carry its loads, it would fracture. Such fractures happen, and include stress or march fractures and spontaneous fractures. Microdamage burdens too small to cause an overt fracture might still cause bone pain during strenuous activity, perhaps due to overstrain of the undamaged parts of a bone (bone does have pain nerve endings, and overstraining it does cause pain (21,62). Nature may offer that pain as bone a warning and an inducement to reduce one's mechanical usage until the microdamage repair processes can catch up to the need.

To sum up: Complete repair of a microdamage locus takes some 6 months in healthy people. During that lag time more microdamage can accumulate. How much accumulates can determine if the bone will fracture, or merely hurt on effort, or continue to function without problems. In some people strenuous activity can cause so much new microdamage during that lag time that fracture or bone pain do occur.

Management of the problem. The above material suggests the beginning of strenuous new activities gradually rather than abruptly, and taking about 6 months rather than a few weeks to develop full athletic endurance and vigor, would prevent fractures and/or bone pain due to microdamage. If bone pain develops it represents a warning that a fracture could follow, so the frequency, intensity and duration of the activity causing it should reduce considerably for several months to let the repair processes catch up to need.

The same philosophy should apply to managing microdamage problems in bone supporting load-bearing endoprostheses, to aseptic necroses including idiopathic aseptic necrosis of the femoral head, (38) and to many bone pain problems in osteoporoses and osteomalacias. The author's personal experience with that philosophy in such problems is encouraging. It worked well and consistently in his orthopaedic practice after 1962-1963, when the basic facts underlying it first became understood.

Similar ideas might extrapolate to microdamage phenomena in fibrous tissue organs such as ligaments and tendons, and in articular cartilage.

Dicussions elsewhere deal with how our new understanding of microdamage pathophysiology bears on the degisn and endurance of joint, bone and dental replacements and vascular, ligament and tendon grafts. (38) Those important matters in modern surgical practice involve much of the new physiology summarized above.

VIII: Conclusion

This text provides a "minicourse" on some of the new bone biology that concerns some clinical problems. Recent articles, meetings and discussions show growing numbers of respected international authorities concur, and that the problem with the "old" bone biology lay less in its errors than in the fact that, like Galileo's physics when seen through the eyes of Einstein's, it was incomplete, and in 1988 we must move on to more and better things.

The absence above of discussions of the functions, regulation and roles of individual cells and their biochemical processes has a simple explanation. The matters discussed earlier stem from previously unknown but important special multicellular mechanisms that have no counterparts in individual cells, but that provide the immediate causes of most disease. It is not yet known which of those mechanisms' cells ultimately account for their properties and malfunctions, nor how they do so. The author believes that ignorance has three major causes: restricted past interdisciplinary communication in this field; the belatedly recognized intermediary organization that provides the mechanisms and responses described earlier; (38) and the persisting afterglow of some early controversies and uncertainties that further evidence and research have resolved. It is a credit to its organizers that this meeting addresses some of those matters.

In 1988 we know the bone mass and fragility effects described earlier depend on how special multicellular <u>mediator mechanisms</u> responsible for tissue and organ level growth, modeling and remodeling, respond to mechanical and nonmechanical influences, and in doing so decide <u>if, when, where, how many</u> and <u>how long</u> 'clasts and 'blasts will be produced, and <u>how active</u> they will be during their short functional lifespans. It is becoming quite clear that those bone mass effects depend minimally on direct actions of those influences on already existing 'clasts and 'blasts.

<u>ACKNOWLEDGEMENTS</u> The author would like to express his appreciation to Mrs. Betty Uhernik who typed the many drafts of this article, to colleagues of the Southern Colorado Clinic who provided the necessary facilities, to Dr. David Gavin who supplied its drawings, and to Dr. A.M. Parfitt who provided the opportunity to present it via this conference to the skeletal sciences field at large. It seems also noteworthy that the Southern Colorado Clinic is one of a few private medical groups in the U.S.A. and Canada that encourage and support the kinds of scientific work and writing that can help to advance medical knowledge and expertise without receiving any income or other financial return for their generosity.

REFERENCES

1. Aegerter E, Kirkpatrick JA Jr. (1975) Orthopaedic Diseases. W.B. Saunders, Philadelphia.

2. Albright JA, Brand RA. (1987) The Scientific Basis of Orthopaedics, eds. 2nd Ed. Appleton-Century Crofts, New York.

3. Aloia JF, Aswani AN, Yeh JK, Cohn SH. (1986) Physical activity as a determinant of bone mass in premenopausal women. Abstr. J Bone Min Res 8:236.

4. Anderson C, Cape RDT, Crilly RG, Hodsman AB, Wolfe BMJ. (1984) Preliminary observations on a form of coherence therapy for osteoporosis. Calc Tiss Int 36:341-343.

5. Anderson WAD, Kissane JM. (1977) Pathology, Ed. 7. Eds. C.V. Mosby Co., St. Louis.

6. Arnold JS. (1970) Focal excessive resorption in aging and senile osteoporosis. In Osteoporosis; ed. U.S. Barzel. Grune and Stratton, New York, pp. 80-113.

7. Ascenzi AA, Bonussi E. (1967) The tensile properties of single osteons. Anat Rec 158:375-386.

8. Biewiener AA, Taylor R. (1986) Bone strain: A determinant of gait and speed? J Exp Biol 123:383-400.

9. Bloom W, Fawcett DW. (1975) A textbook of Histology. 10th ed. W.B. Saunders, Philadelphia.

10. Briancon D, Meunier PJ. (1979) Le Traitement de l'Ostéoporose par l'Association Fluorure de Sodium, Calcium, Vitamine D. Univ. Claude Bernard, Lyon.

11. Broman GE, Trotter M, Peterson RR. (1958) The density of selected bones of the human skeleton. Am J Phys Anthrop 16:197-206.

12. Burnstein AH, Reilly DT. (1976) Aging of bone tissue: Mechanical properties. J Bone and Jt Surg. 58A:82-86.

13. Carter DR, Orr TE, Fyrhie DP, Schurman DJ. (1987) Influences of mechanical stress on prenatal and postnatal skeletal development. Clin Orthop Rel Res 219:237-250.

14. Carter DR. (1891) The relationship between in vivo strains and cortical bone remodeling. C.R.C. Critical Reviews of Biomechanical Engineering. 8:1-28.

15. Carter DR, Hayes WC. (1977) Compact bone fatigue damage; A microscopic examination. Clin Orth Rel Res 135:192-205.

16. Chakkalaka Da, Johnson MW. (1981) Electrical properties of compact bone. Clin Orthop Rel Res 161:146-153.

17. Cochran G, Van B. (1982) A Primer of Orthopaedic Biomechanics. Churchill-Livingstone, Edinburgh.

18. Cowin SC. (1986) Wolff's Law of trabecular architecture at remodeling equilibrium. J Biomechan Eng 108:83-88.

19. Currey J. (1984) The Mechanical Adaptations of Bones. Princeton University Press, Princeton.

20. Doyle F, Brown J, Lachance C. (1970) Relation between bone mass and muscle weight. Lancet 1:391-393.

21. Duncan CP, Shim S. (1979) The autonomic nerve supply of bone. J Bone and Jt Surg 59B:323-324.

22. Enlow DH. (1963) Principles of Bone Remodeling. Charles Thomas, Springfield.

23. Epker BN, Frost HM. (1965) Correlations of patterns of bone resorption and formation with physical behavior of loaded bone. J Dent Res 44:32-42.

24. Eriksen EF. (1986) Normal and pathological remodeling of human trabecular bone. Three-dimensional reconstruction of the remodeling sequence in normals and in metabolic bone disease. End Rev 7:327-408.

25. Eriksson C. (1976) Bone morphogenesis and surface change. Clin Orthop Rel Res 121:295-302.

26. Evans FG. (1957) Stress and Strain in Bones. Charles Thomas, Springfield.

27. Flora L, Hassing GS, Parfitt AM, Villanueva AR. (1981) Comparative skeletal effects of two diphosphonate drugs. In Osteoporosis, eds. H.F. DeLuca, H.M. Frost, W.S.S. Jee, C.C. Johnston, Jr. and A.M. Parfitt. University Park Press, Baltimore, pp. 389-407.

28. Frost HM. (1964) The Laws of Bone Structure. Charles Thomas, Springfield.

29. Frost HM. (1966) Bone Dynamics in Osteoporosis and Osteomalacia. Charles Thomas, Springfield.

30. Frost HM. (1973) Orthopaedic Biomechanics. Charles Thomas, Springfield.

31. Frost HM. (1973) The origin and nature of transients in human bone

remodeling dynamics. In: Clinical Aspects of Metabolic Bone Disease. Eds. B. Frame, A.M. Parfitt and H. Duncan. Excerpta Medica, Amsterdam, pp. 124-137.

32. Frost HM. (1973) Bone Remodeling and Its Relation to Metabolic Bone Disease. Charles Thomas, Springfield.

33. Frost HM. (1979) Treatment of osteoporoses by manipulation of coherent bone cell populations. Clin Orthop Rel Res 143:227-244.

34. Frost HM. (1983) The minimum effective strain: A determinant of bone architecture. Clin Orthop Rel Res 175:286-292.

35. Frost HM. (1985) The pathomechanics of osteoporoses. Clin Orthop Rel Res 200:198-225.

36. Frost HM. (1986) Pathogenetic mechanisms of the osteoporoses. In: Current Concepts of Bone Fragility, ed. H. Uhthoff. Springer-Verlag, Berlin, pp. 329-361.

37. Frost HM. (1986) Bone microdamage: Factors that impair its repair. In: Current Concepts of Bone Fragility, ed. H.K. Uhthoff, Springer-Verlag, Berlin, pp. 123-148.

38. Frost HM. (1986) Intermediary Organization of the Skeleton. C.R.C. Press, Boca Raton.

39. Frost HM. (1986) Osteogenesis imperfecta: The setpoint proposal. Clin Orthop Rel Res 216:280-297.

40. Frost HM. (1987) The mechanostat: A proposed pathogenic mechanism of osteoporoses and the bone mass effects of mechanical and nonmechanical agents. Bone and Mineral 2:73-85.

41. Frost HM. (1987) Structural adaptations to mechanical usage. A proposed "three-way rule" for lamellar bone modeling. Comp Vet Orth and Trauma; in press.

42. Fyrhie DP, Carter DR. (1986) A unifying principle relating stress to trabecular bone morphology. J Orthop Res 4:304-317.

43. Garn SM. (1970) The Earlier Gain and Later Loss of Cortical Bone. Charles Thomas, Springfield.

44. Gillespie JA. (1954) The nature of the bone changes associated with nerve injuries and disuse. J Bone and Jt Surg 36B:464-473.

45. Hasling C, Eriksen EF, Charles P, Mosekilde L. (1987) Exogenous triiodothyronine activates bone remodeling. Bone 8:65-69.

46. Hert J, Liskova M, Landgrut B. (1967) Influence of long term continuous bending on the bone. Folia Morph 17:389-399.

47. Hori M, Takahashi H, Konno T, Inoue J, Haba T. (1985) A classification of in vivo bone labels after double labeling in canine bone. Bone 6:147-154.

48. Jaffe HL. (1972) Metabolic, Degenerative and Inflammatory Disease of Bones and Joints. Lea and Febiger, Philadelphia.

49. Jaworski ZFG, Liskova-Kiar M, Uhtoff H. (1980) Effects of long term immobilization on the pattern of bone loss in older dogs. J Bone and Jt Surg 62B:104-110.

50. Jaworski ZFG, Duck B, Sekaly G. (1981) Kinetics of osteoclasts and their nuclei in evolving secondary haversian systems. J Anat 133:397-405.

51. Jaworski ZFG, Uhthoff HK. (1986) Reversibility of nontraumatic disuse osteoporosis during its active phase. Bone 7:431-440.

52. Jee WSS. (1983) The skeletal tissues. In: Histology, 5th Ed. Ed, L. Weiss. Elsevier-North Holland, pp. 200-255.

53. Jerome T. (1987) Effects of ovariectomy on trabecular bone remodeling in young and old rats. Reported at the University of Utah-sponsored Bone Biology Workshop, Sun Valley, ID., August.

54. Johnson MW. (1984) Behavior of fluid in stressed bone and cellular stimulation. Calc Tiss Int Suppl 36:72-76.

55. Johnson LC. (1964) The kinetics of skeletal remodeling. In: Structural Organization of the Skeleton. Eds, R.A. Milch and R.M. Robinson. National Foundation March of Dimes, New York pp. 66-142.

56. Johnston CC, Jr., Norton JA, Khair MEA, Longcope C. (1979) Age related bone loss. In: Osteoporosis II, ed. U.S. Barzel, Grune and Stratton, New York pp. 91-100.

57. Kadaba MP, Dell DSG, Palmieri V, Johnson MW, Cochran GVB. (1987) Frequency analysis of bone strains and strain-induced potentials *in vitro* and *in vivo*. Abstr. Orthopaedic Research Society, American Academy Orthopaedic Surgery, Chicago, 12:190.

58. Lanyon LE. (1984) Functional strain as a determinant for bone remodeling. Calc Tiss Int Suppl 36:56-61.

59. Liskova M, Hert J. (1971) Reaction of bone to mechanical stimuli. Part II: Periosteal and endosteal reaction of tibial diaphysis to intermittent loading. Folia Morphol 19:301-315.

60. Martin RB, Burr DB. (1982) A hypothetical mechanism for the stimulation of osteonal remodeling by fatigue damage. J Biomech 15:137-139.

61. McLean FC, Urist MR. (1955) Bone: An Introduction to the Physiology of Skeletal Tissue. Univ Chicago Press, Chicago.

62. Miller MR, Kasahara M. (1963) Observations on the innervation of human long bones. Anat Rec 145:13-23.

63. Nilsson BE, Andersson SM, Hardrup T, Westlin NE. (1978) Ballet dancing and weight-lifting-effects on BMC. Am J Roentgen 131:541-542.

64. Nunamaker DM, Butterweck DM, Black J. (1987) Fatigue fractures in thoroughbred race horses. Relationship with age and strain. Abstr Orth Research Society, American Academy Orthopaedic Surgeons, Chicago 12:72.

65. Owen M. (1978) The histogenesis of bone cells. Calc Tiss Res 25:205-207.

66. Parfitt AM. (1980) Morphologic basis of bone mineral measurements: transient and steady state effects of treatment in osteoporosis. Min and Elect Metab 4:273-287.

67. Parfitt AM, Mathews HE, Villanueva AR, Kleerekoper M, Frame B, Rao DS. (1984) Relationships between surface, volume and thickness of iliac trabecular bone in aging and in osteoporosis. J Clin Invest 72:1396-1409.

68. Parfitt AM. (1963) The physiologic and clinical significance of bone histomorphometric data. In: Bone Histomorphometry: Techniques and Interpretation. Ed, R.R. Recker, C.R.C. Press, Boca Raton pp. 143-224.

69. Pedrini-Mille A, Pedrini Va, Maynard JA, Vailas JC. (1986) Effects of strenuous exercise on physes and bones of growing animals. Abstr Orthopaedic Research Society; American Academy of Orthopaedic Surgeons, Chicago 11:164.

70. Popou EP. (1952) The Mechanics of Materials. Prentice-Hall, Englewood Cliffs.

71. Putschar WGJ. (1960) General pathology of the musculoskeletal system. In: Handbuch der Allgemeinen Pathologie. Eds, F. Buchner, E, Letterer and F. Roulet. Springer-Verlag, Berlin pp. 361-488.

72. Radin EL. (1972) Trabecular microfractures in response to stress: The possible mechanism of Wolff's Law. In: Orthopaedic Surgery and Traumatology. Excerpta Medica, Amsterdam pp. 59-65.

73. Radin EL, Parker HG, Pugh JW, Steinberg RS, Paul IL, Rose RM. (1973) Response of joints to impact loading--III. Relationship between trabecular microfractures and cartilage degeneration. J Biomech 6:51-57.

74. Rasmussen H, Bordier P, Marie P, Auquier L, Eisinger JB, Kuntz D, Caulin F, Argemi B, Gueris J, Julien A. (1980) Effect of combined therapy with phosphate and calcitonin on bone volume in osteoporosis. Bone 2:107-112.

75. Recker RR. (1983) Bone Histomorphometry. Techniques and Interpretation (ed). C.R.C. Press, Boca Raton.

76. Recker RR. (1981) Continuous treatment of osteoporosis. Current status. Orthop Clin N Amer 12:611-627.

77. Recker RR, Saville PO, Heaney RP. (1977) Effect of estrogens and calcium carbonate on bone loss in postmenopausal women. Ann Int Med 87:649-655.

78. Reilly DT, Burnstein AH. (1974) The mechanical properties of cortical bone. J Bone and Jt Surg 36A:1001-1022.

79. Rubin CT. (1984) Skeletal strain and the functional significance of bone architecture. Calc Tiss Int Suppl 36:11-18.

80. Rutishauser E, Majno G. (1950) Lésions par surcharge dans le squelette normale et pathologique. Bull Schweiz Akad der Med Wiss 5:333-342.

81. Schaffler MD. (1985) Stiffness and fatigue of compact bone at physiological strains and strain rates. Thesis, West Virginia Univ School of Med pp. 1-217.

82. Schnitzler CM, Solomon L. (1986) Histomorphometric analysis of a calcaneal stress fracture: A possible complication of fluoride therapy for osteoporoses. Bone 7:193-198.

83. Sedlin ED. (1964) Uses of bone as a model system in the study of aging. In: Bone Biodynamics, ed. H.M. Frost. Little-Brown, Boston pp. 655-666.

84. Slovik DM, Rosenthal DI, Doppelt SH, Potts JT, Jr., Daly MA, Campbell JA, Neer RM. (1986) Restoration of spinal bone in osteoporotic men by treatment with human parathyroid hormone (1-34) and 1,25-dihydroxy vitamin D. J Bone Min Res 1:377-381.

85. Smith RW, Walker RR. (1964) Femoral expansion in aging women: Implications for osteoporoses and fractures. Science 145:156-157.

86. Snapper I. (1957) Bone Diseases in Medical Practice. Grune and Stratton, New York.

87. Talmage RV, Stinnett SS, Landwehr JT, Vincent LM, McCartney WH. (1986) Age-related loss of bone mineral density in non-athletic and athletic women. Bone and Min 1:115-125.

88. Trotter M, Peterson RR. (1955) Ash weight of human skeletons in percent of dry, fat free weight. Anat Rec 123:341-352.

89. Tschantz P, Rutishauser E. (1967) La surcharge mechanique de 'l'os vivant. Annales d'Anat et Path 12:223-248.

90. Turner RT, Bell NH. (1986) The effects of immobilization on bone histomorphometry in rats. J Bone Min Res 1:399-407.

91. Turner RT, Vandersteenhoven JJ, Bell NH. (1987) The effects of ovariectomy and 17B-estradiol on cortical bone histomorphometry in growing rats. J Bone Min Res 2:115-122.

92. Uhtoff HK, Jaworski ZFG. (1978) Bone loss in response to long term immobilization. J Bone and Jt Surg 60B:420-427.

93. Uhtoff HK. (1986) Current Concepts of Bone Fragility (ed). Springer-Verlag, Berlin.

94. Urist MR, Hudak R, Hud Y-K, Rasmussen J, Hirota W, Lietze A. (1985) Bone morphogenetic protein (BMP) and anti-BMP immunoassay in patients with osteoporosis. In: The Chemistry and Biology of Mineralized Tissues. Ed, W.T. Butler, EBSCO Media, Birmingham pp. 62-69.

95. Villanueva AR, Frost HM. (1970) Evaluation of features determining the tissue-level haversian bone formation rate in man. J Dent Res 49:836-846.

96. Weinmann JP, Sicher H. (1955) Bone and Bones, 2nd Ed. C.V. Mosby, St. Louis.

97. Wolff J. (1982) Das Gesetz der transformation der knochen. A. Hirschwald, Berlin.

98. Woo SL-Y, Kuei SC, Amiel D, Gomez MA, Hayes WC, White FC, Akeson WH. (1981) The effect of prolonged physical training on the properties of long bone. A study of Wolff's Law. J Bone and Jt Surg 63A:780-787.

99. Wronski TJ, Walsh CC, Iganaszewski LA. (1986) Histologic evidence for osteopenia and increased bone turnover in ovariectomized rats. Bone 7:119-124.

100. Wronski TJ, Morey ER. (1983) Inhibition of cortical and trabecular bone formation in the long bones of immobilized monkeys. Clin Orthop Rel Res 181:269-276.

101. Young DR, Niklowitz WJ, Brown RJ, Jee WSS. (1986) Immobilization-associated osteoporosis in primates. Bone 7:109-118.

(Editors' note: At short notice, illness prevented Dr. Frost from attending the symposium to present this paper. DR. GIDEON A. RODAN, Department of Bone Biology and Osteoporosis, Merck Sharp & Dohme, West Point, PA, and, at the time of the symposium, President of the American Society for Bone and Mineral Research, made a presentation on this same topic. This discussion pertains to Dr. Rodan's presentation. We remain most grateful to Dr. Rodan for his assistance.)

Discussion:

DR. KLEEREKOPER (Detroit): Dr. Rodan, have you tried any other inhibitors of resorption in your model?
DR. RODAN (West Point, PA): Diphosphonates were equally effective; one dose given before the tenotomy or neurectomy inhibited about 50 percent of the bone loss at ten days.
DR. RECKER (Omaha): The effects that you showed were very rapid, but in the Jaworski and Uhtoff studies on the dog, it took some time for bone loss to occur. How much of the phenomenon you demonstrated was due to a RAP (regional acceleratory phenomenon)? Did you do a sham operation on any of the animals?
DR. RODAN: Sham operated control animals did not show bone loss. I believe that rats lost bone more rapidly in the subepiphyseal cancellous bone of the tibia because of the higher rate of bone turnover.
DR. RECKER: Well, the RAP is roughly proportionate to the degree of the biological insult, and a sham operation is not as big an insult as sectioning a tendon.
DR. RODAN: I agree; after tenotomy, the initial bone loss at ten days was slightly larger than after neurectomy, which is a lesser insult. But at 42 days, the two were very comparable.
DR. REEVE (England): I find your data fascinating, Michael. What are the possible similarities or differences between the group with osteoporotic crush fractures and normal women immediately after the menopause?
DR. PARFITT (Detroit): The patients who have fracture probably underwent the same immediate changes at menopause. They started with the high remodeling osteoclast-dependent bone loss that is characteristic of all clinically important modes of bone loss, whether due to immobilization, as Gideon showed, or whatever. But then some of them undergo transition to low turnover. Another way of stating my point is that there are some patients in whom osteoporosis is a real disease, which involves remodeling defects in one region of the skeleton and not in other regions. The nature of that disease is for people like Gideon to find out; the purpose of histomorphometry is to define the questions that the cell biologists have to find answers for.
Why are the surfaces different? I can only speculate. There may be gradients in the cellular composition of the bone marrow adjacent to the endocortical surface and adjacent to the cancellous surface, and there is some evidence for that. It's also possible that the blood supply is different. Dr. Burkhardt in Germany has pioneered the study of the blood supply of the marrow; we normally ignore it completely because with the way sections are prepared in most labs, you don't see the blood vessels. But obviously they're there and are critically important. And they could change differently with age in different regions of the bone. Finally, as a development of what Gideon said, different parts of the bone may be differentially sensitive to mechanical influences because the cancellous bone in the middle is much more isolated from the direct effects of muscular action than the bone closer to the periosteum.

DR. DEQUEKER (Belgium): Are the same surface specific responses found in Type 2 osteoporosis with femoral neck fractures?

DR. PARFITT: Hip fracture patients are very unsuitable for study by the same kinds of methods as vertebral fracture patients. They're much sicker, and have all kinds of other medical problems. You can't study pathogenesis at the time of the fracture because of transient changes in mineral metabolism that are due to the fracture, rather than to the conditions that occurred before the fracture, and a lot of them die before you can get to study them.

I'm not aware of any good steady state histomorphometric data using tetracycline labeling in hip fracture patients.

DR. JOHNSTON (Indianapolis): Could there be some mechanism that reduces remodeling activity in relation to the amount of bone that's present, so that, after you've lost some critical amount, it shuts off?

DR. PARFITT: There could be such a non-specific protective mechanism, but in healthy people with similar amounts of cancellous bone as the osteoporotic patients the remodeling pattern is still quite different.

DR. JOHNSTON: But most osteoporotics have less bone than normal subjects.

DR. PARFITT: I agree. Another point is that looking at the bone in someone 20 years past menopause doesn't tell you why they lost bone 15 years earlier.

DR. GLORIEUX (Montreal): There is a clinical parallel to Dr. Rodan's presentation. In two first cousins with Caffey's disease a short course of indomethacin significantly reduced the excessive periosteal bone formation. So, in this condition, there is probably a local dysregulation of periosteal bone formation that is related to prostaglandin synthesis.

DR. KLEEREKOPER: I now bring to a close our formal tribute to the late Boy Frame, recognizing that informal tribute will continue through the whole week.

II
Bone Remodeling

Overview: Bone Remodeling

A.M. PARFITT

Bone & Mineral Research Laboratory
Henry Ford Hospital
Detroit, MI

INTRODUCTION AND OVERVIEW:

The supracellular organization of bone remodeling, aptly referred to by Frost as the skeletal intermediary organization (1), is the essential link between the macroscopic changes in bone mass and the microscopic changes in bone structure that occur with ageing and disease, the adaptations of bone to mechanical loading, and the cell and molecular biology of bone. Since remodeling occurs in temporally and spatially discrete packets or quanta (2), total skeletal remodeling represents the summation of contributions by a large number of focal events, each at a different stage of evolution. In general, the direction of change in bone volume and mass at a surface, whether gain or loss, is determined by the focal balance between the depth of resorption and the thickness of new bone within each individual cycle of remodeling, but the magnitude of change depends mainly on the rate of remodeling activation.

Whole body rates of resorption and formation can be measured by radio-calcium kinetics (3) and estimated by retention of labeled disphosphonate (4) and by the serum levels and urinary excretion rates of a wide variety of biochemical markers. The clinical utility of these markers was reviewed by Marcus (5). Urinary excretion of hydroxyproline in the fasting state remains the most widely used marker of whole body bone resorption rates, but little new has been learned since our last clinical conference in 1983 (6). A new marker of bone resorption, reflecting the number of resorbing cells rather than the quantity of resorbed bone, is tartrate resistant acid phosphatase (TRAP), an enzyme found only in osteoclasts and in abnormal derivatives of the hematopoietic stem-cell such as the Gaucher cell (5). TRAP correlates well with urinary hydroxyproline but has not yet been compared with bone histomorphometry or evaluated in the management of osteoporosis.

A major recent development has been the discovery of osteocalcin and the measurement of its serum level as an index of bone formation. Marcus reviewed the accumulated evidence in detail and pointed out the precautions that must be taken in interpretation. Serum osteocalcin is relatively insensitive to changes in bone formation rate in Paget's disease, but identifies with reasonable precision the direction and magnitude of change in bone formation in a wide variety of other disorders. In osteoporosis the data are conflicting, but most groups have found no correlation between serum osteocalcin and histologically determined bone formation rate. Like other markers, osteocalcin is a significant but weak predictor of the subsequent rate of bone loss in perimenopausal women. For physicians and patients who are unconvinced about the cardio-protective effect of estrogen replacement therapy, the combination of a low measurement for bone mass and a high value for some biochemical marker may help select women for such therapy who are at greatest risk of osteoporosis and have most to gain from preventing bone loss (5).

Most patients with metabolic bone disease, particularly osteoporosis, are white women, so that most studies of normal bone remodeling have focused on the effects of age in this group. But white men and blacks also experience age-related bone loss and suffer from fractures, albeit less frequently. Studies of bone remodeling in these groups are important not only in themselves but because differences between sexes and between races may provide important clues to fracture pathogenesis. Recker reviewed the available data on the demographics of bone remodeling (7). The main effect of age is a modest increase in remodeling activation in both sexes, that has been shown by histologic, biochemical and kinetic measurements but is of smaller magnitude than the effects of estrogen deficiency in women. In addition, there is a decline in the work efficiency of osteoclast and osteoblast teams (7). Bone fragility is increased by the removal of whole trabecular elements and the resultant disruption of architecture, a change more evident in women than in men. Trabecular perforation must result from the cumulative effect of some combination of decreased initial trabecular thickness, increased frequency of remodeling activation, increased resorption depth or decreased wall thickness, but the relative importance of these factors is unknown.

In the US, Blacks have more bone than whites, both because of higher peak adult bone mass and slower age-related bone loss. The frequency of remodeling activation, estimated both by histologic and biochemical methods, is lower than in whites and osteoblast work efficiency is reduced (7,8). Reduced remodeling activation has two consequences with opposite effects on fracture risk - conservation of mass and increased bone age. Fracture risk is lower in Blacks than in Whites so that the former effect predominates. Both increased bone age and slower osteoblast work are postulated to increase bone fragility, the former by increasing the accumulation of fatigue damage and microfractures and the latter by depressing their repair (1). The presence of both of these abnormalities in a group with lower fracture risk is a challenge to those who believe that qualitative factors are important (9). It is of particular interest that South African Blacks, who differ ethnically from US Blacks, have increased rates of bone remodeling and a much lower fracture rate than US Blacks (C. Schnitzler, Discussion in this session). It seems clear that the study of bone remodeling in different ethnic groups has much more to teach us about the interplay between quantitative and qualitative factors in fracture pathogenesis.

Many hormones affect bone remodeling and are implicated in the pathogenesis of metabolic bone diseases, including osteoporosis. The classic endocrinopathies are easily recognized; their effects on bone are complex and the available knowledge was reviewed by Melsen (10). Although not able to distinguish between direct and indirect effects of hormone excess, or deficiency, bone histomorphometry is the only way of determining the cumulative long-term summation of all effects. It may be difficult to separate the effects of age-related changes in hormone secretion from the effects of ageing along, but for increases in function the former explanation is more likely and for decreases in function the latter is more likely. Estrogen deficiency increases remodeling activation and estrogen replacement decreases it; whether these changes result from a direct effect of estrogen on bone lining cells of osteoblast lineage, or are mediated indirectly by a different cell type or a different hormone is unknown. Nevertheless other age-related changes in bone cell function are not corrected by estrogen replacement (10).

One of the most important lessons from bone histomorphometry, superficially paradoxical but important for cell biologists to explain, is that the total quantity of resorption or formation (determined by the frequency of remodeling activation), the amount of work performed by an individual team of osteoclasts or osteoblasts, and the rate at which the work is performed can each vary independently (2). For example, in primary hyperparathyroidism bone formation rate per unit of bone surface is increased, but the mineral apposition rate is decreased. A more surprising finding is that in hypothyroidism osteoblasts work more slowly but eventually make more bone than normal (10). Increased wall-thickness in hypothyroidism must result from some combination of increased osteoblast recruitment and increased lifetime work capacity. Could a profound reduction in the number of teams recruited make more precursor cells available for each team? This and many other unanswered questions arise from the study of bone remodeling in the intact organism. A base is useful only to the extent that it provides support for the super-structure above, and no science can claim to be basic to clinical medicine unless it eventually comes to grips with the questions posed by clinical investigators.

REFERENCES:
1. Frost HM. Intermediary organization of the skeleton. Vols I, II. CRC Press, Boca Raton, 1986.
2. Parfitt AM. Bone remodeling: Relationship to the amount and structure of bone and the pathogenesis and prevention of fractures. In: Riggs BL, Melton LJ, eds. Osteoporosis - Etiology, Diagnosis and Management. New York, Raven Press, 1988.
3. Reeve J, Arlot M, Hesp R, Tellez M, Meunier PJ. Tracer measurements of bone remodelling and their significance in involutional osteoporosis. In: Frame B, Potts JT Jr, eds. Clinical Disorders of Bone and Mineral Metabolism. Excerpta Medica, Amsterdam, 1983:99-104.
4. Fogelman I, Bessent RG, Citrin DL, Boyle IT, Greig WR. The use of whole body retention of Tc-99m diphosphonate in the diagnosis of metabolic bone disease. J Nucl Med 1978;19:270.
5. Marcus R. Biochemical markers of bone remodeling. In: Kleerekoper M, Krane S, eds. Clinical Disorders of Bone and Mineral Metabolism. Mary Ann Liebert Publishers, Inc, New York, 1988 (in press).
6. Kivirikko KI. Excretion of urinary hydroxyproline peptides in the assessment of bone collagen deposition and resorption. In: Frame B, Potts JT Jr, eds. Clinical Disorders of Bone and Mineral Metabolism. Excerpta Medica, Amsterdam, 1983:105-107.
7. Recker RR. The effects of age, sex and race on bone remodeling. In: Kleerekoper M, Krane S, eds. Clinical Disorders of Bone and Mineral Metabolism. Mary Ann Liebert Publishers, Inc, New York, 1988 (in press).
8. Weinstein RS, Weinstein DL, Bell NH. Evidence for diminished rates of mineralization and bone formation in normal blacks. In: Program and Abstracts: Clinical Disorders of Bone and Mineral Metabolism, 1988;18.
9. Parfitt AM. Surface specific bone remodeling in health and disease. In: Kleerekoper M, Krane S, eds. Clinical Disorders of Bone and Mineral Metabolism. Mary Ann Liebert Publishers, Inc, New York, 1988 (in press).
10. Melsen F, Mosekilde L, Eriksen EF, Charles P, Steinicke T. In vivo hormonal effects on trabecular bone remodeling, osteoid mineralization and skeletal turnover. In: Kleerekoper M, Krane S, eds. Clinical Disorders of Bone and Mineral Metabolism. Mary Ann Liebert Publishers, Inc, New York, 1988 (in press).

Biochemical Markers of Bone Remodeling

ROBERT MARCUS

Department of Medicine
Stanford University School of Medicine
and Geriatric Research, Education and Clinical Center
Veterans Administration Medical Center
Palo Alto, CA

Over the past twenty years, considerable insight regarding the fundamental processes and derangements of bone remodeling has been obtained through the pioneering work of Frost and others on bone histomorphometry. Unfortunately, iliac crest biopsy is an invasive procedure, requiring sophisticated laboratory support that is not readily available. The potential for biopsy to achieve general use in diagnosis or as a means to monitor the progress of individual patients is therefore limited. Consequently, there has been widespread interest in validating biochemical markers which accurately reflect the elements of remodeling, and which are easily measured in urine or plasma. This presentation addresses the current status of several of these potential markers.

For the purposes of discussion, I define "marker" as an entity whose concentration or activity in plasma or urine reflects, but does not modulate remodeling events. Although the circulating levels of parathyroid hormone, estrogens, and vitamin D regulate bone turnover, they are not, strictly speaking, "markers." I shall consider this topic from the perspective of clinical utility. The particular needs of investigators who are concerned with fundamental bone biology are sufficiently diverse that the utility of any marker will be highly individual and not usefully addressed here.

For clinical purposes, an ideal marker might fulfill several functions. It could be a surrogate for bone biopsy, permitting the specific diagnosis of bone disorders. It could also be an accurate predictor of the rate of bone loss, assisting the clinician identify patients most likely to benefit from therapy. To be of greatest use, it should permit subtle distinctions in difficult areas of diagnosis, for example, to distinguish low- from high-turnover osteoporosis. Conversely, it would not be useful to develop markers that are indicative only of florid, otherwise obvious disease.

From the start, the degree to which any biochemical marker can ever perfectly reflect the standard remodeling indices of iliac crest biopsies is highly constrained. Since 80% of the skeleton is cortical bone, important contributions to whole-body turnover will come from the cortical skeleton, whereas standard histomorphometry is directed primarily at trabecular bone. Furthermore, the whole body production of a marker is determined by factors other than the relative balance of resorption and formation within a given bone remodeling unit. These include the relative abundance of active bone remodeling elements per unit of bone mass as well as the total mass of skeleton available for remodeling. As one obvious example, it may be impossible to use simple urinary excretion data to distinguish 3% annual bone loss from an initial total body calcium of 600 g from 6% loss in a person with 1200 g total calcium.

In light of the above, I believe that no current single biochemical marker, alone or in combination, constitutes a satisfactory alternative to iliac crest biopsy for the specific diagnosis of bone disease. Osteomalacia cannot be distinguished from low-turnover osteoporosis without tetracycline-assisted histomorphometry. Aluminum deposition osteomalacia requires specific histologic confirmation. Even in myeloma, where abnormal tumor products are generally present in urine or plasma, only a biopsy is diagnostic in the patient whose tumor is truly non-secretory.

With respect to prediction of rates of bone loss, there is evidence that some markers may be useful, and I will discuss these below. Because remodeling is a coupled process, markers of resorption and formation should change in parallel. Although this may frequently be true, considerable variation exists in the degree of coupling inefficiency among individuals and from one condition to the next, so for proper understanding of remodeling dynamics, it is crucial to develop biochemical measures of both processes.

RESORPTION MARKERS: Biochemical measures of bone resorption are listed below:

Table 1. Indices of bone resorption:

Traditional	Potentially useful
Urine hydroxyproline	Acid phosphatase
Urine Ca/creatinine ratio	Calcitonin challenge

Traditional indices of bone resorption activity include urinary excretion of calcium and hydroxyproline. Both allow reasonable estimates of overall bone turnover and correlate with rates of bone loss. Neither accurately reflects individual osteoclastic function.

Urinary hydroxyproline Hydroxylation of proline is a post-translational modification to collagen. Since hydroxyproline is not incorporated into new collagen, its appearance in biological fluids is a reflection only of collagen breakdown. It is not specific for bone, and, in fact, only a small fraction of total hydroxyproline production appears in urine, the major fraction having been metabolized in the liver. Day to day variation of hydroxyproline excretion is small, although the measurement is confounded by the hydrolysis of dietary collagen and gelatin. Patients must therefore consume a meat and gelatin-free diet for two days prior to urine collection. Two-hour fasting specimens are a satisfactory alternative to 24 hour collections, and permit normalization of hydroxyproline excretion per mg creatinine or per dl of glomerular filtrate.

Total urinary hydroxyproline excretion increases with age. Delmas et al (7). Recently showed this rise to be significant when corrected for renal function. Elevated ratios of urinary hydroxyproline/creatinine are easily demonstrated in groups of patients with conditions of high bone turnover compared to normals or low turnover patients. This finding is not diagnostically specific, since equivalent increases may be seen regardless of the cause of increased turnover, be it hyperparathyroidism, thyrotoxicosis, Paget's disease, etc. Hydroxyproline excretion increases at menopause and decreases with estrogen therapy. This effect may be due in part to alterations in collagen turnover in tissues other than bone. Not all reductions in bone turnover are accompanied by reductions in hydroxyproline excretion. Progestins of the 19-nor testosterone class decrease urinary calcium and protect bone mass in menopausal women, although reductions in hydroxyproline excretion have not generally been reported.

Most patients with osteoporosis have normal urinary hydroxyproline excretion. Joly et al (13) found increased values in patients with increased circulating immunoreactive PTH. Although good correlations between hydroxyproline excretion and kinetic assessments of bone turnover are reported, hydroxyproline excretion correlates poorly with traditional histomorphometric assessments in osteoporotics.

Nordin and Polley (15) evaluated the hydroxyproline/creatinine ratio as a predictor of forearm mineral loss in a large group of women at menopause and found a correlation (-.16) which was highly significant, although of relatively low magnitude.

Urinary calcium excretion reflects the net contributions of dietary intake, renal handling, and bone resorption. Nordin has shown that the effects of a calcium containing meal on urine calcium have dissipated by 6 hours. Therefore, following overnight fast, a 2 hour calcium/creatinine ratio offers a reasonable index of bone resorption. One cannot evaluate the renal contribution from this ratio alone, and in many conditions, such as estrogen deficiency, glucocorticoid administration, or hyperparathyroidism altered reabsorption efficiency substantially modulates calcium excretion. Calcium/creatinine ratios increase at menopause and decrease following estrogen replacement. Nordin and Polley (15) found a significant correlation between Ca/Cr and forearm bone loss in menopausal women, but neither the magnitude nor significance of this correlation was as strong as that for hydroxyproline.

Tartrate-resistant acid phosphatase. Major sources of circulating acid phosphatase activity are bone, prostate, and hematopoietic tissues. L-Tartrate-inhibitable activity is characteristic of prostatic enzyme, and is routinely used to evaluate patients with prostatic adenocarcinoma. Tartrate-resistant acid phosphatase (TR ACP) is considered to originate in osteoclasts, and high levels obtain in Paget's disease and hyperparathyroidism. Enzyme activity in serum correlates highly with the urinary hydroxyproline/creatinine ratio (19). Plasma TR ACP increases shortly after menopause, and appears to correlate with the rate of bone loss (19). To date, there has not been sufficient published experience with this marker in normal subjects or in osteoporotic patients to know whether it will confer any advantages over the traditional measures.

Calcitonin challenge tests

Blanc et al. (1) reported that the hypocalcemic response to calcitonin injection correlated with bone turnover: higher rates of turnover were associated with deeper and more sustained hypocalcemia. Since the osteoclast is the major target cell in bone for this hormone, the response is presumed to reflect osteoclastic resorption. This test clearly distinguished normal individuals from patients with major clearcut disorders of mineral metabolism, such as myeloma, however it has not been useful to distinguish subtle differences among normal subjects or in osteoporotics. It appears that subjects with lower turnover rates experienced minimal drops in serum calcium, sometimes in the same range as the error of the measurement. In addition, the test requires 24 hours of sequential blood samples, and is therefore cumbersome to perform.

We recently showed that calcitonin administration acutely elevates plasma levels of cyclic AMP, and that this rise is significantly greater in patients with hyperparathyroidism and Paget's disease than in normal subjects (14). It is not known whether this test will be useful in predicting bone loss or resorption activity in other settings.

BONE FORMATION: Biochemical correlates of osteoblastic function are listed below:

Table 2. Indices of bone formation.

Traditional	New	Potentially useful
Total Alkaline P'tase	Osteocalcin (Bone Gla protein)	Bone Alkaline P'tase Procollagen I extention peptide

For many years, the only clinically applicable marker of osteoblastic function has been serum alkaline phosphatase activity (AP). AP is easy to measure, reasonably stable over time in individuals, and inexpensive. Its major drawback is lack of specificity for bone. In normal, non-pregnant humans, serum AP represents approximately equal amounts of enzyme from liver and bone. These isoenzymes are produced by a single "bone-liver-kidney" gene, with post-translational glycosylation introducing subtle differences in the circulating enzyme species. In pregnancy and certain malignancies, other isoenzymes of AP contribute to total activity, but under ordinary circumstances the primary differential must be made between liver and bone enzyme. Several methods have been described, but the most useful appears to be based on the relative thermolability of bone enzyme.

AP activity reflects overall skeletal turnover, and is considerably higher during years of growth and development than in young adults. With continued aging, AP rises again, particularly in women, with a notable increase at menopause.

Total AP is quite elevated in some bone disorders, such as Paget's disease and vitamin D deficiency osteomalacia. In these settings, it provides a reasonable guide to therapy over time. In other conditions, such as most patients with primary hyperparathyroidism, AP is in the normal range or only slightly elevated, and correlates poorly, if at all, with degree of hypercalcemia or PTH levels (8). AP is generally within the normal range in uncomplicated osteoporosis, and significant elevations should lead the physician to consider the presence of osteomalacia. Delmas et al (6) assessed total AP in a large group of osteoporotic women, and found that mean values were moderately higher than would have been predicted from age, with 22% of patients beyond two standard deviations above the mean. However, there was no correlation between AP and lumbar spine density. Brown et al. (2) measured total AP activity in 26 postmenopausal women who underwent iliac crest biopsy. No significant correlation was found between AP and any index of bone formation. Similar results were reported by Whyte et al (21). Nordin and Polley (15) showed a significant relationship between AP and forearm bone loss in menopausal women, although the correlation was only 0.12.

Bone alkaline phosphatase. Distinguishing hepatic from skeletal AP has been approached by immunologic and chromatographic techniques, but one of the more successful approaches has been to exploit the differential thermolability of these isoenzymes. Used in tandem, heat and specific inhibition permit the measurement of skeletal AP in plasma. These methods confirm a rise in skeletal AP during normal aging, and suggest a rise in patients with osteoporosis (11). Skeletal AP correlates well with urinary hydroxyproline, but much more experience with this activity is required before it can be embraced as a useful clinical marker.

Procollagen I extension peptide. A cleavage product of type I collagen in bone, the procollagen extension peptide is released into the circulation. Since it is a product of osteoblasts, pcoll I-C levels may provide a marker of bone forming activity. Initial studies confirm a relationship with other measures of bone turnover, but conclusions regarding its ultimate role as a remodeling marker are premature.

Osteocalcin. The gamma-carboxyglutamic acid-containing peptide, osteocalcin or BGP, is the major non-collagen protein synthesized by osteoblasts. Secretion of this 5700 Dalton peptide is under regulatory control by 1,25 dihydroxyvitamin D. Although the majority of synthesized BGP associates with bone matrix, some appears in circulating blood, where it reflects overall osteoblastic activity. It is not clear that the binding of newly synthesized BGP to bone matrix is identical in all situations or at all ages. Theoretically, therefore, high levels of BGP might not always indicate increased synthesis. For example, Poser et al (17) found that osteocalcin extracted from bone from an elderly man had a complement of gamma carboxy glutamate less than the expected 3 residues per mole. If an aberrant osteocalcin molecule bound less readily to matrix, artifactually high levels in serum could be observed.

Before assessing the clinical utility of osteocalcin, it is important to make a few technical points. Osteocalcin is measured by radioimmunoassay. Most assay methods to date employ antisera generated against bovine osteocalcin, but some work has been done with fragments of human BGP. Although parallel dilution of human serum against antisera to bovine osteocalcin is reported with several well-validated research assays, problems in this area have been described with commercially available osteocalcin kits. A second point concerns timing of samples. Gundberg et al (12) have shown substantial diurnal variation in osteocalcin levels in man, so sample collection time must be standardized. Osteocalcin survives fairly well in the freezer, but activity is reduced with multiple thawing. Thus, it is important to thaw samples only once, immediately prior to assay.

Unlike AP, circulating osteocalcin is derived exclusively from bone, and reflects osteoblastic activity. Many (7,10), but not all (4), investigators report a rise in osteocalcin levels with normal human aging. The basis for discrepancies on this point is not clear. There may be important differences of assay technology, although systematic differences in population characteristics have not been adequately explored. Since bone is lost with age, it may seem paradoxical that a measure of bone formation would rise. However, one must remember that, in a coupled system, the overall rate of bone formation reflects to some degree an antecedent episode of resorption. Thus, elevations in BGP are clues to a general level of bone turnover, which, by its inefficient nature will be predictive of bone loss.

Circulating levels of BGP correlate well with bone turnover in a variety of physiologic and pathologic states. They are elevated in hyperthyroidism, hyperparathyroidism, and Paget's disease, and reduced in hypoparathyroidism. In hyperparathyroidism, the elevation in BGP correlates with the presence or absence of clinically evident bone disease, and there is a strong negative correlation between BGP and forearm bone mineral content (22).

Where efficient coupling or osteoblast function has been impaired, BGP is low. Examples include hypercalcemia of malignancy and glucocorticoid osteopenia. Estrogen withdrawal raises BGP levels; estrogen therapy reduces them (20). Some discrepancies in this general scheme have been observed. Several groups have found that BGP in Paget's disease is not as consistently elevated as the alkaline phosphatase activity. Papapoulos et al (16) reported that treatment of Paget's disease with diphosphonate reduced AP and hydroxyproline, but gave transient elevations in BGP. The diphosphonate may have displaced preformed BGP from mineral, or the rise may have been due to a treatment-induced increase in PTH or calcitriol.

Excellent correlations are found between serum osteocalcin and indices of bone formation on iliac crest biopsy of patients with a variety of bone disorders, including osteoporosis (2,6). Whether BGP correlates as well in normal subjects is not clear. Administration of 1,25D quickly leads to increases in circulating osteocalcin. Duda et al (9) showed that the response to exogenous 1,25D is more exuberant in patients with osteoporosis than in age-matched non-osteoporotic women. They interpreted these results to indicate that primary osteoblastic failure is not the major cause of bone loss in postmenopausal osteoporosis.

Biochemical Predictors of Bone Loss

Several groups have used biochemical markers alone or in combination to rationalize selection of patients for therapy aimed at protecting bone mass. In particular, concern has been expressed that decisions regarding estrogen replacement therapy should be based on an individual woman's risk for "rapid" bone loss at menopause, and that this strategy will maximize the beneficial effects of estrogen while minimizing potential toxicity. Christiansen et al (5) reported that determination of body fat mass, urine calcium and hydroxyproline, and serum alkaline phosphatase correctly identified the majority of "fast" and "slow" bone losers in a large group of menopausal women. However, this model awaits prospective validation in a separate, independent group of women. Slemenda et al (18) recently showed that BGP is a stronger predictor of menopausal bone loss ($r=-.48$) than are circulating levels of endogenous estrogens, androgens, or androgen-estrogen conversion parameters.

Although these relationships have been evaluated within a short period of menopause, if they are validated they might also find application to older women who are traditionally felt no longer to be suited for estrogen. Evidence for increased turnover even at advanced ages might identify estrogen-responsiveness. However, recent evidence raises questions about the entire strategy of selecting patients for estrogen therapy on the basis of skeletal risk. A considerable emerging literature now supports the conclusion that estrogen replacement confers important cardiovascular risk protection on menopausal women (3). Since ischemic heart disease is the leading cause of hospitalization and mortality in older women, such protection would far outweigh other considerations, and suitability for estrogen would properly be determined with little regard for the skeleton.

With recent discovery of new substances unique to bone, the search for markers remains an exciting, fruitful area of investigation. Turning again to the question of clinical utility, it is reasonable to ask whether, among the choices available, does any current marker stand out as the universally most accurate index or predictor ? For the present, I think the answer is no. From considerations outlined above, it appears that great potential lies with osteocalcin. Even though there remain some clinical situations, such as Paget's disease, in which osteocalcin may be less accurate than other markers, for most purposes a single measurement of osteocalcin offers a more accurate prediction of bone turnover than the other markers discussed in this presentation. However, for osteocalcin to be generally useful, assay technology will require additional improvement and standardization, and high quality assays will need to become widely available.

References

1. Blanc D, Chapuy MC, Meunier P. Evaluation de l'activite osteoclastique par le test d'hypocalcemie provoquee par la calcitonine de saumon. Nov Presse Med 1977, 6:2489-2494.

2. Brown JP, Delmas PD, Malaval L, Edouard C, Chapuy MC, Meunier PJ. Serum bone gla-protein: a specific marker for bone formation in postmenopausal osteoporosis. Lancet 1984, i:1091-1093.

3. Bush TL, Barrett-Connor E, Cowan LD, Criqui MH et al. Cardiovascular mortality and noncontraceptive use of estrogen in women: results from the lipid Research Clinics program follow-up study. Circulation 1987, 75:1102-1109.

4. Catherwood BD, Marcus R, Madvig P, Chelling AJ. Determinants of bone gamma-carboxyglutamic acid-containing protein in plasma of healthy aging subjects. Bone 1985, 6:9-13.

5. Christiansen C, Riis BJ, Rodbro P. Prediction of rapid bone loss in postmenopausal women. Lancet 1987 i:1105-1107.

6. Delmas PD, Wahner HW, Mann KG, Riggs BL. Assessment of bone turnover in postmenopausal osteoporosis by measurement of serum bone gla-protein. J Lab Clin Med 1983, 102:470-476.

7. Delmas PD, Stenner D, Wahner HW, Mann KG, Riggs BL. Increase in serum bone gamma-carboxyglutamic acid protein with aging in women. Implications for the mechanism of age-related bone loss. J Clin Invest 1983, 71:1316-1321.

8. Delmas PD, Demiaux B, Malaval L, Chapuy MC, Edouard C, Meunier PJ. Serum bone gamma carboxyglutamic acid-containing protein in primary hyperparathyroidism and in malignant hypercalcemia. comparison with bone histomorphometry. J Clin Invest 1986, 77:985-991.

9. Duda RJ, Kumar R, Nelson KI, Zinsmeister AR, Mann KG, Riggs BL. 1,25-dihydroxyvitamin D stimulation test for osteoblast function in normal and osteoporotic postmenopausal women. J Clin Invest 1987, 79:1249-1253.

10. Epstein S, Poser J, McClintock R, Johnston CC Jr, Bryce G, Hui S. Differences in serum bone gla protein with age and sex. Lancet 1984, i:307-310.

11. Farley J Jr., Chesnut CJ, Baylink DJ. Improved method for quantitative determination of serum alkaline phosphatase of skeletal origin. Clin Chem 1981, 27: 2002-2007.

12. Gundberg CM, Markowitz ME, Mizruchi M, Rosen JF. Osteocalcin in human serum: a circadian rhythm. J Clin Endocrinol Metab 1985, 60:736-739.

13. Joly R, Chapuy MC, Alexandre C, Meunier PJ. Osteoporoses `a haut niveau de remodelage et fonctione parathyroidienne. Pathol. Biol. 1980.

14. Minkoff JR, Grant BF, Marcus R. Plasma cyclic AMP response to calcitonin: a potential clinical marker of bone turnover. Bone 1986, 6:285-290.

15. Nordin BEC, Polley KJ, Metabolic consequences of the menopause. Calcified Tissue Intl, 1987 (Suppl. 1), 41:S1-S59.

16. Papapoulos SE, Frolich M, Mudde AH, Harinck HIJ, vd Berg H, Bijvoet OLM. Serum osteocalcin in Paget's disease of bone: basal concentrations and response to bisphosphonate treatment. J Clin Endocrinol Metab 1987, 65:89-94.

17. Poser JW, Esch FS, Ling NC, Price PA. Isolation and sequence of the vitamin K-dependent protein from human bone: undercarboxylation of the first glutamic acid residue. J Biol Chem. 1980, 255:8685-8690.

18. Slemenda C, Hui SL, Longcope C, Johnston CC. Sex steroids and bone mass. a study of changes about the time of menopause. J Clin Invest 1987, 80:1261-1269.

19. Stepan JJ, Pospichal J, Presl J, Pacovsky V. Bone loss and biochemical indices of bone remodeling in surgically induced postmenopausal women. Bone 1987, 8:279-284.

20. Stock JL, Coderre JA, Mallette LE, Effects of a short course of estrogen on mineral metabolism in postmenopausal women. J Clin Endocrinol Metab 1985, 61:595-600.

21. Whyte MP, Bergfeld MA, Murphy WA, Avioli LV, Teitelbaum SL. Postmenopausal osteoporosis: a heterogenous disorder as assessed by histomorphometric analysis of iliac crest bone from untreated patients. Am J Med 1982, 72:193-202.

22. Yoneda M, Takatsuki K, Oiso Y, Takanao T, Kurokawa M, et al. Clinical significance of serum bone gla protein and urinary gla as biochemical markers in primary hyperparathyroidism. Endocrinol Japon 1986, 33:89-94.

Discussion:

DR. JOHNSTON (Indianapolis): In the short term, for three to five years after menopause, the major determinant of future bone mass is bone mass at menopause; the contribution of differences in remodeling rate is small. Looking at individual patients rather than at groups, we find little contribution from measurement of osteocalcin to estimation of future bone mass compared to the contribution of current bone mass. Obviously, the longer after menopause, the more will the rate of loss contribute. But we don't know whether people who are losing relatively rapidly right after menopause are the ones who will continue to lose rapidly and ultimately develop osteoporosis.

DR. REEVE (England): Another problem with hydroxyproline excretion is that in our experience, it's quite variable from day-to-day. As a predictor of bone resorption, which was measured simultaneously using kinetic techniques, the mean of three consecutive measurements is much better than a single examination.

DR. MARCUS (Palo Alto, CA): We have found less day-to-day variation if one uses a two-hour overnight fasted collection, rather than a 24-hour collection. The coefficient of variation for repeated measures on the two-hour specimen was under six percent in a group of ten women who were tested six times.

DR. RODAN (West Point, PA): To what extent can the increase in osteocalcin with age be attributed to altered handling by the kidney?

DR. MARCUS: Well, you're opening up a Pandora's box, because we don't know what exactly it is we are measuring. There are a variety of fragments that may contribute to total osteocalcin measurements; it depends on the antiserum that you're using. With most assays, the renal contribution is trivial unless there is a severe deficit in glomerular filtration rate. With Catherwood's assay, there is a more robust inverse relationship with glomerular filtration rate, so the serum level rises at an earlier stage of renal insufficiency than with other assays.

DR. PARFITT (Detroit): How certain are you that urinary hydroxyproline goes up with age? Some investigators in Italy found that it only went up when related to urinary creatinine, because the absolute rate of hydroxyproline excretion does not change but the absolute creatinine excretion goes down.

DR. MARCUS: This is a generic problem that applies not only to urinary hydroxyproline, but to every measurement that I discussed. I reviewed essentially all the English language literature dating back several decades. And for every statement I made it was possible to find contrary observations. Nevertheless, I think the weight of evidence is that there is a rise in hydroxyproline excretion with age.

Effects of Age, Sex, and Race on Bone Remodeling

ROBERT R. RECKER and ROBERT P. HEANEY

Creighton University
Omaha, NE

INTRODUCTION

The purpose of this discussion is to explore some of the differences in bone remodeling associated with age, sex and race in the search to explain some of the known differences in skeletal fragility. "Excessive skeletal fragility" may be preferable to the term "osteoporosis" which tends to imply that the fracture syndrome is due to bone loss. Of course, most investigators believe that reduction in bone mass does play a role in the fracture syndrome of the elderly however, recent work suggests that it is not the whole story. For example, change in the geometric arrangement of trabecular elements and inefficient repair of microdamage are two factors that could also be involved. Errors in bone remodeling would have to be present to account for any one or all three, bone loss, maldistribution of trabecular elements and inefficient repair of microdamage. It is thus appropriate to examine bone remodeling for some of the answers to the clinical problem of excessive skeletal fragility.

DEFINITION OF BONE REMODELING

Frost (1) has described and defined the phenomenon of bone remodeling as the surface-based removal and replacement of bone tissue in the adult human which follows a lock-step sequence of events. It occurs in quantum packets called Basic Multicellular Units (BMU's) at foci on the Haversian surfaces of compact bone or on the quiescent surfaces of trabeculae. The volume of bone replaced is equal to the volume removed under normal circumstances. There are about 1.125×10^6 BMU actively engaged at any one time in a healthy adult (2), and each one replaces about 0.05 mm3 of bone tissue during a remodeling cycle. Each cycle takes on average about five months to complete (3).

It is important to distinguish remodeling as it is defined here from modeling which is a different phenomenon (1). Modeling is the process by which the skeleton sculpts and molds itself in response to the elongation of growth. It is characterized by drifts of bone surface through space, accomplished by continuous osteoclast work on a resorption surface, along with continuous osteoblast work on a formation surface. Thus while the work of modeling is done by osteoclasts and osteoblasts, the regulation and control of this work is entirely different. The capacity for modeling is essentially lost after childhood while remodeling takes place continuously throughout life. Many authors have confused these functions and have included both under the definition of remodeling.

METHODS OF MEASURING REMODELING

HISTOMORPHOMETRY

The most direct method of sampling the remodeling system in the human is by transilial biopsy after double tetracycline labeling (4). Undecalcified biopsy cores can be embedded in a hard plastic such as methyl methacrylate and stained thin sections can be used for examination of static features while unstained sections can be examined under blue light fluorescence for analysis of remodeling dynamics from the tetracycline labels (5). The wall thickness of osteons can also be measured by several methods from these sections along with measures of trabecular connectivity such as trabecular spacing, trabecular thickness and trabecular number (6).

The important variables (7) that will be discussed are the following. Bone volume (TV/BV), wall thickness (W.Th) osteoid surface (OS/BS), eroded surface (ES/BS), osteoid thickness (O.Th), trabecular thickness (Tb.T), trabecular separation (Tb.S), trabecular number (Tb.N), mineralizing surface (MS/BS), mineral apposition rate (MAR), bone formation rate (BFR), lag times (MLT), and remodeling periods (Rm.P).

CALCIUM KINETICS

These methods (8) make use of calcium isotope tracer methodology wherein a tracer quantity of 45-calcium or 47-calcium is injected into the circulation and the plasma (or urine) specific activity curve is analyzed by one of several mathematical models. Concomitant measures of endogenous losses of calcium in the stool and urine are needed to calculate bone mineral accretion, and of calcium absorption from the gut to calculate bone mineral resorption.

The kinetic method permits measurement of the total entry and exit of calcium from the skeleton and thus it is a close approximation of bone turnover summed over the entire skeleton.

WHOLE BODY RETENTION

Whole body retention (WBR) of technetium-labeled diphosphonate has been used to estimate global skeletal remodeling (9) and has given results comparable to other methods. The diphosphonate adsorbs onto mineral crystal surfaces and thus preferentially accumulates at bone formation sites. The amount retained in the body is proportional to the number and extent of formation sites present. The agent also accumulates to some extent at surfaces other than formation sites and this confounds the results to a variable degree. It is also confounded by variation in kidney function and by the presence of focal bone lesions such as Pagets disease. Nevertheless, the method has been convenient, inexpensive and useful.

BIOCHEMICAL MARKERS OF REMODELING

Several methods have been put forth and each has enjoyed some usefulness in certain circumstances. The major advantages of these methods are their low cost and convenience, and some provide specific information of value such as in the case of urinary hydroxyproline and bone resorption rates. This discussion will include information on the following variables: serum levels of alkaline phosphatase (ALP) and bone GLA-protein (BGP), and urine levels of hydroxyproline corrected for glomerular filtration (OHPr/CR).

AGE-RELATED CHANGES IN BONE REMODELING

Most of the data on age-related changes in bone remodeling come from studies in women and will be discussed here. Later on, information on sex-differences will be presented.

HISTOMORPHOMETRY

Morphologic and geometric changes

There are several important structural changes in trabecular and cortical bone that are age-related. Reduction in trabecular bone volume and cortical thickness have been well described but there are other changes that are not necessarily apparent from examination of bone cell function by any of the methods mentioned above. These changes can only be seen by histomorphometric examination of trabecular microstructure or by high-resolution computed tomography.

The reduction in trabecular and cortical bone combines with an still another structural change, age-related reduction in the wall thickness (W.Th) of completed osteons. At least 7 authors have reported finding this (3,10-15) change in W.Th with several different methods in healthy living volunteers and in autopsy samples. Further, the mechanism for this seems to be reduced osteoclast work since Erikson (16) has found an age-related reduction in resorption depth at remodeling sites. Coupled with these is the finding that trabecular thickness does not decline with age (3,6). Instead, the distance or separation between trabeculae increases and the number of trabecular elements per unit volume of bone tissue decreases with age while leaving trabecular thickness unchanged (3,6,17). These findings indicate that bone loss occurs as a loss of trabecular elements with age rather than global thinning of trabeculae. Further, it can be inferred that the average age of bone tissue increases since the central or interstitial parts of the trabeculae tend to remain unremodeled, and this can be expected to result in accumulation of excessive microdamage with resultant reduction in mechanical strength. Changes in the dynamics of bone remodeling must be interpreted in light of these findings.

Age-related change in mineral apposition rate (MAR)

The MAR has been shown to decrease with age both in cortical bone (18) and in trabecular bone (3). However, Frost (18) also reported an increase in the rate of activation of new remodeling sites (activation frequency). This would tend to offset the effect of reduced MAR in measurements of global bone formation rates. The trabecular measurement that comes closest to the activation frequency as measured in cortical bone is the mineralizing surface (MS/BS) and it has been found to exhibit no change with age (3,10,13,15), or an increase (20) or decrease (21) with age. The most likely scenario is that there is an age-related decrease in MAR in both cortical and trabecular bone, coupled with an increase in the activation frequency of new remodeling sites in cortical bone (and perhaps in trabecular bone), and either no net change or a slight increase in global bone formation rates as will be seen in some of the reports described below.

The net result of these changes would be a reduction in the efficiency of repair of microdamage, an increase in the mean age of the bone tissue and perhaps an increase in the remodeling space with its accompanying reduction in bone volume. All of these would be expected to reduce the mechanical strength of the skeleton, particularly when accompanied by the overall net reduction in trabecular bone volume which is well known to occur.

Other histomorphometric changes

The various tetracycline-based histomorphometric expressions of bone formation rates have either not shown any age-related change or have shown mixed results. For example, in a study (3) of 34 healthy normal postmenopausal women none of the bone formation variables showed a change with age whereas in Melsen's study (21) of a younger group, bone formation at the BMU-level and at the tissue-level showed a decline with age in women (but not in men).

The mineralization lag-time (Mlt) showed a non significant increase with age in those reports on trabecular bone from the iliac crest (3,15,20,21). However, the variation in this expression was considerable, and so a fairly strong trend could have been masked. The same problem occurred in Frost's report (18) on cortical bone of the rib and thus the question of whether there is a secular trend in MLT remains open. A prolonged MLT could be important as a component of the overall reduction in mechanical strength of the skeleton with age because it could contribute to inefficient repair of microdamage.

Frost's report (18) on cortical bone seems to show an increase in the formation period (FP) (formerly called "sigma") but he did not supply a formal regression of that variable on age. In Recker's report (3) there was an increase in FP with age, but it was not statistically significant because of considerable variation in the expression. A prolonged FP could also be important as a component of the overall reduction in mechanical strength of the skeleton with age because it too could signify inefficient repair of microdamage. It should be pointed out that prolongation of MLT and/or FP would be compatible with unchanged or slightly increased global bone remodeling rates provided the activation frequency of new remodeling sites was sufficiently increased.

The static measures of bone remodeling taken from transiliac bone biopsies have been confusing. Osteoid surface (OS/BS) has been demonstrated to increase with age (20) or remain unchanged (3,15,17,21,22). Resorption surface (ES/BS) has also been demonstrated to increase with age (16,17,20,22) or remain unchanged (3,21). The only comprehensive evaluation of static variables in cortical bone was done by Frost (13) and showed an increase in the number of osteoid seams and in the number of resorption sites with age.

SUMMARY OF SECULAR TRENDS IN HISTOMORPHOMETRIC DATA

The strongest secular trends revealed in the iliac histomorphometric data seem to be in the trabecular microstructure. There is a well documented reduction in wall thickness along with a reduction in trabecular number, and an increase in trabecular spacing. Trabecular thickness does not change. The reduction in trabecular bone volume is brought about by loss of trabecular elements and not by global thinning of trabeculae. The tetracycline data show a reduction in mineral apposition rate and a weak trend toward a prolonged mineralization lag time and prolonged formation period. In addition, there is a small increase in the activation frequency of new remodeling sites in cortical bone which results in a slight increase in global bone remodeling rates.

RADIOCALCIUM KINETICS AND AGE-RELATED CHANGES

There are few data available on age-related changes in bone remodeling in normal subjects as measured by radiocalcium kinetics. Heaney et. al. (24) demonstrated an increase in accretion and resorption at menopause with resorption increasing more than accretion. That report did not include observations extending long enough past menopause to judge whether the transmenopausal increase was sustained or whether another change in remodeling occurred which was age-related.

Unpublished data from Omaha reveal an interesting age-related effect on remodeling which is modulated by the presence or absence of estrogen. A total of 428 radiocalcium kinetic studies were performed over a period of 21 years on 191 normal females between ages 35 and 65 from a prospective study of subjects at risk for osteoporosis. Two hundred thirty one studies were performed on 110 subjects who were estrogen replete and 197 studies were performed on 104 subjects who were estrogen deprived. Some subjects appeared in both groups. Mean accretion in the estrogen replete group was 0.338 ± 0.089 gm/d and in the estrogen deprived group was 0.403 ± 0.093 gm/d.

Bone mineral accretion rates adjusted for variation in body surface area were regressed on age. In the estrogen replete group there was a weak but statistically significant negative correlation with age and in the estrogen deprived group there was a weak but statistically significant positive correlation with age. The increase in remodeling was about 28% over the age span of 35-65, or about 0.95% per year. This is in the same range as found with other methods described in this article.

WHOLE BODY RETENTION OF RADIOLABELED BONE-SEEKING AGENTS

The 24-hour retention (WBR) of 99m-Tc-methylene-diphosphonate (99m-Tc-MDP) was measured in a large group of normals reported by Fogelman et al (25) and in another group by Hyldstrup et al (26). In the latter study there was a slight decline in retention during the second and third decades followed by a slight rise with age after the fourth decade. Retention increased from 0.33 at age 50 to 0.41 at age 80. This represents a 24% change over a period of 30 years or about 0.8% per year. Similar age-related changes were also noted in the measurements of ALP and OHPr\Cr in this study. Similar findings had been reported earlier by Fogelman et al (25). A significant rise in WBR has been shown at menopause (27) but few data on secular trends are available using this method.

BIOCHEMICAL MARKERS OF BONE REMODELING

There are three biochemical markers of bone remodeling that are important, serum alkaline phosphatase (ALP), serum bone GLA-protein (BGP) and urinary excretion of hydroxyproline per unit glomerular filtration rate (OHPr\Cr). ALP and BGP are related to global bone formation rates and OHPr\Cr is related to global bone resorption rates although there are confounding factors causing these measurements to be less than perfectly correlated with bone formation or resorption.

The most comprehensive study of ALP and OHPr\Cr in postmenopausal women (28) found that ALP rose immediately after menopause and then remained at that level or rose slightly over the next two decades. The OHPr\Cr also rose immediately after menopause and then seemed to drift downward slightly over the next two decades.

Podenphant et. al. (27) showed similar findings but also demonstrated that ALP correlated with tetracycline-based measurements of bone remodeling while OHPr\Cr did not. The reason for the lack of correlation in the case of OHPr\Cr was not clear. The sharp rise at menopause and plateau or slight rise thereafter is a pattern that has been demonstrated by several authors (26,29,30).

Bone GLA-protein (BGP), a vitamin K-dependent peptide unique to bone, is another marker for bone turnover that has been studied more recently (31). It is a sensitive test for bone turnover (32) and most of serum BGP is produced by osteoblasts during bone formation rather than by bone resorption (33). Delmas (30) showed a rise in BGP with age from 30-90 which roughly paralleled a rise in ALP and OHPr\Cr. The serum BGP rose about 1.58% per year, ALP about 0.5% per year and OHPr\Cr about 0.93 % per year over this age span. Other reports have shown similar results (27,34).

In summary, the biochemical markers of bone remodeling show a weak age-related rise in bone remodeling and a sharp rise at the time of menopause with resumption of the weak rise afterwards.

SUMMARY OF AGE-RELATED CHANGES IN BONE REMODELING

Taken as a whole, the measures of bone remodeling seem to suggest the following. There is a sharp rise in global remodeling rates at the time of menopause followed by a weak rise after that. There is a reduction in both osteoclast and osteoblast work at the level of the BMU but this is offset by an increase in the activation frequency of new remodeling sites. There is a concomitant change in trabecular microstructure characterized by a reduction in the number of trabecular elements with no change in their thickness. Wall thickness of completed osteons is reduced. Along with this is a reduction in trabecular number per unit area and an increase in trabecular spacing. The effect of these changes would be reduction in mechanical strength of the skeleton through reduction in bone mass, inefficient repair of microdamage and unfavorable microstructure.

SEX DIFFERENCES IN BONE REMODELING

HISTOMORPHOMETRIC DIFFERENCES

Age-related change in trabecular microstructure seems to be different in men compared to women. Parfitt (6) demonstrated loss of trabecular elements rather than global thinning of trabeculae in women, but in men there was a tendency for thinning to occur. Aaron (17) found a more striking sex difference in that trabecular thinning was much more prominent in men. This sex difference could explain some of the reduced skeletal fragility found in men compared to women.

Other sex differences have been reported in bone histomorphometry, most of them in the static measures. Melsen (21) showed higher OS\BS, ES\BS, MS\BS and BFR\BMU in men in transiliac biopsies. Others have shown increased OS.Th, MLT (15), OS\BS, dLS\BS, and BFR\BS (20). Several authors have reported a decline in W.Th in men similar to what is found in women (11,12,14,15). No one has reported a sex difference in MAR. Frost (18) did not show sex differences in his study of the rib.

BIOCHEMICAL MARKERS

The biochemical markers of bone remodeling have shown some sex differences. For example, OHPr\Cr remains relatively stable throughout life in men (26) while it rises abruptly in women at menopause and continues to rise albeit more slowly after that in women (28). Bone GLA-protein was shown to be higher in men by Epstein (34). There are relatively few reports comparing sex differences in biochemical markers and those that are available show few differences.

WHOLE BODY RETENTION OF 99M-TC-LABELED DIPHOSPHONATE

Reports of whole body retention of 99m-Tc-labeled diphosphonate have shown no sex differences (29), or have shown modestly higher values in young men, and except for a peak increase at menopause in women, similar values thereafter (25). As in the case of the biochemical markers, few data are available.

ETHNIC DIFFERENCES IN BONE REMODELING

It is a bit surprising that there have been few studies of bone remodeling in racial groups other than whites, since it has been generally known for some time that bone mass is greater in blacks (35) and the incidence of fractures is much reduced. Bell et al (36) studied adult blacks comparing them to adult whites and found serum PTH and 1,25 dihydroxyvitamin D levels to be higher in the blacks while BGP levels were much lower (14 ± 2 vs 24 ± 3 ng/ml).

Bone biopsies have been compared in blacks and whites and an update on these studies has appeared in an abstract (37). The blacks demonstrated a lower MS/BS, MAR and BFR/BS. There were no differences in the static bone histomorphometric measures. These findings fit with the earlier finding of reduced BGP levels and suggest that the intrinsic remodeling rate in the skeleton of blacks is lower than in whites. It is difficult to understand how the lower bone remodeling rate is associated with greater bone mass and reduced fragility in blacks since remodeling is thought to be the mechanism of repair of bone tissue microdamage. These findings would indicate that repair of microdamage is less efficient in blacks. Since blacks do not suffer more skeletal fragility, we must conclude that these remodeling changes are unrelated to skeletal fragility in blacks and that the remodeling mechanism which is responsible for repair of microdamage is intact.

SUMMARY OF AGE-, SEX- AND RACE-RELATED CHANGES IN BONE REMODELING

Reduction in TB/BV with age does not come about by simple thinning of trabeculae. Instead, there is loss of trabecular elements with reduction in their number, increase in their spacing and maintenance of their thickness. In men this tendency is less pronounced, with less bone loss and some thinning of trabeculae. Reduction in W.Th occurs in both sexes, a finding that is very well documented. It is due to reduced resorption depth at remodeling sites.

The MAR decreases with age both in cortical and trabecular bone. This is offset by an increase in the activation frequency of new remodeling sites mostly in Haversian bone.

Measurements of age-related changes in bone remodeling rates have given remarkably similar results whether by radiocalcium kinetics, whole body retention, or biochemical markers. In general, they all show a sharp rise at menopause and a very gradual rise thereafter. The magnitude of changes are very similar by all these methods. In men the changes are similar except the menopausal change is absent.

The ethnic difference in remodeling between blacks and whites is that bone formation at the BMU is slower and there are fewer remodeling sites active at any one time. The histomorphometry data that show this are supported by the finding of reduced BGP levels in blacks.

WORKING MODEL

How might these changes in bone remodeling account for increased bone fragility with age and in women? A working model would be that bone is lost during remodeling and in the case of the trabeculae, there is loss of trabecular elements rather than thinning of trabeculae which exaggerates the fragility because of loss of connectivity. In addition, there is inefficient remodeling. Wall thickness declines while trabecular thickness does not which means that there is more unremodeled interstitial tissue and the mean age of the skeletal tissue is increased. This would lead to more accumulation of microdamage and in turn to more fragility. The sluggish repair of microdamage is augmented by the reduced MAR which is accompanyed by an increase in the activation frequency in cortical bone. This would enlarge the remodeling space and hasten the erosion of the cortical endosteal surface. These changes would tend to be self-accelerating because they would tend to increase strain on the remaining skeleton thereby further increasing the microdamage and the fragility.

The challenge to research in this area is to acquire a better understanding of the mechanisms of control of bone remodeling so that the seemingly unrelenting increase in skeletal fragility with age can be halted and even reversed. Unless there is concentrated effort in this area the answer to the problem of excessive skeletal fragility will remain as elusive as it has been for the past several decades.

REFERENCES

1) Frost HM. Bone modeling and skeletal modeling errors. Springfield: Charles C. Thomas, 1973.

2) Parfitt AM. The Physiologic and clinical significance of bone histomorphometric data. in: Recker RR, ed. Bone histomorphometry: techniques and interpretation. Boca Raton: CRC Press, 1983:143-224.

3) Recker RR, Kimmel DB, Parfitt AM, Davies KM, Keshawarz N, and Hinders S. Static and tetracycline-based bone histomorphometric data from 34 normal postmenopausal females. J Bone Min Res 1988;3:133-144.

4) Frost HM, Villanueva AR, and Roth H. Measurement of bone formation in a 57 year old man by means of tetracyclines. Henry Ford Hospital medical bulletin. 1960;8:239-254.

5) Baron R, Vignery A, Neff L, Silverglate A, and Santa Maria A. Processing of undecalcified bone specimens for bone histomorphometry. in: Recker RR, ed. Bone histomorphometry: techniques and interpretation. Boca Raton: CRC Press, 1983:13-36.

6) Parfitt AM, Mathews CHE, Villanueva AR, Kleerekoper M, Frame

B, and Rao DS. Relationships between surface, volume, and thickness of iliac trabecular bone in aging and in osteoporosis. J Clin Inves 1983;72:1396-1409.

7) Parfitt AM, Drezner MK, Glorieux FH, Kanis JA, Malluche H, Meynbier PJ, Ott SM, and Recker RR. Bone histomorphometry:standardization of nomenclature, symbols, and units. J Bone Min Res 1987;2:595-610.

8) Heaney RP. Calcium kinetics in plasma: as they apply to the measurements of bone formation and resorption rates. In Bourne GH, ed. The biochemistry and physiology of bone. New York: Academic Press Inc, 1976;4:105-133.

9) Fogelman I, Bessent RG, Citrin DL, Boyle IT and Greig WR, The use of whole body retention of Tc-99m diphosphonate in the diagnosis of metabolic bone disease. J Nucl Med 1978;19:270.

10) Meunier PJ, Courpron P, Edouard C, Alexandre C, Bressot C, Lips P, and Boyce BF. Bone histomorphometry in osteoporotic states. In: Barzel US, ed. Osteoporosis II. New York: Grune & Stratton,1978:27-47.

11) Lips P, Courpron P, and Meunier PJ. Mean wall thickness of trabecular bone packets in the human iliac crest: changes with age. Calcif Tiss Res 1978;26:13-17.

12) Courpron P, Lepine P, Arlot M, Lips P, and Meunier PJ. Mechanisms underlying the reduction with age of the mean wall thickness of trabecular basic structure unit (BSU) in human iliac bone. In: Jee WSS, and Parfitt AM, eds. Bone Histomorphometry, Third international workshop. Paris: Armour Montagu-4, 1981:323-330.

13) Darby AJ, and Meunier PJ. Mean wall thickness and formation periods of trabecular bone packets in idiopathic osteoporosis. Calcif Tissue Int 1981;33:199-204.

14) Kragstrup J, Melsen F, and Mosekilde L. Thickness of bone formed at remodeling sites in normal human iliac trabecular bone: variations with age and sex. Metab Bone Dis & Rel Res 1983;5:17-21.

15) Vedi S, Compston JE, Webb A, and Tigh JR. Histomorphometric analysis of dynamic parameters of trabecular bone formation in the iliac crest of normal British subjects. Metab Bone Dis & Rel Res 1983;5:69-74.

16) Erikson Ef, Mosekilde L, and Melsen F. Trabecular bone resorption depth decreases with age: differences between normal males and females. Bone 1985;6:141-6.

17) Aaron JE, Makins NB, and Sagreiya K. The microanatomy of trabecular bone loss in normal aging men and women. Clin Orth and Rel Res 1987;215:260-271.

18) Frost HM. Tetracycline-based histological analysis of bone remodeling. Calcif Tiss Res 1969;3:211-237.

19) Dahl E, Nordal KP, Halse J, and Attramadal A. Histomorphometric analysis of normal bone from the iliac crest of Norwegian subjects. Bone and Mineral 1988;3:369-377.

21) Melsen F, and Mosekilde L. Tetracycline double-labeling of iliac trabecular bone in 41 normal adults. Calcif Tiss Res 1978;26:99-102.

22) Malluche H, Meyer W, Sherman D, and Massry S. Quantitative bone histology in 84 normal American subjects. Calcif Tissue Int 1982;34:449-455.

24) Heaney RP, Recker RR, and Saville PD. Menopausal changes in bone remodeling. J Lab Clin Invest 1978;92:964-970.

25) Fogelman I, and Bessent R. Age-related alterations in skeletal metabolism--24-hr whole-body retention of diphosphonate in 250 normal subjects: concise communication. J Nucl Med 1982;23:296-300.

26) Hyldstrup L, McNair P, Jensen GF, Mogensen NB, and Transbol IB. Measurements of whole body retention of diphosphonate and other indices of bone metabolism in 125 normals: dependency on age, sex and glomerular filtration. Scand J Clin Lab Invest 1984;44:673-8.

27) Podenphant J, Johansen JS, Thomsen K, Riis BJ, Leth A, and Christiansen C. Bone turnover in spinal osteoporosis. J Bone Mineral Res 1987;2:497-503.

28) Nordin BEC, and Polley KJ. Metabolic consequences of the menopause. Calcif Tissue Int 1987;41:(Suppl 1).

29) Hyldstrup L, McNair P, Jensen GF, Nielsen HR, and Transbol I. Bone mass as referent for urinary hydroxyproline excretion: age and sex-related changes in 125 normals and in primary hyperparathyroidism. Calcif Tissue Int 1984;36:639-644.

30) Delmas PD, Stenner D, Wahner HW, Mann KG, and Riggs BL. Increase in serum bone gamma-carboxyglutamic acid protein with aging in women. J Clin Invest 1983;71:1316-1321.

31) Price PA, and Nishimoto SK, Radioimmunoassay for the vitamin K-dependent protein of bone and its discovery in plasma. Proc Natl Acad Sci 1980;77:2234-2238.

32) Price PA, Parthemore JG and Deftos LJ, New biochemical marker for bone metabolism, J Clin Invest 66: 878-883, 1980

33) Price PA, Williamson MK, and Lothringer JW. Origin of the vitamin K-dependent bone protein found in plasma and its clearance by kidney and bone. J Biol Chem 1981;256:12760-12766.

34) Epstein S, Poser J, McClintock R, Johnston CC, Bryce G, and Hui S. Differences in serum bone GLA protein with age and sex. Lancet 1984;1:307-310.

35) Trotter MG, Broman E, and Peterson RR, Densities of bones of white and negro skeletons. J Bone Jt Surg Am 1960;42A:50-58.

36) Bell NH, Greene A, Epstein S, Oexmann MJ, Shaw S, and Shary J. Evidence for alteration of the vitamin D-endocrine system in blacks. J Clin Invest 1985;76:470-473.

37) Weinstein RS, Weinstein DL, and Bell NH. Rates of bone formation and mineral apposition are diminished in normal black man and women. (Abstract) ASBMR, 1988.

Discussion:

DR. DREZNER (Raleigh-Durham): A question about nomenclature; we talk about trabecular number decreasing, but in fact it increases, because if you split one into two, you have two trabecular elements. Are we really measuring trabecular number or density?

DR. RECKER (Omaha): What we're actually measuring is the odds that a line transecting a section is going to encounter a trabecula.

DR. PARFITT (Detroit): Dr. Drezner, what goes up is the number of isolated profiles in a two-dimensional section.

DR. DREZNER: Isn't that more a density measurement, then?

DR. RECKER: There might be a better term, but I don't know what it might be.

DR. SCHNITZLER (Johannesburg): We examined trabecular architecture in a number of specimens from Black and White subjects, and trabecular thickness and cancellous bone volume were greater in Blacks than in Whites. With age, bone loss was mainly due to trabecular thinning in Blacks, but due to disappearance of trabeculae in Whites.

Perhaps if you start with thick trabeculae, they become thinner as bone is lost, but if there are thin trabeculae already, perforation is more likely. That might also explain the difference between white females and males.

DR. RECKER: Connectivity is an important element of the overall strength of bone as a material, and loss of connectivity would exaggerate loss of strength out of proportion to the total amount of bone that's lost.

DR. REEVE (England): I'm attracted by the idea that damage may occur in interstitial bone, but it may be a little too simple. At individual remodeling sites there will be differences between the amounts of bone resorbed and the amount of bone formed, and there will be a random element to this. If individual trabecula drift through space, there will be some remodeling of the interstitial bone.

DR. RECKER: The bone left by penetration of a trabecula will be unaffected by drift.

DR. PARFITT: Dr. Reeve, what is the evidence that trabeculae do undergo drift during normal aging?

DR. REEVE: I have no evidence, but I suggest we study it.

DR. PARFITT: If you look at hand x-rays in individuals taken many years apart, the trabecular structure in each bone remains exactly the same, but each bone is different from every other bone in that person's hand. So I doubt that drift of trabeculae occurs except in response to some drastic change in mechanical loading.

DR. RECKER: On the other hand, you can find very old labels in the interstitial bone that are distant from and not parallel to the current surface, which suggests that there is some trabecular drift.

DR. PARFITT: I agree that a systematic study of that phenomenon would be worthwhile.

DR. REEVE: The amount of drift I was contemplating was equivalent to half the thickness of a trabecula.

DR. PARFITT: So, you wouldn't see it on an x-ray; good point.

DR. POTTS (Boston): Once this postulated rupture in a trabeculum had occurred, will there be metabolic consequences as well as structural consequences, such as accelerated resorption?

DR. RECKER: I would speculate that an increase in strain on remaining bone would accelerate microdamage and accelerate repair by remodeling, but a decrease in strain would favor resorption.

DR. PARFITT: Dr. Weinstein, would you care to expand on or update any of the data you have on Black/White differences?

DR. WEINSTEIN (Augusta, GA): Our study was not on autopsies, but on normal healthy volunteers, who provide the best comparison with our patients. We found no structural differences between Whites and Blacks, but in both the cancellous bone and cortical bone tissue, there was a significant decrease in labeled perimeter and formation rate. These findings have been confirmed in twice as many subjects and will be presented this evening.

In Vivo Hormonal Effects on Trabecular Bone Remodeling, Osteoid Mineralization, and Skeletal Turnover

FLEMMING MELSEN, LEIF MOSEKILDE, ERIK FINK ERIKSEN,
PEDER CHARLES, and TORBEN STEINICKE

University Departments of Endocrinology and Pathology
Aarhus Amtssygehus
and Department of Clinical Physiology and Nuclear Medicine
Aarhus Kommunehospita
Denmark

INTRODUCTION

Bone remodeling constitutes the cellular processes going on throughout life that allow continuous replacement of old bone with new in order to adjust trabecular structure to mechanical forces, to repair microfractures and to secure the viability of the embedded osteocytes. Besides mechanical forces the remodeling processes are influenced by local concentrations of ions, paracrine factors and hormones. Typical changes in bone remodeling will therefore occur in diseased states characterized by excess or lack of calcitropic and other hormones. These in vivo effects cannot be deduced from in vitro studies on the effect of different hormones on isolated cells or organ cultures. In vivo the hormonal effects are modulated by adaptive changes in ions, local tissue factors and other hormones. Furthermore, the specific intermediate organization (1) of cortical as well as trabecular bone will modulate the tissue and organ level response to a hormonal challenge. Finally, three anatomical areas or envelopes have been defined, where remodeling takes place: 1) the periosteal envelope, 2) the Haversian envelope, and 3) the endosteal envelope. Variable responses might be expected from these envelopes due to differences in their physiological properties (2,3).

The introduction of in vivo tetracycline double labeling by Frost (4) and the development of suitable techniques for routine bone biopsies by Bordier (5) made it possible to study the effects of hormonal disturbances on bone mass and bone remodeling in humans. Recently, advanced stereological methods have facilitated accurate measurements of all elements in trabecular bone remodeling and allowed a three-dimensional reconstruction of the remodeling sequence in normals and in metabolic bone diseases (6,7). Furthermore, methods are now available for studying the influence of age and hormonal changes on the biomechanical competence of trabecular bone and to relate structural changes to variations in bone strength (8).

The aim of the present survey is to describe some of the effects of endocrine disturbances on trabecular bone remodeling, osteoid mineralization and bone mass in vivo. Furthermore, relations between tissue level and organ level mineralization and resorption rates are described, together with the effects of selected hormones on organ level bone turnover.

BONE REMODELING

Bone remodeling was first studied in cortical bone (1,9). From these studies emerged the concept of remodeling being initiated by **A**ctivation of certain cells to become resorptive cells at a given locus. These cells, mainly osteoclasts, then begin bone **R**esorption. Later, osteoblasts invade the area and start bone **F**ormation. This **A-R-F** sequence is most easily demonstrated in cortical bone, where longitudinal sections of complete remodeling systems can be obtained (10). During the last few years, it has been obvious that trabecular bone is renewed in the same way as cortical bone (6,7). Resorption takes place at discrete sites at the marrow-bone interface (endosteal surface), forming scalloped interruptions of the lamellar system, the Howships lacunae. At a given site, the **resorption period** lasts for about 4-6 weeks. The first part of the resorptive phase is dominated by osteoclasts (6). Later, the resorption rate is slower and the process is dominated by mononuclear cells. The end result of the resorptive process is a resorption lacuna with a certain **final resorption depth**. Subsequently, the lacunae are refilled with lamellar bone by osteoblasts invading the lacunae. The duration of the **bone formation period** is about three months. The end result is a new **bone structural unit (BSU)**, characterized by a certain **mean wall thickness**. The BSU in trabecular bone is also called a **packet** or a **wall**. When no net bone loss or gain is occurring, the final resorption depth equals the mean wall thickness.

The frequency by which a given place on the trabecular bone surface undergoes remodeling is termed the **activation frequency** (11). This quantity, which shows a great variability under hormonal influence, is of paramount importance for the final results of the remodeling processes. Activation is the process by which osteoclast precursors are transformed to multinuclear osteoclasts and attracted to the bone surface, where they start resorbing bone. Since the purpose of the remodeling process is to renew old bone, it is natural to look for some kind of signal from the bone, or the cells on the bone surface, to the osteoclasts or osteoclast precursors. These local signals are probably prostaglandins or lymphokines. Moreover, activation is influenced by several systemic hormones, including thyroid hormones, PTH, 1,25-dihydroxy Vitamin D, calcitonin, sex hormones and growth hormone (Table 1). Excess thyroid hormones increases and lack of thyroid hormones decreases the activation frequency (12,13). It is unknown whether the effects are mediated directly by T_3 or T_4 or indirectly through local stimulation of growth factor production. Chronic excess of PTH, as in primary hyperparathyroidism, stimulates the activation frequency (14), as do injections of PTH(1-34) to dogs for 15 weeks (15). Osteoclasts do not have PTH receptors (16), and in vivo isolated osteoclasts do not respond to PTH. It has therefore been postulated that PTH stimulates bone activation and osteoclast recruitment indirectly through surface cells and local T-lymphocytes (17). 1,25-dihydroxyvitamin D, on the other hand, seems to stimulate the transformation of mononuclear osteoclast precursors, probably of the monocyte-macrophage lineage, to multinucleated osteoclasts (17). This model for bone activation explains the well known synergistic effect of PTH and 1,25-dihydroxyvitamin D on osteoclast number and activity. Calcitonin, on the other hand, acutely reduces the activity of the osteoclasts by a direct effect on the cells (18).

The activation frequency, the coupling between resorption and formation, and the balance between the final resorption depth and the mean wall thickness are of paramount importance for the understanding of changes in trabecular bone mass, structure and strength. **Uncoupling** with resorption without formation may occur during normal remodeling due to perforation of trabecular structures (see below). The occurrence of formation without previous resorption can be considered negligible in normal bone. Discrepancies in the extent of formative and resorptive surfaces do not provide evidence for uncoupling (19).

REVERSIBLE AND IRREVERSIBLE CHANGES IN BONE MASS

In order to preserve bone mass and skeletal integrity, the amount of bone removed during bone resorption should equal the amount of bone laid down during the subsequent bone formation. This precondition should theoretically be secured by a quantitative coupling between resorption and formation. In trabecular bone, however, a net decrease in bone volume, ash weight and bone strength with age has been demonstrated in males, as well as females, indicating that average resorption exceeds average formation after the age of 20-30 years (20,21).

The following mechanisms may be operative and need to be evaluated when dealing with spontaneous or induced changes in bone mass (22,23).

<u>Reversible bone loss</u>: A deficit in bone and bone mineral due to ongoing bone resorption leading to expansion of the **remodeling space** (the total amount of bone resorbed and not yet reformed during the ongoing remodeling cycles) will result in an increased porosity in cortical bone and an increased area of Howships lacunae at the trabecular surface. Expansion of the remodeling space will occur if a) the activation frequency is increased with an increased number of ongoing remodeling cycles, b) the final resorption depth is increased, c) the resorptive period is prolonged, and d) the formative period is prolonged. If bone remodeling returns to normal the holes will be refilled during the following formative phase. The bone loss, therefore, is reversible.

<u>Irreversible bone loss</u>: In trabecular bone irreversible bone loss may occur by two mechanisms. 1) An imbalance between the thickness of bone resorbed (final resorption depth) and formed (mean wall thickness) per remodeling cycle will result in a net loss or gain of bone per remodeling cycle. The bone changes due to this mechanism are accelerated with increased activation frequency (accelerated irreversible bone loss). 2) Disintegration of the trabecular structure due to **perforation** of trabeculae. The average resorption depth in trabecular bone is 50-60 um in normal individuals but the final depth exhibit a wide scatter from 15-250 um (6). Trabecular thickness show wide variability from 10 to 400 um. Therefore, the possibility exists that a deep resorption cavity can hit a narrow trabecular structure and penetrate it completely or that two resorption cavities from each site of the trabecular structure meet each other. This will remove the structural basis for the subsequent bone formation (uncoupling) resulting in a hole in the trabecular network.

The risk of trabecular perforations increase with a) increased final resorption depth, b) decreased trabecular thickness, c) enhanced activation frequency. Figure 9 illustrates the effect of repeated perforations on trabecular bone volume and integrity and on intertrabecular distance in sections from iliac crest biopsies. Since trabecular perforations are unavoidable, even during normal trabecular bone remodeling, a certain amount of bone loss with age will always occur, unless completely new trabeculae are formed to replace those which disappear. Due to the decrease in intertrabecular support perforation will result in a more marked reduction in bone strength than in bone mass.

OSTEOID FORMATION AND MINERALIZATION

The amount of unmineralized bone (osteoid) depends on the average thickness and the surface extent of the osteoid seams. In a steady state situation with regard to osteoid thickness the **osteoid appositional rate** equal the average **bone formation rate**, which can be determined by tetracycline double labeling (4). The average **osteoid thickness** equals the thickness of osteoid laid down per day (the osteoid appositional rate) multiplied by the number of days between osteoid formation and mineralization (**the mineralization lag time**) (24). The surface extent of osteoid is proportional to the **activation frequency** of new remodeling cycles and the average length of the **formation period** (24). Variations in the amount of osteoid or in the shape of the osteoid seams are found in many endocrine diseases. It appears from the relations described above that changes may be caused by disturbances in osteoid formation or mineralization lag time, which will result in altered osteoid seam thickness, or in activation frequency and length of formative period, which will affect the surface extent of osteoid.

METHODS

Histomorphometry

Transcortical iliac crest bone biopsies are obtained from the standard region 2 cm below and 2 cm behind the anterior superior iliac spine (24) after intravital double labeling (interval 10 days) with tetracycline. The undecalcified methylmetacrylate-embedded biopsies are cut on a heavy duty microtome (Jung Model K). Then 7-8 um thick sections are stained with Masson trichrome, Goldner trichrome and toluidine blue for light microscopy, and 20 um thick sections are mounted for fluorescent microscopy.

The histomorphometric analyses and the applied stereologic transformations have previously been described in detail (6,7,23). The following parameters were measured or calculated:

Trabecular bone volume (BV/TV, %) as the volume of mineralized bone and osteoid to total bone volume (bone + marrow).

Lamellar thickness (LT, um) as the mean of the expected distribution of lamellar orthogonal intercept length multiplied by pi/4.

Eroded surface (ES/BS, %) as the extent of resorption lacunae to total trabecular bone surface.

Final resorption depth (R.D, um) as the number of lamellae eroded from the trabecular bone surface to the bottom of resorption lacunae covered by preosteoblast-like cells, multiplied by the lamellar thickness.

Osteoid surface (OS/BS,%) as the extent of osteoid covered surfaces to total trabecular bone surface.

Mean wall thickness (W.Th) as the number of lamellae between cement line and quiescent trabecular bone surface multiplied by the lamellar thickness.

Mean osteoid thickness (O.Th, um) as the mean of the expected distribution of osteoid orthogonal intercept length multiplied by pi/4.

Labeled surfaces (LS/BS,%) as the extent of tetracycline labeled surfaces in fraction of trabecular bone surface.

Mineral appositional rate (MAR um/d) as the mean distance between the tetracycline lines in all double labeled zones divided by the labeling interval and multiplied by pi/4. This variable describes the cellular level mineralization rate.

Adjusted appositional rate (Aj.AR, um/d as:
$$Aj.AR = (LS/BS * MAR)/ (OS/BS).$$
This variable gives the amount of new bone mineralized per day per unit osteoid covered surface, which in a steady state with regard to osteoid seam thickness equals the osteoid appositional rate.

Bone formation rate (BFR/BS um3/um2/day) as:
$$BFR/BS = (LS/BS * MAR).$$
This variable gives the amount of new bone mineralized per day per unit trabecular bone surface and reflects the turnover of trabecular bone.

Mineralization lag time (Mlt, days) as:
$$Mlt = O.Th/Aj.AR,$$
which gives the average time lag between the formation and subsequent mineralization of osteoid.

Quiescent surfaces (QS/BS,%) as:
$$QS/BS = 100 - (ES/BS + OS/BS),$$
which gives the extent of surfaces not involved in resorption or formation.

Formative period (FP, days) as:
$$FP = W.Th / Aj.AR.$$

Resorptive period (RP, days) as:
$$RP = ((ES/BS)/(OS/BS)) * FP.$$
Remodeling period (Rm.P, days) as:
$$Rm.P = RP + FP.$$
Quiescent period (QP, days) as:
$$QP = ((QS/BS)/(OS/BS)) * FP.$$
Activation frequency (Ac.f, days-1) as:
$$Ac.f = 1/(RP+FP+QP),$$
which gives the frequency by which a new remodeling cycle is initiated at a random location on the trabecular surface.
  Balance per remodeling cycle (B.rc, um) as:
$$B.rc = W.Th - RD,$$
which gives the thickness of bone gained or lost per remodeling cycle.

^{47}Ca-kinetics

The patients, after an equilibrium period of one week were studied while on a diet as similar as possible to their daily fare. The serving was doubled, one part for the patient, the other for analysis. Carmine red was given orally at the start and end of the study to demarcate the faecal collection period. In order to correct the faecal calcium output ^{51}Cr-tablets were given three times a day with the meals as a non-absorbable faecal marker. The day the calcium balance study was initiated 0.74 MBq (20 uCi) of ^{47}CaCl$_2$ was given intravenously. Blood samples were then withdrawn after 5, 10, 15, 20, 30, 45, 60, 120, 180 and 360 minutes and after 1, 2, 3, 4, 5, 6, and 7 days. The ^{47}Ca-radioactivity was determined in serum samples and in daily urinary and fecal samples using a scintillation well counter. The ^{47}Ca-kinetic data were analyzed according to a previously described (25) modification of the expanding calcium pool model (26).

  Calcium balance, (B mmol/d) was calculated as the difference between dietary calcium and the total loss of calcium through faeces, urine and skin.
  Bone mineralization rate (m, mmol/d) was computer-calculated according to the model.
  Bone resorption rate (r, mmol/d) was calculated as m - B.

RESULTS

Table I summarizes the main effects of selected endocrine disturbances on essential trabecular bone remodeling parameters. Estimates of final resorption depths and mean wall thicknesses are not yet available from patients with acromegaly and medullary thyroid carcinoma and from patients in prednisone treatment.

Hyperthyroidism (13,24)

Table II compares trabecular bone and organ level remodeling in untreated hyperthyroidism with normal age- and sex-matched controls. The activation frequency is increased to around 160% of normal. Both resorption and formation periods are shortened to respectively 38 and 79% of normal mean because of stimulation of osteoclastic and osteoblastic activity. The final resorption depth is normal as is the completed mean wall thickness. However, due to the often short duration of the hyperthyroid state before investigation the measured completed mean wall thickness may not be representative for the hyperthyroid state. When growth curve based data are used for estimation of completed wall thickness (13) a net negative balance per remodeling cycle of 9.6 um can be demonstrated due to a reduced wall thickness. For the total skeleton the mineralization rate was increased. The resorption rate was slightly increased but the difference did not reach significance.

Table I. Deviations in main parameters of trabecular bone remodeling in selected endocrine disturbances.

	Activation Frequency	Resorption Period	Formation Period	Resorption Depth	Wall Thickness	Balance Per Remodl. Cycle	Trab. Bone Volume	Resorption Rate	Mineralization Rate
Hyperthyroidism	↑	↓	↓	-	-	↓	↓	↑	↑
Hypothyroidism	↓	↑	↑	↓	↑	↑	↑	↓	↓
Hyperparathyroidism	↑	-	-	↓	↓	-	-	↑	↑
Medullary Thyroid Carcinoma	(-)?	?	?	?	?	(-)?	-	?	?
Acromegaly	(↑)?	?	?	?	(↑)?	(↑)?	↑	?	?
Estrogen Treatment	↓	-	-	-	-	-	-(↑?)	↑	↑
Prednisone Treatment	(↓)?	?	?	?	(-)?	( )?	↓	↓?	↓

↑ = increased;   ↓ = decreased;   - = unchanged;   ( ) = estimated;   ? = unknown

78

Table II. Trabecular and organ level bone remodeling (mean or median (#) and 95% confidence limits) in hyperthyroidism and normal sex- and age-matched controls.

	Patients	Controls	p
TISSUE LEVEL, n	15	13	
Activation frequency, #/year	.78 (.55-1.01)	.50 (.26-.73)	<0.01
Resorption period, days*	22 (18-38)	58 (42-95)	<0.01
Formation period, days*	109 (96-124)	151 (132-172)	<0.05
Final resorption depth, um	62 (56-67)	60 (53-68)	N.S.
Wall thickness, um	58 (56-61)	61 (58-63)	N.S.
Balance/Remodeling cycle, um	-8 (-15-2)	-1 (-2-1)	<0.001
ORGAN LEVEL, n	10	10	
Resorption rate, mg Ca/d*	390 (109-1207)	316 (89-612)	N.S.
Mineralization rate, mg Ca/d*	497 (213-997)	192 (36-418)	<0.05

The amount of trabecular bone is reduced in hyperthyroidism (Table III). This is caused by a reversible as well as an irreversible bone loss. The increased activation frequency will expand the remodeling space and induce a reversible bone loss, which to some extent is mitigated by the shortened remodeling period. The negative net balance will in combination with the enhanced activation frequency induce an accelerated irreversible bone loss. Furthermore, the high activation frequency will increase the risk of trabecular perforations.

Table III. Trabecular bone volume, osteoid formation and mineralization (mean (SE)) in hyperthyroidism and normal sex- and age-matched controls.

	Patients n	Patients X(SE)	Controls n	Controls X(SE)	p
Bone volume um3/um3	36	0.18(0.01)	30	0.22(0.01)	<0.05
Osteoid surfaces um2/um2	37	0.19(0.02)	30	0.14(0.01)	<0.002
Seam width, um	31	7.2 (0.4)	19	9.0 (0.3)	<0.05
Appositional rate, um/day	20	0.86(0.08)	20	0.44(0.04)	<0.01
Mineralization lag time, days	20	11.7 (1.2)	20	23.7 (2.3)	<0.01

The surface extent of osteoid is increased (Table III) because of the increased activation frequency and in spite of the shortening of the formative period. On the other hand, the osteoid seam thickness is reduced because of a marked shortening of the mineralization lag time. The osteoid appositional rate is markedly increased indicating an increased osteoblastic activity.

Hypothyroidism (12,24)

Table IV compares trabecular bone and total skeleton remodeling in untreated hypothyroidism with normal age- and sex-matched controls. The activation frequency is decreased to about 28% of normal. Both resorption and formation periods are markedly prolonged to respectively 238 and 411% of normal mean because of reduced activity of osteoclasts and osteoblasts. The final resorption depth is significantly reduced whereas the completed mean wall thickness is increased. The reduction in resorption rate and the increase in mean wall thickness result in a positive balance per remodeling cycle. Bone turnover at organ level is reduced with a significant decrease in resorption rate and mineralization rate.

Table IV. Trabecular and organ level bone remodeling (mean or median (*) and 95% confidence limits) in hypothyroidism and normal sex- and aged-matched controls.

	Patients	Controls	p
TISSUE LEVEL, n	19	16	
Activation frequency, #/year	.15 (.12-.18)	.53 (.30-.76)	<0.001
Resorption period, days*	76 (52-110)	32 (22-43)	<0.001
Formation period, days*	620 (521-780)	151 (132-172)	<0.001
Final resorption depth, um	42 (38-47)	53 (47-59)	<0.01
Mean wall thickness, um	60 (58-62)	54 (51-57)	<0.01
Balance/remodeling cycle, um	17 (13-20)	-1 (-3-1)	<0.001
ORGAN LEVEL, n	8	10	
Resorption rate, mg Ca/d*	49 (0-373)	316 (89-612)	<0.02
Mineralization rate, mg Ca/d*	83 (0-232)	192 (36-418)	<0.05

The amount of trabecular bone is normal in hypothyroidism (Table V) or slightly increased (27). The reduced activation frequency will per se decrease the remodeling space but this effect will be counteracted by the considerable prolongation of the remodeling period. The positive net balance per remodeling cycle will per se increase the amount of trabecular bone, but the effect will be small due to the low activation frequency. Theoretically, the reduced activation frequency and the decrease in resorption depth will decrease the risk of trabecular perforations.

Table V. Trabecular bone volume, osteoid formation and mineralization (mean (SE)) in hypothyroidism and normal sex- and age-matched controls.

	Patients n	X(SE)	Controls n	X(SE)	p
Bone volume um3/um3	13	0.20(0.02)	27	0.20(0.01)	N.S.
Osteoid surfaces um2/um2	13	0.14(0.02)	27	0.17(0.01)	N.S.
Seam width, um	14	6.4 (0.7)	27	8.7 (0.4)	<0.01
Appositional rate, um/day	10	0.12(0.05)	10	0.38(0.06)	<0.01
Mineralization lag time, days	10	92.1 (26.9)	10	29.9 (3.0)	<0.05

The surface extent of osteoid is normal in hypothyroidism (Table V) because of the decrease in activation frequency and the prolongation of the formative period. The osteoid seam thickness is reduced because of a marked reduction in the osteoid appositional rate and in spite of a prolongation of the mineralization lag time.

Hyperparathyroidism (14,24)

Table VI compares trabecular and organ level bone remodeling and turnover in untreated hyperparathyroidism with normal age- and sex-matched controls. The activation frequency is increased to around 148% of normal. Resorption and formation periods are normal. The final resorption depth is decreased as is the completed mean wall thickness. The balance between resorption depth and formation thickness is normal. At organ level the resorption and mineralization rates are increased.

Table VI. Trabecular and skeletal bone remodeling (mean or median (*) and 95% confidence limits) in primary hyperparathyroidism and normal sex- and age-matched controls.

	Patients	Controls	p
TISSUE LEVEL, n	19	16	
Activation frequency, #/year	.62 (.52-.86)	.42 (.25-.60)	<0.05
Resorption period, days*	31 (21-47)	39 (27-56)	N.S.
Formation period, days*	172 (128-229)	134 (115-154)	N.S.
Final resorption depth, um	45 (42-49)	57 (51-63)	<0.01
Mean wall thickness, um	51 (48-53)	56 (53-59)	<0.02
Balance/remodeling cycle, um	4 (0-8)	1 (-4-5)	N.S.
ORGAN LEVEL, n	14	10	
Resorption rate, mg Ca/d*	640 (151-1207)	316 (89-612)	<0.01
Mineralization rate, mg Ca/d*	455 (202-933)	192 (36-418)	<0.01

The amount of trabecular bone is normal in hyperparathyroidism (Table VII). The increased activation frequency will expand the remodeling space and induce a reversible bone loss. On the other hand the study disclosed a tendency towards a positive balance per remodeling cycle, the effect of which will be enhanced by the increased activation frequency. The high activation frequency will increase the risk of trabecular perforations. This effect will, however, be counteracted by the reduction in resorption depth. Hence, the amount of trabecular bone is affected by several opposing factors, resulting in an unchanged trabecular volume.

Table VII. Trabecular bone volume, osteoid formation and mineralization (mean (SE)) in hyperparathyroidism and normal sex- and aged-matched controls.

	Patients n	X(SE)	Controls n	X(SE)	p
Bone volume um3/um3	23	0.18(0.01)	25	0.19(0.01)	N.S.
Osteoid surfaces um2/um2	23	0.23(0.02)	25	0.21(0.02)	<0.01
Seam width, um	24	10.0 (0.6)	25	9.9 (0.5)	N.S.
Appositional rate, um/day	18	0.40(0.03)	31	0.55(0.04)	<0.01
Mineralization lag time, days	18	28.6 (2.8)	29	21.6 (2.1)	<0.05

The surface extent of osteoid is increased (Table VII) because of the increased activation frequency in combination with a normal formative period. The osteoid seam thickness and the mineralization lag time are normal in spite of a slight decrease in osteoid appositional rate.

Estrogen Treatment in Osteoporosis

Table VIII compares trabecular bone remodeling in postmenopausal crush fracture spinal osteoporosis before and after one year of cyclic estrogen/gestagen treatment. Following treatment the activation frequency decreases to about 52% of pretreatment values. Resorption and formation periods are unchanged as are the final resorption depth, the completed mean wall thickness and the balance between resorption depth and formation thickness.

Table VIII. Trabecular bone remodeling in 10 patients with spinal crush fracture osteoporosis before and after estrogen treatment for one year.

	Before n=10 X(SE)	After n=10 X(SE)	p
Activation frequency, #/year	0.51 (0.07)	0.27 (0.05)	<0.01
Resorption period, days*	60 (21)	45 (7)	N.S.
Formation period, days*	207 (45)	281 (72)	N.S.
Final resorption depth, um	47 (1)	52 (3)	N.S.
Mean wall thickness, um	47 (1)	45 (2)	N.S.
Balance/remodeling cycle, um	2 (2)	-3 (3)	N.S.

The amount of trabecular bone is unchanged in these 10 patients after one year of estrogen treatment (Table IX). The decrease in activation frequency, however, will reduce the remodeling space leading to a small increase in bone mass and bone mineral content. This increase is probably too small to be detected in this limited population. Furthermore, the decrease in activation frequency will theoretically reduce the risk of perforations. The osteoid surfaces decreased because of the reduction in activation frequency. The mean osteoid seam width also decreased. The reason for this is less obvious. It may be caused by a non-steady state with a reduction in the number of young broad osteoid seams secondary to the reduced activation frequency. No alteration was observed in osteoid appositional rate or mineralization lag time.

Table IX. Trabecular bone volume, osteoid formation and mineralization (mean (SE)) in postmenopausal spinal crush fracture osteoporosis before and after one year of cyclic estrogen/gestagen treatment.

	Before		After		p
	n	X(SE)	n	X(SE)	
Bone volume um3/um3	10	0.13(0.01)	10	0.12(0.02)	N.S.
Osteoid surfaces um2/um2	10	0.16(0.02)	10	0.09(0.02)	<0.05
Seam width, um	10	10.3 (0.3)	10	8.3 (0.7)	<0.05
Appositional rate, um/day	10	0.46(0.09)	10	0.46(0.11)	N.S.
Mineralization lag time, days	10	44 (14)	10	49 (19)	N.S.

Medullary Thyroid Carcinoma (28)

We have no data on activation frequency, mean wall thickness, resorption depth or resorptive and formative periods in this patient group of chronic calcitonin excess. However, Table X gives the data for bone volume, osteoid formation and mineralization and resorption surfaces.

Table X. Trabecular bone volume, osteoid formation and mineralization and resorption surfaces (mean (SE)) in medullary thyroid carcinoma and sex- and age-matched controls.

	Patients		Controls		p
	n	X(SE)	n	X(SE)	
Bone volume um3/um3	10	0.25(0.02)	20	0.21(0.02)	N.S.
Osteoid surfaces um2/um2	10	0.30(0.04)	10	0.20(0.02)	<0.05
Seam width, um	10	10.6 (0.8)	10	9.8 (0.7)	N.S.
Appositional rate, um/day	9	0.39(0.01)	10	0.48(0.06)	N.S.
Mineralization lag time, days	9	27.9 (3.5)	10	21.7 (1.9)	N.S.
Resorption surfaces	10	0.08(0.01)	10	0.04(0.01)	<0.01

The amount of trabecular bone is unchanged. Resorptive and osteoid covered surfaces are increased indicating an enhanced activation frequency or/and a prolongation of the resorptive and formative periods of the remodeling cycle. Exact data interpretation is impossible without information on resorption depth and mean wall thickness. It is expected that chronic calcitonin excess should reduce the activation frequency. However, receptor down regulation and stimulation of renal 1-alpha-production may modulate the chronic response on calcitonin (28).

Acromegaly (29)

We have not yet precise data describing trabecular bone remodeling in this patient group of chronic somatotropin excess. However, Table XI gives the data for bone volume, osteoid formation and mineralization and resorption surfaces.

Table XI. Trabecular bone volume, osteoid formation and mineralization and resorption surfaces (mean (SE)) in patients with acromegaly and sex- and age-matched controls.

	Patients		Controls		p
	n	X(SE)	n	X(SE)	
Bone volume um3/um3	18	0.26(0.01)	17	0.20(0.02)	<0.01
Osteoid surfaces um2/um2	18	0.28(0.03)	17	0.19(0.02)	<0.01
Appositional rate, um/day	9	0.66(0.13)	9	0.36(0.06)	N.S.
Resorption surfaces	18	0.07(0.01)	17	0.04(0.01)	<0.05

The amount of trabecular bone is increased in acromegaly. Resorptive and osteoid covered surfaces are increased indicating an enhanced activation frequency or/and a prolongation of the resorptive and formative periods of the remodeling cycle. Exact data interpretation is impossible without information on resorption depth and mean wall thickness. The reason for the altered trabecular bone thickness is unclear. The most likely explanation, however, is that excess somatotropin creates a positive balance per remodeling cycle.

Conclusion

Quantitative bone histomorphometry is an efficient tool for the evaluation of the effects of chronic excess or lack of hormones on bone remodeling **in vivo**. It is also the only way to get this information. It should be stressed, however, that it is important to estimate qualities like activation frequency, length of resorptive and formative periods and balance between resorption depth and formation thickness in order to give precise descriptions of changes in bone remodeling and to understand variations in bone mass. Furthermore, in the future structural changes in trabecular thickness and intertrabecular distance should be evaluated in the different metabolic states in order to deduce variations in the risk of trabecular perforations, which will severely affect bone strength.

Since trabecular and cortical bone may show different reactions to hormones it is important to study the effects of different hormones on the whole skeleton. Previous studies (30) have indicated that in thyroid and hyperthyroid disorders significant correlations exist between tissue level and organ level bone turnover parameters. This, however, has not been proven for the other hormonal disturbances. Furthermore, calcium kinetic studies on skeletal turnover are important for testing the significance of biochemical markers of bone resorption and formation.

References

1. Frost HM: Mathematical Elements of Lamellar Bone Remodeling. Charles C. Thomas, Springfield, IL, 1964.

2. Garn SM, Rohmann CG, Wagner D, Ascol W: Continuing bone growth throughout life: A general phenomenon. Am J Phy Anthropol 26:313, 1967.

3. Sedlin ED, Frost HM, Villanueva AF: Variations in cross-section area of rib cortex with age. J Gerontol 18:9, 1963.

4. Frost HM: Tetracycline-based histological analysis of bone remodeling. Calcif Tiss Res 3:211, 1969.

5. Bordier P, Matrajt H, Miravet L, et al.: Mesure histologique de la masse et de la resorption des travees osseuses. Pathol Microbiol 12:1238, 1964.

6. Eriksen EF, Melsen F, Mosekilde L: Reconstruction of the resorptive site in iliac trabecular bone: A kinetic model for bone resorption in 20 normal individuals. Metab Bone Dis Rel Res 5:235, 1984.

7. Eriksen EF, Gundersen HJG, Melsen F, Mosekilde L: Reconstruction of the formative site in iliac trabecular bone om 20 normal individuals employing a kinetic model for matrix and mineral apposition. Metab Bone Dis Rel Res 5:243, 1984.

8. Mosekilde L: Normal vertebral body size and compressive strength: Relations to age and to vertebral and iliac trabecular bone compressive strength. Bone 7:207, 1986.

9. Frost HM: Bone Remodeling and Its Relationship to Metabolic Bone Diseases. Charles C. Thomas, Springfield, IL, 1973.

10. Jaworski ZFG, Lok F: The effect of moderate uremia and high phosphate-normal calcium diet on the linear erosion rate measured in the Haversian turnover sites in the rib of the adult dog. In: Jaworsky ZFG (ed) Bone Histomorphometry. University of Ottawa Press, Ottawa, 1976, pp 148-152.

11. Frost HM: Dynamics of bone remodeling. In: Frost HM (ed) Bone Biodynamics. Little, Brown and Co., Boston, 1964.

12. Eriksen EF, Mosekilde L, Melsen F: Kinetics of trabecular bone resorption and formation in hypothyroidism: Evidence for a positive balance per remodeling cycle. Bone 7:101, 1986.

13. Eriksen EF, Mosekilde L, Melsen F: Trabecular bone remodeling and bone balance in hyperthyroidism. Bone 6:421, 1985.

14. Eriksen EF, Mosekilde L, Melsen F: Trabecular bone balance and remodeling in primary hyperparathyroidism. Bone 7:213, 1986.

15. Podbesek RD, Stevenson R, Zanelli GD, et al.: Treatment with human parathyroid hormone fractment (hPTH 1-34) stimulates bone formation and intestinal calcium absorption in the greyhound: Comparison with data from the osteoporosis trial. In: Cohn DV, et al. (eds) Hormonal Control of Calcium Metabolism. Excerpta Medica. Amsterdam, 1981, pp. 118-123.

16. Jilka RL, Cohn DV: Role of phosphodiesterase in the parathormone stimulated adenosine 3,5-monophosphate response in bone cell populations enriched in osteoclasts and osteoblasts. Endocrinol 109:743, 1981.

17. Baron R, Bignery A, Horowitz H: Lumphocytes, macrophages and the regulation of bone remodeling. In: Peck WA (ed) Bone and Mineral Research Annual 2, Elsevier, Amsterdam, 1984, p. 175.

18. Chambers TJ, Magnus CJ: Calcitonin alters behavior of isolated osteoclasts. J Pathol 27:1236, 1982.

19. Parfitt AM: The coupling of bone formation and bone resorption: A critical analysis of the concept and of its relevance to the pathogenesis of osteoporosis. Metab Bone Dis Rel Res 4:1, 1982.

20. Courpron P: Donnees histologiques quantitaties sur le vieillesment osseux humain. Ph.D. thesis, University of Lyon, Lyon, France, 1971.

21. Melsen F, Melsen, B, Mosekilde L, Bergman S: Histomorphometric analysis of normal bone from the iliac crest. Acta Path Microbiol Scand (A) 86:63, 1978.

22. Parfitt AM: Age related structural changes in trabecular and cortical bone. Cellular mechanisms and biomechanical consequences. Calcif Tiss Int 26:123, 1984.

23. Parfitt AM: Quantum concept of bone remodeling and turnover: Implications for the pathogenesis of osteoporosis. Calcif Tiss Int 28:1, 1979.

24. Melsen F, Mosekilde L: The role of bone biopsy in metabolic bone disease. Orthop Clin North Amer 12:571, 1981.

25. Jensen FT, Charles P, Mosekilde L, Hansen HH: Calcium metabolism evaluated by Calcium-kinetics: A physiological model with correction for fecal lag time and estimation of dermal calcium loss. Clin Phys 3:187, 1983.

26. Burkinshaw LD, Marshall DH, Oxby CB, Spiers FW, Nordin BEC, Young MM: Bone turnover model based on a continuously expanding exchangeable calcium pool. Nature (London) 222:146, 1969.

27. Rasmussen H, Bordier P: The Physiological and Cellular Basis of Metabolic Bone Disease. Williams & Wilkins, Baltimore, 1974.

28. Emmertsen K, Melsen F, Mosekilde L, Lund B, Sorensen OH, Nielsen HE, Solling H, Hansen HH: Altered Vitamin D metabolism and bone remodeling in patients with medullary thyroid carcinoma and hypercalcitoninemia. Metab Bone Dis Rel Res 4:17, 1981.

29. Halse J, Melsen F, Mosekilde L: Iliac crest bone mass and remodeling in acromegaly. Acta Endocr 97:18, 1981.

30. Charles P, Eriksen EF, Mosekilde L, Melsen F, Jensen FT: Bone turnover and balance evaluated by a combined calcium balance and Calcium kinetic study and dynamic histomorphometry. Metabolism 36:1118, 1987.

Discussion:

DR. LANG (New Haven): Dr. Melsen, it has been suggested that women without estrogen are more susceptible to PTH mediated bone resorption. What was the estrogen status of your patient with hyperparathyroidism?

DR. MELSEN (Denmark): They were all postmenopausal and untreated; selected on these criteria from a larger group of 140 patients.

DR. BONE (Detroit): Patients with medullary thyroid carcinoma may have an increase in parathyroid hormone as a secondary response to the calcitonin level.

DR. MELSEN: We interpret our results to indicate that parathyroid hormone is overwhelming the effect of calcitonin on bone.

DR. PARFITT (Detroit): At our first symposium in 1972 data were presented from Dr. Bordier's laboratory that bone remodeling was very low in medullary thyroid carcinoma. That was the prevailing dogma for many years until Dr. Melsen's group studied a sufficient number of cases to refute that misconception, which still lingers in the literature in a few places.

You've shown us a lot of changes that occur as a result of different hormonal abnormalities. Where do you think the action of these different hormones is located?

DR. MELSEN: I think the most important effect of all these hormones is to increase or decrease the activation frequency.

III
Allied Disciplines

Overview: Allied Disciplines

STEPHEN M. KRANE

Arthritis Unit
Massachusetts General Hospital
Boston, MA

In the course of planning this symposium several of us thought it would be valuable to discuss certain problems of the skeleton that might not be considered as related to what have been perhaps arbitrarily defined as metabolic bone diseases. We reasoned that principles are emerging from recent research that eventually might be applicable to the care of patients with these diseases or understanding pathogenesis.

There is little question that in order to maintain exquisite control of skeletal metabolism, it will be necessary to establish what factors regulate the function of bone cells and their interactions. For example, regulation of the rate at which osteoblasts deposit bone matrix and effect its mineralization is critical for maintenance of adequate bone mass during remodeling and the degree and quality of repair in response to injury or tumor. The quality and amount of the organic matrix deposited in bone are critical as demonstrated by the profound pathological consequences of single amino acid substitution in the helical portion of the type I collagen chains in instances of osteogenesis imperfecta.

We chose to discuss several topics that illustrate some new approaches that are of interest with respect to skeletal metabolism. Dr. Tsipouras from the University of Connecticut presented an analysis of the genetic approach to understanding collagen structure and synthesis in human disease, particularly the use of analysis of restriction fragment length polymorphisms. This technique has made it possible to demonstrate linkage in several kindreds with multiple members affected with some forms of osteogenesis imperfecta. Dr. Tsipouras' talk is entitled "Application of Molecular Genetics to Osteopenic Bone Disease".

Dr. Glowacki from the Children's Hospital in Boston and Harvard Medical School described what is known about some of the mechanisms that govern induction of new bone, particularly the system in which the endochondral sequence is induced by implantation of fragments of demineralized bone. This model, described first by Urist and Huggins, not only permits dissection of controls at each phase in the sequence but application of some of the principles derived from its study also provides new therapeutic approaches to such clinical problems as non-union of fractures and reconstitution of various types of skeletal discontinuity.

Considerable progress has now been made in understanding what governs proliferation and differentiation of hematopoietic precursor cells. Not only have several of the specific growth factors involved been isolated, the cDNAs cloned and expressed and their receptors characterized but sufficient quantities of the recombinant polypeptides are available to specifically treat some anemias and neutropenias. Sufficient promise has now been shown using some of these colony stimulating-factors to relieve the bone marrow failure after irradiation or chemotherapy. Osteoclasts are also derived from hematopoietic precursors and knowledge of factors that govern the differentiation of these cells is critical to understanding physiological and pathological bone resorption. Dr. Roodman from the University of Texas in San Antonio presented an up-to-date general description of "Hematopoietic Growth Factors" particularly in the context of therapeutic potential and the relationship to osteoclast differentiation.

Certainly, introduction of computerized tomography and magnetic resonance imaging has revolutionized clinical care by providing more accurate means for assessing the type and extent of all sorts of pathological lesions in soft tissues. The application of magnetic resonance imaging techniques to analysis of musculoskeletal disorders has recently been achieved. Dr. Murphy from the Mallinkrodt Institute of Radiology at Washington University in St. Louis discussed some of his experience with "Musculoskeletal Magnetic Resonance Imaging" to illustrate the power of the method.

Bone tumors are rare and physicians who care for adults with metabolic bone diseases usually do not have the chance to develop any experience in the diagnosis or management of these neoplasms. Even in patients with Paget's disease, osteosarcomas develop as a complication of the skeletal lesions with a frequency of well under 1%. Nevertheless, these are still important cancers in pediatric orthopedic practice, and there has been considerable improvement in outlook as a result of better procedures to evaluate the lesions and proper appreciation of the usefulness of surgery and chemotherapy. Understanding the biology of osteosarcomas will certainly provide us with useful information about the biology of osteoblasts, since in these tumors the malignant cells are certainly related to osteoblasts. Dr. McGuire from the St. Louis University discussed "Surgical Management of Patients With Skeletal Tumors," particularly from the point of view of management but also described his attempts to identify specific components on the surface of the malignant cells using monoclonal antibodies.

These presentations provide a flavor of the research accomplishments in disciplines that relate in some way to metabolic bone disease. The application of principles and methodology of modern cell and molecular biology to these clinical problems will be even more widespread in the future. Other technologies particularly derived from the physical sciences will continue to offer new approaches to diagnosis and management of skeletal disorders. Further development of some of these and the introduction of new surprises will certainly influence the program of the next Henry Ford Hospital International Symposium.

Application of Molecular Genetics to Osteopenic Bone Disease

PETROS TSIPOURAS[1] and DAVID W. ROWE[2]

Divisions of [1]Genetics and [2]Endocrinology
Department of Pediatrics
University of Connecticut Health Center
Farmington, CT

INTRODUCTION

Much of the current research into the etiology of idiopathic osteoporosis has focused on hormonal and environmental factors that affect the rate of bone loss. There is an increasing appreciation that heritable factors that modulate peak bone mass are also important determinants of the residual bone mass in the postmenopausal years. Osteoporosis may constitute a subset of osteopenic bone disease which consists of a heterogeneous collection of syndromes of diminished bone mass without fractures in which environmental and genetic factors play a contributing role in pathogenesis. The purpose of this discussion is to formulate the rationale and propose a strategy for applying principles of molecular genetics to identify genetic factors which play a role in this complex disorder. We believe that the information gained from this approach will have practical clinical implications for diagnosis and therapy.

A. Heterogeneity of atherosclerotic heart disease

Atherosclerotic heart disease (ASHD) is a paradigm of a heterogeneous condition in which a number of single gene disorders have been identified. The work of Brown and Goldstein has demonstrated that ASHD can result from different mutations to the LDL receptor (1). This is an excellent example of how a single gene disorder can result in a phenotype similar to "nongenetic" heart disease. Other single gene disorders have been identified using molecular genetic techniques. Restriction fragment length polymorphisms (RFLPs) linked to some of the apolipoprotein genes have been associated with an increased prevalence of ASHD (2). In these disorders the precise mutation or dysfunction of the apolipoprotein as well as how the mutation leads to ASHD is not as well defined as in the LDL receptor mutations. Imposed on this background of single gene disorders are other genetically determined diseases, such as adult onset diabetes mellitus and hypertension, that contribute to the susceptibility of blood vessels to ambient cholesterol levels. Similarly, environmental or lifestyle factors are other contributors to lipid deposition into vessel walls.

The example of ASHD clearly illustrates how a single gene disorder can cause disease and how the disease can be potentiated by lifestyle choices or other genetically determined diseases (figure 1). The age at which the disease

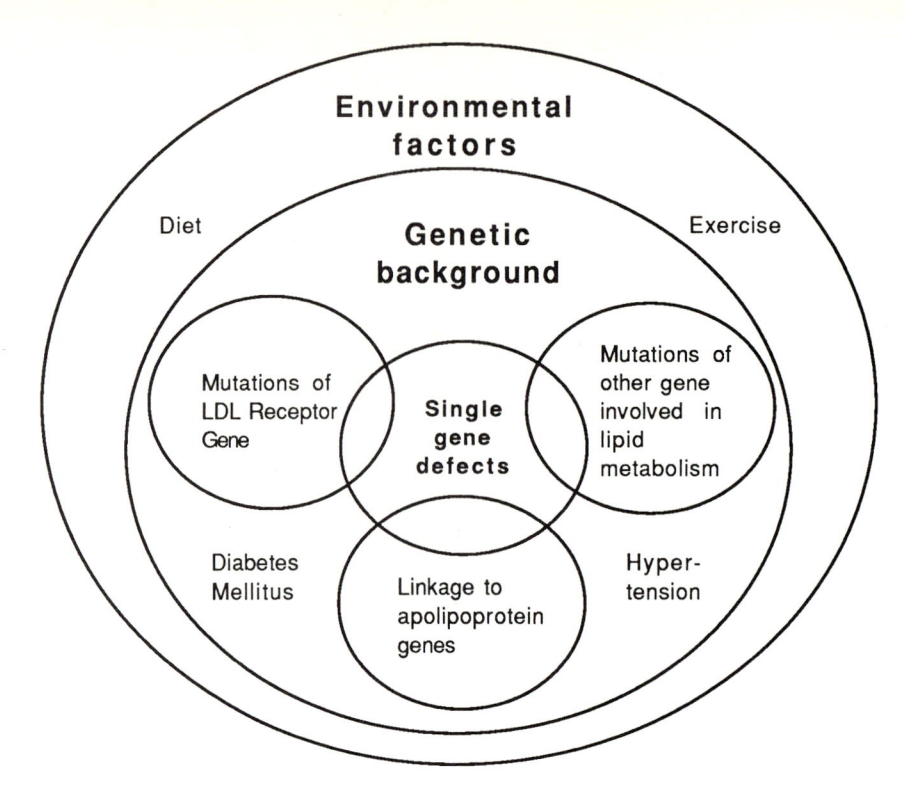

Figure 1: Heterogeneous nature of ASHD. Well-defined single gene defects as well as others which are only recognized by RFLPs of specific candidate genes exist within a background of other genetic and environmental factors, all of which determine the extent of ASHD.

presents is the sum of all the underlying genetically determined risk factors and environmental factors. The strategy for therapy for this disease is to identify during their childhood those individuals with single gene disorders that predispose to heart disease and to provide them with aggressive preventive management to control secondary genetic and environmental factors which contribute to the appearance of the disease.

B. Heterogeneity of osteopenic bone disease

The interaction of single gene disorders and other genetically determined traits with environmental factors to result in diminished bone mass is not as well appreciated in osteopenic bone disease as it is in ASHD. However, the same principles apply. Osteogenesis imperfecta (OI) is the best example of a single gene disorder which is a clear form of heritable osteopenic bone disease. In this disorder, mutations of the type I collagen gene, which interfere with the stability of the collagen fibrils, lead to accumulation of bone which is diminished in mass and is structurally compromised.

In a manner similar to ASHD, other genetically determined traits can affect the rate of bone formation or loss and thus contribute to the overall severity of osteopenia in adulthood (figure 2). Genetic disorders such as Turner syndrome and vitamin D resistant rickets are two examples, as are the genetic factors inherent in a particular race and sex. Finally, lifestyle and other environmental factors such as exercise, cigarette smoking, alcohol intake, and diet may also affect bone mass. Whether or not an individual exhibits osteopenic bone disease is a composite of all the single gene disorders affecting bone matrix genes, other genetically determined traits which might affect bone mass, and non-genetic factors. If the combination of these factors exceed a certain threshold then clinically significant osteoporosis will become apparent.

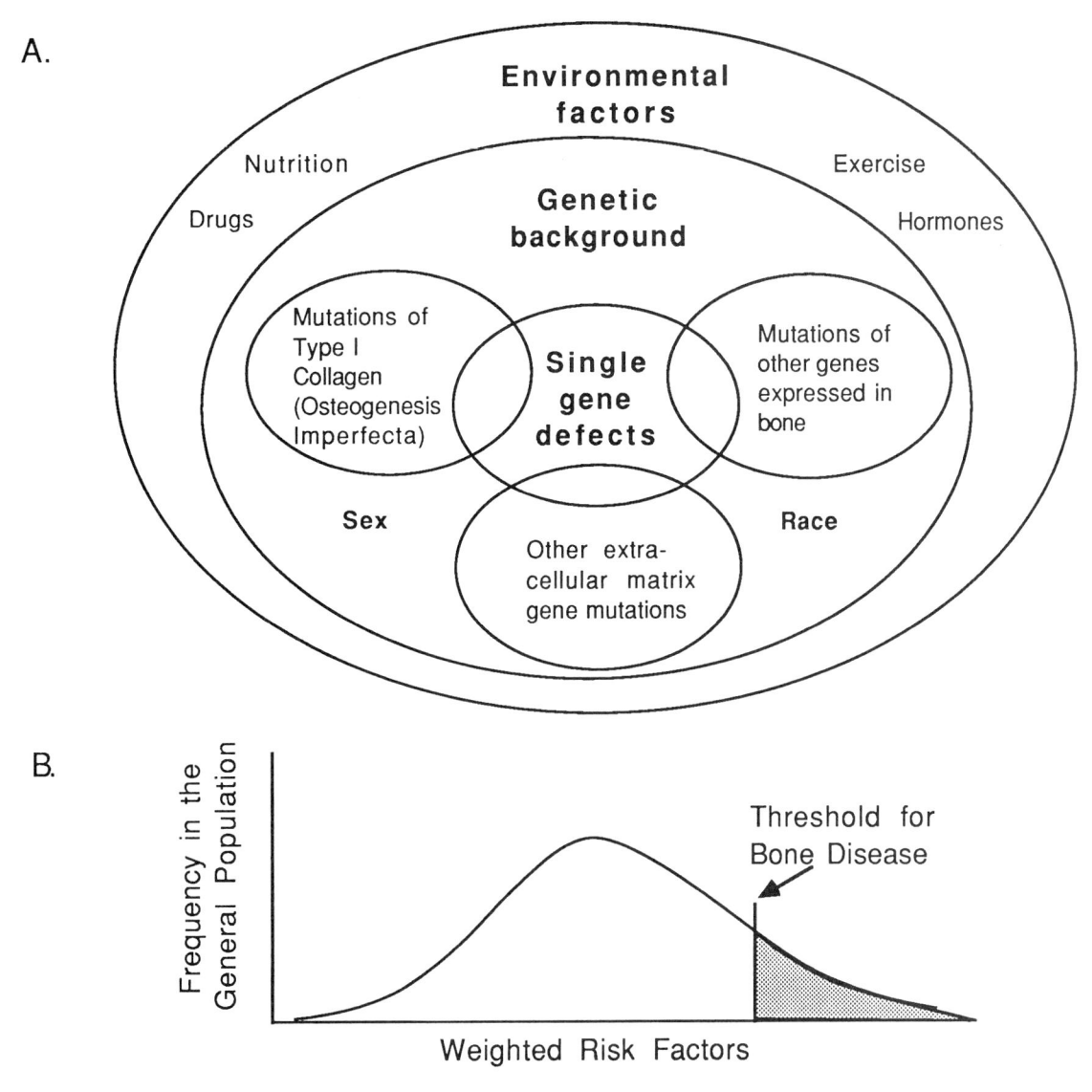

Figure 2: <u>A.</u> Heterogeneous nature of osteopenic bone disease. In a manner analogous to ASHD, genetic and environmental factors determine the presence of clinically apparent bone disease.

<u>B.</u> Concept of a threshold for bone disease. Whether an individual manifests bone disease is dependent on the number and severity of the genetic and environmental factors that are present.

C. Molecular defects of type I collagen associated with OI

Molecular studies of individuals with OI have revealed the wide variety of mutations at two separate loci (the $\alpha 1$ or $\alpha 2$ genes of type I collagen) that can give rise to a spectrum of bone fractures which may be evident at infancy or not until the postmenopausal period (3). Although the mutations found in the perinatal lethal form of OI (type I) are unlikely ever to be found in adults, the principles learned from studying this disorder are applicable. The structure of a normal collagen fiber is dependent on the close interactions of three peptide chains (α chains) that are assembled into the triple helix in an ordered manner (4). In the perinatal lethal form, mutations that disrupt the stability of the helical domain of the triple helical collagen molecule have been demonstrated (5). These studies have revealed that a single amino acid substitution in a collagen α chain not only damages the helical structure of the collagen molecule but also adversely affects collagen molecules composed of normal alpha chains because the entire extracellular matrix is dependent on interactions between adjacent extracellular matrix is dependent on interactions between adjacent extracellular matrix molecules. Thus, these mutations are inherited as dominant traits because the abnormal collagen chain can adversely affect molecules that are made from the normal allele (6).

Analysis of other forms of OI (types I, III, and IV) have shown that the degree of clinical severity correlates with the location of the helix-disrupting mutation: those which disrupt the helix through its entirety are more severe than those which are disrupted near the N-terminal end of the helix. Furthermore, mutations located in the α2(I) chain are better tolerated than those in the α1(I) chain (7). The other major type of mutation that results in a mild form of OI (type I) appears to be an error of mRNA processing such that the amount of mRNA derived from the mutant allele is reduced. The result is underproduction of an otherwise normal collagen molecule which probably accounts for the relatively mild phenotype (8,9).

Thus, variability in expression of disease severity in OI is dependent on the site where a mutation is located within the triple helical structure, or the degree of underproduction of a normal molecule. All of these examples represent single gene disorders, any one of which results in osteopenia and could be aggravated by other genetic disorders or environmental factors that adversely affect bone mass. An excellent example of this interaction is a study by Paterson who found that women with mild OI showed a recurrence of fractures at the menopause. Fractures occurred earlier and with greater frequency in women than men but both sexes showed an enhanced rate over individuals without OI (10).

D. Identification of other single gene disorders causing osteopenic bone disease (figure 3)

Insights into the abnormalities of type I collagen in OI was possible because investigators had access to cultured fibroblasts which express the same type of collagen that is present in bone. Unfortunately, other disorders of bone may involve genes which are only synthesized by bone cells and thus are not accessible to analysis using cultured fibroblasts. One way to overcome this problem is the use of restriction fragment length polymorphisms (RFLP) as markers to test for linkage of a specific gene to a heritable phenotype. This approach has proved to be successful in dominantly inherited OI in which linkage has been demonstrated, both to the α1(I) and the α2(I) collagen genes (11,12).

Although 95% of cases of dominantly inherited OI show linkage to the type I collagen genes, approximately 5% do not, suggesting that other genes are likely to cause an OI-like phenotype (13). Potential candidate genes for which linkage needs to be either demonstrated or excluded in OI and other osteopenic bone disorders include the minor chain collagens associated with type I collagen (type V and type XII), and the noncollagenous proteins that are unique to bone (14). As these genes are cloned they will become important for establishing RFLP analysis in families with heritable osteoporosis. It is unlikely that all forms of heritable osteoporosis are due to a structural abnormality of one of the matrix proteins of bone. Other candidates may include genes necessary for differentiation of pre-osteoblastic, maintenance of an osteoblastic phenotype or factors that might regulate osteoclastic degradation of bone. Thus, as genes for growth and differentiation factors, hormone receptors and integrins on bone cells are cloned, these too, will be useful probes to determine if linkage can be established or excluded in specific pedigrees.

It is unlikely that all potential single gene disorders will be identified by specifically probing with genes coding for known matrix or cellular proteins.

Identification of Pedigrees with Clearly Defined Forms of Heritable Osteoporosis
- Multigenerational affected and unaffected members
- Willingness of many family members to participate

↓

Develop Filters with Restriction Endonuclease Digests of DNA from Each Pedigree
- Probe with gene to known connective tissue proteins
- Probe with unknown genes obtained from osteoblast specific cDNAs
- Probe with anonymous chromosome-specific probes

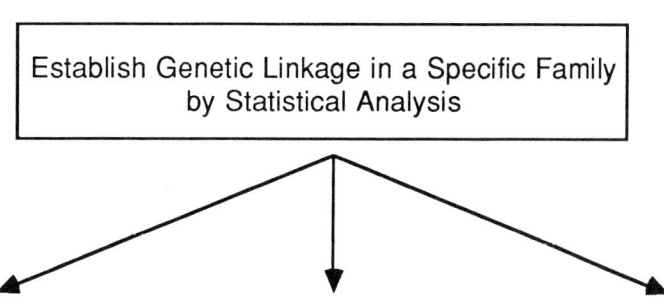

↓

Establish Genetic Linkage in a Specific Family by Statistical Analysis

↙   ↓   ↘

To a Known Gene
- define abnormal nucleotide sequence
- show same mutation is present in other affected members
- examine children harboring same mutation

To an Osteoblast cDNA
- characterize and sequence the normal DNA
- establish function, tissue distribution and regulation of the normal gene
- identify the mutation site in the abnormal gene

To an Anonymous Gene
- localize gene with adjacent chromosomal probes
- "chromosomal walking" to identify DNA fragment that hybridizes with bone mRNA
- clone and characterize the identified mRNA

Figure 3: Strategy for identification of "osteoporosis genes." Once informative pedigrees are established, then linkage studies can be carried out. Depending on the source of the linked DNA probe, a number of subsequent steps will follow.

This raises the problem of how osteoporosis genes can be located when the abnormal proteins are yet to be discovered. This situation has been circumvented in other genetic disorders using linkage studies with random DNA probes (15). In this approach small sequences of DNA, whose exact chromosomal locations are known, are used as random probes. If genetic linkage is found between a probe and heritable osteoporosis in the family under study, then it is likely that there is an abnormal gene contributing to the disorder which is located near the probe on that chromosome. These probes are randomly distributed over the entire human genome at an approximate range of 10 centimorgans (16). Once linkage is established to one of these markers, then further studies can be carried out to localize the trait to either a previously identified gene (which by its nature is a candidate "osteoporosis gene", such as the type I collagen genes), or to a new, as yet unrecognized gene, which could underlie heritable osteoporosis. This use of anonymous probes has been most successful in finding DNA markers for Huntington's chorea and cystic fibrosis. The strategy of establishing linkage prior to identifying the mutant gene or understanding how its mutation causes a disorder is referred to as reverse genetics (17), and has been particularly successful in defining the mutant protein that results in Duchenne's muscular dystrophy (18). These same principles should be applicable to heritable osteoporosis.

E. Practical implications of molecular studies in heritable osteoporosis

This is an exciting time for human genetics as efforts grow to map the human genome and determine its sequence (19). This information will allow investigators to rapidly characterize those genes that linkage studies identify candidate disease-causing genes. Knowing the location of the abnormal gene and the precise mutation resulting in the disease phenotype not only can give insight on the pathophysiology of the disease, but also can be used for precise diagnosis and institution of preventive therapy. In the case of heritable osteoporosis, if a family is found to harbor a specific mutant gene that is known to lead to osteoporosis in adulthood, then children inheriting such a gene would be evaluated for the earliest signs of abnormality of bone mass. If a child has the gene and already has a subnormal bone mass, then hormonal or other manipulations could be evaluted as potential therapeutic agents to forestall the onset of osteoporosis. Once it is known which osteoporosis genes can, by acting alone, result in the disorder, it will become possible to examine smaller pedigrees and even single individuals for the presence of the abnormal gene(s). Additionally it will be possible to determine whether an affected individual has inherited two or more abnormal genes that acted in concert to increase the magnitude of bone loss.

Although establishing the family pedigrees and performing linkage studies may at first appear to be a prolonged and arduous task, the speed at which mutant genes have been identified in other less common genetic disorders is breathtaking, and should encourage investigators to apply these successful techniques to well-defined pedigrees with heritable osteoporosis.

References

1. Goldstein, J.L. and Brown, M.S. (1986). A receptor-mediated pathway for cholesterol homeostasis. Science 232:34-39.
2. Berg, K. (1987). Genetics of coronary heart disease and its risk factors. Ciba Found. Symp. 130:14-33.
3. Byers, P.H. and Bonadio, J.F. (1985). The molecular basis of clinical heterogeneity in osteogenesis imperfecta: mutations in type I collagen genes have different effects on collagen processing. In Genetic and Metabolic Diseases in Pediatrics. Eds. Lloyd, J.K. and Scriver, C.R. Butterworth International Medical Reviews, London. pp. 56-90.
4. Prockop, D.J. (1984). The synthesis of type I collagen fibers and potential inhibitors of the process. Prog. Clin. Biol. Res. 154:81-88.
5. Byers, P.H., Tsipouras, P., Bonadio, J.F., Starman, B.J. and Schwartz, R.C. (1988). Perinatal lethal osteogenesis imperfecta (OI type II): A biochemically heterogeneous disorder usually due to new mutations in the genes for type I collagen. Am.J.Hum. Genet. 42:237-248.
6. Prockop, D.J. (1984). Osteogenesis imperfecta: phenotypic heterogeneity, protein suicide, short and long collagen. Am.J.Hum.Genet. 36:499-50.
7. Tsipouras, P., Boresen, A.L., Dickson, L.A., Berg, K., Prockop, D.J. and Ramirez, F. (1984). Molecular heterogeneity in the mild autosomal dominant forms of osteogenesis imperfecta. Am.J. Hum. Gent. 36:1172-1179.
8. Barsh, G.S., David, K.E., and Byers, P.H. (1982). Type I Osteogenesis Imperfecta: A Nonfunctional Allele for pro $\alpha 1(I)$ Chain of Type I Procollagen. Proc. Natl. Acad. Sci. 79:3838-3842.
9. Rowe, D.W., Shapiro, J.R., Poirier, M. and Schlessinger, S. (1985). Diminished type I collagen synthesis and reduced $\alpha 1(I)$ collagen mRNA in cultured fibroblasts from patients with dominantly inherited (type I) osteogenesis imperfecta. J. Clin. Inves. 76:604-611.
10. Paterson, C.R., McAllion, S., and Stellman, J.L. (1984). Osteogenesis imperfecta after the menopause. New Engl. J. Med. 310:1694-1696. 607

11. Tsipouras, P., Myers, J.C., Ramirez, F. and Prockop, D. (1983). RFLP associated with the pro $\alpha2(I)$ gene of human type I procollagen. J. Clin. Inves. 72:1262-1267.
12. Sykes, B., Oglivie, D., Wordsworth, P., Anderson, J., and Jones, N. (1986). Osteogenesis imperfecta is linked to both type I collagen structural genes. Lancet 69-72, 1986.
13. Tsipouras, unpublished data.
14. Fisher, L.W., Denholm, L.J., Conn, K.M. and Termine, J.D. (1986). Mineralized tissue protein profiles in the Australian form of bovine osteogenesis imperfecta. Calcif. Tissue Int. 38:16-20.
15. Landers, E.S. and Botstein, D. (1986). Strategies for studying heterogeneous genetic traits in humans by using restriction fragment length polymorphisms. Proc. Natl. Acad. Sci. 83:7353-7357.
16. Donis-Keller, H. et al. (1987). A genetic linkage map of the human genome. Cell 51:319-337.
17. Orkin, S.H. (1986) Reverse genetics and human disease. Cell 47:845-860.
18. Monaco, A., Neve, R., Colletti-Feener, C., Bertelson, C., Kurnit, D. and Kunkel, L. (1986). Isolation of candidate cDNAs for portions of the Duchenne muscular dystrophy gene. Nature 323:646-650.
19. Levin, R. (1988) Genome projects ready to go. (Research News) Science 240: 602-604.

Discussion:

DR. RAISZ (Connecticut): Could the failure to find a linkage in that last family that you showed be due to a recombination very close to the defect in the collagen gene? I didn't follow the whole thing, but it looked to me that only one family skipped out of it.

DR. TSIPOURAS (Connecticut): It's a very good point. These particular markers are within the gene. And therefore one would have to postulate recombination between intragenic recombination, in other words the mutation side in the alpha-1 or the alpha-2 collagen genes, and the marker (we know that they're in introns) in both genes.

DR. RAISZ: But it's a very long gene with a lot of introns. So, conceivably, it could happen.

DR. TSIPOURAS: The alpha-1 is about 17,000 base pairs. The alpha-3 is 42. It is possible, but rather unlikely, to have intragenic recombination in humans.

DR. CHESNUT (Seattle): A very lucid presentation of something that's difficult for most of us clinicians to follow. You whetted our appetite a little bit, in that we might have hoped that there might have been more data on osteoporosis, per se. I'm aware of what Peter Byers is doing at our institution.

Do you have a working hypothesis at this time to weight the genetic factors that could contribute to such things as peak bone mass and resultant fractures, presumably later, in comparison to such things as nutrition and other environmental factors? You must have something you're looking at for your study to be done.

DR. TSIPOURAS: At this point, what we're really interested in, by following this random anonymous DNA probe approach, is to come up with at least a foci that could be found linked to the osteoporosis phenotype. Now, what that will uncover is not going to be the same as in single gene disorders. In osteogenesis imperfecta, you have a marker, you link it to a phenotype. If you have tight linkage, then you can presume that the mutation is going to be close by to that marker. So, you know what you have to do next.

In multifactorial traits, like osteoporosis -- and, in fact, this is a model that we try to develop and evolve to study multifactorial traits -- what we really have to find out is whether we have additive epistatic effects. And by that I mean, we have multiple genes which contribute a little bit, each one of those, or whether we have a major single gene which is influencing -- or, is influenced in its expression by the genetic background.

Now, the additive epistatic effects obviously are going to be influenced by environmental factors. And at this point, what I'm saying is that there are too many different factors that are entering in the equation. And, depending on the kind of families we have, I can't answer your question.

Obviously, it's something which we have in mind, but we do not have the data yet to analyze or think about it. You know, what I'm saying is that we may start seeing many different single genes. And that's why osteogenesis imperfecta is very useful.

Let's say that we find osteonectin, just for an example. If we find osteonectin linked to a form of osteogenesis imperfecta, then obviously we're going to use osteonectin in our studies in osteoporosis.

So, if we find different single genes -- and when we start identifying what these genes are, questions like the ones you asked are going to be obvious: what are the interactions of those genes with other factors.

DR. REBUCK (Detroit): Have there ever been any affected identical twins? That would help.

DR. TSIPOURAS: They have been used extensively, not in osteogenesis imperfecta, but obviously twin studies have been used extensively in genetic linkage studies. But identical twins are not necessarily helpful. Fraternal twins are more useful. Identical twins is one individual. So, really, it doesn't help you. They use the same genetic background. If you have fraternal twins, then it's better. You have two siblings.

DR. KRANE: What we're pleading for is identification of large kindreds with osteoporosis where there are suggestions of more than one individual affected; the larger the kindred, the easier the data are going to be to obtain.

Hematopoietic Growth Factors

G. DAVID ROODMAN

*University of Texas Health Science Center
and Audie Murphy Veterans Administration Hospital
San Antonio, TX*

HEMATOPOIETIC GROWTH FACTORS

One of the most exciting developments in hematology has been the availability of hematopoietic growth factors in sufficient amounts and purity for clinical use. The availability of hematopoietic growth factors provides the means for tapping the immense reserve of hematopoietic cells present in a patient's marrow.

White cells, platelets, and lymphocytes are derived from a pluripotent hematopoietic stem cell present in the marrow. This stem cell is usually not in active cycle, and only a small percentage of these cells go into active cycle at any given time. These cells then differentiate in a stocastic manner to give rise to the committed progenitor cells for each of the hematopoietic lineages. Development of in vitro marrow culture techniques have allowed identification, characterization and partial purification of these committed progenitor cells, as well as identification and characterization of hematopoietic growth factors which can affect both the growth and differentiation of hematopoietic progenitors. Hematopoietic progenitors are termed CFUs, colony forming units, so named because they form colonies when cultured in semi-solid media. They are further identified by the type of differentiated progeny which they form. For example, CFU-GM, the granulocyte macrophage colony forming cell, is the progenitor for both granulocytes and macrophages and probably the osteoclast. Similarly, in the erythroid series there are CFU-E, erythroid colony forming cells, and for megakaryocytes there are CFU-Meg. All these committed progenitor cells can be grown in semi-solid media and give rise to differentiated progeny in the presence of the appropriate growth factor. Each colony is derived from a single progenitor cell so that one can quantify the number of progenitor cells present in marrow simply by counting the number of colonies formed.

TABLE 1
HEMATOPOIETIC GROWTH FACTORS

Name	Protein Size (kD)	Cellular Sources	Sites/Cell
IL-3 (multi)	14-28	T cells	1000-5000
G-CSF	18-22	Monocytes Fibroblasts	1000-5000
GM-CSF	14-35	T cells Endothelial cells Fibroblasts	1000-5000
M-CSF	35-45 (x2) 18-26 (x2)	Monocytes Fibroblasts Endothelial cells	3000-15,000
Ep	18-39	Proximal tubule	600

This table lists five different hematopoietic growth factors which have been identified and are currently being tested *in vivo*. Interleukin-3, or multi-CSF stimulates the growth of multipotent progenitors which in turn give rise to all the myeloid cell lines; erythroid, megakaryocytic, granulocyte-macrophage, eosinophil, etc. This protein is about 14-28,000 daltons, depending on the degree of glycosolation. It is produced by T-lymphocytes. There are about 1,000-5,000 sites per cell for this molecule. GM-CSF, the granulocyte macrophage colony stimulating factor affects predominately CFU-GM, the granulocyte macrophage progenitor cell, but it can also affect multipotent stem cells, erythroid cells, eosinophils and megakaryocytes. G-CSF is a factor with a restricted activity and only stimulates the growth of granulocyte progenitors. M-CSF only acts on monocytes and myelomonocytic cell lines. Erythropoietin's (Ep) action is restricted to the erythroid series, and Ep acts only on erythroid progenitors. Some recent data suggests Ep also can affect megakaryopoiesis. As can be seen from this table most of these factors have molecular weights in the range of 18,000-25,000 and their target cells contain very few receptors, approximately 500-1,000 receptors per cell. They are produced by a variety of cells sources and all these factors occur in very trace amounts in the plasma.

GM-CSF has multiple effects on granulocytic and eosinophilic function as well as stimulating proliferation and differentiation of the precursor. For example, it can stimulate: 1) the antibody dependent cellular cytotoxicity activity of both these cell types against tumor cells, 2) enhance phagocytosis and superoxide production, 3) degranulation with lysosome release , 4) increase expression of functional antigens, and 5) increase neutrophil and eosinophil survival *in vitro* and probably *in vivo*.

Table 2
CSF-GM Increases Granulocytic and Eosinophilic Function

1. ADCC of tumor cells
2. Phagocytosis
3. Superoxide production
4. Degranulation
5. Expression of functional antigens
6. Survival in vitro

Similarly, GM-CSF also affects macrophage activity. It induces antibody dependent cellular cytotoxicity toward tumor cells, enhances killing of schistosomula, enhances intracellular killing of Leishmania and induces macrophage tumoricidal activity in the absence of endotoxin.

CSF's also stimulate the growth of malignant myeloid cells as well as normal myeloid cells. G-CSF, GM-CSF, and IL-3 will stimulate the growth of acute myeloid leukemia colony forming cells in vitro and in some cases, even induce their differentiation.

Table 3
Possible Uses of CSF's In Vivo

1. Increase neutrophil production
2. Adjunct in treatment of infections
3. Increase neutrophil survival
4. Stimulate leukemic cells into cell cycle
5. Differentiation of leukemic cells

Therefore, there are several possible uses for CSF's in vivo (Table 3). They can be used to increase neutrophil production after bone marrow transplantation or following chemotherapy. They can be used as an adjuvant in treating infections, since they stimulate neutrophil and macrophage activity and increase neutrophil survival. They can also stimulate leukemic cells into cell cycle, making them more responsive to chemotherapy, and can induce leukemic cells to differentiate into functional cells. Based on these types of data, clinical trials are now underway testing the effects of erythropoietin and several of the colony stimulating factors in vivo.

Patients with glomerulonephritis have decreased erythropoietin production, and their hematocrits are directly proportional to their erythropoietin levels. Therefore, Adamson and coworkers undertook a Phase I-II study to test the effects of erythropoietin in vivo in patients with end-stage renal disease. There were 25 patients of which 7 were anephric. Twelve of the 25 were transfusion dependent. They all had elevated creatines, elevated BUN's and hematocrits of about 20%. The reticulocyte counts were only 1% which was inappropriate for the degree of their anemia.

The results of this trial showed that patients who received greater than 15 units per kg of erythropoietin 3 times per week, had increases in their hematocrits. Patients who were receiving 150 units per kg body weight had hematocrits of about 40%, and these hematorcrits could be maintained on lower doses of erythropoietin. Therefore, in patients who follow medical management, erythropoietin appears to be safe, effective therapy for patients with chronic renal failure on dialysis. The side effects that have been noted in clinical trials with erythropoietin include: 1) development of functional iron deficiency which can be treated with iron; 2) exaccerbation of pre-existing hypertension because of their increased blood volume secondary to their increased red cell mass; 3) increased creatine and BUN because the increased viscosity of their blood which decreased the efficiency of their dialysis, and 4) hyperkalemia in patients not adhering to a low potassium diet.

Similarly, colony stimulating factors have also been used in vivo. To date, the majority of these studies have been in animal models, although several very recent human trials have been reported. Nathan and coworkers reported the results of GM-CSF administration to primates undergoing autologous marrow transplantation. Three groups of animals were transplanted: those that were treated both with GM-CSF prior to and after irradiation, those which were only treated with GM-CSF after irradiation, and a nontreatment control group. Controls had white counts of about 3600 prior to transplantation and required about 17-24 days to recover their white counts and their platelet counts. In contrast, animals treated before and after transplantation with GM-CSF achieved white counts as high 40,000 prior to transplantation and recovered both their neutrophils and platelets earlier than the control animals. Neutrophil recovery was seen as early as 9 days in these animals and platelet recovery was also significantly decreased.

GM-CSF administration also aided neutrophil recovery in animals showing delayed engraftment. Animals who showed delayed engraftment were given GM-CSF 40-50 days after transplantation. They had a prompt increase in the neutrophil counts and recovery of their neutrophil function. Their platelet counts also increased after GM-CSF administration.

Groopman and coworkers have examined the effects of GM-CSF administration to patients with AIDS who have neutropenia. Administration of GM-CSF induced a brisk increase in neutrophils in these patients, but more markedly increased eosinophilia which resolved with the cessation of GM-CSF. These data show that GM-CSF can increase neutrophil production in patients with AIDS as well as in subjects undergoing autologous marrow transplantation. Of interest, lymphocyte counts also increased in these patients.

Recombinant GM-CSF can be given by the subcutaneous route as well as the intravenous route and still obtain similar results. Administration by intermittant subcutaneous injection of GM-CSF results in a greater increase in the white count than intravenous GM-CSF. The white counts are maintained for longer period of time consistent with the increase half-life of the material given by the subcutaneous route. Therefore, it appears that long-term outpatient administration of GM-CSF may be possible by the subcutaneous route.

G-CSF has been used to ameliorate the neutropenia seen in patients receiving chemotherapeutic agents. Because of the specificity of the G-CSF in inducing only neutrophil production, several investigators have concentrated their studies on the effects of G-CSF on chemotherapy induced neutropenia.

Intravenous infusion of G-CSF in patients who received high doses of Melphalan chemotherapy, resulted in a marked shortening of the duration of their leukopenia after chemotherapy. Therefore, it appears that these growth factors may be able to decrease the neutropenia and morbidity of many chemotherapeutic agents.

Recently Gutterman and coworkers have shown that GM-CSF can induce differentiation of leukemic cells or pre-leukemic cells in vivo. They treated patients with GM-CSF who had myelodysplastic syndrome and pancytopenia. Several of the patients had increased myeloblasts in their bone marrow. Many of these dysplastic syndromes are pre-leukemic states in which patients frequently have hypocellular marrows, chromosomal abnormalities in these cells, as well as increased immature cells in their bone marrow. Approximately 20% of them will eventually evolve into acute myelogenous leukemia.

Treatment of these patients with GM-CSF resulted in an increase in their peripheral blood neutrophils, their platelet counts and hematocrits, without affecting their lymphocytes. Interestingly, it did not increase the percentage of immature cells in their marrow. This was a major concern because GM-CSF can increase leukemic cell growth in vitro. However, it appeared that GM-CSF was inducing differentiation since the marrow became hypercellular and contained a marked increase in the number of mature cells. Of interest though, was that the cells which were still present in the marrow contained chromosomal abnormalities. The results demonstrate that the abnormal cells were still present but had been induced to differentiate to functional granulocytes with GM-CSF.

Therefore, we are entering an exciting time in which we can use hematopoietic growth factors to enhance engraftment of neutrophils and platelets in patients. We can treat anemia with erythropoietin and possible even treat leukemia or infections with these agents. The CSF's activate macrophages and neutrophils as well as stimulate their production, so that these factors may also be important in treating patients with overwhelming infections. In the next few years these hematopoietic growth factors will undoubtedly be used in a variety of clinical studies and their use will continue to increase exponentially.

In summary, the cloning, purification, and availability of large amounts of recombinant hematopoietic growth factors is opening new vistas in the treatment of patients with a broad spectrum of disease processes and may provide important information on the regulation of hematopoiesis and relatedly bone cell biology.

SELECTED REFERENCES
1. Clark SC, Kamen R. The human hematopoietic colony-stimulating factors. Science 236:1229-1237, 1987.

2. Eschbach JW, Egrie JC, Downing MR, Browne JK, Adamson JW. Correction of the anemia of end-stage renal disease with recombinant human erythropoietin. N Engl J Med 316:73-78, 1987.

3. Grabstein KH, Urdal DL, Tushinski RJ, Mochizuki DY, Price

VL, Cantrell MA, Gillis S, Conlon PJ. Induction of macrophage tumoricidal activity by granulocyte-macrophage colony-stimulating factor. Science 232:506-508, 1986.

4. Griffin JD, Lowenberg B. Clonogenic cells in acute myeloblastic leukemia. Blood 68:1185-1195, 1986.

5. Kelleher C, Miyauchi J, Wong G, Clark S, Minden MD, McCulloch EA. Synergisms between recombinant growth factors, GM-CSF and G-CSF, acting on the blast cells of acute myeloblastic leukemia. Blood 69:1498-1503, 1987.

6. Lopez AF, Williamson J, Gamble JR, Begley CG, Harlan JM, Kiebanoff J, altersdorph A, Wong G, Clark SC, Vadas MA. Recombinant human granulocyte-macrophage colony-stimulating factor stimulates in vitro mature human neutrophil and eosinophil function, surface receptor expression, and survival. J Clin Invest 78:1220-1228, 1986.

7. Metcalf D, Begley CG, Johnson GR, Nicola NA, Vadas MA, Lopez AF, Williamson DJ, Wong GG, Clark SC, Wang EA. Biologic properties in vitro of a recombinant human granulocyte-macrophage colony-stimulating factor. Blood 67:37-45, 1986.

8. Metcalf D, Begley CG, Nicola NA, Johnson GR. Quantitative responsiveness of murine hemopoietic populations in vitro and in vivo to recombinant multi-CSF (IL-3). Exp Hematol 15:288-295, 1987.

9. Nienhuis AW, Donahue RE, Karlsson S, Clark SC, Agricola B, Antinoff N. Recombinant human granulocyte-macrophage colony-stimulating factor (GM-CSF) shortens the period of neutropenia after autologous bone marrow transplantation ina primate model. J Clin Invest 80:573-577, 1987.

10. Sieff CA. Hematopoietic growth factors. J Clin Invest 79:1549-1557, 1987.

Discussion:

DR. KRANE (Boston): Could you tell us whether that patient who received M-CSF and had repeated marrow aspirations, was there the opportunity to look at the bone? We know that in mice, the administration of M-CSF does not induce increased numbers of osteoclast. How about in humans?

DR. ROODMAN (San Antonio, TX): I don't think there's any data. They've looked at marrow cellularity, predominantly marrow differentials. And they've only reported increased cellularity. No one has commented on osteoclasts, and I would predict they probably are not increased, though I don't think there's any data available on this point.

DR. KRANE: How about patients with some of the various osteopetrosis phenotypes. Have you or anybody else started to think about the use of some of these hematopoietic growth factors in a selected group of those patients?

DR. ROODMAN: I think, personally, that because there is such a heterogeneity of the etiology of osteopetrosis, it may be difficult to pick the appropriate patient to give the CSF's to. Lyndon Keyes looked at calcitriol and it was shown that in a subgroup of patients, he can get some osteoclast resorbing bone. But in other ones, he can't.

So, I think it may be premature to start thinking about using these agents in those types of patients.

DR. KRANE: Do you think we're going to come up with a colony-stimulating factor for osteoclasts that you haven't yet identified?

DR. ROODMAN: Elsburger thinks she has identified one and has, at least in abstract form, reported that she can extract from bone a factor which increases osteoclast-like cell formation in her mouse marrow culture system. I may be incorrect because I don't like to quote her data, but I don't think she's characterized what that factor is, or purified it. So, it may be one that's already known or it may be a new factor. I think that awaits further study.

DR. SUTTON (Vancouver): I just wanted to ask if non-glycosolated erythropoietin is effective subcutaneously by analogy with GM-CSF? Because that would have enormous economic implications, if it were.

DR. ROODMAN: I do not know. I don't think it's been tried. So, I can't tell you. I know that the cost of erythropoietin, if you're going to do in vitro studies, is $350 for 500 units. But I predict, and I think it's reasonable, that the cost is really going to come way down. There are at least four different molecular biology companies that are fighting to market erythropoietin. Competition alone is going to drive down the price, I think, so that it's going to be reasonable at some time.

DR. REEVE (England): Going back to the earlier part of the talk, I was interested in the replenishment of the stem cell pool. And drawing a perhaps slightly fanciful analogy, it seems to me that when patients are treated with fluoride, that after five years, they run out of steam and the osteoblasts aren't really responding, at least if you go by the Danish results.

Now, what happens when you simulate these more mature derivatives? Does the feedback to the stem cell keep the stem cells replenished or do you run the risk of running out of stem cells? How is that controlled?

DR. ROODMAN: Well, I think that's a very good question. It's actually been looked at by treating animals with repeated courses of GM-CSF. It turns out you enhance the number of progenitors as well as to differentiate progeny, so that the immense proliferative capacity and self-renewal capacity of the bone marrow gives you an upper hand. So, that, it appears you will not really exhaust the bone marrow, at least in the studies that have been reported. No one has looked at, you know, years of treatment with GM-CSF to answer that question correctly. But in short-term repeated dosages, there still is a brisk leukocytosis every time you do it.

Now, the other thing I didn't mention, which I'll do quickly, is that the leukocyte response is very rapid, within 24 hours of the GM-CSF. And there is no way that you can go from a progenitor cell to a mature granulocyte in less than a week. So, what it also is doing is, it's probably causing demargination, early release from the marrow, and increased neutrophil survival in the circulation to account for the early effects you're seeing with GM-CSF.

Then, after the stem cells get cranked up, then that would explain how you maintain that level of neutrophilia after several days.

DR. KRANE: Could you comment about whether a CFU osteoblast will be identified?

DR. ROODMAN: Well, my knowledge on osteoblasts is fairly limited. My understanding is that osteoblasts are not hematopoietic, though other people have argued that they may be. There are CFU fibroblasts, that is, colony-forming units that give rise to fibroblast. Also, stromal cells in long-term cultures are alk-phos positive and they make different types of collagen. But I do not know if you're going to be able to do that or not. I really don't know.

DR. KRANE: You show your prejudices. Just because the osteoblast is not a hematopoietic cell it still can have a precursor and go through the similar business of differentiation utilizing its own set of growth factors.

DR. ROODMAN: Very true.

Bone Induction

JULIE GLOWACKI

Department of Orthopedic Surgery
Brigham and Women's Hospital
and Harvard Medical School
Boston, MA

Introduction

When faced with osseous reconstruction problems, surgeons (including orthopedic, hand, craniofacial, oral, periodontal, and plastic) have a variety of materials to consider. The material of choice is fresh autogenous particulate bone marrow, which includes viable osteoblasts and preosteoblasts that survive the transplantation procedure. Iliac crest provides a large volume of grating material. Segments of cortical bone can be successfully transplanted by maintaining the vascular supply either by microsurgical reanastomoses or by repositioning of the bone on a vascular pedicle. Due to limited availability and suitability of such fresh, living grafts for solving all osseous problems, surgeons are frequently forced to consider alternatives or supplemental implant material. There are several types of banked bone materials that are available, including frozen or lyophilized allogeneic and xenogeneic bone and demineralized bone implants. In addition to these bone-derived materials, there are many alloplastic materials that have been used successfully for particular applications. These include the resorbable ones, such as plaster of Paris or crystalline hydroxyapatite, and the non-resorbable ones, such as ceramic hydroxyapatite. A complete understanding of the biological mechanisms of healing that is promoted by these different materials will afford the surgeon with a more rational basis for deciding which material is most suitable for different applications.

New bone can be formed by three basic mechanisms of healing: osteogenesis, osteoconduction, and osteoinduction. In osteogenic transplantation, viable osteoblasts and preosteoblasts are moved to a different part of the body, where they establish centers of bone formation. Cancellous bone and marrow grafts provide such viable cells. The term "graft" applies only to transplantation of living tissue. Maintenance of viability of large pieces of corticocancellous bone can be achieved by transplantation of vascularized segments of bone.

In the transplantation of large segments of non-vascularized cortical bone or with allogeneic banked bone, direct osteogenesis by the transplant does not take place. In these cases, osteoconduction occurs; the dead bone acts as a scaffold for the ingrowth of vessels, followed by the resorption of the implant and deposition of new bone derived from the edges of the defect. This process is very slow and may require years to unite a large segmental defect. Failure of incorporation of the bone is attributed to resorption of the bone exceeding the ingrowth of new bone. This is frequently encountered in onlay or contour augmentation procedures or in attempts to fill large defects. Alloplastic materials support bony ingrowth by this same osteoconductive mechanism.

<u>Osteoinduction</u> is the phenotypic conversion of connective tissue into bone by an appropriate stimulus. This concept implies that formation of bone can be demonstrated in nonskeletal sites. Demineralized bone and dentin are such osteoinducers[1,2].

After implantation into subcutaneous pockets[3] or into osseous defects[4] in rats, demineralized bone powders induce the conversion of connective tissue into cartilage, which becomes calcified, invaded by host vessels, and replaced by bone. This highly synchronous sequence of events is analogous to normal endochondral ossification. This principle is exemplified in the clinical use of demineralized bone implants in osseous repair, reconstruction, and construction.

Preparation of Demineralized Bone

We have shown the importance of complete removal of all potentially inflammatory or antigenic materials from bone powder to be implanted in experimental animals or to be used clinically[5]. This method has been used successfully for donor bone from rats, humans, calves, chickens, rabbits, cats, and both the exoskeleton and endoskeleton of an armadillo. In brief, allogeneic bone for clinical use is obtained from an Interhositol Organ Bank, as part of a multiple organ donor program. The bones are cleaned of marrow, adherent periosteum, and connective tissue, and washed in cold water. Extraction with absolute ethanol and anhydrous ether is accomplished at room temperature. The bones are cut into segments or coarse chips, or sieved into powder (75-450 μm). The demineralization is carried out in the cold with 0.5 M HCl. The acid and dissolved minerals are washed away by copious changes of distilled water until the pH is neutral. The demineralized implants are double-wrapped, sterilized, and stored at room temperature. Initially we sterilized with cathode ray irradiation (2 x 10^6); more recently we have been using ethylene oxide on the cold cycle.

Induced Endochondral Osteogenesis

The initial reaction to subcutaneous implants of demineralized bone powder in rats is the ingrowth of connective tissue type cells surrounding each particle. Chondroblasts and cartilage matrix are evident by 9 days after implantation. This phase is followed by cartilage mineralization, vascularization, resorption, and its replacement by bone and marrow. This sequence is highly synchronous when a narrow range of particle size, such as 75-250 μm, is used[4]. Particulate material is not always useful clinically because it needs to be contained and does not provide immediate stability. Demineralized cancellous bone blocks also stimulate osteogenesis within its porous structure at a slower, less synchronous pace[6], but is suitable for onlay procedures or for filling large cysts or gaps.

Clinical Uses of Demineralized Bone

We have used demineralized bone implants in three forms for different clinical situations. Because fine powders provide the maximum surface area for interaction with target cells in the recipient bed[4], powdered cortical bone is preferred to fill small defects. When rehydrated with Ringer's lactate at the time of implantation, demineralized bone powder can be used to caulk irregular gaps[7,8] and fill periodontal defects[9]. Cancellous blocks are soft and rubbery after demineralization; they can be carved to exact specifications after rehydration at the time of the operation.

Demineralized bone powder has been used for a variety of congenital and acquired osseous defects. To date we have treated over 90 patients with maxillocraniofacial deformities, 60 with orthopedic problems such as nonunion fractures, cysts, and scoliosis, and 70 with advanced periodontal lesions. Healing is monitored by standard procedures: clinical examination, roentgenographic evaluation, occasionally by computed tomography or ultrasonography, and by biopsy when appropriate. There have been no complications during surgery, four instances of infection during the immediate postoperative period, and inadequate bone formation only when large demineralized cortical segments were used. We no longer use large cortical pieces because they are not as osteoinductive as implants with greater surface area.

In general, demineralized bone implants stimulate healing with 3-6 months. No resorptions of demineralized bone onlays have been seen in patients followed for 3-4 years. We find this consistent with the experimental studies that showed that the obligatory resorption seen with conventional mineral-containing (osteoconductive) grafts is bypassed with osteoinductive implants. Biopsies of craniofacial recipients have revealed new bone united to particles of the demineralized bone. In the biopsies of orthopedic cases, it has been difficult to identify the original implant material. According to Wolff's Law, this may be attributable to the faster metabolism of tissue in long bones that in the non-weight-bearing craniofacial sites.

We have reported a successful case using demineralized bovine bone, that is, xenogeneic. With careful preparation of bovine bone, in order to remove all cellular and potentially antigenic components, xenoimplants may provide an unlimited supply of banked material for osseous surgery. A limitation to the use of demineralized bone implants is that they provide no immediate strength or rigidity and thus require fixation in segmental or weight-bearing defects.

The major advantages of the use of demineralized bone implants are the avoidance of the harvesting procedure and thus shortened operative time, the potentially umlimited supply of banked material, rapidity of the osteoinductive process, and the potential avoidance of late graft resorption, a problem especially in contour augmentation in the craniofacial region.

We prepare our own material for hospital-side use, according to protocols approved by our internal review board. Until demineralized bone implants become commercially available with FDA approval, hospitals could consider preparing material for in-house use. Cadaver bone from kidney donors would be appropriate starting material. Preparative procedures should be monitored for bioactivity. In vitro assays may be useful in the future, but at the moment the rat bioassay is the most reliable indicator of proper processing.

References

1. Ray, R.D., and Holloway, J.A.: Bone implants. J. Bone Joint Surg., 39A:1119, 1957.
2. Urist, M.R.: Bone: formation by autoinduction. Science 150:893, 1965.
3. Reddi, A.H., and Huggins, C.B.: Biochemical sequences in the transformation of normal fibroblasts in adolescent rats. Proc. Natl. Acad. Sci. U.S.A. 69:1601, 1972.
4. Glowacki, J., Altobelli, D., and Mulliken, J.B.: Fate of mineralized and demineralized osseous implants in cranial defects. Calcif. Tissue Int. 30:71, 1981.
5. Glowacki, J., Mulliken, J.B.: Demineralized bone implants. Clin Plastic Surg. 12:233, 1985.
6. Mulliken, J.B., and Glowacki, J.: Induced osteogenesis for repair and construction in the craniofacial region. Plast. Reconstr. Surg. 65:553, 1980.
7. Glowacki, J., Kaban, L.B., Murray, J.E., et al.: Application of the biological principle of induced osteogenesis for craniofacial defects. lancet 1:959, 1981.
8. Upton, J., Boyajian, M., Mulliken, J.B., and Glowacki, J.: The use of demineralized bone implants to correct phalangeal defects: A case report. J. Hand Surg. 9A:388, 1984.
9. Sonis, S.T., Kaban, L.B., and Glowacki, J.: Clinical trial of demineralized bone powder in the treatment of periodontal defects. J. Oral Med. 38:117, 1983.

Discussion:

DR. KAYE (Montreal): Thank you for a fascinating paper. You partially touched on my question just at the end. I wonder if you could expand on it. Is this purely a local phenomenon? For example, in experimental animals, if they have no PTH or no vitamin D, what happens when you put in your demineralized bone?

DR. GLOWACKI (Boston): In all of the experiments that we've done and that Hari Reddy and others have published on the hormonal influence of bone induction, what happens is what you would expect by these factors, that bone active factors act upon the induced bone just the way that they act upon the intact skeleton.

And just to amplify that a bit, the induced bone also grows commensurate with the skeleton. We were concerned about whether there would be overgrowth of the bone or it would fail to grow in correspondence with the growth of the child. But it seems to be under the same mechanical and systemic factors that the entire skeleton is playing.

DR. RAISZ (Connecticut): Do you have any idea whether the pseudo bone or the cultured bone that's formed as nodules in cell cultures is equally inductive? In other words, can matrices that are made in vitro by osteoblastic cells cultures be demineralized and transplanted in induced bone? Has anybody tried that experiment?

DR. GLOWACKI: I hear, within the lines of your question, what is causing all of this, you know, is it an osteoblast -- whether it's an osteoblast product.

DR. RAISZ: Can osteoblast make the whole thing?

DR. GLOWACKI: Yes, I think the only data on that is from Marshall Urist and his colleagues, who show that osteogenic sarcomas produce a material that is capable of mimicking the entire endochondral sequence when implanted.

DR. RAISZ: You haven't tried that?

DR. GLOWACKI: No.

DR. KRANE (Boston): In the dramatic example of that child with the craniofacial disorder, are osteoblasts that made the new bone that filled in the defect derived from the local tissue or from the blood? Was the local cellular defect corrected by having cells migrate into the lesion?

DR. GLOWACKI: Well, we think that, because of the rapidity with which we saw ossification by x-ray, that the target cells there were from the dura and that they certainly ended up being normal, that probably what was going on in utero was that it was suture defect rather than an osteoblast defect.

DR. KRANE: On the basis of a discussion with Dr. Michael Parfitt this morning, perhaps some of the cells that are functioning in the cancellous bone predominantly affected in patients with osteoporosis may represent a population of cells of a different phenotype than osteoblasts in other portions of the skeleton.

We generally don't consider this possibility but why not? I mean, who would have said 25 years ago that there were T and B lymphocytes, no less subsets of these cells? Now we have antigenic and functional markers to distinguish one population from the other. Perhaps markers will be developed to distinguish among osteoblasts as well.

DR. GLOWACKI: One aspect related to that is that, even though one implants the demineralized bone into a membranous bone, the inductive process always occurs by the endochondral route. And, so, that may suggest a different subset of cells that are responding to it.

Surgical Management of Patients with Skeletal Tumors

MICHAEL H. McGUIRE

Creighton University
Omaha, NE

GENERAL CONSIDERATIONS

Tumors arising primarily from the skeleton represent an interesting and certainly a challenging aspect of the practice of orthopedic surgery. Fortunately, the number of sarcomas diagnosed each year in the United States is miniscule compared to the more common carcinomas. Of approximately 7000 new sarcomas diagnosed in this country each year, 2000 arise from the skeleton, whereas others develop from the soft tissues. By comparison, over 100,000 new cases each of colon, breast, lung, and prostate carcinoma occur annually in the United States.[7] This chapter will outline those methods used to evaluate patients who are found to have a bone lesion that may represent one of these rare tumors. These methods usually allow (often prior to biopsy) separation of the primary malignant bone tumors from those lesions found to be benign, metastatic, infectious, developmental, or even metabolic in nature. The applications of these principles to the surgical management of bone tumors will be discussed.

Diagnosis. The staging of skeletal tumors is somewhat of a misnomer in that the goal is the thorough evaluation of a patient with a symptomatic complaint, a physical finding, or a radiographic appearance of a potentially serious skeletal lesion. As in all of clinical medicine, the cornerstone of diagnosis remains the taking of the patient's history and the performance of a physical examination.

History. Certainly the most common presenting complaint is that of pain. Unfortunately, this observation on the patient's part does not usually separate neoplastic processes from other afflictions of the musculoskeletal system. Equally confusing is the frequency with which the onset of pain is associated with some incident of trauma, which may have been minimal in nature. In fact, the nature of the onset, the duration of symptoms, and the severity of the complaints often do not suggest the diagnosis. Pain associated with tumors may characteristically be persistent and occasionally is considered worse at night; it should not be relieved by rest.

Of more importance is a general review of the patient's health with special reference obviously to any history of previous or other more common malignancies. A history of recent or past infection, systemic immune suppression, unusual cultural or dietary practices, or even trauma can perhaps provide a clue to either the etiology of the lesion or at least to the appropriate direction in which the workup should proceed. The patient's age is of prime importance in that different skeletal lesions so consistently appear in characteristic age groups. Certainly lesions appearing during the patient's fifth decade or beyond are most likely to represent multiple myeloma or a metastatic carcinoma. This is true even if there is no known primary carcinoma (i.e., it has yet to be discovered). Perhaps 20 to 25% of patients dying of metastatic carcinoma do so without identification of the primary cancer.

Physical Examination. The physical examination of a patient with skeletal tumor (like the history) should include a general survey. The involved areas of patients with tumors of the extremity is often found to be tender. A mass may or may not be present. Swelling in an adjacent joint may suggest extension of the tumor or may be sympathetic in nature. Any evidence of neurologic or circulatory compromise by the tumor mass should be noted. The skin and associated soft tissues may or may not be "fixed." Careful neurologic examination of patients with spinal column lesions is mandatory to discover any evidence of cord compression.

Laboratory Tests. The evaluation of the patient continues with a somewhat routine set of basic laboratory investigations. A complete blood count with a differential white blood cell determination and an erythrocyte sedimentation rate will suggest or usually rule out an infectious process. The diagnosis for the occasional child with a skeletal presentation of leukemia may be established by this simple investigation. In a similar fashion the elderly patient with multiple myeloma may be identified by the combination of anemia and an elevated sedimentation rate. The serum calcium, phosphorus, and alkaline phosphatase levels will suggest the possibility of one of the metabolic diseases of bone. A routine urinalysis, blood sugar, blood urea nitrogen, and perhaps liver and thyroid function tests complete the laboratory screening process. The clinical situation may dictate other investigations such as serum acid phosphatase (prostate carcinoma), serum immunoglobulin electrophoresis (multiple myeloma), urinary hydroxyproline (Paget's disease), or even urinary vanillylmandelic acid (VMA) in a young child with suspected metastatic neuroblastoma. Little time is spent on these investigations, which may clarify (or nearly so) the differential diagnosis.

Imaging Modalities. The clinician must next make a decision as to which, if any, of several imaging modalities should be used for the necessary evaluation of the patient. For purposes of discussion we will assume that routine radiographs of the affected region in at least two projections have been obtained by this juncture in the evaluation. The single imaging modality most likely to establish the diagnosis of a skeletal tumor is conventional high-quality radiography. The recognition of this fact is of utmost importance and therefore requires that the clinician and the radiologist have clear, sharp radiographs prior to extending their diagnostic opinion. In choosing from additional x-ray studies, computed tomography (CT) scans, nucelar scans, magnetic resonance images (MRI), and special invasive studies such as arteriography, the clinician must decide what information is required. Conceptually, one should realize that in the evaluation of a primary malignant bone tumor, the imaging modalities are meant to define either the local problem or the possibility of systemic spread or involvement. Likewise, for a bone tumor felt to represent metastasis from a primary carcinoma, the studies listed above can be considered either to document the extent of local destruction or to identify the primary (in cases where it is yet to be discovered) or to note the routine radiographs to be benign in nature, the proper selection of additional studies can usually establish the diagnosis without needing to resort to biopsy.

The patient with a lesion that is found on radiographic examination can be further evaluated in a number of ways. CT of the lesion can demonstrate the degree of cortical destruction, any evidence of trabecular host bone response, and the volume of the soft tissue mass if present. Experience accumulated over the past decade suggests that the relationship of the associated neurovascular structures to the tumor's soft tissue mass can be confidently predicted by CT. Our experience with MRI of sarcomas arising in long bones has led to the conclusion that MRI is the most accurate and sensitive measure of the exact extent of medullary involvement by a tumor.[8]

The technetium nuclear bone scan is pivotal in this evaluation because it provides information about the local problem and because it is part of the systemic evaluation. A lesion arising in either the axial or the appendicular skeleton that is producing bone, destroying bone or eliciting a response from the host bone will be, as expected, "hot" on nuclear scanning. The scan of the remainder of the skeleton, however, is critical to the evaluation. If the lesion is found to be solitary and have normal uptake, and if the remainder of the skeleton is also negative, it must be a benign process. However, if multiple "hot" lesions are found, then metastatic disease must be most likely. It should be noted that the skeleton itself represents the second most common site (following the lungs) of metastatic involvement of primary skeletal sarcomas. Multiple myeloma, which is both very common (five times more frequent than all bone sarcomas combined[7]) and common in the spine, is notorious for being either hot or cold or even negative on bone scan.

It is difficult to imagine a patient with a bone tumor who does not require or at some time obtain a chest x-ray. Certainly a patient coming to surgery or one in whom a malignancy is suspected must be so examined. Chest CT is commonly used to supplement the radiograph in an effort to find the primary carcinoma or to rule out pulmonary metastases from a sarcoma as part of the systemic evaluation. Abdominal, retroperitoneal, and pelvic CT scans are use in a similar systemic manner. These are especially important in metastatic lesions of the skeleton and in the lymphomas. Generating and summarizing all this information is necessary prior to considering biopsy of a skeletal lesion in order to avoid errors.[4]

Biopsy of the Lesion

Finally the evaluation of the patient and the tumor is completed by the performance of a biopsy and the appropriate examination of the tissue obtained. The clinician needs to make several decisions at this time, i.e., several questions need to be answered prior to proceeding. Which lesions need to be biopsied? How should the biopsy be performed? Who should perform the biopsy? These issues have been addressed by the members of the Musculoskeletal Tumor Society.[4] Perhaps the greatest service one can perform is to recognize those benign or inactive lesions and processes that by their self-limiting nature do not require biopsy. In these cases, reassurance of the patient and appropriate follow-up can avoid an "unnecessary" procedure. In other cases (again in both the axial and appendicular skeleton) the information generated to this point will dictate a biopsy to establish the exact diagnosis in a difficult case.

Schajowicz[6] and others[4] have discussed the problems and considerations associated with a biopsy. As the members of the team (orthopedists, radiologists, and pathologists) at an institution gain experience, I suspect that fewer biopsies are performed, and those patients who do undergo biopsy have smaller procedures. This certainly applies to benign self-limiting lesions (as mentioned above) and probably also to malignant ones. A large destructive lesion of a long bne with a huge associated soft tissue mass in a young patient must be a primary malignancy and can often be so established by a "puncture biopsy," where a small (2-3 mm) core of tissue is easily obtained from the mass by any of several small needles (e.g., Tru-cut). An experienced pathologist, who is accustomed to preparing and examining these limited tissue specimens, and who has been given the courtesy of full pre-biopsy presentation and discussion of the case, is required for successful use of this technique for histologic examination of the tumor. Conversely, a small reactive lesion within the bone and confined by a thickened cortex is inaccessible to such flexible needle devices. This lesion, which would require drilling of the cortex with a Craig needle or other trochar device or even creating a cortical window and accepting the risk of fracture, probably is benign and does not need biopsy, unless excision is necessary for treatment (e.g., osteoid osteoma). Our experience suggests (fortunately) that the malignant lesions are easiest to biopsy because of their size and the extraosseous extent of soft, tumor tissue. We are investigating the use of fine-needle apspiration and cytologic examination of material from bone tumors, and we are especially interested in this technique in lesions of the axial skeleton and other relatively inaccessible locations. Obviously, many cases still come to open incisional biopsy.

Finally the question of who should do the biopsy must be addressed. The surgeon who will be responsible for the patient's care regardless of diagnosis or of outcome is certainly the most appropriate one to do the biopsy. This is most important in primary malignancies arising from the skeleton, especially considering modern-day treatment options. Treatment of a skeletal neoplasm requires an accurate diagnosis, and in most cases a definitive diagnosis requires histologic confirmation.

STAGING

The information generated by carefully following the patient evaluation scheme that has been described is enormous and important, but does not, of itself, indicate the stage of the tumor. The combination of a history and physical examination, appropriate imaging studies, and the biopsy generates the information usually needed to determine the diagnosis, the histopathologic grade, and the local extent of the lesion, and to determine whether any evidence of systemic involvement (metastases) exists. However, it is the orderly grouping of these separate factors that determines a surgical staging system. The clinician must realize that a surgical staging system is neither a tumor classification system nor a histopathologic grading system. Rather it is a process for understanding the nature and extent of a patient's neoplastic process. In this manner, patients can be grouped according to the stage of their lesion and information concerning types of treatment and outcomes can be compared. Additionally, decisions as to appropriate surgical procedures and other treatments can be based on the stage of the lesion.

Phemister is usually given credit for developing a classification of bone tumors based on the type of neoplastic tissue produced. Both benign and malignant categories exist for each of the tissue types of lesions arising from bone. This has been refined by the World Health Organization under the direction of Schajowicz and others. This classification represents an important contribution to our understanding but is not a surgical staging system.

Broders et al.[1] in 1939 published a pathologic grading system devised from the study of carcinomas and used it to evaluate the features of 152 soft tissue fibrosarcomas. Broders Grades 1 and 2 are lesions that are well-differentiated (or moderately so) and have few mitotic figures and little cytologic atypia. The higher grade lesions (Broders 3 and 4) are proportionately less differentiated and more cellular. These lesions have frequent mitotic figures and usually areas of necrosis. This work has persisted as a pathologic grading system. While obviously the surgical stage is tied to the pathologic grade, they are different in that the pathologic grade does not address anatomic consideration or, in fact, the real natural history of each diagnostic category.

The American Joint Committee for Cancer Staging and End Results Reporting[5] developed a staging system that has been used extensively for carcinomas. The system considers the pathologic grade (Broders 1 to 4) and the TNM system, where T is the size of the primary tumor, N determines the presence of local lymph node involvement, and M represents distant metastases. This system has not been useful in the evaluation of patients with bone sarcomas, however, because of the size of the lesion is not necessarily important and because the bone sarcomas rarely metastasize to or via regional lymph nodes. Hematogenous spread to lungs and other bones are much more common.

Surgical Staging System

Finally, the Musculoskeletal Tumor Society has adopted a system for the surgical staging of musculoskeletal sarcomas. This system was developed by Enneking and coworkers[3] over the past decade to apply to those lesions arising from mesenchymal connective tissues and to address the problems mentioned above with other systems. Marrow and reticuloendothelial lesions (i.e., round cell origin) are not formally included; but practically speaking, most such lesions are now "staged" in a similar fashion. The staging system is designed to help define the probability of success for surgical procedures that achieve defined surgical margins during the local treatment of sarcomas. It applies to lesions arising in soft tissues and in bone and has now been expanded to include both benign and malignant connective tissue tumors.[2] The staging system combines three factors: grade (G), site (T), and metastases (M) (Tables 1 and 2).

1. Surgical Grade. The surgical grade (G) is a description of the biologic behavior of a lesion that is gleaned from the histology, the natural history, and the radiographic appearance of the tumor.[2] All benign lesions are consisered G_0 (e.g., simple bone cyst); low-grade malignancies, G_1 (e.g., chondrosarcoma arising in old enchondroma); and high-grade malignancies, G_2 (e.g., conventional osteosarcoma).

2. Site. The site (T) is a statement generated by the preoperative imaging studies of the local exent of the tumor. If the lesion is benign, confined to a compartment, and surrounded nicely by a reactive rim, it is a T_0. Low-grade malignant (and aggressive benign) lesions confined to the anatomic compartment (bone or fascial-lined soft tissue space) in which they arose are T_1. High-grade malignancies that escaped their compartment of origin or those lesions arising from anatomic locations without fascial borders are considered T_2 in nature. Lesions may go through cortical bone and across fascial planes due to their aggressive nature or as a result of surgery.

3. Metastases. Metastases (M) simply indicate whether there is any evidence of metastatic involvement. M_0 indicates no evidence and M_1 means either regional lymph node or distant systemic metastases.

All benign tumors are surgical grade G_0 and their stage is designated by Arabic numbers 1, 2 and 3 corresponding to lesions that are latent,

TABLE 1. STAGES OF BENIGN MUSCULOSKELETAL LESIONS*

	1	2	3
Grade	G_0	G_0	G_0
Site	T_0	T_0	T_{1-2}
Metastases	M_0	M_0	M_{0-1}
Clinical course	Latent, static, self-healing	Active progressing expands bone or fascia	Aggressive, invasive, breaches bone or fascia
Isotope scan	Background uptake	Increased uptake in lesion	Increased uptake beyond lesion
CT	Crisp, intact margin, well defined capsule homogeneous	Intact margin "expansile" thin capsule homogenous	Indistinct broached margin extracapsular and/or extra-compartmental extension

* Modified from Enneking WF: Staging of muculoskeletal neoplasms. Skeletal Radiol 13:187, 1985.

active, and aggressive. Examples would be a Stage 1 small non-ossifying fibroma, a Stage 2 large active simple bone cyst, and a Stage 3 destructive giant cell tumor of bone.

The malignancies are divided also into three stages and given Roman numerals I, II, and III. All low-grade (by history and histology) malignancies are Stage I; all high-grade malignancies are Stage II; and any malignancy with evidence of metastatic disease is Stage III. Stages I and II are further divided into A and B subgroups, depending on their anatomic site and whether they extend beyond the comparmtent of origin. (See site (T) in the description above.) Most Stage I lesions will be intracompartmental (A) lesions, whereas most Stage II lesions will have extended beyond the compartment of origin and will be (B) lesions, i.e., T_2. In this manner, a low-grade chondrosarcoma arising secondarily in relationship to an old enchondroma and remaining confined by the host bone cortex is a Stage I-A. Conversely, a conventional high-grade osteosarcoma with a large soft tissue mass is a Stage II-B. Evidence of metastatic disease in either of these cases converts them to Stage III. Enneking has recently provided an excellent discussion of the development and value of the staging system.[2]

Surgical Margins. This staging system has defined surgical margins in reference to the oncologic relationship of the tumor to the surroudning tissues. Intralesional, marginal, wide and radical margins are defined. Intralesional surgery is done when the tumor is entered, as in a biopsy.

TABLE 2. STAGES OF MALIGNANT MUSCULOSKELETAL LESIONS*

	I_A	I_B	II_A	II_B	IIIA	IIIB
Grade	G_1	G_1	G_2	G_2	G1-2	G1-2
Site	T_1	T_2	T_1	T_2	T1	T2
Metastases	M_0	M_0	M_0	M_0	M1	M1
Clinical course	Symptomatic indolent growth	Symptomatic indolent growth	Symptomatic rapid growth	Symptomatic rapid growth fixed mass pathologic fracture	Systemic symptoms palpable nodes pul. symptoms	
Isotope scan	Increased uptake	Increased uptake	Increased uptake beyond radiographic limits	Increased uptake beyond radiographic limits	Pulmonary lesions no increased uptake	
CT	Irregular or broached capsule but intracompartmental	Extracompartmental extension or location	Broached (pseudo) capsule-intracompartmental	Broached (pseudo) capsule-extracompartmental	Pulmonary lesions or enlarged nodes	

* Modified from W. F. Enneking, Skeletal Radiology (1985) 13:188

Marginal surgery is the "shelling out" procedure through reactive tissue, and certainly includes the risk of local persistence of tumor tissue. A wide surgical margin is obtained when one layer of uninvolved tissue exists between the tumor and the plane of dissection. With unusual exceptions (skip metastases), this procedure accomplished local control. Finally, a radical margin is obtained by removal of the entire compartment or compartments involved by the tumor. This procedure should guarantee local control and no recurrence of the neoplastic process, even for the most high-grade lesion. It is occasionally difficult for the clinician to accept that each of these surgical margins can be obtained by either resections or by amputations. However, it is important to recognize that the margin (not the procedure) dictates the oncologic success of the operation. Obviously, if an amputation is chosen, at least a wide surgical margin is desirable.

SURGICAL MANAGEMENT

Osteosarcoma of the distal femoral metaphysis can be considered a prototype of modern surgical management. Most of these lesions will have an associated soft tissue mass at time of presentation, but will be free of evidence of metastatic disease and therefore be Stage II-B, i.e. high-grade, extra-compartment, localized disease. The goal of the surgical procedure is to produce a wide surgical margin. As discussed, a wide surgical margin exists when a cuff of uninvolved normal tissue (usually bone or muscle) exists between the tumor and the surgeon's plane of dissection at the time of amputation or resection. Many distal femoral osteosarcomas with limited soft tissue extensions can be managed surgically without resorting to amputation. In these cases a wide surgical margin can be obtained by leaving a cuff of muscle (quadriceps) about the tumor at the time of local resection. Most surgeons desire at least 5 cm. of normal marrow and femoral cortex above the lesion and the knee joint is likewise usually included in the resection. Reconstruction is accomplished according to the surgeon's preference. We have most commonly chosen an allograft bone transplant to bridge the defect and to produce an arthrodesis at the knee. Other options include a variety of bone and prosthetic devices with or without an attempt to preserve the joint. Adjuvant chemotherapy is now considered routine.

We[9] have been interested in the prospects for immunomodulation of human osteosarcomas. Monoclonal antibodies generated against our human osteosarcoma cell lines have proven to be selective, stable, and sensitive to both fresh osteosarcoma tissue and cultured cell lines. The monoclonal antibody that we named TMMR-2 has been found to exert a biologic suppression of our human osteosarcoma cell lines as measured by incorporation of ^{3}H-thymidine. This observation suggests possible clinical application and is being studied in an ongoing manner.

REFERENCES

1. Broders AC, Hargrave R, Myerding HW: Pathological features of soft tissue fibrosarcoma with special reference to the grading of its malignancy. Surgery, Gynecology & Obstetrics 69:267-280, 1939.

2. Enneking WF: Staging of musculoskeletal neoplasms. Skeletal Radiology 13:183-194, 1985.

3. Enneking WF, Spanier SS, Goodman MA: A system for the surgical management of musculoskeletal sarcoma. Clinical Orthopaedics and Related Research 153:106-120, 1980.

4. Mankin HJ, Lange TA, Spanier SS: The hazards of biopsy in patients with malignant primary bone and soft-tissue tumors. Journal of Bone and Joint Surgery 64-A:1121-1127, 1982.

5. Manual for Staging of Cancer 1977. American Joint Committee on Cancer Staging and End Results Reporting, Chicago, 1977.

6. Schajowicz F: Tumors and tumorlike lesions of bone and joints, pp. 1-24. New York, Springer-Verlag, 1981.

7. Silverberg BS, Lubera BBA: Cancer Statistics, 1987. Ca - A Cancer Journal for Clinicians 37:2-19, 1987.

8. Sundaram M, McGuire MH, et al: Magnetic resonance imaging in planning limb-salvage surgery for primary malignant tumors of bone. Journal of Bone and Joint Surgery 68-A:809-819, 1986.

9. Tsai CC, McGuire MH, Roodman ST: Production and characterization of monoclonal antibodies to human osteosarcoma: Flow cytometric and immunocytochemical studies. Lab Invest, 56(80A):477, 1987.

Discussion:

DR. RAISZ (Connecticut): The last slide reminded me of a concern that we all have in the, thank God, rare case of Paget's with osteogenic sarcoma. What is the status of that? Should we be trying to do more, either surgically or with chemotherapy or radiation in these patients?

DR. McGUIRE (Worcester, MA): Well, fortunately, as you know, it's a very rare complication. I guess I don't know how many people in this country have Paget's disease. I get a few sent my way. But it must be that, you know, less than one percent of the people develop Paget's.

Now, I thought I was sort of safe from that until two months ago. I know that in ten years there had been no Paget's sarcomas in St. Louis. Now, there have been two in the last month. So, maybe it caught up with us. But I guess I was happy to see, in one of the talks last night, a sort of listing of the things that cause pain in Paget's and the author didn't bother to put sarcoma down. And I think that's appropriate. I mean, there just aren't very many Paget's sarcomas.

They inevitably are recognized. The five-year survival remains zero, partly because of the age group. We treat them by surgical resection and appropriate reconstruction of their disease. But they are not candidates for the aggressive chemotherapy programs because of their age. And I showed you a perfectly healthy 14-year-old kid with cardiomyopathy.

So, for this group, if everyone is aware of that, that's enough. Hopefully you won't find it.

DR. RAISZ: You are staging them and operating on them?

DR. McGUIRE: Sure.

DR. POTTS (Boston): That was a very impressive review for some very tough management cases.

DR. McGUIRE: Thank you.

DR. POTTS: I just wanted to ask a question about the monoclonal antibody to be sure I understood it. Obviously, you're excited about that as an adjunct for therapy. You said that it stopped DNA synthesis. Was it not cytotoxic to the tumor cells or not cytotoxic to normal cells?

DR. McGUIRE: To the tumor cells.

DR. POTTS: So, it's only static on the tumor cells.

DR. McGUIRE: Exactly. Because it doesn't recognize the normal cells. So, at this point, it seems specific for the osteosarcoma cell. Now, we are working on the antigen. It seems to have a molecular weight of around 100,000 to, perhaps, 114,000 daltons. But we're not too far on that, yet.

DR. POTTS: Are you combining it with any cellular toxins?

DR. McGUIRE: Yes. The difference here is that this one, by whatever mechanism happened to end up in our hands, is more specific than those few reports in the literature. And I don't think anyone has shown me, at least, a graph of starting off DNA synthesis. We may never get past that, but that's where we are right now.

IV
Clinical Case Presentations

Overview:
Clinical Case Presentations

LOUIS V. AVIOLI[1] and HENRY G. BONE III[2]

[1]The Jewish Hospital of St. Louis
St. Louis, MO
[2]Henry Ford Hospital
Detroit, MI

This was an interesting session, presenting a spectrum of clinical disorders of bone and mineral metabolism, which provided for ample discussion and was most instructive to those in attendance.

The first presentation, "Familial Expansile Osteolysis," by Drs. Wallace, Osterberg, and Mollan from Musgrave Park Hospital, Belfast, Northern Ireland, focused on an autosomal dominant disorder of bone which produced progressive dysplasia and hearing loss. Great pain is suffered by the affected patients in the limbs which are afflicted with the disease. These patients have expansile focal lesions in the peripheral skeleton, which typically begin in the third decade, resulting in deformities which resemble those of Paget's disease, but are much more severe and progressive in many cases. Deafness due to unique middle ear changes is manifested early in life, as is a loss of dentition due to a characteristic pattern of resorption of the teeth. Second generation bisphosphonate treatment has produced only transient benefit, and in most cases, amputation is required to relieve the pain when it is severe.

The paper on "Endemic Multiple Epiphyseal Dysplasia-Epidemiological, Radiological and Genealogical Study," by Drs. Teotia and Teotia of the LLRM Medical College, Meerut, India, described extensive studies in several hundred patients who were clinically affected. Most patients had either a subnormal or a short stature and presented with limping, pain and stiffness in the hips and knees, hip flexion, genu valgum, genu varum, and rotational deformities of the legs. There was considerable heterogeneity in the clinical and radiological presentation, but various patterns of the multiple epiphyseal dysplasia have been characterized by the authors. Epidemiologic data suggest an autosomal dominant form of inheritance in most cases of this disease, which is called "Handigodu syndrome" by the authors, after the name of the village where the disease was first described.

"Paget's Bone Disease and Heredity: Case Report," authored by Drs. Agnusdei, Civitelli, Camporeale, and Gennari of the University of Siena, Italy, and the Jewish Hospital of St. Louis, Missouri, concerned a young woman referred for evaluation of an elevated serum alkaline phosphatase level and a family history of Paget's disease of bone in the patient's father and paternal grandmother which suggested an autosomal dominant inheritance pattern. An extensive evaluation revealed generalized osteopenia, coupled with a high bone turnover rate, but without focal lesions. The authors suggest that this case may indicate the presence of a "Pagetic trait" of Paget's disease of bone which was already established in the older family members.

"Clinical and Radiological Improvement During High Dose Oral Calcium Treatment in 4 Patients with Hereditary Resistance to 1,25 Dihydroxycholecalciferol," authored by Drs. Woodhouse, Sakati and Marx of the King Faisal Specialist Hospital in Riyadh, Saudi Arabia, and the National Institutes of Health in Bethesda, Maryland, focused on four male children of related parents who presented with severe rickets and alopecia. They were hypocalcemic, but had elevated circulating 1,25-dihydroxycholecalciferol levels. Only one of the four responded with a calcemic effect to ergocalciferol treatment at doses of 80,000 to 6 million units per day. High doses of oral calcium were then prescribed for periods of 1/2 to five years. This produced a striking improvement. The patients' height and weight increased and they had significant radiological improvement as well. They remained mildly hypocalcemic. The authors concluded that high dose oral calcium therapy was of potential benefit in patients who are unresponsive to calciferols.

In "Rickets Due to Calcium Deficiency," by Drs. Proesmans, Legius, Eggermont and Bouillon of Leuven, Belgium, three young children were described with rickets in whom the 1,25-dihydroxy Vitamin D levels were elevated and the 25-hydroxy Vitamin D levels were normal. These patients also had generalized hyperaminoaciduria and two had low tibial phosphate reabsorption. Urinary calcium was low to very low in all patients. These patients were found to have been fed with a commercial soya drink which was not adapted for infant feeding, but was their principal source of calories for at least six months. This drink has a very low calcium content in comparison to either milk or to commercial infant feeding formulas. The authors interpretation of the pathophysiology is that the insufficient calcium intake caused secondary hyperparathyroidism and hypophosphatemia. The stimulated 1,25-dihydroxy Vitamin D production coupled with the low intestinal calcium intake, resulted in the bone lesions.

In a paper entitled, "Ectopic Calcification in a Patient with Hypophosphatemic Rickets," Drs. Suh and Jones of the University of Hawaii, Honolulu, a young girl with hypophosphatemic rickets was presented. She was born with calcification of the aorta and the subclavian arteries which resolved by four months of age. She also had a calcification in the right hand, which was surgically removed during her infancy. She had impaired hearing due to fixation of the ossicles by abnormal calcification. She had calcification affecting the ear lobes which was shown on biopsy to be heterotopic ossification. Treatment with calcitriol and phosphate was instituted for the next 11 months. She then began to have pain in the right ankle and shoulders where x-ray revealed soft tissue calcification. Laboratory studies demonstrated improvement of the rickets, but also demonstrated hypercalciuria and a decreased creatinine clearance. The calcitriol and phosphate were discontinued with resolution of the soft tissue calcifications, but reactivation of the rickets. The clinical status of the patient remains precariously balanced between treatment of the rickets, which produces the abnormal calcification, and the withdrawal of Vitamin D and phosphate, which permits resolution of the calcification, but reactivation of the metabolic bone disease.

Dr. Yoshimoto and his colleagues, Drs. Ohno, Fukase, Chiba, Tsunenari, Ogawa, Tsutsumi, Nakata, Kishi, Fujita, Ushida and Katsura, from Kobe University in Japan, described "Hypercalcemia and Generalized Osteopenia with a Myelodysplastic Syndrome." The patient was a 65 year old man who presented with weakness, pain, lower extremity edema, nausea, fatigue and thirst. He was found to have severe hypercalcemia (18.5 mg/dl) in the presence of mild renal dysfunction and a normal serum phosphate level. The serum magnesium level was slightly decreased and the alkaline phosphatase was quite elevated. Leukocytosis of 11000 cells/mm^3 was noted. The patient was treated with saline infusions and prednisolone and calcitonin. He had an improvement of his hypercalcemia and renal function over the next two weeks. He was noted to have generalized loss of bone mass in a number of areas which were examined. Bone biopsy showed a fibrous change with hypervascularity and increased bone formation and resorption without tumorous invasion. Additional studies found no evidence for Paget's disease, primary hyperparathyroidism, or other non-hematologic disorders. Bone marrow aspiration revealed abnormal myeloblasts, megakaryocytes and megaloblasts and there was increased activity of natural killer cells among peripheral lymphocytes. The authors suggest that humoral factors generated by stem cells may be the cause of this syndrome.

In the paper entitled, "Abnormal Bone Density Following Treatment for Childhood Acute Lymphoblastic Leukemia (ALL)", Drs. Gilsanz, Ortega, Gibbens, Carlson and Boechat of the Childrens Hospital of Los Angeles and the University of California at Los Angeles described a series of 25 survivors of treatment for ALL. As a group, these patients whose bone density was measured by quantitative computed tomography had lower trabecular, integral and cortical vertebral bone densities than control children who underwent CT examination because of trauma. Although all patients had been treated with methotrexate and prednisone, the low bone density was only noted in children who had also received prophylactic central nervous system radiation. Five of the nine children who received 2400 rads to the central nervous system had vertebral densities more than two standard deviations below the normal range.

In the paper entitled, "Parenteral Fluoride Therapy in a Patient with Chronic Malabsorption Markedly Increases Spinal Bone Density," Drs. Tudtud-Hans, Ament, Baylink, and Pettis of Loma Linda California, described a 60 year old woman with osteopenia associated with malabsorption and chronic steroid therapy who was treated with intravenous fluoride. This was undertaken because individuals with gastrointestinal disease may not tolerate oral fluoride therapy well. This patient had received total parenteral nutrition via Broviac catheter and sodium fluoride 5 mg IV per day was added to the TPN solution. She also received calcium supplements and monthly injections of estradiol. Serum fluoride levels were adjusted until they were stable at about 15.7 mM. After one year, the patient was found to have a 100% increase in trabecular vertebral density by quantitated computed tomography. Subsequently, the fluoride dose was decreased to 8 mg IV every other month. This study suggested that intravenous fluoride therapy could be quite useful in patients on total parenteral nutrition.

In the final presentation, Drs. Weinstein, Weinstein and Bell, of the Medical College of Georgia and Medical University of South Carolina, presented evidence for diminished rates of mineralization and bone formation in normal black individuals. In this histomorphometic study, double tetracycline labelled trans-ilial bone biopsies were carried out in six black and nine white subjects. The mean cortical bone width and porosity, cancellous bone area, trabecular width and spacing, wall width, osteoid area, osteoid perimeter, osteoid seam width, and osteoblastic, osteoclastic, and reversal perimeters were not significantly different between the two groups. However, the mineralizing perimeter, mineral appositional rate, and bone formation rate were all significantly lower in the blacks as compared to the white subjects. In addition, there was a negative correlation between mean wall width and mineral appositional and bone formation rates in the black, but not in the white subjects. It was suggested that a reduction in the rate of skeletal remodeling may contribute to the greater bone mass and lower incidence of fractures in black adults.

V
Spinal Osteoporosis

Overview:
Spinal Osteoporosis

CHARLES H. CHESNUT III

Osteoporosis Research Center
University of Washington School of Medicine
Seattle, WA

Osteoporosis remains the most common of the metabolic bone diseases. Nevertheless, it is only in the past two decades that the academic community, the practicing physician, the patient, and the media have recognized the morbidity and economic health care costs of this disease, particularly to the aging population. An example of the evolution of osteoporosis' recognition in the academic sphere is the relative time and space allotment for previous Henry Ford Hospital International Symposia. In the first (1972) International Symposium, Clinical Aspects of Metabolic Bone Disease, a three-hour afternoon session with eight presented papers was devoted to osteoporosis; the subsequent publications occupied 62 pages of the 694-page volume of the Proceedings. At the second (1983) International Symposium, Clinical Disorders of Bone and Mineral Metabolism, osteoporosis occupied four hours of the program, with 11 presented papers encompassing 59 pages of the 552-page Proceedings. For the current 1988 International Symposium, an entire day was directed towards information on osteoporosis, with a morning session devoted to spinal osteoporosis, and an afternoon session to metabolic bone disease of the hip. A total of 17 presented papers comprised the osteoporosis presentations; undoubtedly a major portion of the Proceedings will be devoted to this disease. In 1988, it would appear that appropriate recognition of osteoporosis and its complications has occurred.

Dr. Peck provided a timely introduction to the morning Session on spinal osteoporosis; timely in that this Session corresponded to the beginnings of National Osteoporosis Week. He gave an informative overview of progress in the field during the 1980's, noting particular advances in understanding the regulation of bone-remodeling, in developing techniques for quantitating bone mass (particularly the new x-ray based procedures), and in devising preventative therapeutic programs. He noted that prevention is currently the most important therapeutic strategy in osteoporosis; estrogen therapy remains the major prophylactic modality, but cannot and should not be utilized by all women. Alternative anti-resorptive strategies are available, such as calcitonin and possibly the diphosphonates; in addition, on the horizon are numerous other anti-resorptive and even bone-restorative approaches. The

1980's have been a most productive time for osteoporosis research, but quite obviously much remains to be accomplished.

Dr. Melton, and his co-author Dr. Riggs, then offered an innovative epidemiological approach in support of their hypothesis of two heterogeneous osteoporosis syndromes: Type I, and Type II. Dr. Melton noted the similarity of the Type II osteoporosis to a Gompertzian disease model; i.e., a degenerative disease with: an exponentially increasing incidence rate with aging; an early-onset, insidious progression and later symptomatic threshold; a multifactorial etiology; a common occurrence in the population at large; and a lack of response to treatment. Type I osteoporosis, on the other hand, resembles a non-Gompertzian disease model: a lack of an exponential increase with age; an acute onset after the menopause; a less common occurrence in the population at large; a specific pathophysiology or pathogenesis: estrogen deficiency; and a greater potential response to treatment. While currently available data does not definitively prove the heterogeneity of osteoporosis, and the presence of Type I and Type II osteoporosis syndromes, such an obviously thoughtful and intellectually challenging approach to the epidemiological pathogenesis of osteoporosis was most stimulating, and led to an invigorating discussion.

Dr. Genant reviewed the current status of bone densitometry, noting the technical capabilities of the three non-invasive techniques for quantitating bone mass: single and dual photon absorpiometry, computerized tomography, and the new x-ray dual energy technique. He particularly noted the controversy regarding bone mass quantity as a primary determinant of fracture risk, noting that while the areas of controversy are under clinical and epidemiological investigation, critical management decisions must be made for the current female population at risk for, or already affected with, osteoporosis. In this regard, he noted, as Wasnich et al have indicated, that bone mass is a continous variable with fracture the primary outcome. Individuals with low bone density may not have yet fractured, but this does not mean that they are free of osteoporosis; the probability of fracture is increased, and fractures indeed display a probabilistic nature. Dr. Genant noted that most investigators would accept usage of bone mass quantitation in detecting low bone mass, and presumably an increased risk for fracture, in individuals with secondary osteoporosis (athletic amenorrhea, chronic steroid therapy, etc.), but that there would be a lack of consensus regarding their use in assessing the need for estrogen therapy, and in assessing the presence and severity of osteoporosis generally. In terms of screening for osteopenia (either "mass screening" or "selective screening"), a definitive recommendation could not be made; this remains an area of considerable medical, political and financial controversy. Even "selective screening" of individuals with a suggestive history of osteopenia, and the presence of multiple risk factors, is not universally accepted as a reasonable clinical tool, due to some evidence suggesting that historically-based risk factors, alone or in combination, have limited predictive value for fracture risk in the individual patient. Lastly, Dr. Genant noted appropriately that the progress in improving precision with rectilinear SPA scanning, x-ray based DPA, and automatic image analysis QCT, have enabled the clinician to monitor efficacy of treatment intervention with a higher degree of certainty than was possible in the past.

The presentations and discussions then shifted to a consideration of female populations not usually thought of in the context of osteoporosis (i.e., the teenager, the young adult, and the pre- and perimenopausal female), and the determinants of bone mass within these premenopausal populations. Dr. Matkovic led off with a reiteration of the hypothesis noting peak bone mass at skeleton maturity (age 10-20) to be a major determinant of postmenopausal bone mass; a low bone mass at skeleton maturity presumably contributes to low postmenopausal bone mass, and presumably increases the risk for subsequent fracture. In addition, data was presented from multiple sources noting that the demands for skeletal calcium are highest during the adolescent growth spurt period (the time of peak bone mass attainment), that calcium deficiency at this time can decrease the degree of positive calcium balance and presumably the amount of bone mass, and that calcium intake is deficient (below the RDA) in many American adolescent females. While such observations are validated by current data, it was noted in subsequent discussion that no definitive data currently exist demonstrating that increasing and/or repleting calcium intake in adolescent females increases bone mass over control groups not increasing or repleting calcium. Nevertheless, the concept of developing maximal peak bone mass in adolescence to protect against further osteoporosis appears most reasonable.

From a consideration of factors contributing to the development of adequate bone mass, the Symposium then turned to factors for preserving peak bone mass. Dr. Drinkwater agreed that failure to achieve one's maximal potential bone mass during the young adult years is a risk factor for subsequent osteoporotic fracture, but she also noted that a genetic component to maximal attainable bone mass precludes all women being equally successful in reaching bone mass levels presumed to be protective. She did, however, point out that all women can make changes in their lifestyles to maximize their potential bone mass gain, and minimize their bone mass loss. In this regard, she noted that alcohol, coffee, and tobacco are three possible negative risk factors for preserving bone mass in the premenopausal years. More importantly, she described three variables known to have a positive effect on premenopausal bone mass, including the maintenance of a normal menstrual cycle, adequate calcium intake, and adequate physical activity. In terms of the menstrual cycle, she presented data demonstrating that normal levels of estrogen (as determined by normal menstrual cycles) are necessary for maintenance of bone mass during a woman's young adult years. The role of calcium in preserving bone mass remains controversial, as does the overall effects of increasing physical activity, although the current data do support physical activity increases being effective in increasing bone mass in women across a wide range of ages. However, her studies in amenorrheic athletes raises questions about the abilities of exercise to preserve bone if estrogen levels are inadequate. Quite obviously, normal menses, adequate calcium intake, and adequate exercise are important in preserving bone mass; it also appears that the lack of any single factor cannot be completely compensated for by increasing the other two factors. Preserving bone mass prior to the menopause is an area that will receive much attention in the future.

The Session then considered perimenopausal and immediately postmenopausal bone loss. Dr. Heaney noted four components of perimenopausal bone loss, including age-related bone loss, bone loss associated with estrogen deficiency, bone loss associated with calcium deficiency, and bone loss associated with other factors, such as alcoholism, etc. A hypothetical model incorporating the first three of these factors was presented by Dr. Heaney; he concluded from the model that, while estrogen deficiency is a major contributor to bone loss immediately after the menopause (in the "young elderly"), it is a less prominent contributor later on (10-20 years postmenopausal, the "old elderly"). In the later years, calcium intake may be a more important contributor to bone loss than estrogen deficiency. Indeed, when evaluated in the Heaney model (assuming a 20 mgm per day calcium loss) calcium deficiency accounts for 50% more bone loss than does estrogen deficiency over 20-30 years postmenopause.

Dr. Heaney also reiterated the current concerns regarding the absorbability of calcium from various calcium sources, noting that most food sources have readily absorbable calcium, but that a number of calcium supplements and pills may have difficulties with dissolution and resultant absorbability.

Dr. Heaney pointed out that despite the current controversies regarding the importance of calcium in the prevention of immediately postmenopausal bone loss, an intake of 1000 mgm of calcium per day for estrogen-replete perimenopausal women, and 1500 mgm per day for estrogen deprived postmenopausal women, is "safe and prudent". He also reiterated the fundamentally sound observation that, while not all postmenopausal bone loss is due to calcium deficiency, such a deficiency does contribute to some bone loss; since there is no way to distinguish individuals whose bone loss is due to calcium deficiency from those whose loss is due to other contributing factors, it is quite reasonable to ensure a calcium intake at the NIH recommendations noted above. Calcium deficiency, then, does appear to be a significant contributor to bone loss, with, however, its greatest effects later in the postmenopausal period.

Undoubtedly, estrogen deficiency is the main contributor to significant bone loss immediately (1-10 years) after the menopause, and this was again reinforced by Dr. Christiansen, who reviewed the data from his laboratory and other centers, designating estrogen deficiency as the most important variable in immediately postmenopausal bone loss. He then reinforced the now well-documented conclusions that estrogen and/or progesterone replacement therapy can prevent the progression of bone mass loss after the menopause, at all skeletal sites studied to date. However, defining the woman's individual risk for subsequent bone loss, as well as her need for estrogen replacement therapy, remains difficult; definitive identification of at-risk women by various blood and urine parameters, and bone mass quantitating techniques, has not yet been possible. Nevertheless, the current data presented by Dr. Christiansen certainly support estrogen replacement therapy as the primary therapeutic modality for the prophylaxis of osteoporosis.

Dr. Chesnut next considered alternatives to calcium and estrogen for optimizing bone mass in the perimenopause: calcitonin and the diphosphonates (bisphosphonates) are additional therapeutic agents for preventing bone loss, primarily by an inhibition of bone resorption. Synthetic salmon calcitonin possesses safety and has proven efficacy in osteoporotic individuals; in addition, one study by Stevenson et al has shown it to be equivalent to estrogen in prevention of bone loss in immediately postmenopausal women without osteoporosis. However, the drug is currently available in most countries as an injectable agent, which is unsuitable for prophylactic use; a nasal spray is available, and some, but not all, preliminary studies with this preparation appear promising. Expense for the calcitonin preparations currently available remains a problem. The bisphosphonates (such as etidronate) are certainly reasonable candidates for prophylactic usage in that they are relatively safe when given intermittently, are relatively inexpensive, and are orally administered; their therapeutic efficacy, however, remains unproven. Studies in osteoporotic females are inconclusive with these agents, and there are no studies currently available in the immediately postmenopausal women in whom the biphosphonates are utilized for prophylaxis. Nevertheless, these two potential prophylactic therapies, biphosphonates and calcitonin, have the attribute of safety; such safety is a significant asset when compared to estrogen. Estrogens can prevent bone loss over an extended period of time, but occasionally at a high cost in terms of side effects.

Treatment of the osteoporotic woman was addressed next; here, the presentations were confined to a discussion of vitamin D therapy (calcitonin and biphosphonates had been covered by Dr. Chesnut, and sodium fluoride and parathyroid hormone were covered in the other Sessions). Dr. Gallagher noted a therapeutic rationale for the vitamin D congeners: a correction of the calcium malabsorption present in many osteoporotic patients, a subsequent improvement of calcium balance, and, possibly, in high dosage, a stimulation of bone formation. He reviewed the currently somewhat disparate data regarding usage of $1\alpha(OH)D_3$ and $1,25(OH)_2D$ in the osteoporotic individual, concluding that the vitamin D metabolites may have a beneficial effect on bone mass, but unfortunately at dosage levels frequently associated with significant renal toxicity. The role of the D metabolites in the therapy of osteoporosis remains undefined.

The morning Session was then concluded with consideration of a somewhat different topic: corticosteroid-induced osteopenia. Dr. Raisz confronted this difficult problem, noting that this clinical entity is not "an unsolveable problem" as was intimated in his title, but, on the other hand, was certainly unsolved at present. He reviewed the current understandings regarding the mechanism of corticosteroid action on bone, and considered the therapeutic dilemma confronting the clinician in treating steroid-induced osteopenia, including the major problem of reversing the inhibitory effects of glucocorticoids on bone formation. The dilemma is compounded by the inability to accurately predict which steroid-treated patients will develop osteoporosis and fractures. As Dr. Raisz noted however, progress is being made in the laboratory in learning more about the pathogenesis of corticosteroid-induced osteopenia, including regulation of bone cells, and about new classes of factors stimulating bone growth; nevertheless, at the present time, it is unfortunately necessary to consider alternatives to corticosteroids when possible, or to utilize the lowest possible dosage of cortisone to both treat the underlying problem and to spare the skeleton.

The Session closed with a final discussion of the topics considered; the new and innovative data presented, particularly by Drs. Melton, Drinkwater and Heaney, received much attention. Again, the obvious increased interest developing in osteoporosis over the past two decades was much in evidence throughout the morning Spinal Osteoporosis Session.

Osteoporosis: 1988 and Beyond

WILLIAM A. PECK

Department of Medicine
Washington University School of Medicine
and The Jewish Hospital of St. Louis
St. Louis, MO

I am grateful to the organizing committee for affording me this time to editorialize about our decade of progress in osteoporosis and our needs for the future. It is of course a particular honor to do this on the third day of the presidentially ordained National Osteoporosis Prevention Week.

Let us examine six of the most important tasks that have been undertaken: (a) understanding the nature and regulation of bone growth and remodeling; (b) understanding the micro- and macromolecular structure of bone; (c) understanding the biomechanics of bone as an organ; (d) developing acceptable methods for measuring bone mass, strength, and turnover; (e) understanding the causes of and risk factors for osteoporosis, falling and fracture; and (f) developing acceptable methods for preventing and treating osteoporosis and fractures. I will emphasize three of these: the nature and regulation of bone growth remodeling; the development of methods for measuring bone mass, and the development of strategies for preventing osteoporosis.

There has been great progress in delineating the local cellular and humoral events involved in the regulation of bone remodeling. Activation involves site preparation and transduction: osteoclasts arise from an early branch point in marrow mononuclear cell lineage; local humors modifying marrow cell development also influence the emergence of osteoclasts; osteoclasts act by creating an extracellular lysosomal vacuole; candidate bone growth and coupling factors have been identified, including transforming growth factor ß (TGFß); and a plausible coupling mechanism has emerged. It appears that remodeling involves a complex interplay of events among four related compartments--bone, surface cells, nearby marrow cells, and regional and systemic forces. The need for the future is to advance these lines of investigation. Of particular importance will be an enhanced understanding of the cell and molecular biology of locally elaborated and stored factors and their interactions with systemic factors.

Great strides have been made in developing methods for quantifying bone mass and density. Engineering breakthroughs have yielded equipment which can define bone mass in the axial skeleton with a high degree of accuracy, precision, safety and convenience. The recent emergence of dual energy radiography represents another important step forward; it (a) reduces the precision error of vertebral mass measurement to an almost unimaginably low level--thus permitting frequent monitoring of bone loss in an individual; (b) standardizes measurements so that inter-equipment variations are minimized and multicenter studies are facilitated; (c) lowers the potential cost per test dramatically (thus increasing accessibility) by shortening scan time significantly and by obviating the need for frequent source changes.

There are also advances in other arenas of bone densitometry--computed axial tomography has come of age in the bone field, and its use has yielded new information about preventive strategies and the nature of changes in trabecular microarchitecture with advancing age. Alterations in trabecular structure via preferential loss, effacement and microdiscontinuity play a crucial role in mechanical failure of trabecular bone.

With the capacity to measure bone mass effectively has come a powerful research tool. It is in fact the research mainstay of the clinical investigator. As technology becomes available to populations outside of the United States, we will have to rely less and less on fracture frequency data for vitally needed epidemiological information.

Prevention has justifiably emerged as the most important strategy in osteoporosis. Osteoporosis must be prevented, preventive strategies are available, and new ones are on the horizon. Therapy with fluoride, with the regimen known as Activate-Depress-Free-Repeat (ADFR), and with growth factors notwithstanding, there is yet no safe, effective therapy for osteoporosis which can be placed in the hands of the primary care physician. Among the preventive strategies that have been promulgated are: calcium nutrition, physical exercise, estrogens, and calcitonin.

Few believe that maintenance of a high-calcium intake will in itself prevent bone loss in postmenopausal women. The bulk of evidence accumulated over the past decade, however, indicates that long-term calcium nutrition is one determinant of peak bone mass and a high calcium intake can contribute to reductions in aging-associated bone loss. The issue is not "calcium or no calcium," but how much and what kind. The need for calcium to achieve that threshold above which bone stores are spared varies among individuals and in the same individual at different times. It is a great challenge to our scientific community to quantify these needs for calcium; in fact, it is a trust.

Mounting evidence points to physical exercise as a determinant of bone structure and mass--but, like calcium nutrition, it has been difficult to quantify. Except for the totally immobilized, everyone exercises, compounding the problem of study design. We don't know how it works--an important line of investigation--and we don't know much about dose response or interactions with other factors, such as calcium intake and hormonal status.

Although it has been known for nearly a half a century that estrogen therapy reduces postmenopausal bone loss, we now realize that estrogen works at a low dose and that its use decreases fracture risk. An important advance has been the discovery of estrogen receptor activity and message in bone cells, paving the way toward understanding the impact of estrogen on bone remodeling. Safety concerns and inconvenience continue to limit estrogen acceptance, and less than 10% of eligible subjects receive it. Used properly by compliant patients at risk for osteoporosis under the care of knowledgeable physicians, low-dose estrogen therapy is safe and cost-effective.

Estrogen therapy will not and should not be accepted by all women, and does not help men at risk for osteoporosis nor the large number of patients with secondary disease. Alternative antiresorptive strategies are available and more are on the horizon. Short-term studies have disclosed calcitonin to reduce bone loss, not only in subjects with established osteoporosis but also in non-osteoporotic postmenopausal women. Long-term studies, fracture frequency data, and enterally active and lower-cost preparations are needed. Still, the emergence of calcitonin in the marketplace is the culmination of major basic and clinical science thrusts in recent years.

On the horizon are antiresorptive and bone restorative approaches that were only imagined ten years ago. Cyclic therapy, third generation diphosphonates, parathyroid hormone analogues and growth factors typify strategies that have progressed beyond the concept stage. To eliminate osteoporosis, our research must be vigorous. At the same time we must keep the public informed of our progress and problems--they pay the bills for science and for health. This is the essence of National Osteoporosis Prevention Week.

Discussion:

DR. CHESNUT (Seattle): Obviously, you, the National Osteoporosis Foundation, and other institutions have put forth education about osteoporosis over the past five years. Are we seeing increasing awareness of this particular disease at the practitioner level?

DR. PECK (St. Louis): It's difficult to teach old dogs new tricks. I think that there is increased physician awareness about osteoporosis as a problem. But I'm not sure that there is increased impact of that awareness in terms of patient management. Certainly, estrogen therapy use has not increased markedly over the past several years, although it has risen somewhat.

I think part of the problem is that we need safer, more effective preventive and therapeutic strategies to put in the hands of individuals such as the practicing physician. Also, I point out that one of the strategies to prevent fracture is to prevent falling. And I think there is increased physician awareness of the necessity to induce strategies to reduce falling and home accidents, particularly. In my travels, I see them more interested in this. We have much to do.

Further Characterization of the Heterogeneity of the Osteoporotic Syndromes

L. JOSEPH MELTON III[1] and B. LAWRENCE RIGGS[2]

[1]Section of Clinical Epidemiology
Department of Health Sciences Research
[2]Division of Endocrinology and Internal Medicine
Mayo Clinic
Rochester, MN

Intuitive recognition of heterogeneity in osteoporosis is reflected in the original names, "postmenopausal" and "senile". Characterization of these two syndromes has been refined on the basis of clinical, laboratory and epidemiological evidence, and they have been relabelled with the less prejudicial terms, Type I and Type II osteoporosis (1). Type I (postmenopausal) osteoporosis, which occurs in a relatively small proprotion of postmenopausal women and even less commonly in men, is characterized by accelerated and disproportionate loss of trabecular bone, resulting in vertebral and distal forearm (Colles') fractures. The vertebral fractures usually occur within the first 15-20 years after menopause, commonly present with back pain and may be of the crush type associated with major deformity of the vertebra. Type II (senile) osteoporosis, on the other hand, occurs commonly in elderly women and men and is manifested by hip and vertebral wedge fractures. It is characterized by proportionate loss of both cortical and trabecular bone at a rate similar to that in the general population. Vertebral fractures in the latter syndrome are often painless but may lead to progressive loss of height and dorsal kyphosis.

Because of disagreement regarding details of pathophysiology, some question the existence of more than one syndrome of osteoporosis, although variation in the patterns of bone loss with aging must still be explained. More importantly perhaps, it is necessary to account for dramatic differences in the epidemiology of specific osteoporosis-related fractures. This report reviews evidence for heterogeneity in osteoporosis and adapts a conceptual model, Gompertz' law (2), to account to the differences observed.

Heterogeneity in bone loss. Osteoporosis is the end result of a long period of slow age-related bone loss, combined with postmenopausal bone loss in women and with bone loss due to specific diseases and drugs in both sexes. All of these changes occur in the context of the peak adult bone mass that each person achieves. With so many factors involved, it is not surprising that bone mass varies widely in the population, even in subgroups of a given age and sex. It is less obvious why bone mass should vary substantially at different skeletal sites in the same person--site-specific correlation coefficients are usually less than 0.7 or so.

The imperfect concordance of bone mass measurements at various sites may be explained, in part, by differences in the patterns of bone loss with aging, although this remains controversial. Cross-sectional studies, for example, generally show little bone loss in the midradius prior to menopause but large losses afterwards. Studies of the lumbar spine are less consistent; many but not all investigators find evidence for substantial premenopausal bone loss with a trend toward midlife acceleration. These cross-sectional estimates are somewhat difficult to interpret due to the relatively small sample size in most studies and the consequent inability to choose reliably among competing statistical models of bone loss. However, extensive longitudinal data now show significant premenopausal bone loss in individual women that is greater in the lumbar spine than in the midradius (3). More importantly, there is a complete lack of correlation between rates of loss in these two areas (Figure 1), raising the possibility of a different natural history of bone loss from each skeletal site.

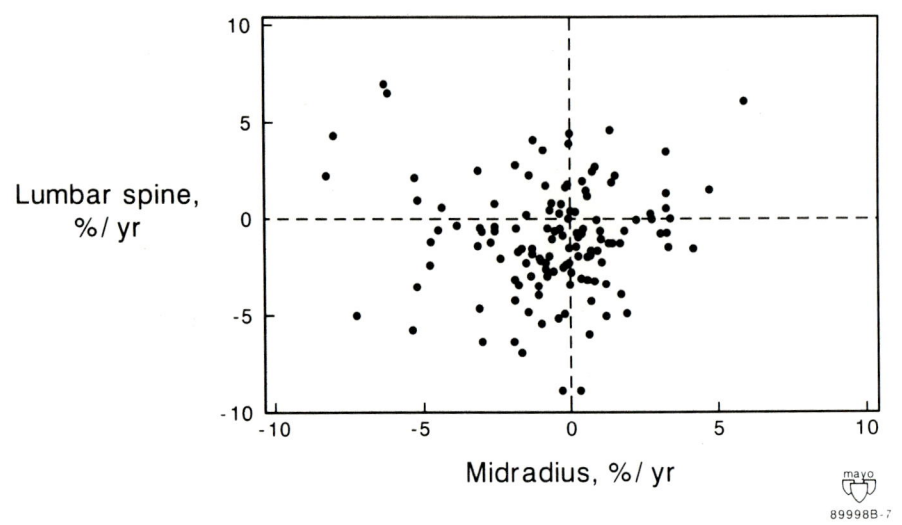

Figure 1. Relationship between longitudinal rates of change in BMD of midradius (99% cortical bone) and lumbar spine (<70% trabecular bone) in 139 normal women. There is no suggestion of a relationship (r = -0.04, NS) (3).

These observations regarding bone loss from the axial and appendicular skeletons have been attributed to differences in the behavior of trabecular and cortical bone. In the femoral neck, for example, age-related bone loss appears to be greater for trabecular than for cortical components, the latter more closely resembling bone loss in the femoral shaft (4). These effects may be due, in turn, to differences between trabecular and cortical bone in response to fast and slow forms of bone loss (Table 1).

Table 1. Comparison of two morphologic types of bone loss (5)

Characteristic	Osteoclast-mediated	Osteoblast-mediated
Cellular defect	Lack of restraint	Lack of number
Remodeling mechanism	Deeper resorption	Shallower formation
Structure		
trabecular	Perforation + disconnection	Simple thinning
cortical	Subendosteal cavitation	Simple thinning
Reduction in strength	More than predicted[a]	As predicted[a]
Timing	Early	Late
Rate	Rapid	Slow
Magnitude	Usually greater	Usually less
Activation	Often increased	Often decreased

[a]From reduction in mass or mineral content.

Because of its large surface area and relatively thin network of structures, trabecular bone is believed to be especially sensitive to rapid, osteoclast-mediated bone loss (5), which may underlie Type I osteoporosis. Trabecular plates may be perforated or lost completely so that the resulting loss of strength is disproportionately greater than the loss of mass, and vertebral fractures may result. Cortical bone, with its greater mass and relatively smaller surface area, may be affected as well but the biomechanical consequences are not as great except in the thin metaphyseal shell at the ends of long bones. Thus, increased endosteal trabeculation, or transiently increased cortical porosity in the perimenopausal period (6), could account for the association of Colles' fracture with Type I osteoporosis. The slower, osteoblast-mediated bone loss continues with aging (5) and may underlie Type II osteoporosis.

Heterogeneity in clinical manifestations. While the nature of these differences in bone loss remains to be fully resolved, empirical evidence for heterogeneity lies in the relatively low concordance of age-related fractures within individuals. As reviewed elsewhere (7), about twice as many patients with hip fracture have had a prior fracture of the proximal humerus or distal forearm and three to ten times as many (depending on age) have had a prior vertebral fracture than would be expected by chance alone. Likewise, patients with vertebral osteopenia (roentgenographic density grades 0 or 1) may have a higher risk of hip fracture than those with more normal (grades 2 or 3) vertebrae. Patients with a Colles' fracture seem to have about one and one-half times the usual risk for a subsequent hip fracture, but closer inspection reveals a major discrepancy. Among women under age 70 years at the time of Colles' fracture, the relative risk of a subsequent hip fracture is 1.0, no different from the risk in the general population (8). Only among the small number of women 70 years old and over at the time of Colles' fracture is there an increased risk of hip fracture. This observation suggests a closer relationship among fractures within Type I or Type II osteoporosis than across types.

Heterogeneity in fracture risk. Incidence rates for Colles' fracture, are very much higher around the time of menopause than are those for hip fracture (Figure 2). However, Colles' fracture rates level off around age 50 years in men and age 60 years in women. Hip fracture incidence rates, on the other hand, rise exponentially throughout life. The pattern for vertebral fractures is intermediate. As noted, Colles' fracture and postmenopausal crush fractures of the thoracic and lumbar vertebrae are hypothesized to be manifestations of Type I osteoporosis, while hip fractures and vertebral wedge fractures are associated with Type II osteoporosis (1). The overall incidence of vertebral fractures shown in Figure 2 may, thus, represent a composite of the two types. Direct evidence for this is provided by a random sample of 70-year-old Danish women, one-fifth of whom had vertebral fractures; 20% of them had collapse fractures, while 80% had vertebral wedging (9).

Numerous efforts have been made to explain these discrepancies (7). The plateau in Colles' fracture incidence, for example, has been attributed to an age-related decline in protective reflexes, with less tendency to break the impact of a fall with an outstretched arm. However, there is no direct evidence that this accounts for the pattern seen, nor would this appear to explain the postmenopausal increase and subsequent decline in ankle fracture incidence in women or the low Colles' fracture rates in men. There is little more evidence for the hypothesis that the exponential increase in hip fracture incidence (which is much greater than the increased frequency of falling with aging) is due to spontaneous fractures related to fatigue failure. Moreover, it seems unlikely that fatigue failure could account for the similar incidence trends of proximal humerus and pelvic fractures. Indeed, these are all post hoc explanations, which appear to have little generalizability. Little atten-

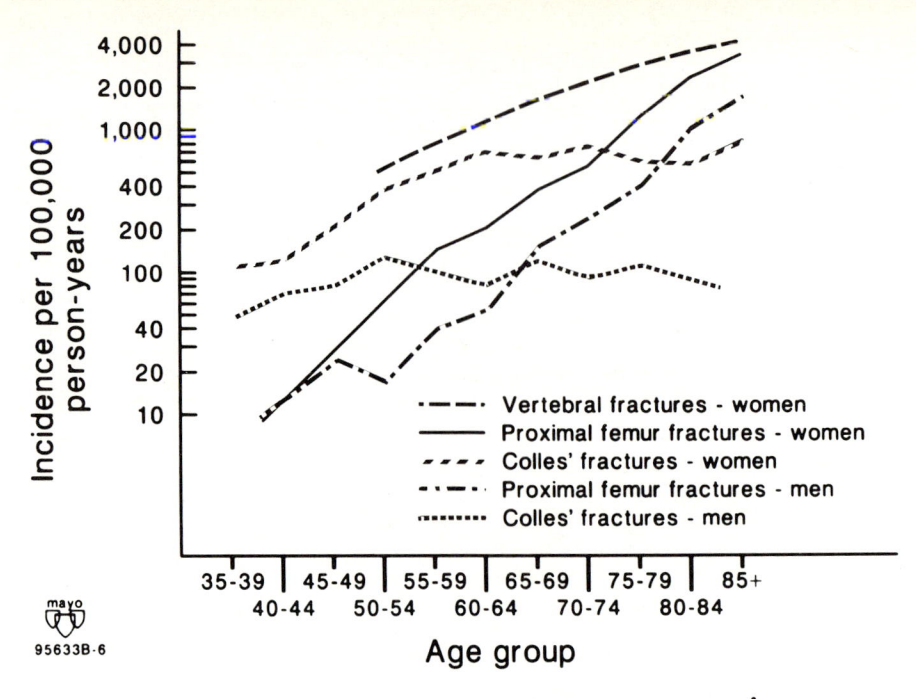

Figure 2. Age- and sex-specific incidence of Colles' fractures contrasted with that for vertebral and hip fractures among Rochester, Minnesota, residents (10).

tion has been given to the possibility that the epidemiologic patterns observed might reflect some more global phenomenon.

Gompertz' law. The exponential increase in hip fracture incidence in both sexes recalls similar exponentially increasing incidence rates with aging for other complex chronic diseases (Table 2). These conditions have been termed "Gompertzian" (after the British actuary, Benjamin Gompertz, who first described the exponential nature of mortality) and they have certain characteristics in common: 1) They are degenerative diseases with early onset and insidious progression until a symptomatic threshold is reached late in life; 2) The majority of the population is affected, although many never experience the final clinical event; 3) These diseases have no single cause but multiple risk factors which influence the rate of progression; and 4) The underlying pathophysiology is generally unamenable to therapy (2).

Table 2. Comparison of two types of chronic disease (2)

Gompertzian (exponential increase with age)	Non-Gompertzian (non-exponential with age)
Cancer of the lung, breast, colon, stomach, kidney	Hodgkin's disease
	Acute leukemia
	Wilms' tumor
Arteriosclerosis	Rheumatic heart disease
Atherosclerosis	Rheumatoid arthritis
Osteoarthritis	Systemic lupus
Alzheimer's disease	Multiple sclerosis
Stroke	Amyotrophic lateral sclerosis
Emphysema	Asthma
Cirrhosis	Hepatitis
Diverticulitis	Crohn's disease
	Ulcerative colitis

The other diseases listed in Table 2 follow a different pattern. Like Colles' fractures, incidence rates for these disorders do not increase exponentially with aging (non-Gompertzian). They, too, have some characteristics in common: 1) These are diseases with more acute onset and variable progression, often marked by remissions; 2) A minority of the population is affected; 3) A specific pathophysiology is more likely to be involved that may have a genetic, toxic or infectious basis; and 4) Because the condition is more likely to have an identifiable "cause", therapeutic efforts are generally more successful (2).

Based on these empirical observations, Type II osteoporosis (Gompertzian) and Type I osteoporosis (non-Gompertzian) are different diseases, even though they operate through the final common pathway of low bone mass and individual patients may be affected by both conditions. Hypotheses of pathophysiology are consistent with the Gompertzian model (Table 3).

Table 3. Comparison of two types of involutional osteoporosis (11)

	Type I	Type II
Age (yr)	51-75	>70
Sex ratio (F:M)	6:1	2:1
Type of bone loss	Mainly trabecular	Trabecular and cortical
Rate of bone loss	Accelerated	Not accelerated
Fracture sites	Vertebrae (crush) and distal radius	Vertebrae (multiple wedge) and hip
Parathyroid function	Decreased	Increased
Calcium absorption	Decreased	Decreased
Metabolism of 25-OH-D to $1,25(OH)_2D$	Secondary decrease	Primary decrease
Main causes	Factors related to menopause	Factors related to aging

Thus, Type I osteoporosis is generally considered to be more closely linked with a specific factor, estrogen deficiency, which somehow leads to increased bone turnover and accelerated bone loss. The slower age-related bone loss of Type II osteoporosis, on the other hand, is related to a complex set of age-related physiologic changes. It is currently thought that impaired renal conversion of vitamin D to its most active form, $1,25(OH)_2D$, may lead to decreased intestinal calcium absorption and secondary hyperparathyroidism (11). However, it is also possible, as noted previously, that impaired osteoblast function plays a role since remodeled bone is not completely replaced. The extent to which these processes represent primary defects or secondary effects of decreased muscle mass, reduced activity, dietary deficiencies, or other behavioral or physiologic correlates of aging has not been determined. In any event, the Gompertzian analogy suggests that the search for etiologic explanations in Type I and Type II osteoporosis might be broadened to consider explanations for features held in common with diverse other chronic diseases.

Clinical implications of heterogeneity. Despite the absence of agreed upon pathophysiologic explanations for heterogeneity in osteoporosis, the clinical implications are considerable: First, heterogeneity in bone metabolism may partially explain the low concordance of fractures at various skeletal sites, although biomechanical factors and differences in traumatic exposures undoubtedly play a role as well (10). The correlation between different fractures is much less than one would expect if all were simply manifestations of the same disorder. Indeed, the practical result is that most patients with one age-related fracture will not have any other specific fracture, even though the risk may be statistically significantly increased on average.

Second, if age-related fractures at various sites are not well correlated, then the rationale of evaluating bone mass at one site for determining bone mass at another may also be suspect. Bone mass measurements at one site do not predict bone mass at other sites in individual patients with sufficient accuracy to be very useful in patient care; but if heterogeneity is responsible, rather than methodologic problems in bone mass measurement, hopes will be further dampened for the practical utility of peripheral bone mass screening in predicting vertebral or hip fracture risk.

Third, heterogeneity may have an influence on the relevance of specific risk factors. Corticosteroids, for example, represent a powerful risk factor for vertebral fractures in men and clinical studies suggest that the same is true for women (12). The risk of hip fractures associated with corticosteroid use appears to be substantially less (13). Likewise, oophorectomy prior to natural menopause is associated with accelerated bone loss and an increase in vertebral fractures (14) but not consistently with hip fractures (13,15,16).

The latter observation, finally, raises questions about treatment and prevention of osteoporosis. It is generally accepted that long-term postmenopausal estrogen replacement reduces the risk of hip fracture by about half (17). Data on vertebral fractures are sparse, but it has been suggested that the beneficial effect of estrogen is even greater, reducing fracture risk by as much as 90% (18). The exact figures vary widely from study to study but, when all three pertinent sites have been evaluated simultaneously, postmenopausal estrogen therapy has been more effective in preventing vertebral and Colles' fractures than hip fractures (19). Such results would be consistent with the Gompertzian model, which predicts that risk factors unrelated to estrogen deficiency should be much more prominent in the etiology of hip fractures. As Fries (2) points out "These distinctions are important because they clarify a perceived conflict between those steeped in the traditional biomedical search for cause and cure, and those most enthusiastic about a new need for effective health promotion and life-style based disease prevention. In fact, there are specific areas in which each approach is more likely [to be effective]."

Summary
Hip fractures, the characteristic clinical manifestation of Type II osteoporosis, increase exponentially in incidence with aging in men and women, reflecting the Gompertzian model of a degenerative disease with early onset and insidious progression until a symptomatic threshold is reached after a long latent period. Such diseases are typically multifactorial and affect the majority of the population. In contrast, Colles' fractures and postmenopausal vertebral crush fractures, which are most closely associated with Type I osteoporosis, reveal a plateau in incidence rates around age 65 years. This is consistent with non-Gompertzian conditions that have relatively early onset and a variable clinical course often marked by remission. Such diseases affect a smaller proportion of the population, often have a specific etiology, and may be more amenable to treatment. These epidemiologic observations provide empirical support for the existence of two distinct syndromes of involutional osteoporosis.

Acknowledgments
The authors would like to thank Miss Mary Ramaker for help in preparing the manuscript.

This work was supported in part by research grants AR-27065 and AR-30582 from the National Institutes of Health, U.S. Public Health Service.

References
1. Riggs BL, Melton LJ 1983 Evidence for two distinct syndromes of involutional osteoporosis. Am J Med 75:899-901.

2. Fries JF 1984 The compression of morbidity, Benjamin Gompertz, the two types of chronic disease, and health policy. In: Proceedings, Exploring New Frontiers of U.S. Health Policy, Graduate Program in Public Health, University of Medicine and Dentistry of New Jersey-Rutgers Medical School and Rutgers, The State University of New Jersey. October 12, 1984.
3. Riggs BL, Wahner HW, Melton LJ III, Richelson LS, Judd HL, Offord KP 1986 Rates of bone loss in the appendicular and axial skeletons of women: Evidence of substantial vertebral bone loss before menopause. J Clin Invest 77:1487-1491.
4. Bohr H, Schaadt O 1985 Bone mineral content of the femoral neck and shaft: Relation between cortical and trabecular bone. Calcif Tissue Int 37:340-344.
5. Parfitt AM 1988 Chapter 2: Bone remodeling: Relationship to the amount and structure of bone, and the pathogenesis and prevention of fractures. In: Riggs BL, Melton LJ III (eds) Osteoporosis: Etiology, Diagnosis, and Management. Raven Press, New York, pp. 45-93.
6. Parfitt AM 1984 Age-related structural changes in trabecular and cortical bone: Cellular mechanisms and biomechanical consequences. Calcif Tissue Int 36:S123-S128.
7. Melton LJ III 1988 Chapter 5. Epidemiology of fractures. In: Riggs BL, Melton LJ III (eds) Osteoporosis: Etiology, Diagnosis, and Management. Raven Press, New York, pp 133-154.
8. Owen RA, Melton LJ III, Ilstrup DM, Johnson KA, Riggs BL 1982 Colles' fracture and subsequent hip fracture risk. Clin Orthop 171:37-43.
9. Jensen GF, Christiansen C, Boesen J, Hegedus V, Transbol I 1982 Epidemiology of postmenopausal spinal and long bone fractures: A unifying approach to postmenopausal osteoporosis. Clin Orthop 166:75-81.
10. Melton LJ, Cummings SR, Johnston CC 1987 Heterogeneity of age-related fractures: Implications for epidemiology. Bone Min 2:321-331.
11. Riggs BL, Melton LJ 1986 Medical progress: Involutional osteoporosis. N Engl J Med 314:1676-1686.
12. Melton LJ III, Riggs BL 1988 Chapter 6: Clinical spectrum. In: Riggs BL, Melton LJ III (eds) Osteoporosis: Etiology, Diagnosis, and Management. Raven Press, New York, pp 155-179.
13. Paganini-Hill A, Ross RK, Gerkins VR, Henderson BE, Arthur M, Mack TM 1981 Menopausal estrogen therapy and hip fractures. Ann Intern Med 95:28-31.
14. Lindsay R, Hart DM, Forrest C, Baird C 1980 Prevention of spinal osteoporosis in oophorectomised women. Lancet 2:1151-1154.
15. Weiss NS, Ure CL, Ballard JH, Williams AR, Darling JR 1980 Decreased risk of fractures of the hip and lower forearm with postmenopausal use of estrogen. N Engl J Med 303:1195-1198.
16. Kreiger N, Kelsey JL, Holford TR, O'Connor T 1982 An epidemiologic study of hip fracture in postmenopausal women. Am J Epidemiol 116:141-148.
17. Johnston CC Jr 1985 Chapter 8: Studies on prevention of age-related bone loss. In: Peck WA (ed) Bone and Mineral Research/3. Elsevier, New York, pp 233-257.
18. Lindsay R 1988 Chapter 12: Sex steroids in the pathogenesis and prevention of osteoporosis. In: Riggs BL, Melton LJ III (eds) Osteoporosis: Etiology, Diagnosis, and Management. Raven Press, New York, pp 333-358.
19. Ettinger B, Genant HK, Cann CE 1985 Long-term estrogen replacement therapy prevents bone loss and fractures. Ann Intern Med 102:319-324.

Discussion:

DR. RAISZ (Connecticut): Have you looked at the relative risk of a hip fracture in people who've had a vertebral fracture and also, of course, the one we expect to see, the Colles' fracture leading to the vertebral fracture? How do those ratios compare?

DR. MELTON (Rochester, MN): Yes, that's a thing that you would have thought we would have done by now. And, in fact, that study is under way. The difficulty has been, for us, the ability to identify vertebral fractures because many don't come to clinical attention. And, so, we didn't have a lot of confidence in our ability to find these patients. Many of you don't know about the data system in Rochester, but we can identify all the Rochester residents with any diagnosis or surgical procedure by any provider. But that presumes, of course, that a diagnosis has been made. And, if you have things that are only findings or things that are not found, then you can't do the study.

But we have identified a cohort of women, less than 70, who have had symptomatic vertebral fractures. And we're following them now through the record system in a retrospective cohort study, looking at their hip fracture risk. Unfortunately, we didn't get far enough along in that study to present that today, but my early indications are that they may be at increased risk of intertrochanteric fractures and not cervical fractures. So, it seems that something is going on there, but I'm not sure, overall, whether or not their risk of hip fractures will be increased or not.

DR. PARFITT (Detroit): If Type 1 osteoporosis is a non-Gompertzian disease, that affects only specific individuals, why is it so closely related in various ways to menopause, which is a universal phenomenon in women?

DR. MELTON: Well, of course, I don't know the answer to that. But one statement we always make is that the interesting thing about vertebral fractures is, every woman has a menopause, but relatively few women have symptomatic vertebral fractures. That's been presented as a paradox and perhaps it's related to this kind of process.

DR. RIGGS (Rochester, MN): I might just add, that, as you know, we have postulated that Type 1 osteoporosis is a combination of menopause plus some additional factor that makes certain women particularly susceptible to estrogen deficiency.

DR. MELTON: You know, one piece of information is missing and one we're trying to develop right now is a sense of how common Type 1 osteoporosis and postmenopausal vertebral fractures are. Most of the literature that you read comes from centers of excellence in managing metabolic bone disease. And, so, it's certainly not surprising that large numbers of their patients have this problem.

But I, as an epidemiologist, don't have a strong sense of how common this problem is in the general community. And the suspicion that we have is that perhaps it's not as common as we thought. And, so, on a community-wide basis, if symptomatic vertebral crush fractures are a relatively uncommon condition, then that would be what you would expect with a Type 1 non-Gompertzian sort of problem.

Appropriate Use of Bone Densitometry

HARRY K. GENANT,[1,2] JON E. BLOCK,[1] PETER STEIGER,[1]
CLAUS C. GLUEER,[1] BRUCE ETTINGER,[1,3] and STEVE T. HARRIS[2]

Departments of [1]Radiology and [2]Medicine
University of California
San Francisco, CA
[3]Department of Medicine
Kaiser Permanente Medical Center
San Francisco, CA

The evolution of techniques to non-invasively quantitate the skeleton has progressed rapidly over the past fifteen years and has been responsible, in part, for the expanded research, clinical and public interest in osteoporosis. We currently have at our disposal the ability to inspect and evaluate the peripheral skeleton, the central skeleton, the entire skeleton as well as the trabecular and cortical bone envelopes with a high degree of accuracy and precision. Bone densitometry, as a research tool, has led us to appreciate more fully the vast complexity of osteoporosis and, as a clinical tool, has provided an important first-step toward ameliorating this syndrome.

Technical Capabilities

Essentially three techniques are currently employed for the non-invasive assessment of the skeleton on a clinical basis: single photon absorptiometry (SPA), dual photon absorptiometry (DPA), and quantitative computed tomography (QCT). Certainly other techniques such as neutron activation analysis and compton scattering exist, but these methods do not have widespread clinical potential. SPA can be used to assess bone mass in the peripheral skeleton at sites of principally cortical bone such as the mid-shaft radius. Quantification by SPA is relatively fast, inexpensive, has a low associated radiation dose, and is accurate and precise. Rectilinear scanning (SPA-R) has the additional capability of assessing sites of proportionately greater trabecular bone such as the calcaneus or the ultra-distal radius. DPA is an evolutionary bi-product of SPA, and allows for the quantification of total body bone mass or any designated segment thereof; although the more traditional spine and hip assessment procedures are more widely employed. Standard DPA scanning is somewhat time-consuming but this inconvenience is offset by low associated radiation dose and good accuracy and precision. QCT allows for the direct measurement of trabecular or integral bone density in the spine; however, QCT techniques have also been applied to quantification of the peripheral skeleton and the hip but principally on a research basis.

Several new developments in bone densitometry are in the early stages of clinical application; preliminary results thus far are promising. Recent software and hardware advances in QCT have substantially improved performance characteristics by controlling technical parameters and automating the procedure (QCT-A) [1,2,3]. Resultant decreases in scanning time, reduction in associated radiation dose, and semi-automated analysis approaches will likely substantiate this technique as a powerful clinical tool. On a similar front, technical modifications in DPA such as the use of a dual energy x-ray source in place of an isotope source, improvements in detector configuration, and automation of analysis procedures have greatly enhanced the speed and precision of this technique (DPA-X). In both cases, substantial reduction in costs are being realized due to the greater ease, facility and time efficiency of these innovations. Tables I and II summarize various parameters as they apply to each technique and illustrates the impact of recent improvements on the performance characteristics of these newer modalities.

The terms sensitivity, precision and accuracy are used to describe the performance characteristics of the different bone mass measurement techniques. By **sensitivity** we mean the capacity to readily separate an abnormal from a normal population or to readily detect changes with time in a patient or a population. By **precision** we mean longitudinal reproducibility in serial studies, while **accuracy** refers to the reliability that the measured value reflects true mineral content. A further distinction among techniques might also be made based upon their respective abilities to predict fracture and/or monitor treatment interventions or the natural course of disease. Care should be taken in selecting the measurement technique or combination of techniques in relation to individual patients so that appropriate information can be gathered to strengthen management decisions. For example, while a measure of radial cortical bone, as a surrogate of total skeletal mass, may have adequate predictive ability for certain fractures, it may be relatively insensitive for detecting early postmenopausal bone loss and for monitoring changes in bone density [4,5,6]. In contrast, measurement of the ultra-distal radial site provides improved sensitivity for monitoring serial changes [7,8]. Quantification of calcaneal bone mass has been shown to provide excellent predictive value for a variety of fractures both in terms of prevalence and incidence data [9,10,11,12], but its capacity to monitor changes has not been established. Direct assessment of the spine detects early menopausal bone loss, is a sensitive site for serial assessment, and is a strong predictor of vertebral fracture; however, this site is less predictive of hip fracture risk than is direct measurement of the proximal femur [13,14,15,16,17,18].

Table I

STANDARD TECHNIQUES

TECHNIQUE	SPA	DPA	QCT
SITE	Prox Radius (Cortical)	Spine, Hip, (TB) (Integral)	Spine (Trabecular)
SENSITIVITY	1X	2X	3-4X
PRECISION	2-3%	2-4%	2-5%
ACCURACY	5%	4-10%	5-20%
TIME	15 min	20-40 min	10-20 min
DOSE	10 mrem	5 mrem	100-1000 mrem
CHARGE	$75	$100-150	$100-200

Recommended Clinical Applications

The question now remains as to whether we are currently at a point where bone densitometry, by any method, should be recommended widely and become standard medical practice. We know more today about each technique's

Table II

NEWER DEVELOPMENTS

TECHNIQUE	SPA-R	DPA-X	QCT-A
SITE	Dist Rad, Calcaneous (Integral)	Spine, Hip, (TB) (Integral)	Spine, (Hip) (Trabec/Integ)
SENSITIVITY	2X	2X	3-4X
PRECISION	1-2%	1-2%	1-2%
ACCURACY	5%	3-5%	5-10%
TIME	10-20 min	5 min	10 min
DOSE	5-10 mrem	2-5 mrem	100-300 mrem
COST(PROJECTED)	$50	$75	$100

advantages and their respective shortcomings than we ever have, and certainly the field continues to move rapidly in a positive direction via the improvement of current technology and the development of additional and exciting new modalities. But in the midst of all this development and improvement, and while we await the results of numerous ongoing and planned clinical and epidemiologic investigations, we are faced with critical management decisions involving the current population of women already afflicted with osteoporosis or at risk for developing it. We must, therefore, rely on sound expert opinion and available technology to guide our clinical approach to patient management.

Previously, the prevailing notion was that osteoporosis, by clinical definition, could be reduced to a simple distinction between atraumatic fracture and non-fracture; indeed, this philosophy led some researchers [19,20,21,22] to suggest that bone density, per se, is not a sensitive predictor of fracture because only modest separation was obeserved between fracture patients and non-fracture comparison subjects of the same age. The suggestion was based, in part, upon early densitometry studies showing considerable overlap between hip fracture subjects and matched controls. However, a more recent study [18] suggests better hip fracture discrimination when measurement of the Ward's triangle region of the hip is evaluated. Certainly, many investigators have shown that direct quantitative assessment of the spine by QCT or DPA satisfactorily discriminates spine fracture from non-fracture subjects [23,5,17]. Additionally, all bone densitometry techniques illustrate a progressive and substantial loss of bone from all skeletal sites (albeit at different rates and to different degrees) over the life span [24,25,26], and it is this systematic bone loss that contributes most significantly to fractures in old age. In fact, several studies [27,16,12] have shown that osteoporotic fractures do not become likely until a certain threshold of bone density is crossed, and that high density values independent of age confer significant protection against fracture. Most importantly, these recent findings have convinced many researchers to no longer consider osteoporosis as a fracture/non-fracture dichotomy but rather to now consider osteoporosis as the lower part of a continuum of bone density, with greatest risk among those with lowest absolute density values. Wasnich [28] recalls a parallel situation in regard to the use of blood pressure monitoring to predict stroke risk. Bone mass, he points out, like blood pressure must be treated as a continuous variable with fracture analogous to stroke as a primary outcome. Indeed most individuals with hypertension will not have suffered a stroke, yet they are nonetheless at great risk.

Similarly, because of the probabilistic nature of fractures many individuals with low bone density will not have fractured, but they should likewise not be considered normal or free of osteoporosis.

While controversy exists and will likely always exist in regard to the standard use of bone densitometry [20,21,29,30], we currently consider a number of clinical applications valid. Only the first of these four recommendations, however, could have consensus support among all investigators in the field. Nonetheless, a growing body of literature is being accumulated to support wider applications for the individual patient.

1. Assessment of patients with metabolic diseases known to affect the skeleton: Many metabolic disorders have profound influences on calcium metabolism and adversely affect the skeleton resulting in secondary forms of osteopenia/osteoporosis. Included among these disorders are hyperparathyroidism, renal insufficiency, Cushing's syndrome, chronic immobilization with acute spinal cord injury, ammenorrhea among pre-menopausal women, as well as chronic steroid or thyroid therapy. Some of these disorders such as Cushing's syndrome differentially affect the trabecular bone envelope, with relative sparing of cortical bone, making an assessment of trabecular sites advisable. On the other hand, renal osteodystrophy may result in dramatic appendicular cortical demineralization in the presence of low, normal or even high spinal trabecular bone, suggesting an assessment by a combination of techniques may be appropriate. Bone mass measurements have considerable importance in these secondary forms of osteoporosis as they can aid the physician in clinical management such as reducing corticosteroids in the case of steroid-induced osteoporosis, providing subtotal parathyroidectomy in hyperparathyroid bone disease, or initiating estrogen replacement therapy in the case of amenorrhea/oligomenorrhea [29].

2. Assessment of Perimenopausal women regarding the initiation of estrogen replacement therapy: The distinct loss of bone due to accelerated resorption is a universally accepted phenomenon in women at the menopause. However, the magnitude of this loss is site and technique dependent; typically 1-2% per year from appendicular cortical regions and 4-6% from spinal trabecular regions [13,31,32]. This finding has led some investigators [33] to differentiate a form of osteoporosis specifically associated with this rapid, menopause-related trabecular resorption (Type I) from a relatively slower, age-related cortical atrophy (Type II). These details aside, it is clear that the natural loss of ovarian function has a profound influence on a woman's risk for the development of osteoporosis.

Most women who initiate estrogen replacement therapy at the time of menopause or soon thereafter are spared the normal skeletal degradation that would otherwise occur at this point in the life cycle [31]. Discontinuation of therapy results in resumption of the normal menopausal bone loss phase [34]. Perhaps more important, long-term estrogen replacement therapy also reduces the likelihood of fracture among users two-fold [35].

While estrogen replacement therapy is known to be an effective anti-resorbing agent for bone, it does have side effects and is likely not required for all menopausal women [36]. Decisions about initiation of estrogen therapy, therefore, are contingent upon a number of factors including the current level of bone density, laboratory evidence of rapid bone loss, and possibly the long-term risk of cardio-vascular disease [37]. Many experts would agree that compliance to estrogen therapy may be enhanced by quantitative information concerning fracture risk and efficacy of treatment.

The absolute level of bone density at the menopause and the magnitude of subsequent bone loss are important considerations in assessing the risk for subsequent fracture. Even considering menopausal and subsequent age-related decrements in bone mass, the sub-group of women who have high absolute bone density at the menopause will most likely be conferred significant protection by virtue of their relatively dense skeleton, and may not require estrogen or any other intervention. By the same token, women with low to moderate levels of bone density may, in fact, be at increased risk for fracture if therapy is not initiated early [29]. Decisions about initiation of therapy in the context of osteoporosis, therefore, can most appropriately be made in conjunction with an objective assessment of the skeleton and in consultation with a physician knowledgeable not only in the administration of appropriate therapy but also informed on which quantitative methods will be necessary to guide the medical decision making process.

3. Establishing a diagnosis of osteoporosis or assessing its severity in the context of general clinical care: A growing number of postmenopausal women are concerned about their current skeletal status and their future risk of fracture. Some authorities [29,38,36] have recommended a comprehensive approach for managing these patients whereby an initial risk factor analysis is performed followed by a determination of skeletal status if a number of these risk factors are found. We agree that if known factors predisposing to secondary forms of osteoporosis are found, then bone density should be measured (see #1); however, we must caution that while this clinical approach may appear to be prudent, some recent evidence suggests that historically based risk factors (eg. low calcium diet, smoking, family history of osteoporosis) either taken singly or in combination have limited predictive value in the individual patient for fracture risk or for bone density [39,40]. On the other hand, a large body of evidence has been accumulated to show that the absolute level of bone density is closely related to the risk of fracture. First, most of the variance in bone strength is attributable to bone mass [41]. Second, several recent studies have shown a gradient of increasing fracture risk corresponding to absolute declines in bone density [16,12]. Third, prophylactic agents, such as estrogen, that abbreviate bone loss and reduce the occurrence of hip and spine fractures, undoubtedly do so through a mechanism affecting skeletal involution. It should be recommended, therefore, that in individuals where there is a suspicion of osteoporosis or where there is a confirmed diagnosis of osteoporosis based upon x-ray evidence, that a quantitative evaluation be performed to determine where they fall in the spectrum of bone density values. If fracture risk is low, conservative management with calcium and exercise may be employed, while if fracture risk is severe, aggressive treatment with calcitonin or estrogen may be prescribed.

4. Monitoring the efficacy of treatment interventions or the natural course of disease: Bone mass measurement techniques have been criticized in the past for their inability to monitor individual changes in bone mass due to high associated precision errors relative to estimated rates of change. Tremendous progress has been made in the past two years in response to this criticism, and current precision errors for SPA with rectilinear scanning, for the new high-speed, x-ray based DPA, and for QCT with automatic image analysis approach 1-2%. Precision levels of this degree, however, are highly dependent upon adherence to strict quality assurance measures and careful technical monitoring.

Several authors [42,20] raised appropriate cautions about the interpretation of serial bone density measurements. They showed that for the individual patient, based upon two-point measurements and 2% precision error, bone density changes must be greater than 5.6% to be detected with 95% confidence. These authors used a two-tailed estimation of confidence intervals which may be inappropriate for assessing individual changes in bone density. The important clinical questions under consideration are whether an individual is losing bone at a rate considered clinically significant (eg. at the time of menopause) or whether they are gaining bone as a result of some treatment intervention (eg. calcitonin therapy in osteoporotic patients); effects to the contrary are of limited clinical importance. Thus, monitoring bone mass changes in the individual patient can be satisfactorily accomplished using one-tailed tests of significance, and perhaps 90% confidence is adequate for purposes of clinical decision making [43]. For example, using two-point serial measurements, a technique with a 2% precision error can detect changes in bone mass greater than 3.6% with 90% confidence; likewise, with 1.5% precision, changes of 2.7% can be detected. The measurement times should be appropriately spaced and the measurement site appropriately selected such that the changes to be detected match the precision capabilities of the technique. Numerous studies have observed large annual losses from sites rich in trabecular bone among women undergoing surgical or natural menopause [13,31,32], patients initiating high dose corticosteroid treatment [44,45], and individuals with complete immobilization [46,47]. Similarly, large annual gains have been observed in osteporotic patients receiving calcitonin treatment [48,49] or investigational agents such as sodium fluoride [50], diphosphonates [51], or parathyroid hormone [52].

Given these continued improvements in measurement precision, the speed at which bone mass measurements can now be performed, and their reduced cost, coupled with the marked effect of some interventions, it is difficult to pose convincing arguments against monitoring individual patients when important therapeutic decisions are to be made.

The dilemma of Mass Screening

The purpose of any screening instrument is to identify from among populations at risk those individuals who should receive further assessment or treatment. The technique should be reliable, easily administered, and an inexpensive measure of a variable that has practical significance. Bone mass measurements, in general, qualify on all these counts. The term "mass screening", however, has a negative connotation among researchers and clinicians. Many experts have recommended so-called "selective screening" to include white and Asian women, at the age of menopause and beyond, with several presumed risk factors for osteoporosis, and in consultation with their physician [29,53,38,36]. It has been suggested [54] that this "selective screening" process intimates mass screening in as much as most postmenopausal women have low enough bone desnity values to place them at risk and thus would be candidates for "selective screening". However, while we agree that most postmenopausal women are at risk for osteoporosis, those with lowest absolute density values are at greatest risk for fracture and should be targeted accordingly for appropriate medical intervention. Therefore, we wish to avoid non-productive nomenclature battles over the terms "mass screening" or "selective screening" and proceed with the most efficient approach to ameliorate osteoporosis and its sequelae. If this means examining most patients with underlying disorders of bone metabolism, then we must do this. If this means examining most peri-menopausal women to assess their requirement for estrogen replacement therapy, then we must do this. If this means confirming a diagnosis of osteoporosis and establishing fracture risk in older individuals, then we must do this and so on. In reality, of course, we are well aware that these recommendations cannot be followed without major contigencies.

Knowledge about the proper use and interpretation of bone densitometry as well as an understanding of the appropriate medical interventions is not universal or consistent across all physicians nor is there a uniformly high quality of instrumentation and technical performance for providing bone density studies to all potential patients. Indeed, this deficiency of medical and technical cognizance is the principal deterrent to the widespread implementation of our recommended clinical applications at this time. Given the current impetus to disseminate information about osteoporosis, to make newer instrumentation more readily available, and to constrain the costs associated with these techniques, we anticipate that our recommended clinical applications may soon become standard medical practice.

References

1. Steiger P, Steiger S, Ruegsegger P, Genant HK: Two-and three-dimensional quantitative image evaluation techniques for densitometry and volumetrics

in longitudinal studies.In: Genant HK (ed):Osteoporosis Update 1987. University of California Press, 1987:171-180.
2. Kalender WA, Klotz E, Suess C: Vertebral bone mineral analysis: An integrated approach with CT. Radiology 1987;164:419-423.
3. Kalender WA, Brestowsky H, Felsenberg D: Automated determination of the midvertebral CT slice for bone mineral measurements. Presented at the 73rd annual meeting of the RSNA, Chicago, November 1987, paper no. 876. Submitted to Radiology.
4. Mazess RB, Peppler WW, Chesney RW, Lange TA, Lindgren U, Smith E: Does bone measurement on the radius indicate skeletal status? Concise communication. J Nucl Med 1984;25:281-288.
5. Reinbold WD, Genant HK, Reiser UJ, Harris ST, Ettinger B: Bone mineral content in early-postmenopausal and postmenopausal osteoporotic women: Comparison of measurement methods. Radiology 1986;160(2):469-478.
6. Pocock NA, Eisman JA, Yeates MG, Sambrook PN, Eberl S, Wren BG: Limitations of forearm bone densitometry as an index of vertebral or femoral neck osteopenia. J Bone and Min Res 1986;1(4):369-375.
7. Christiansen C, Riis BJ: Comparison of noninvasive techniques for measurements of bone mass in postmenopausal women. In: Genant HK (ed):Osteoporosis Update 1987. University of California Press. 1987:81-85.
8. Riis BJ, Christiansen C: Measurement or spinal or peripheral bone mass to estimate early postmenopausal bone loss? Am J Med 1988;84:646-653.
9. Wasnich RD, Ross PD, Heilbrun LK, Vogel JM: Prediction of postmenopausal fracture risk with bone mineral measurements. Am J Obstet Gynecol 1985;153(7):745-751.
10. Wasnich RD, Ross PD, Heilburn LK, Vogel JM: Selection of the optimal skeletal site for fracture risk prediction. Clin Ortho Rel Res 1987;216:262-269.
11. Ross PD, Wasnich RD, Vogel JM: Definition of a spine fracture threshold based upon prospective fracture risk. Bone 1987;8:271-278.
12. Ross PD, Wasnich RD, Vogel JM: Detection of prefracture spinal osteoporosis using bone mineral absortiometry. J Bone Min Res 1988;3(1): 1-11.
13. Genant HK, Cann CE, Ettinger B, Gordan GS: Quantitative computed tomography of vertebral spongiosa: A sensitive method for detecting early bone loss after oophorectomy. Ann Int Med 1982;97:699-705.
14. Genant HK, Steiger P, Block JE, Ettinger B, Harris ST: Quantitative computed tomography: Update 1987. Calc Tiss Int 1987(Editorial), 41:174-186.
15. Genant HK, Block JE, Steiger P, Glueer CC, Smith R: Quantitative Computed Tomography in assessment of osteoporosis. Sem Nucl Med 1987;17:316-333.
16. Melton III LJ, Wahner HW, Richelson LS, O'Fallon WM, Riggs BL: Osteoporosis and the risk of hip fracture. Am J of Epidemiol 1986;124:254-261.
17. Mazess RB, Barden HS, Ettinger M, et al: Spine and femur density using dual-photon absorptiometry in US white women. Bone Mineral 1987;2:211-9.
18. Mazess RB, Barden H, Ettinger M, Schultz E: Bone density of the radius, spine, and proximal femur in osteoporosis. J Bone Mineral Res 1988;3:13-18.
19. Aitken JM: Relevance of osteoporosis in women with fractures of the femoral neck. Br J Med 1984;288:1084-1085.
20. Cummings SR, Black D: Should perimenopausal women be screened for osteoporosis. Ann Int Med 1986;104:817-823.
21. Hall FM, Davis MA, Baran DT: Bone mineral screening for osteoporosis. N Eng J Med 1987;316:212-4.
22. Ott SM: Should women get screening bone mass measurements? Ann Int Med 1986;104:874.
23. Firooznia H, Golimbu C, Rafii M, et al: Quantitative Computed tomography assessment of spinal trabecular bone in osteoporotic women with and without vertebral fractures. J Comp Assist Tomogr 1984;8:99-103.

24. Garn SM, Rohmann CG, Wagner B: Bone loss as a general phenomenon in man. Feder Proc 1967;6:1729-1736.
25. Mazess RB: On aging bone loss. Clin Ortho 1982;165:239-252.
26. Genant HK, Cann CE, Pozzi-Mucelli RS, Kantner AS: Vertebral mineral determination by QCT: clinical feasibility and normative data. J Comput Assist Tomogr 1983;7:554.
27. Cann CE, Genant HK, Kolb FO, Ettinger BF: Quantitative computed tomography for prediction of vertebral fracture risk. Bone 1985;6:1-7.
28. Wasnich RD: Fracture prediction with bone mass measurements. In. Genant HK (ed) Osteoporosis Update 1987. University of Calif Press 1987:95-101.
29. Riggs BL, Wahner HW: Bone densitometry and clinical decision-making in osteoporosis. Annals of Int Med 1988;108(2):293-295.
30. Slemenda CW, Johnston C: Bone mass measurement: which site to measure. Am J Med 1988;84:643-645.
31. Ettinger B, Genant HK, Cann CE: Postmenopausal bone loss is prevented by low dosage estrogen with calcium. Ann Int Med 1986;106:40-45.
32. Riis B, Thomsen K, Christiansen C: Does calcium supplementation prevent postmenopausal bone loss? N Eng J Med 1987;316:173-177.
33. Riggs BL, Melton LJ: Evidence for two distinct syndromes of involutional osteoporosis. Am J Med 1983;75:899-901.
34. Lindsay R, Hart DM, Forrest C, Baird C: Prevention of spinal osteoporosis in oophorectomized women. 1980;2:1151.
35. Ettinger B, Genant HK, Cann CE: Long-term estrogen replacement therapy prevents bone loss and fractures. Ann Int Med 1985;102:319-324.
36. Tohme JF, Lindsay R: Bone mineral screening for osteoporosis (letter). N Eng J Med 1987;317:316.
37. Hillner BE, Hollenberg JP, Pauker SG: Postmenopausal estrogen in the prevention of osteoporosis: A benefit that is virtually without risk if cardiovascular effects are considered. Am J Med 1986;80:1115.
38. Raisz LG, Lorenzo JA, Smith JA: Bone mineral screening for osteoporosis (letter). N Eng J Med 1987;317:315.
39. Citron JT, Ettinger B, Genant HK: Prediction of peak premenopausal bone mass using a scale of weighted clinical variables: In Christiansen C, Johansen JS, Riis BJ (eds). Osteoporosis 1987. Osteopress ApS, Kobenhavn K, Denmark 1987;1:146-149.
40. Wasnich RD: Screening for osteoporosis: Pro. In Genant HK (ed) Osteoporosis Update 1987. University of California Press 1987:123-127.
41. Melton LJ, Riggs BL: Risk factors for injury after a fall. Clin Geriatric Med 1985;1:525-536.
42. Heaney RP: En recherche de la difference (P<0.05). Bone and Mineral 1986;1:99-114.
43. Steiger P, Glueer CC, Black DM, Block JE, Smith R, Cummings SR, Genant HK: Monitoring change in bone mineral content: Using the dispersion around the regression line as an estimate of precision. In Christiansen C, Johansen JS, Riis BJ (eds). Osteoporosis 1987. Osteopress ApS, Kobenhavn K, Denmark 1987;1:396-398.
44. Montag M, Belter SV, Meyer-Galander HM, Peters PE: BMC of the spongiosa in lumbar spine, measured by QCT: follow-up study in patients suffering from pemphigus and treated with high doses of cortisone. In Proceedings of the Sixth International Workshop on Bone and Soft Tissue Densitometry. Buxton, England Sept 22-25, 1987.
45. Richardson ML, Genant HK, Cann CE, Ettinger B, Gordan GS, Kolb FO, Reiser UJ: Assessment of metabolic bone diseases by quantitative computed tomography. Clin Orthoped 1985;185:224-238.
46. Krolner B, Toft B: Vertebral bone loss: An unheeded side effect of therapeutic bed rest. Clin Sci 1983;64:537-549.
47. Mazess RB, Whedon GD: Immobilization and bone. Calc Tissue Int 1983;35:265-267.
48. Gruber HF, Ivey JL, Baylink DJ, Matthews M, Nelp WB, Sisom K, Chesnut CH: Long-term calcitonin therapy in postmenopausal osteoporosis. Metabolism 1984;33:295.

49. Gennari C, Chierichetti SM, Bigazzi S, Fusi L, Gonnelli S, Ferrara R, Zacchei F: Compararive effects on bone mineral content of calcium and calcium plus salmon calcitonin given in two different regimens in postmenopausal osteoporosis. Cur Ther Res 1985;38(3);455-464.
50. Duursma SA, Glerum JH, Van Dijk A, Bosch R, Kerkhoff H, Van Putten J, Raymakers JA: Responders and non-responders after flouride therapy in osteoporosis. Bone 1987;8:131-136.
51. Genant HK, Harris ST, Steiger P, Davey PF, Block JE: The effect of etidronate therapy in postmenopausal women: Preliminary results. In Christiansen C, Johansen JS, Riis BJ (eds). Osteoporosis 1987. Osteopress ApS, Kobenhavn K, Denmark 1987;2:1177-1181.
52. Slovik DM, Rosenthal DI, Doppelt SH, et al: Restoration of spinal bone in osteoporotic men by treatment with human parathyroid hormone (1-34) and 1,25-Dihydroxyvitamin D. J Bone Min Res 1986;1(4);377-381.
53. Chesnut CH: Report from the NIH consensus conference, 1984, and NIH/NOF Workshop, 1987. I. Genant HK (ed) Osteoporosis Update 1987. University of California Press. 1987:3-6.
54. Hall FM: Bone mineral screening for osteoporosis: reply (letter). N Eng J Med 1987;317:316.

Discussion:

DR. MARCUS (Stanford): I have a concern about the selectivity of patients for estrogen therapy, but it's not the usual one that I'm sure you hear. That is, I'm not going to base it on the issue of cardiovascular risk protection being so overwhelming that everyone should get estrogen. I happen to believe it is close to that.

My concern is more parochial to bone. We have evidence, as outlined by Joe Melton just before you, that a woman's risks in terms of vertebral compression fracture may be independent or only loosely linked to what her subsequent hip fracture risk is. We have what I think is a substantial body of literature which shows compellingly that estrogen replacement therapy is effective in reducing the risk for hip fracture.

I'd like to know how you can, therefore, base your selectivity on vertebral fracture risk and then have a hope of dealing most effectively with the long-term and most lethal complication of osteoporosis, that is, the hip fracture?

DR. GENANT (San Francisco): First of all, let me indicate that I did not go into detail about bone mass measurement in relationship to hip fracture because that subject is going to be covered this afternoon, and I was specifically charged not to get into detail on that matter. But I will comment about several of those aspects.

I do believe, and the data of Horsman and Wasnich would suggest, that there is a substantial concurrence between the various fractures. A woman with a vertebral fracture, for example, has been estimated to have three to ten times a greater likelihood of hip fracture than a woman who does not have a vertebral fracture.

There are similar concurrences between other fractures. And I believe there is evidence that indicates that, while there are some differences in heterogeneity amongst these fracture patterns, bone loss is a systemic process, although occurring at differing rates at differing sites.

So, I do believe that, if one assesses and determines bone loss at a site such as the spine where earliest loss occurs that this result has relevance to fractures at other sites including the hip. And, certainly, the work of Wasnich would suggest that one need not measure the spine or need not necessarily measure the hip to predict future fracture risk. He has shown that all of the measurement sites have capability for predicting fracture, future fracture, although his data are relatively sparing.

DR. KLEEREKOPER (Detroit): I'm interested in the lady who has unequivocal osteoporosis with fractures, let's say two vertebral fractures, where everybody would agree she has osteoporosis. Does bone mass measurement allow you to predict the natural history in that patient?

DR. GENANT: That's a good question. I don't know that we have answers to that issue. We do know that just the presence of vertebral fractures in and of themselves, based, again, upon the data of Wasnich, are relatively strong predictors of future fracture. And to the extent that vertebral bone density is a predictor of vertebral fracture, I would suspect that it also would contribute to that prediction of future fractures.

The extent to which it would, above and beyond the knowledge of severe fractures present, I cannot answer with certainty.

DR. CUSHARD (Sacramento): Is there any validity to a concept of so-called fracture threshold?

DR. GENANT: Yes, that's an important issue and I didn't have time to discuss it. I think that the concept of fracture threshold has importance, although I think it has a lesser importance than the concept of a continuum of low bone mass and a gradient of risk, because one always has to make some arbitrary decision about how one defines the fracture threshold. Fracture thresholds have been defined, typically, as two standard deviations below young normals. They also have been defined as the 90th percentile of fracture patients. It has been described by Wasnich recently as that level at which the relative risk increases to two.

It's interesting that if you compare across the different definitions that have been applied, in general, you come up with relatively comparable values. So, in decision-making, I think that a fracture threshold does have some importance, although I think that the concept of the gradient of risk and greater risk with lower bone mass is more important.

Developing Strong Bones: The Teenage Female

V. MATKOVIC[1] and D. DEKANIC[2]

[1]*Departments of Physical Medicine and Internal Medicine*
The Ohio State University
Columbus, OH
[2]*Institute for Medical Research*
Zagreb, Croatia, Yugoslavia

Treatment of established osteoporosis, so far, does not significantly restore previously lost bone and because the outlook for such patients often is uncertain, there is a growing emphasis on the prevention of age-related bone loss. This is particularly important in the face of expected increase in the number of elderly people in the U.S.A.[1,2]

At present, there are two approaches to the prevention of this disease: to increase peak bone mass at skeletal maturity and/or to reduce the rate of bone loss after the menopause.[3] Since bone mass is the principal (although not the only) determinant of fracture, high bone mass at skeletal maturity is considered the best protection against age-related bone loss.[4] Besides well known factors influencing body stature, very little is known about mechanisms increasing peak bone mass in the population. Peak bone mass is clearly the result of age, sex, and probably other genetically determined factors but, as has been shown recently, it could also be related to nutrition.[5,6] It has been suggested that calcium can be an important determinant of peak bone mass in young adults.[7]

The age between 9 and 20 seems to be critical for achievement of peak bone mass. From birth until about age 20, bones are in a phase of rapid growth and bone modeling. After this period, the skeleton is in a process of constant remodeling throughout life.[8]

Among this, the period of an adolescent growth spurt of rapid bone modeling is probably the most important one. This is the time when bone mineral content is increasing at the rate of about 8.5% per year.[9,10]

The average male begins his growth spurt at around 12 years of age, reaching his maximum velocity in height growth at about 14 years of age. At this time, he will be growing at nearly twice his childhood or preadolescent rate. His growth will be almost completed by age 18. Females begin puberty approximately two years earlier (8-10) and will reach maximum velocity in their height growth around 12 years of age. Cessation of linear growth in girls will be about age 16. There is about a 2% increase in body length thereafter in both boys and girls, extended to the early twenties or the young adult period. This increase is accounted for primarily by continued vertebral growth.[11]

Skeletal bone mass based on skeletal weight measurement is also achieved by the beginning of the third decade.[12] Total body calcium as determined by neutron activation analysis is the highest at the age of 20.[13,14] Total body bone mineral, as well as total body bone density as determined by dual photon absorptiometry technique, is at its peak at the age of 20 and is declining thereafter.[15]

Looking at tubular (cortical) bone envelopes, it can be concluded that the external diameter of tubular bones, as an indicator of periosteal growth, is reaching a plateau by the age of 20 in males and a few years earlier in females. Medullary area is constantly increasing in males up to the age of 20. In females, however, during this adolescent growth spurt, there is an endosteal apposition of cortical bone. Cortical bone mass, as represented by cortical width and cortical area, is at its maximum by the age of 20, at least as reflected in radiogrammetry studies of the second metacarpal bone.[16]

Bone mineral content of the forearm, as assessed by the single photon absorptiometry technique, is also approaching its highest level by the beginning of young adulthood (third decade) indicating, once again, that adolescence could be a critical period for cortical peak bone formation.

There are very few data regarding changes in trabecular bone mass in the adolescent period, but present literature suggests that the peak bone mass at the vertebral column has been achieved by the age of 20. Postmorten data, using bone ash measurements and compressive strength measurements, indicates an increase in those values up to the beginning of the third decade, with a decline thereafter.[18,19] Determination of bone mineral density at the lumbar spine, using the dual photon technique, also indicates that bone mineral content is declining after its maximum at the age of 20 in both males and females.[20] Based on iliac crest bone biopsies, it can be said again that we are reaching trabecular peak bone mass by the age of 20, or even earlier.[21]

To accumulate total body calcium of about 1000 gr during 20 years (7300 days), females need an average daily accretion of calcium into the skeleton of about 140 mg/day and males need 165 mg/day for total body calcium of 1200 gr/20 years.

During the adolescent growth spurt, the required calcium retention (mg/day) is 2-3 times higher than the average value. The calcium accretion to the skeleton can go up to 500 mg/day for males (Fig. 1) and up to 400 mg/day for females (Fig. 2).[16,22]

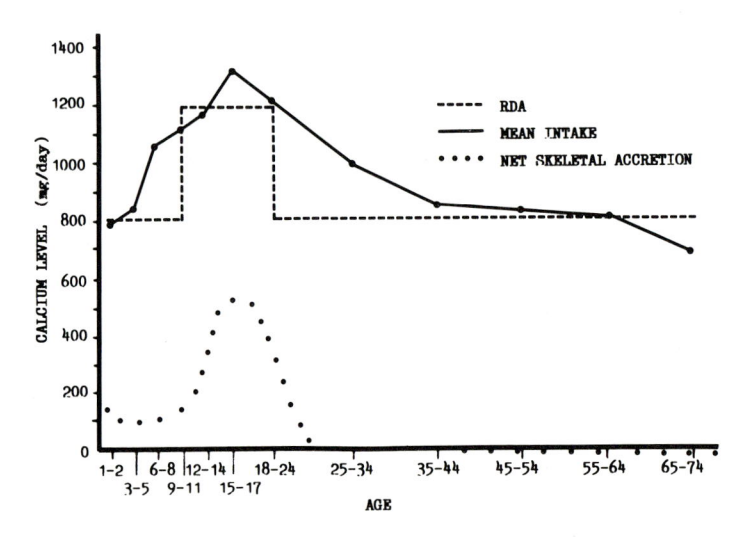

Fig. 1. Recommended Dietary Calcium Allowances (RDA) and calcium intake (mg/day) for males (U.S. Population 1976-1980)[23] and net skeletal calcium accretion (mg/day) according to age.

The ratio of established calcium intake of U.S. population and obligatory calcium accretion into the skeleton is the lowest for adolescent females (Fig. 1,2), indicating that inadequate mineral nutrition can be reached easily during this period.[23] To satisfy such a high skeletal retention, obligatory calcium excretion into the urine and variable absorption efficiency, calcium intake during adolescence should exceed 1000 mg/day.

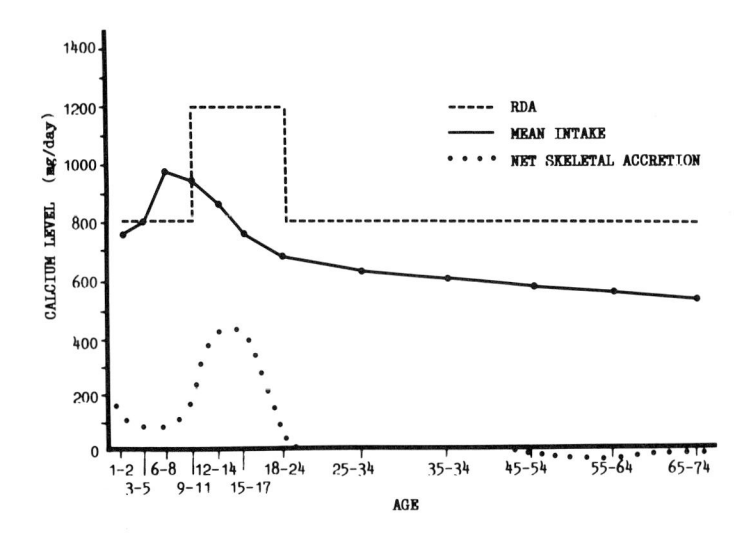

Fig. 2. Recommended Dietary Calcium Allowances (RDA) and calcium intake (mg/day) for females (U.S. Population 1976-1980)[23] and net skeletal calcium accretion (mg/day) according to age.

The calcium metabolism during adolescence is presented in Fig. 3. The average adolescent girl (hydroxiproline [OHPr] excretion 1.5-2 times higher than the average level of excretion during maturity level - 30 mg/24hr) on 1200 mg/day calcium intake (RDA) should have fecal calcium of about 800 mg/day, urine calcium of about 150 mg/day and, depending on the activity level, should have 20-80 mg/day additional calcium loss through the skin.[24] She should absorb about 550 mg of calcium totally to the calcium pool of which 250 will be incorporated into the skeleton. Digestive juice calcium, which depends on body size and dietary phosphorus, should be about 150 mg/day.[25] Exact data

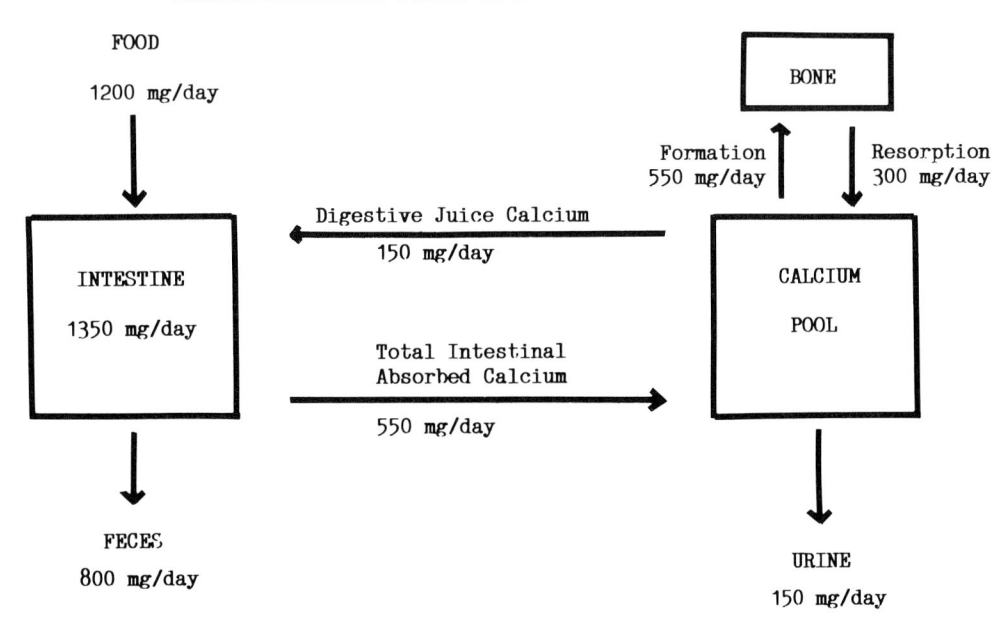

Fig. 3. Schema of calcium metabolism for the normal teenage girl on 1200 mg calcium intake (RDA).

for the amount of calcium which comes to the pool by the process of bone resorption is not known but the values certainly depend on rate of bone modeling. In this case, it was calculated to be 1.5-2 times the adult value as judged by OHPr excretion. In normal metabolic circumstances, this amount of calcium should be matched by bone formation.

If, for example, the calcium intake will be lower than 1200 mg/day with subsequent decrease in calcium retention by 100 mg/day/5 years, this should lower the peak whole body calcium by 182 gr. The same amount of bone calcium will allow the postmenopausal women to be in negative calcium balance of 30 mg/day for 16 years and 15 mg/day for 32 years.

The hypothesis is that residents of a low calcium district in Yugoslavia did not have adequate calcium intake during adolescence and ended bone modeling period with decreased peak bone mass level.[7] It was also recently reported that postmenopausal women who had decreased dairy product consumption during adolescence had decreased bone mass in the postmenopausal period.[26]

Experiments with laboratory animals have established that calcium deficiency can cause osteoporosis. In the majority of the experiments,[27,28] animals were fed low-calcium diets during the growing period, and skeletons were examined when animals reached "adulthood." Results indicate that calcium deficiency can cause osteoporosis by decreasing peak bone mass formation rather than affecting adult bone mass.[29]

Experimental calcium deficiency can cause growth retardation in animals, affecting bone volume and decreasing bone density (bone mass/bone volume). We have no clear-cut evidence that skeletons of growing humans will react to inadequate calcium intake in the same way as laboratory animals, although older growth studies of children suggest that they could. A group of British children at the turn of the century who received milk supplementation grew taller in comparison to a nonsupplemented group.[30]

The Ten-State Nutrition Survey of children of different socioeconomic backgrounds revealed that children of greater affluence had a 5% higher skeletal mass and bone formation rate than children from lower socioeconomic classes.[31] From the above studies, it is not quite clear if those differences were due to inadequate protein and/or mineral nutrition. Malnutrition certainly can lead to growth retardation and, with the correction of nutritional deficit, children can catch-up their growth rapidly.[32] We do not know, at the present time, if there is adequate "catch-up mineralization" of the skeleton, particularly after the growth spurt period. It was also reported recently that some of the children who suffered an accidental fracture have decreased bone mineral density, as determined by single photon absorptiometry technique, as well as decreased calcium intake.[33] Definitive data of the relationship of calcium nutrition and skeletal mineralization, however, have to come from well organized longitudinal studies of bone mass follow-up in children and adolescents on different calcium intakes.[34] The study should cover growth spurt period, as well as the years thereafter up to the age of 20 when peak bone mass formation is ending.

Based on those data, it is apparent that the needs for skeletal calcium are highest during growth spurt period. Mineral deficiency during this period could reduce the degree of positive calcium balance, with a resultant reduction in the level of bone mass reached at skeletal maturity. Presumably, such low bone mass at skeletal maturity would contribute to low bone mass at menopause and subsequent increased risk for fracture. It has recently been shown that, in this critical adolescent period, a substantial proportion of young Americans, particularly females, consume much less than the present recommended dietary calcium allowance.[23]

REFERENCES

1) Concensus Conference: Osteoporosis NIH Concensus Development Conference Statement, Vol. 5, No. 3, 1984.

2) Matkovic, V., Ciganovic, M., Tominac, C., Kostial, K.: Osteoporosis and

epidemiology of fractures in Croatia: an international comparison. Henry Ford Hosp. Med. J. 28:116-126, 1980.

3) Matkovic, V.: Influence of Age, Sex and Diet on Bone Loss in the Population. Ph.D. Thesis. University of Zagreb, Zagreb, 1976.

4) Newton-John, H., Morgan, B.: The loss of bone with age: osteoporosis and fractures. Clin. Orth. 71:229, 1970.

5) Smith, D., Nancy, W., Won Kang, K., Christian, J., Johnston, C.: Genetic factors in determining bone mass. J. Clin. Invest. 52:2800-2808, 1973.

6) Matkovic, V., Kostial, K., Simonovic, I., Brodarec, A., Buzina, R.,: Influence of calcium intake, age and sex on bone. Calcified Tissue Research Suppl. 22:393-396, 1977.

7) Matkovic, V., Kostial, K., Simonovic, I., Buzina, R., Brodarec, A., Nordin, B.E.C.: Bone status and fracture rates in two regions of Yugoslavia. Am. J. Clin. Nutrit., 32:540-549, 1979.

8) Parfitt, A.M.: Quantum Concept of Bone Remodeling and Turnover: Implications for the Pathogenesis of Osteoporosis. Calc. Tiss. Int. 28:1-5, 1979.

9) Mazess, R., Cameron, J.: Skeletal growth in school children: maturation and bone mass. Am. J. Phys. Anthrop.35:399-403, 1971.

10) Christiansen, C., Rodbro, P., Thoger Nielsen, C.: Bone Mineral Content and Estimated Total Body Calcium in Normal Children and Adolescents. Scand. J. Clin. Lab. Invest. 35:507-510, 1975.

11) Tanner, J.M.: Growth at Adolescence. With a general consideration of the effects of hereditary and environmental factors upon growth and maturation from birth to maturity. Blackwell Scient. Publ., Oxford, 1962.

12) Trotter, M., Hixon, B.: Sequential changes in weight, density, and percentage ash weight of human skeletons from an early fetal period through old age. Anat. Rec. 179:1-18, 1974.

13) Ott, S., Murano, R., Lewellen, T.K., Chesnut, C.: Total Body Calcium by Neutron Activation Analysis in Normals and Osteoporotic Populations: A Discriminator of Significant Bone Mass Loss. J. Lab. Clin. Med., 102: 637-645, 1983.

14) Aloia, J., Vaswani, A., Ellis, K., Yuen, K., Cohn, S.: A model for involutional bone loss. J. Lab. Clin. Med., 106:630-637, 1985.

15) Gotfredsen, A., Hadberg, A., Nilas, L., Christiansen, C.: Total body bone mineral in healthy adults. J. Lab. Clin. Med., 110:362-368, 1987.

16) Garn, S.M.: The earlier gain and later loss of cortical bone. In: Nutritional Perspectives, Charles C. Thomas, Publ., Springfield, Illinois, 1970.

17) Mazess, R.B.: On aging bone loss. Clin. Orthop., 165:239-252, 1982.

18) Arnold, J.S.: Amount and quality of trabecular bone in osteoporotic vertebral fractures. Clin. in Endoc. and Metab., 2:221-238, 1973.

19) Weaver, J., Chalmer, J.: Cancellous bone. Its strength and changes with aging and evaluation of some methods of measuring of its mineral content. I: Age changes in cancellous bone. J. Bone Jt. Surg., 48-A, 289-298,1966.

20) Riggs, B., Wahner, H., Dunn, W., Mazess, R., Offord, K., Melton, L.: Differential changes in bone mineral density of the appendicular and axial skeleton with aging: relationship to spinal osteoporosis. J. Clin. Invest. 67:328-335, 1981.

21) Meunier, P., Courpron, P., Edouard, C., Bernard, J., Bringuier, J., Vignon, G. Physiological senile involution and pathological rarefaction of bone. Quantitative and comparative histological data. Clinics in Endocrinol. Metabolism 2:239-256, 1973.

22) Leitch, I., Aitken, F.: The estimation of calcium requirements: reexamination. Nutr. Abstr. Rev., 29:393-411, 1959.

23) Carroll, M., Abraham, S., Dresser, C.: Dietary Intake Source Data: United States, 1976-1980. Vital and Health Statistics 11, No. 231, DHHS Pub. No. (PHS) 83-1681. National Center for Health Statistics, Public Health Services. Washington, D.C.: U.S. Government Printing Office, March 1983.

24) Krebs, J., Schneider, V., Smith, J., LeBlanc, A., Thornton, W., Leach, C.: Sweat calcium loss during running. FASEB J. 2:4667A, 1988.

25) Heaney, R.P. Personal Communication, 1986.

26) Sandler, R., Slemenda, C., LaPorte, R., Cauley, J., Schramm, M., Baresi, M., Kriska, A.M.: Postmenopausal bone density and milk consumption in childhood and adolescence. Am. J. Clin. Nutr., 42:270-274, 1985.

27) Nordin, B.E.C.: Osteomalacia, osteoporosis, and calcium deficiency. Clin. Orthop. 17:235, 1960.

28) Matkovic, V.: Influence of age, sex, and nutrition on the bone of rats. Master of Science Thesis. University of Zagreb, Zagreb, 1974.

29) Matkovic, V., Dekanic, D., Kostial, K.: Calcium, Teenagers, and Osteoporosis. In: Osteoporosis: Current Concepts. Report of the Seventh Ross Conference on Medical Research, Ross Labs, Columbus, Ohio, p 64-66, 1987.

30) Leighton, G., Clark, M.L.: Milk consumption and growth of school children. Lancet 1:40, 1929.

31) Garn, S., Clark, D.: Nutrition, Growth, Development, and Maturation: Findings from the Ten-State Nutrition Survey of 1968-1970. Pediatrics, 56: 306-319, 1975.

32) Ashworth, A., Millward, D.: Catch-up Growth in Children. Nutrition Reviews, 44:157-175, 1986.

33) Chan, G., Hess, M., Hollis, J., Book, L.S.: Bone Mineral Status in Childhood Accidental Fractures. A.J.D.C., 138:569-570, 1984.

34) Heaney, R., Gallagher, J., Johnston, C., Neer, R., Parfitt, A., Whedon, D.: Calcium nutrition and bone health in the elderly. Am. J. Clin. Nutrit. 36:986-1013, 1982.

Discussion:

DR. RAISZ (Connecticut): I wasn't clear about the genetic inheritance of bone mass versus bone density. In other words, if you do bone density measurements either on the forearm or the spine, is there a genetic component to that, as opposed to size of the individual, which I would guess is clearly genetic?

DR. MATKOVIC (Columbus, OH): Size is certainly under genetic influence because we had also bone size parameters in the same relationship. The question is how much you can exclude the effect of bone size on density measurements by single photon and dual photon absorptiometry techniques.

DR. RAISZ: With respect to dual photon, if you measured grams per cm^2 in the lumbar spine, can you say anything about the relative heritability of that from the mother or the father of the daughter, or is there any heritability of that figure?

DR. MATKOVIC: As far as I can say, there is a relationship between the father's values and mother's values and daughter's values at the lumbar spine. The heritability seems to be equal.

DR. RAISZ: It's not more from one parent than the other?

DR. MATKOVIC: I don't believe so.

DR. CHESNUT (Seattle): Both parents gave more significance than either parent alone.

DR. LANG (New Haven): I have two comments and a question. First, regarding the genetic studies, certainly the children are eating the same food that the parents are eating, so nutrition is going to affect those outcomes. Are there any data on twins reared separately?

DR. MATKOVIC: That's the problem when you are doing short-term vertical comparison studies. The longitudinal study over 30 years will certainly solve the problem. I do believe that nutrition influences bone mass formation during the bone growth, so we have to know what was the parents' nutrition during the bone formation.

DR. LANG: Another question or comment about nutrition. Certainly, there are other things in bone besides calcium. And I have a concern, because 20 years ago, very few of us were recommending calcium. And my patients would come back from the health food store where they were being told to take calcium and I would tell them it wasn't any good. Now, they're coming back, being told to take magnesium with their calcium. Do you have any data on magnesium?

DR. MATKOVIC: No, I don't have. We did magnesium balance as well, but did not supplement girls in the study with magnesium.

DR. RIGGS (Rochester, MN): I might just add, at some of the health food stores there's also lead in some of the compounds. So, you have to be careful what you buy.

DR. KLEEREKOPER (Detroit): Is there a level of calcium supplements where you can saturate the beneficial effect on the skeleton, or the more you give, the greater the benefit, and keep going up?

DR. MATKOVIC: When we did our calcium balances, we went to 1700 milligrams/day of calcium intake. So, at that point, we did not see a plateau.

DR. KLEEREKOPER: You did not see a plateau at 1700?

DR. MATKOVIC: No.

DR. KLEEREKOPER: So, you'd expect at 2000 you'd get even better response?

DR. MATKOVIC: It could be that calcium retention will increase, but that is pure speculation.

DR. KLEEREKOPER: And would you care to say something about how we should take our calcium? Should it be milk? Should it be tablets? Should it be coated on our cereal?

DR. MATKOVIC: Well, my recommendation certainly is milk, but if someone cannot tolerate milk I will recommend calcium tablets.

DR. DEQUEKER (Belgium): There is a secular trend in the stature of our teenagers after the Second World War. They get taller, bigger, and they have, also, a larger bone mass. Do you think that the calcium intake changed after the War compared to those before the War and during the War?

DR. MATKOVIC: I don't know. There could be a relationship.

Preserving Strong Bones: The Young Adult Female

BARBARA L. DRINKWATER

Department of Medicine
Pacific Medical Center
Seattle, WA

Investigators may disagree on the exact age when cortical or cancellous bone mass begins to decline in the adult female but there is general agreement that failure to achieve one's maximal potential bone mass during the young adult years is a risk factor for osteoporotic fractures in the future. The observation that some groups, such as males and blacks, have a greater peak mass than women or whites and a lower incidence of osteoporotic fractures suggests that the more bone one can accumulate before the decline in bone mass begins, the longer one may delay the consequences of age-related osteopenia. Since there is a genetic component to the maximal bone mass one can attain, not all women will be equally successful in reaching levels presumed to be protective. However, all women can make changes in their lifestyle that will make the most of their own potential to maximize bone mass and also minimize bone loss as they age.

Factors which affect bone mass can be divided into those which have a negative effect and those which have a positive effect on bone. Among the negative factors listed as risks for osteoporosis are excessive use of alcohol, coffee, and tobacco. While there is no evidence that avoidance of these factors either directly or indirectly affects bone mass during the premenopausal years, all three are frequently found in the medical histories of osteoporotic women.

Variables which have been shown to have a positive effect on bone mass are: 1) maintenance of a normal menstrual cycle, 2) an adequate calcium intake, and 3) increasing one's physical activity. All three factors are important. The lack of any one factor cannot be completely compensated for by increasing the other two. For example, complete inactivity such as bed rest will result in a rapid and marked decrease in bone mass regardless of normal hormone levels or adequate calcium intake. Under more normal circumstances the relative contribution of each factor in maintaining bone mass is not known.

When endogenous estrogen levels in young adult women are decreased following bilateral oophorectomy (1), premature ovarian failure (2), or as a result of hyperprolactinemia (3) there is a concomitant decrease in bone mineral density (BMD) at radial and/or vertebral sites. Regardless of age, it appears that normal levels of estrogen, as represented by the cyclic changes during a normal menstrual cycle, are neccessary for maintenance of bone mass. Decreased endogenous estrogen as a result of pathology is beyond a woman's control, but other conditions leading to similar low levels of estrogen are not. A number of recent studies have reported that the secondary amenorrhea associated with anorexia nervosa or strenuous exercise also results in osteopenia of the lumbar vertebrae (2, 4-8). The lumbar BMD of amenorrheic athletes, for example, averages about 84% that of eumenorrheic controls. The prolonged and intense training regimens of these hypoestrogenic female athletes does not protect them from significant bone loss in spite of their youth.

Both current menstrual status and prior menstrual history appear to have a significant effect on a woman's bone density. When 95 active young women, mean age 27.6 years, were categorized by their present and past menstrual patterns, lumbar bone density was highest in women who had always had regular menstrual cycles (1.28 g/cm^2), lower in women who had had episodes of amenorrhea or oligomenorrhea interspersed with periods of regularity (1.18 g/cm^2), and lowest in those who were currently amenorrheic and had had previous episodes of amenorrhea or oligomenorrhea (1.05 g/cm^2) (unpublished data). A significant negative relationship (r=-0.46, p<0.001) was found between menstrual patterns ranked in terms of their potential estrogenic effect on bone and actual bone density of the lumbar vertebra. The greater the incidence and severity of the menstrual irregularities, the lower the bone density.

Of considerable interest to investigators and to the athletes themselves is the question of whether bone loss can be reversed if normal menses is resumed. Both our group (9) and Lindberg et al. (10) did indeed report an increase in vertebral BMD of 6.3% and 6.7% respectively over a 14 month period after previously amenorrheic women had resumed menses. However, this increase may be limited. We have followed five of our original amenorrheic group over a period of four years since they resumed menses. Lumbar BMD continued to increase during the second year of normal menstrual cycles (+3.2%) but then plateaued over the following two years. Whether a similar pattern would be observed in a larger group of former amenorrheics remains to be seen. However, the significant role of menstrual history in predicting current BMD plus the pattern of changes in lumbar BMD of these five women would suggest that bone lost during periods of decreased endogenous estrogen production may not be completely regained.

Although the etiology of exercise-associated amenorrhea is not yet well-defined, most young athletes regain normal cycles within two or three months when they decrease their training programs by about 10-15% and gain a few pounds. Cessation of menses may be an indication of overtraining. Athletic performance may actually improve by changes in the training regimen and the addition of more lean body mass. It is important to note that eumenorrheic athletes have a significantly higher bone mass than eumenorrheic sedentary women, demonstrating that the combination of normal estrogen levels plus exercise exerts a positive effect on bone. Exercise alone without adequate estrogen levels will not maintain bone mass in young adult women. Therefore, adjusting one's lifestyle to maintain a normal menstrual cycle is one way to prevent premature loss of bone.

CALCIUM

The role of calcium in preserving bone is controversial. Most studies examining the relationship of calcium intake to bone mass have been in the postmenopausal age group. There is almost no data describing the role of calcium in maintaining bone mass during the young adult years. A study by Matkovic et al. (11) did cover a wide age range in describing how differences in calcium intake in two discrete populations affected both peak bone mass and subsequent fractures. Yugoslavian men and women who lived in a high calcium intake district had a higher bone mass by age 30 than another group of Yugoslavians living in a low-intake region. The high-intake group also has a lower incidence of femoral neck fractures among older people. More recently, Sandler et al. (12) retrospectively analyzed milk consumption of older women when they were children and adolescents and reported that women who drank milk with every meal during those years had a higher radial bone density (~4%) as adults.

Using a more detailed retrospective dietary assessment, we examined the influence of daily calcium intake between ages 11 and 14 for a group of 38 eumenorrheic and 26 amenorrheic athletes. While this is preliminary data, the early results are intriguing. The lumbar BMD of the eumenorrheic women was the same regardless of their daily calcium intake as children. However, amenorrheic women who had a calcium intake above 1200 mg/day during those years had a lumbar BMD of 1.172 g/cm^2 compared to 1.042 g/cm^2 for amenorrheic women who had had less than 800 mg calcium per day. The same pattern was observed at the femoral neck. When the women were divided into the nine groups representing current menstrual status and prior menstrual history, there was a highly significant negative correlation (r=-0.73, p<0.001) between lumbar BMD and menstrual pattern for the women who had a low calcium intake during childhood but a much lower relationship for the 40 women who had a high childhood calcium intake (r=-0.324, p<0.05). Neither we nor Sandler et al. (12) found a relationship between current calcium consumption and bone mineral density.

A two year longitudinal study (unpublished data) examining the relationship of calcium intake to changes in bone density in a group of active young women suggests that calcium is indeed a threshold nutrient. Two groups of subjects increased calcium intake to 1500-1700 mg/day by adding either dairy products or a calcium supplement to their diet. A control group maintained their daily calcium intake at the RDA of 800 mg. At the end of two years all three groups had maintained their initial lumbar BMD. Increasing calcium intake to 1500 mg/day or above did not provide any additional benefit to the two experimental groups.

EXERCISE

An increase in physical activity has been shown to be effective in increasing bone mass in women across a wide age range. Female athletes between the ages of 20 to 40, for example, have approximately 10% greater bone density than sedentary women of the same age (4,9). Obervations such as these have led some investigators to suggest that exercise might actually prevent osteoporosis by maintaining bone density above the so-called fracture threshold during the postmenopausal years. However, the studies of amenorrheic athletes raise doubts about the efficacy of exercise in preserving bone in the absence of adequate estrogen levels. The potential of exercise as a prophylaxis for osteoporosis may depend upon a multitude of factors: 1) estrogen status of the individual, 2) genetic limitations to maximal bone mass, 3) risk for Type 1 or Type 2 osteoporotic fractures, 4) presence of other risk factors, and 5) adherence to a physically active lifestyle. There is no longer any doubt that young women with low levels of endogenous estrogen are at risk for premature bone loss. However, within a group of amenorrheic women those who do exercise regularly have a higher BMD than those who are sedentary (1, 5, 8). It appears that physical activity can exert a positive effect on bone even when estrogen levels are low. However, both groups of amenorrheic women, the active and sedentary, have a lower BMD than sedentary women with normal levels of estrogen. The women with the highest BMD are those who are active and who are eumenorrheic.

There have been numerous studies describing how various physiological systems respond to an increase in physical activity. The effect is most striking for those individuals who have previously led sedentary lives. The increase in cardio-respiratory fitness (VO_2max), for example, is much greater for the inactive person just beginning training than for the athlete seeking to improve an already above average aerobic capacity. Judging from bedrest studies, the skeletal system will respond in the same way. However, training studies also show that as training continues the rate of improvement decreases. Finally an upper limit, presumed to reflect one's biological potential, is reached and increasing the training stimulus does not result in additional improvement. One may expect the same response from bone. Sedentary women will increase BMD by increasing their activity levels, but that improvement will be limited by their genetic potential for peak bone mass.

Any gain in bone mass has potential benefits for the individual woman. The problem arises when women assume that increasing BMD through exercise is an alternative to hormone replacement therapy at menopause. At this time there is no evidence that exercise can maintain bone at premenopausal levels. One would be particularly concerned for those women whose skeletal system is particularly susceptible to the abrupt decrease in estrogen levels following menopause and are at risk for early postmenopausal osteoporosis (Type I).

Maintaining an active lifestyle may be most beneficial in preventing the hip fractures typical of Type II or senile osteoporosis. A 5% difference in bone mass between active and sedentary women may postpone a potential hip fracture for an additional ten years in the active group. There are other advantages totally unrelated to bone mass. Active older people have better neuromuscular control, greater strength and flexibility, and better balance. They are less likely to fall and better able to protect themselves if they should fall.

There are, however, a number of unanswered questions about exercise as a means of preserving bone mass in young women. Exercise is quantified in terms of frequency, duration, and intensity and prescribed accordingly. A major difficulty in recommending exercise as a means of maximizing bone mass is that no one knows what type of exercise to suggest or how to quantify it. If female athletes have only a 10% advantage over sedentary women, is the amount of activity necessary to get a meaningful increase in bone mass beyond the capabilities of most women? Compliance is always a major problem in exercise programs. Can we really expect large numbers of women to undertake a strenuous conditioning program for a potential benefit 30 or 40 years in the future? Exercise may indeed be effective in increasing bone mass during the young adult years and attenuating its loss with age, but the threshold level for a beneficial effect must be reasonable or the likelihood of large numbers of women turning to exercise to protect their bones is minimal.

CONCLUSIONS

The most important factor in preserving bone mass during a woman's young adult years is maintenance of normal estrogen levels. Although exercise may attenuate the loss slightly (5,8), the bone mineral density of hypoestrogenic women will be significantly below that of their age group. Weightbearing physical activity and other forms of mechanical stress on bone are also essential. Total inactivity or weightlessness will both result in rapid bone loss in spite of normal estrogen levels and adequate calcium intake. However, the threshold level of activity required to preserve bone mass is unknown at this time. Women who enjoy physical activity and participate in it throughout life may have a 5-15% higher bone density than sedentary women when they reach menopause. The relative importance of calcium in preserving bone during the premenopausal adult years is not well defined. The role of calium may be most important in childhood and adolescence in ensuring that each woman attains her biological potential for peak bone mass. Techniques to maximize and perserve bone mass during the premenopausal years will be useful in reducing the incidence of osteoporosis in the general population and reducing health care costs only if they are accepted and used by large numbers of women.

REFERENCES

1. Cann CE, Genant HK, Ettinger B, Gordon GS 1980 Spinal mineral loss in oophorectomized women: Determination by quantitative computed tomography. JAMA 244: 2056-2059.
2. Klibanski A, Neer RM, Bettins IZ, Ridgway EC, Zervas NT. McArthur JW 1980 Decreased bone density in hyperprolactinemic women. N Engl J Med 303: 1511-1514.
3. Cann CE, Martin MC, Genant HK, Jaffe RB 1984 Decreased spinal mineral content in amenorrheic women, JAMA 251: 626-629.
4. Drinkwater BL, Nilson K, Chesnut CH III, Bremner WJ, Shainholtz S, Southworth MB 1984 Bone mineral content of amenorrheic and eumenorrheic athletes. N Engl J Med 311: 277-281.
5. Marcus R, Cann C, Madvig P, Minkoff J, Goddard M, Bayer M, Martin M, Gaudiani L, Haskell W, Genant H

1985 Menstrual function and bone mass in elite women distance runners. Ann Int Med 102: 158-163.
6. Lindberg JS, Fears WB, Hunt MM, Powell MR, Boll D, Wade C 1984 Exercise-induced amenorrhea and bone density. Ann Int Med 101:647-648.
7. Nelson ME, Fisher EC, Catsos PD, Meredith CN, Turksoy RN, Evans WJ 1986 Diet and bone status in amenorrheic runners. J Clin Nutr 43: 910-916.
8. Rigotti NA, Nussbaum SR, Herzog DB, Neer RM 1984 Osteoporosis in women with anorexia nervosa. N Engl J Med 311: 1601-1606.
9. Drinkwater BL, Nilson K, Ott S, Chesnut CH III 1986 Bone mineral density after resumption of menses in amenorrheic women. JAMA 256:380-382.
10. Lindberg JS, Powell MR, Hunt MM, Ducey DE, Wade CE 1987 Increased vertebral bone mineral in response to reduced exercise in amenorrheic runners. West J Med 146:39-42.
11. Matkovic V, Kostial K, Simonovic I, Buzina R, Broderac A, Nordin BEC 1979 Bone status and fracture rates in two regions in Yugoslavia. Am J Clin Nutr 32: 540-549.
12. Sandler RB, Slemenda CW, LaPorte RE, Cauley, JA, Schramm MM, Barresi ML, Kriska, AM. 1985 Postmenopausal bone density and milk consumption in childhood and adolescence. Am J Clin Nutr 42: 270-274.

Discussion:

DR. RIGGS (Rochester, MN): First, I might just say, Barbara, I don't know if you realize it, but you saved Dr. Genant's life. After he showed several of his slides with scantily-dressed young women as background decoration, several of the feminists in the audience were planning to strangle him at the lunch break. But, since you showed one too, I guess they'll put away their garrotes.

DR. MARCUS (Stanford): That was a wonderful presentation. I wanted to say something about the issue of type of exercise, because I think that in consideration of exercise and amenorrhea, it's clear that we're dealing with an open-circuit type of exercise, primarily aerobic training. I think that one has to consider the possibility that a different type of exercise might actually have a stronger impact on bone density, that is, in particular, resistance training.

In our study, that you so nicely cited, many of our women athletes were weight lifters, not just runners. And I think that that's a potential interaction which has not adequately been addressed.

I'd like to make one further comment on the issue of weight, because we have information that will be presented at ASBMR in a different population, a population of healthy seniors, men and women above the age of 65. We find that strength is a far more potent predictor of lumbar spine and mid-radius density than is weight, per se, in a group of subjects who are of normal weight. I certainly agree with your analysis that, when you lose weight to these almost anorexic levels, weight itself may be more important.

But I think that in a normal, healthy population, it may be that weight itself is more a surrogate for lean body mass, that is, muscle mass and strength, and that strength itself, since it's the muscles which are loading the skeleton, may be a more potent predictor of bone density.

DR. DRINKWATER (Seattle): Yes, Bob, I think you're right there. I think when you're talking about strength in the older population, you're definitely talking about muscle mass. And an older individual who has a higher muscle mass has got to be someone who has been more active and is more active. So, you have an interaction there, not only with muscle mass/body weight, but also previous exercise history and current exercise history.

In terms of the type of exercise, exercise physiologists have a law called the law of specificity. And that means that you only get the benefit from that part of the body that you are exercising. So, yes, weightbearing activity may be fine on the axial skeleton in the lower legs. But if we're going to be concerned, also, about the arms, some type of resistance training for that area of the skeleton is also important.

DR. BERGMANN (Belgium): Do you have data on bone turnover parameters in the amenorrheic athletes? Do they have an increased bone turnover rate as in the postmenopausal period?

DR. DRINKWATER: I'm sorry, we do not have, at this time, information on bone turnover rates.

Optimizing Bone Mass in the Perimenopause: Calcium

ROBERT P. HEANEY

Creighton University
Omaha, NE

INTRODUCTION

It is generally held that the amount of bone a woman has at age 65 or 75 is the resultant 1) of how much bone she has at time of menopause and 2) of how fast she loses bone after menopause. The closer she is to menopause, the stronger is the influence of peak bone mass, and the farther away, the stronger is the influence of rate of loss. Current evidence indicates that there are three principal factors determining bone mass at the time of menopause: 1) the woman's genetic endowment, 2) the amount of bone accumulated during growth, particularly during the second and third decades of life, and 3) the amount and character of the mechanical loading placed upon the skeleton during adult life. These factors are all covered in other papers in this symposium. Because they largely determine how much bone a woman will have at the time of menopause, to a very substantial extent therefore, they determine also what she will have 10, 20, or 30 years later.

There is little or no evidence that a woman can increase bone mass by very much after peak bone mass has been achieved, and so the emphasis in the perimenopause has to be on maintaining the bone mass she has. Specifically that means preventing loss due to controllable factors. Estrogen loss at menopause is one such factor. Estrogen is the single most powerful factor in sustaining bone loss in the immediate perimenopausal period, and its protection is widely recognized. But this factor, too, is covered elsewhere in this volume. So my focus in this chapter will be on the role of nutritional deficiency and on steps that can be taken to minimize its effects - not as a cure-all for osteoporosis or as a substitute for other factors - but as one controllable component of the complex dynamic changes that are occurring in the bone of women at this age.

COMPONENTS OF AGE-RELATED BONE LOSS

There are four identifiable components to the bone loss which is occurring in the perimenopausal period. First is an inexorable, age-related loss which consists in part of topological remodeling errors and which is probably the counterpart of the corresponding decrease in lean body mass which is recognized to occur in senescence. Its magnitude is not known with certainty, but can be estimated to be in the range of 0.2-0.4 percent per year. Although there is some uncertainty about precisely when this loss begins, it is probably not significant before age 35-40. This loss is likely proportional to bone mass and is thus probably exponential.

Table I. Components of Age-related Bone Loss

Cause	Characteristics	Magnitude
gonadal hormone loss	exponential, involving c. 15% of total bone mass	c. 25%/yr
senescence	probably exponential	0.2-0.4%/yr
Ca deficiency	linear	0-1.5%/yr
Other	variable	variable

The second is the loss due to estrogen deficiency. Most studies indicate that this loss is exponential (or some similar formulation) (1,2), and still unpublished analyses by Professor B.E.C. Nordin from the database of his large Adelaide cohort study (3), indicate that the amount of bone affected by estrogen withdrawal is roughly 15 percent of the total skeletal mass, and that the rate constant for loss of that component is about 25 percent per year.

The third component is variable from woman-to-woman, and is due to calcium deficiency, either because calcium intake is low, or because calcium utilization is inefficient, or because endogenous calcium losses are high. Estimates based on data from balance studies performed in our laboratory at Creighton suggest values for bone loss due to this factor in the range of 0 to 1.5 percent per year (4). This loss is linear and is dependent upon extraosseous factors, not on the mass of the skeleton.

Finally there is a group of important, but variable factors including decreased mechanical loading (inactivity), alcohol abuse, smoking, comorbidity, medications taken for a variety of reasons (ranging from corticosteroids to aluminum-containing antacids), and other, as yet inadequately characterized factors, including possibly certain trace elements such as manganese, copper, zinc, and boron (5,6). These four factors are summarized in Table I.

Table II. Bone Mass and Partition of Bone Lost at Varying Ages After Menopause at Age 50

Age	Bone Mass*	Age	Loss due to: Est. def.	Ca def.
10 mg/day Ca deficiency loss				
50	100	--	--	--
55	85.3	1.7	10.7	2.3
60	78.3	3.3	13.8	4.6
65	73.5	4.9	14.6	6.9
70	69.4	6.5	14.9	9.2
75	65.4	8.1	15.0	11.5
80	61.6	9.6	15.0	13.8
20 mg/day Ca deficiency loss				
50	100	--	--	--
55	83.0	1.7	10.7	4.6
60	73.7	3.3	13.8	9.2
65	66.6	4.9	14.6	13.8
70	60.2	6.5	14.9	18.4
75	53.9	8.1	15.0	23.0
80	47.8	9.6	15.0	27.6

*Initial bone mass at age 50 set to 100 units.

The first three can be put together in the form of the following equation:

$$M_t = M_m(.15e^{-.25t} + .85e^{-at}) - dt$$

in which M_t = mass at t years after menopause, M_m = mass at time of menopause, t = years since menopause, a = the exponent for the age-related, inexorable loss of senescence, and d = the coefficient of loss for calcium deficiency.

This equation constitutes a model of age-related bone loss which is consistent with the best information currently available, and which allows an integrated simulation of the effects of these various factors and estimation of their relative contributions to bone loss at various times after menopause.

Table II, for example, presents the data for a menopausal woman with an assumed age-related, inexorable loss of 0.4 percent per year and for two calcium deficiency rates, 0.46 and 0.92 percent per year (amounting to 10 mg and 20 mg/day negative balance, respectively). It sets forth relative contributions of the three sources at ages 50 to 80 (assuming, for purposes of the simulation, that menopause occurred at age 50). Table III presents the same data for the situation in which menopause has been effectively delayed for 10 years by estrogen replacement therapy (ERT) to age 60. (For simplicity's sake, I have assumed in the simulation presented in Table III that the calcium deficiency coefficient is not influenced by estrogen status, which is probably not entirely correct.)

Table III. Bone Mass and Partition of Bone Lost at Varying Ages After Menopause for Estrogen Replacement Through Age 60

			Loss due to:	
Age	Bone Mass*	Age	Est. def.	Ca def.

10 mg/d Ca-deficiency loss

Age	Bone Mass*	Age	Est. def.	Ca def.
50	100	--	--	--
55	96.0	1.7	--	2.3
60	92.1	3.3	--	4.6
65	78.4	4.8	9.9	6.9
70	71.7	6.4	12.7	9.2
75	67.2	7.9	13.5	11.5
80	63.2	9.3	13.7	13.8

20 mg/d Ca-deficiency loss

Age	Bone Mass*	Age	Est. def.	Ca def.
50	100	--	--	--
55	93.7	1.7	--	4.6
60	87.5	3.3	--	9.2
65	72.1	4.8	9.4	13.8
70	63.3	6.3	12.0	18.4
75	56.6	7.6	12.8	23.0
80	50.3	9.1	13.0	27.6

Initial bone mass at age 50 set to 100 units.

The data in these tables show very clearly the important effect on age-related bone loss of even a modest calcium deficiency. Only 10 mg/day negative balance due to calcium deficiency will, by age 75, account for slightly more than one-third of all bone lost to that age, and will have produced nearly 80 percent as much bone loss as estrogen deficiency. And with a 20 mg/day loss, calcium deficiency accounts for 50 percent more bone loss than does estrogen deficiency.

While clearly contributing significantly over the long haul, the calcium deficiency component is relatively much smaller than the estrogen deficiency component in the first few years after menopause. This is because the estrogen deficiency loss is rapid but limited, while the calcium deficiency component is slow but continuous. This simulation also shows forcefully how the estrogen effect is most prominent in the *young* elderly, and is less prominent later on. Even with 10 years of ERT, bone mass at age 75 is only 2 percent higher than without ERT (Tables II and III).

THE EVIDENCE IN REGARD TO CALCIUM

The relative magnitudes of the estrogen deficiency and calcium deficiency components in the early postmenopausal years explain why, in studies performed in women at that age, the effect of calcium deficiency or of calcium supplementation has been found to be less striking than the effect of estrogen replacement therapy in the same women. That, coupled with the fact that not all women are calcium deficient, probably also explains why controversy has arisen in recent years over whether calcium is as important as it had appeared to be at the time of the 1984 NIH Consensus Conference on Osteoporosis (7).

The foregoing analysis makes clear, however, that calcium *is* important, and in fact this conclusion is consistent with the vast majority of cross-sectional, longitudinal, and intervention trials of the effect of calcium on bone mass and bone loss, summarized in a recent review (8). This evidence shows clearly that there is a calcium deficiency component to postmenopausal bone loss in most groups of First World women.

Three intervention trials are worth citing in that regard. A recent report from Denmark (9), widely interpreted in the public media as showing no effect of calcium, is particularly noteworthy. In brief, recently postmenopausal Danish women, receiving a basal intake averaging nearly 1000 mg Ca/day, when given additional calcium, were nevertheless able to reduce loss of diaphyseal (but not metaphyseal or vertebral) bone. The effect was not as striking as the protection conferred by estrogen, but that is hardly surprising, for the estrogen-treated women had all been estrogen-deprived prior to estrogen replacement, while the average basal calcium intake of the women given a calcium supplement had been high by U.S. standards even before supplementation. This study actually showed that an average intake of 1000 mg/day was not sufficient to assure that calcium deficiency would not be contributing to age-related bone loss in some members of the population. The findings of this study are, in fact, entirely consistent with the data from balance studies of postmenopausal women (8), which show that estrogen-deprived early postmenopausal women need calcium intakes in the range of 1500 mg/day.

My colleagues and I at Creighton, in work published ten years before the Danish study, had found essentially the same results for calcium (i.e., protection against diaphyseal but not metaphyseal bone loss) in a similarly designed, randomized trial of estrogen and calcium supplementation (10).

The largest of the calcium intervention studies, just recently published (11), is from Nordin's Adelaide cohort study (3). It shows very clearly a striking cessation in postmenopausal bone loss in forearm bone in women supplemented with calcium in a randomized, placebo-controlled trial.

Thus, at the current state of our knowledge, we can safely conclude that calcium intakes in the range recommended by the National Institutes of Health (1000 mg/day for estrogen-replete perimenopausal women, and 1500 mg/day for estrogen-deprived women) are both safe and prudent. It is also quite clear that, while not all bone loss in postmenopausal women is due to calcium deficiency, some is. Since there are no clinical means for distinguishing women who have a calcium deficiency component to their bone loss from those who are losing bone predominantly for other reasons, it thus makes preeminently good sense to ensure calcium intakes in the range of the NIH recommendations for all perimenopausal and postmenopausal women.

This conclusion becomes particularly important for women who either cannot take estrogen replacement therapy (because, for example, of a family history of breast cancer), or who reasonably choose not to. For, with the inevitability of an estrogen deficiency loss component, they can ill afford a preventable calcium deficiency loss as well.

ASSURING AN ADEQUATE CALCIUM INTAKE

A very practical question immediately arises: what is the best strategy to assure calcium intakes in the recommended range? The answer, of course, is that there is no one best strategy. Still, foods have to be accounted the best source of calcium, both because lifetime compliance is much more likely from dietary sources than from continued, voluntary pill consumption, and second because foods contain many nutrients in addition to calcium, so they more readily provide total nutrition than can single-nutrient supplements. And third, single nutrient supplements are well known to produce imbalances of other nutrients (for example: calcium supplements commonly interfere with iron absorption); whereas that kind of imbalance rarely occurs with food sources.

Finally, foods are to be preferred over pills because calcium pills are regulated in the U.S. as food supplements, not as drugs, and hence they are not subject to the same type of quality control and governmental supervision as is required for drugs. Carr and Shangraw at the University of Maryland have shown clearly that many calcium supplements are so poorly formulated that they do not disintegrate significantly on ingestion, and therefore do not make their calcium available to the body (12). Most food sources, by contrast, have readily absorbable calcium. The richest of these, in the North American diet, are dairy products. While the American Heart Association's "Prudent Diet" limits intake of dairy products, this is quite unnecessary for the vast majority of women. The AHA's concern is for fat intake. But the low fat yogurts and liquid milks can be ingested without limit, and even the fat-rich cheeses can be substituted for other allowed fat sources.

We have accumulated extensive experience in our laboratory at Creighton with the absorbability of calcium from mixed food sources, and find values ranging from 25 to 35 percent absorption in perimenopausal women. This is precisely the same value that we find for isolated dairy products, such as milk, cheese, and yogurt (13). Hence, it is likely that most food sources exhibit absorbability comparable to dairy products. Spinach is a notable exception. Its calcium absorbability is less than 5 percent (14), and most individuals would attribute this poor availability to the presence of oxalic acid in spinach, a substance which is known to form a highly insoluble salt of calcium. By contrast, vegetables such as bok choy, kale, and broccoli, and leafy vegetables such as turnip, beet, and mustard greens, are all good sources of calcium, and have little or no oxalic acid. They have not been explicitly tested in humans, as has spinach, and so one cannot say for certain what their absorbability may be, but small animal nutrition studies indicate that their calcium is probably quite available, and hence that they do not suffer from the same problem as spinach.

Calcium-fortified foods, recently introduced into the market, promise to add significant variety to the types of calcium sources available to the North American consumer. The decrease in total nutrient intake that has occurred in North American society in the last 50 years has resulted in a significant decline in intake of many important nutrients, calcium being only one of them. It becomes an important nutritional strategy, therefore, to increase the nutrient density of various items in the food chain to compensate for decrease in total nutrient intake. Well-recognized examples of this stratagem are the iodination of salt, the enrichment of white bread flour with iron and certain B vitamins, and the fortification of milk with vitamins A and D. Some of this is voluntary, and some mandated by both state and federal laws.

Because it is unlikely that calcium fortification will be required in this country (though calcium fortification of white bread flour *is* mandated in the United Kingdom), we are likely to see only instances of voluntary calcium fortification. Initially stimulated at least in part by commercial motives, such fortification could, nevertheless, become the industry standard, as is now the case with the nearly universal iodination of table salt and vitamin D fortification of both liquid and powdered milks.

One good, recent example of significant calcium enrichment of an already excellent food is calcium fortification of orange juice. Orange juice is regularly consumed by a large fraction of American adults, and is a good alternative beverage for individuals who do not drink liquid milk. At least two orange juice producers have marketed calcium-fortified citrus juices, and one of them (Citrus Hill Plus Calcium®), has been shown to have calcium absorbability at least as good as milk (15). (The other has not, to my knowledge, yet been tested in humans.) Another is the addition of a whey mineral concentrate (MinraLac®) to cottage cheese, thereby greatly improving the calcium content of this otherwise excellent food so often favored by diet-conscious women.

Finally, calcium supplement pills, though strategically less attractive than food sources, will nevertheless be widely used, and are an important component of the therapy of established osteoporosis (where the required calcium intakes will be difficult to achieve from food sources in many cases). As already noted, this is a market in which the ethic of *caveat emptor* is dominant. Preference has to given to sources that disintegrate readily and that have proven bioavailability. Shangraw has recently reviewed his work in this regard, with emphasis dominantly on the calcium carbonate preparations now on the market, and his review can be consulted for product-specific information (16).

REFERENCES

1. Johnston CC Jr, Hui SL, Wiske P, Norton JA Jr, and Epstein S. Bone mass at maturity and subsequent rates of loss as determinants of osteoporosis, pp. 285-291. In: *Osteoporosis: Recent Advances in Pathogenesis and Treatment.* DeLuca HF, Frost HM, Jee WSS, Johnston CC Jr, and Parfitt AM (eds). University Park Press, Baltimore, 1981.

2. Gallagher JC, Goldgar D, and Moy A. Total bone calcium in normal women: effect of age and menopause status. *J Bone Mineral Res* 1987;2:491-496.

3. Nordin BEC and Polley KJ. The Adelaide bone loss risk factor survey. *Calcif Tissue Int* 1987;41:S1-59.

4. Heaney RP, Recker RR, and Saville PD. Calcium balance and calcium requirements in middle-aged women. *Am J Clin Nutr* 1977;30:1603-1611.

5. Heaney RP. Nutritional factors in bone health. In: *Osteoporosis: Etiology, Diagnosis, and Management,* pp. 359-372. Riggs BL and Melton LJ III (eds). Raven Press, New York, 1988.

6. Nielsen FH, Hunt CD, Mullen LM, and Hunt JR. Effect of dietary boron on mineral, estrogen, and testosterone metabolism in postmenopausal women. *Proc Soc Exp Biol Med* 1987;1(5):394-397.

7. Consensus Conference, Osteoporosis. *JAMA* 1984;252:799-802.

8. Heaney RP. The calcium controversy: A middle ground between the extremes. *Public Health Reports* 1988 (in press).

9. Riis B, Thomsen K, and Christiansen C. Does calcium supplementation prevent postmenopausal bone loss? *N Engl J. Med* 1987;316:173-177.

10. Recker RR, Saville PD, and Heaney RP. The effect of estrogens and calcium carbonate on bone loss in postmenopausal women. *Ann Intern Med* 1977;87:649-655.

11. Polley KJ, Nordin BEC, Baghurst PA, Walker CJ, and Chatterton BE. Effect of calcium supplementation on forearm bone mineral content in postmenopausal women: a prospective, sequential controlled trial. *J Nutr* 1987;117:1929-1935.

12. Carr CJ and Shangraw R. Nutritional and pharmaceutical aspects of calcium supplementation. *Am Pharmacy* 1987;NS27(2);49-57.

13. Recker RR, Bammi A, Barger-Lux J, and Heaney RP. Calcium absorbability from milk products, an imitation milk, and calcium carbonate. *Am J Clin Nutr* 1988;47:93-95.

14. Heaney RP, Weaver CM, and Recker RR. Absorbability of calcium from spinach. *Am J Clin Nutr* 1988;47(4):707-709.

15. Smith KT, Heaney RP, Flora L, and Hinders S. Calcium absorption from a new calcium delivery system (CCM). *Calcif Tissue Int* 1987;42:351-352.

16. Shangraw R. Factors to consider in the selection of a calcium supplement. *Public Health Reports* 1988 (in press).

Discussion:

DR. KHAIRI (Indianapolis): I'd like you to comment whether the dose of 1500 milligrams supplement for women -- is there a difference if we give it in three doses, or one dose or two doses?

DR. HEANEY (Omaha): There is a pretty good body, but not entirely solid body, of evidence that suggests that absorption is better in three doses than in one. And, if I had to guess right now, that's where I'd put my money.

DR. PARFITT (Detroit): Hegsted recently analyzed some epidemiologic data, making comparisons between countries, which suggested to him that there was a positive correlation between the average dietary consumption of calcium in a country and the hip fracture risk in that country. How can you reconcile that with the benefits of calcium within a single community that you are suggesting?

DR. HEANEY: Well, when one goes across different countries with different food intake patterns and different exercise patterns, it's extremely difficult, as you know, to try to track that kind of nutritional information. I alluded very briefly to the importance to the obligatory calcium losses as one of the components of calcium deficiency, but didn't have the time to talk about that.

Both Nordin's data in Leeds and Adelaide and our data in Omaha show very clearly that there is a better correlation between obligatory calcium loss and bone mass than there is between calcium intake and bone mass. But, of course, they're all components of this calcium balance question.

And North American women, at least, have very high obligatory calcium losses, in the range of 180 milligrams per day, which is about the lowest the average a postmenopausal woman can cut her excretion. That's a very significant problem. And that clearly is not true in some Third World countries, for example.

DR. JOHNSTON (Indianapolis): Your model certainly is an interesting one, Bob. And I presume that the calcium deficiency that you show would include the added burden placed on it by malabsorption.

One thing that's always been a bit puzzling is why one doesn't see the senescent loss in the two long-term estrogen replacement studies, Bob Lindsay's and Nachtigall's. Even though many of those women were younger when they started, I think they still should have extended into that area. And we don't seem to see any loss on estrogen replacement for 10 to 13 years.

DR. HEANEY: Thank you for your comment. I think the Lindsay data do show a senescent loss, as a matter of fact. When they reach about the age you would expect, those numbers begin to decline. But the problem with it is that you begin to lose numbers out of the cohort. So, when you begin to compare mean values at subsequent data points, you have different "n's" and you don't know where those same individuals were at earlier points. So, I don't know the answer to that question.

But I think you do see that senescent loss. The problem is, four-tenths of a percent per year is not very much. You have to see it cumulatively, as you know.

DR. BELL (Charleston): We've observed an interesting phenomenon, Bob, and I wondered if you had seen it. We've done balance studies in adolescents and young adults. And what we found is that, if we increase the calcium intake from 400 to 1000 milligrams a day, we see an expected decrease in serum 1,25 dihydroxy vitamin D. In these individuals, we've increased the calcium intake further to 1600 milligrams a day. And in a number of individuals, we see that the serum 1,25 levels stay down and it doesn't improve the calcium balance very much.

But in some individuals, when we go to the higher intake, 1,25 levels go back up again and we see a more positive calcium balance. So, it looks to be biphasic in individuals. And I wondered if you'd seen that phenomenon in any of the balance studies that you conducted at your place?

DR. HEANEY: Those are fascinating observations. We haven't looked at that end of the age spectrum. I'll look forward to talking with you about them. There's some interesting peculiarities about the 1,25 response that I don't thoroughly understand. But I know Munro Peacock has thought about these issues for some time and has some interesting thoughts on that matter.

DR. HARRIS (San Francisco): In your list of considerations about various calcium supplements, you mentioned the safety of the accompanying anion. Would you like to comment upon any implications of the different anions?

DR. HEANEY: Well, very frankly, I don't know that there is any significant risk there. But we need to bear in mind that, if we're talking about a lifetime therapy to get a gram of calcium into somebody's body every day, we're getting a lot more of the accompanying anion than we are of the calcium. And for preparations, such as, say, calcium citrate, for which I have no particular information one way or the other, what are we dealing with? About 13 percent calcium by weight, so that you are getting, roughly, seven times as much citrate as you are getting calcium.

I don't have any reason to think that that's going to be particularly harmful. But somebody needs to look at this issue, whether that kind of a chronic high anion intake is entirely safe.

Optimizing Bone Mass in the Perimenopause: Estrogen

CLAUS CHRISTIANSEN and BENTE JUEL RIIS

Department of Clinical Chemistry
Glostrup Hospital
University of Copenhagen
Glostrup, Denmark

Introduction
In 1900, the average life expectancy of women in the Western world was below 50 years; today, it is 79 years. In the same period, the average age at the menopause has virtually remained unchanged. As we live longer, age-related diseases become an increasing problem, as do diseases related to the menopause. Osteoporosis is a prime example. It is characterized by an age-related and especially a menopause-related universal, gradual, and relentless reduction in bone mass. This loss compromises the mechanical competence of the skeleton to such an extent that even minor trauma may result in fracture. Figure 1 illustrates the decrease in bone mass and increase in fracture incidence as a function of age in women and demonstrates the rapid rise in fracture incidence that begins in the fourth decade in women. Figure 2 shows the distribution of fractures sustained after the menopause, and caused by minor traumas, in a Danish population of 70-year old women. More than 40% of women of that age have had a fracture attributable to low bone mass (1). The three main fracture sites associated with osteoporosis are the vertebrae (particularly lower thoracic and lumbar), distal radius (Colles' fracture), and, by far the most serious, femoral neck fracture (transcervical and intertrochanteric), but other sites may be affected.
The magnitude of the public health problem posed by osteoporosis is substantial. In the United States, there are about 210,000 femoral neck fractures each year (2), and approximately 20% of patients die within 3 months (3), i.e., the deaths are attributable to fracture complications. Figure 3 shows a cross-section of the distal part of the radius in an osteoporotic and non-osteoporotic person. It is clear that the osteoporotic bone has not only lost bone mass, but also the original architecture. Obviously, no kind of intervention will ever be able to restore the osteoporotic bone to its original non-osteoporotic state. It will therefore always be preferable to intervene before the damage has occurred.

Risk factors for developing osteoporosis
From a theoretical point of view there are two major important factors that are determining the risk of osteoporosis: peak bone mass and rate of bone loss. Peak bone mass is probably mostly determined by genetic factors (4), but environmental factors, such as diet (5) and exercise, may also play a role (6). Men have on the average a 20% higher peak bone mass than women (7). It is generally believed that both men and women start to lose bone mass some

Cumulated number of fractures and bone mineral content in women after the menopause

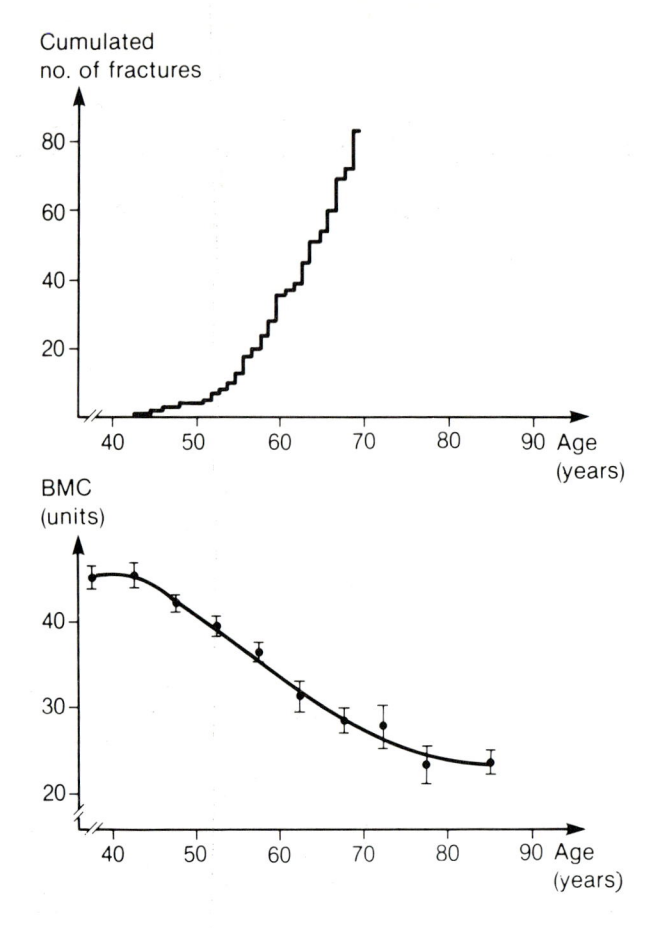

Figure 1
Cumulated number of fractures and bone mineral content (BMC) as a function of age in postmenopausal women.
(Copyright C Christiansen, used with permission).

time after peak bone mass has been reached (7-9). This loss is small (3-5% per decade) and has been compared with the age-related loss of other functions, such as muscle mass (7).
Figure 4 shows cross-sectional data on bone mass as a function of age in men and women. The bone mass is divided by total body potassium, which is an estimate of muscle mass. Compared with muscle mass, men and women have the same peak bone mass; men do not lose more bone mass than muscle mass.
In men this slow bone loss continues throughout life. The pathogenesis of the age-related bone loss is not clarified, and both genetic and environmental factors may play a role.
Whereas bone is lost at the same rate in men throughout life, in women it is accelerated in the years around the menopause (8-11). Figure 5 shows that the postmenopausal bone loss is independent of the age-related loss of muscle mass. All women are exposed to this accelerated bone loss, but the individual variation is wide (12). On the average, postmenopausal women lose approximately 2% of their bone mass a year, but more than a quarter of all postmenopausal women lose above 3% a year. The postmenopausal bone loss follows an exponential curve, and will thus level off after about 8 years (9,13). The pathogenesis of the postmenopausal bone loss is still not understood, although its close relation to female sex hormones is widely established. Re-

Prevalence of fractures in 70 years old females

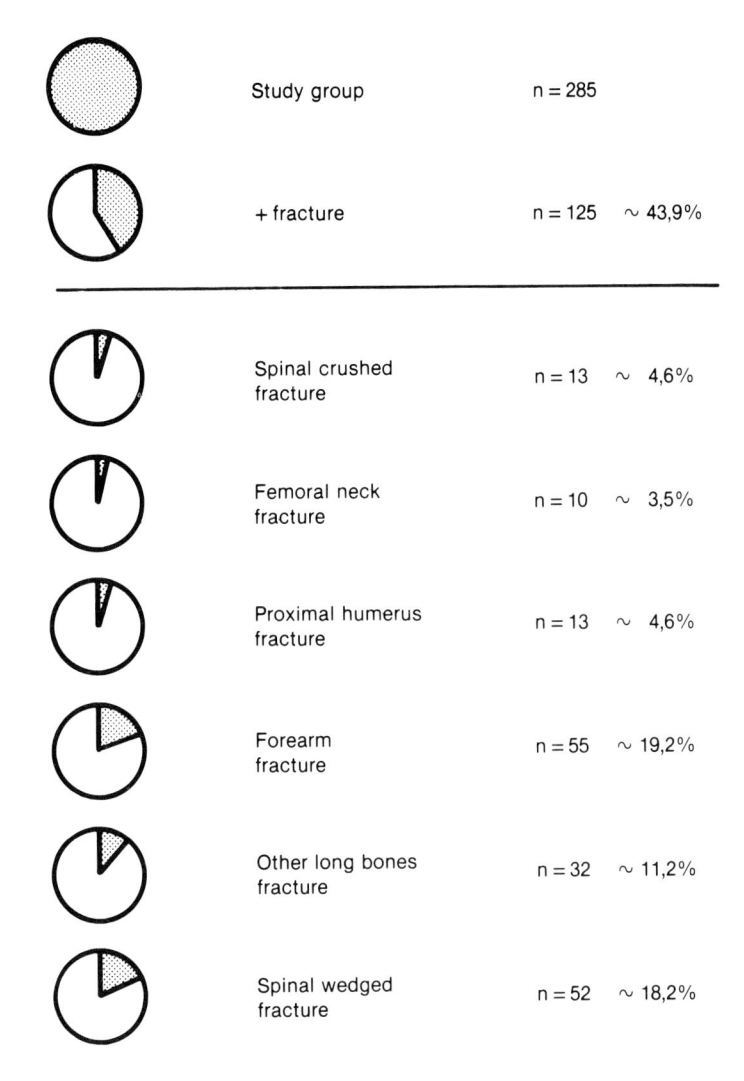

●	Study group	n = 285	
◓	+ fracture	n = 125	∼ 43,9%
○	Spinal crushed fracture	n = 13	∼ 4,6%
○	Femoral neck fracture	n = 10	∼ 3,5%
○	Proximal humerus fracture	n = 13	∼ 4,6%
◔	Forearm fracture	n = 55	∼ 19,2%
○	Other long bones fracture	n = 32	∼ 11,2%
◔	Spinal wedged fracture	n = 52	∼ 18,2%

Figure 2
Distribution of fracture occurring at the menopause as a result of minor traumas in a Danish population of 70-year old women.
(Copyright C Christiansen, used with permission).

cent studies have furthermore suggested that estrogens have a direct action on bone via estrogen-receptors (14,15).
The difference in peak bone mass and bone loss between men and women explains why osteoporosis is much more common in women than in men. The individual variation in both peak bone mass and in the postmenopausal bone loss may further explain why some, but not all women develop osteoporosis.

Preventive treatment?
It is now well established that the postmenopausal bone loss is prevented by estrogen replacement therapy (16,17). Other treatment modalities may be on their way (18). However, it does not seem to be cost effective to treat all postmenopausal women. A number of proposals have therefore been made to find an easy and inexpensive way to detect the women at risk.
It is obvious that the optimum and most expensive screening procedure is one

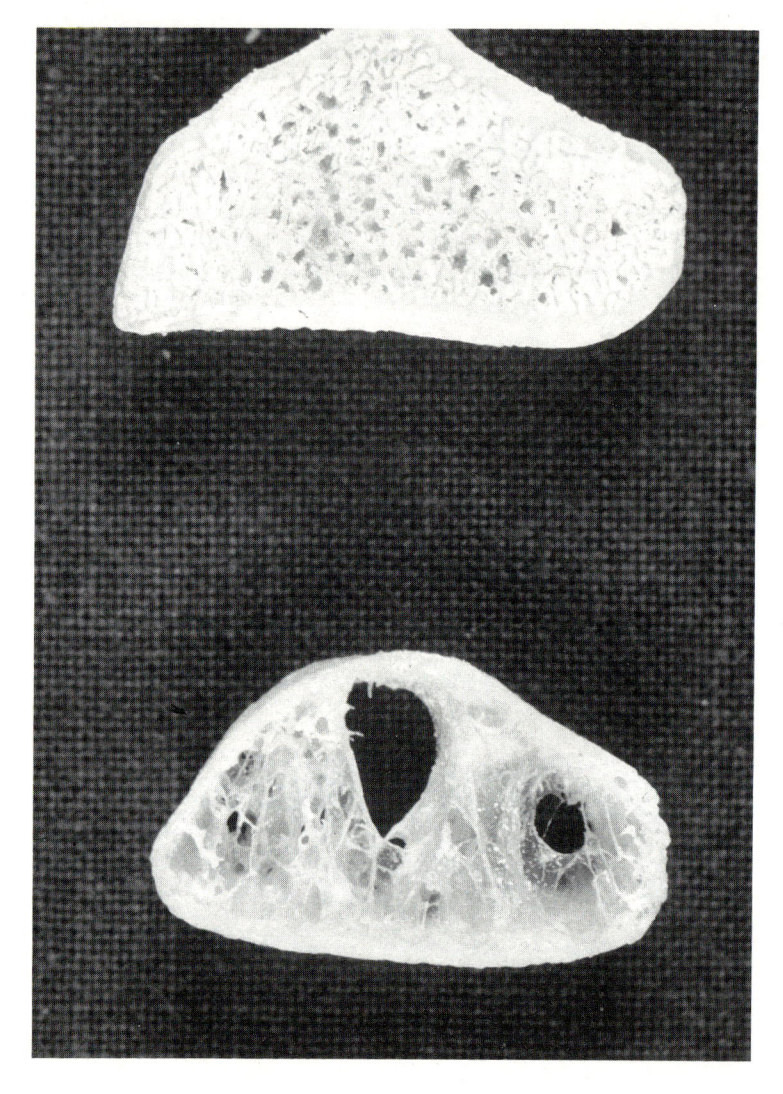

Figure 3
Cross-section of the distal part of the radius in an osteoporotic and non-osteoporotic person.
(Copyright C Christiansen, used with permission).

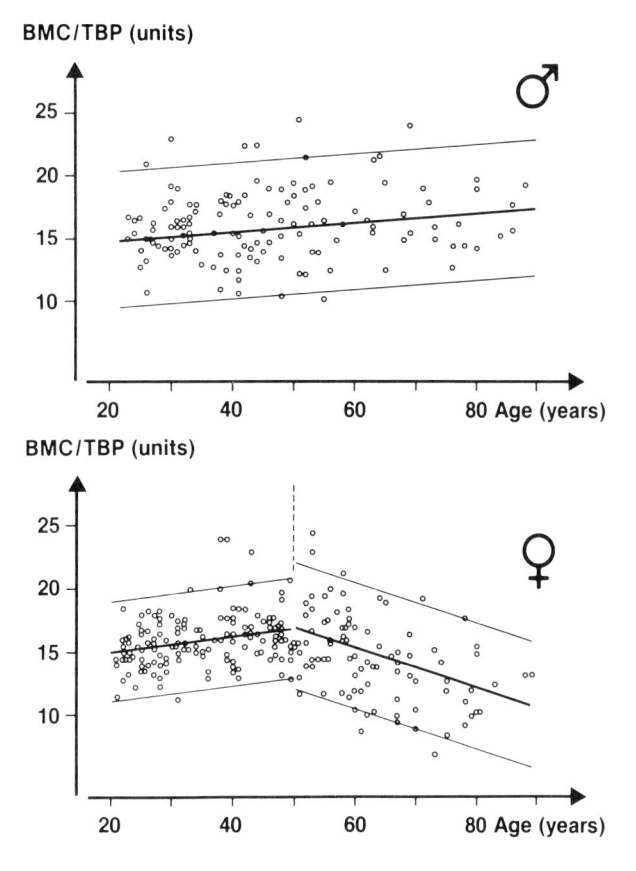

Figure 4
Bone mineral content divided by total body potassium (as an estimate of muscle mass) as a function of age in normal men and women (Mean±2SD).
(Copyright C Christiansen, used with permission).

bone mass measurement and one determination of rate of bone loss (19) at the time of menopause. Both the major risk factors would thus be covered. If the physician has to chose between one of the procedures, it is not clear which one is the most predictive.
Several investigators have reported that the peak bone mass is the most determining factor for amount of bone mass later in life (20,21, Lindsay R and Johnston CC Jr; personal communications). Due to the individual difference in rate of bone loss (19), the correlation between peak bone mass and future bone mass will probably become weaker as a function of time, although it will exist for many years. Bone mass is obviously an important factor for osteoporotic fractures, although a "fracture-threshold" never has been established. However, other factors may play a role (22,23).
From figure 3 it appears that loss of bone quality may be as important as bone quantity. It is not clear which factors deteriorates the bone architecture, but from a theoretical point of view rate of bone loss may be important. This could thus explain why a person with a high peak bone mass, but with a postmenopausal high rate of bone loss will develop symptomatic osteoporosis, even with a bone mass that is within "the normal limit". Correspondingly, a woman with a peak bone mass in the very low end of the "normal range", and with a low rate of postmenopausal bone loss, may not develop osteoporosis (fractures) even if she finally has a bone mass below the normal range.

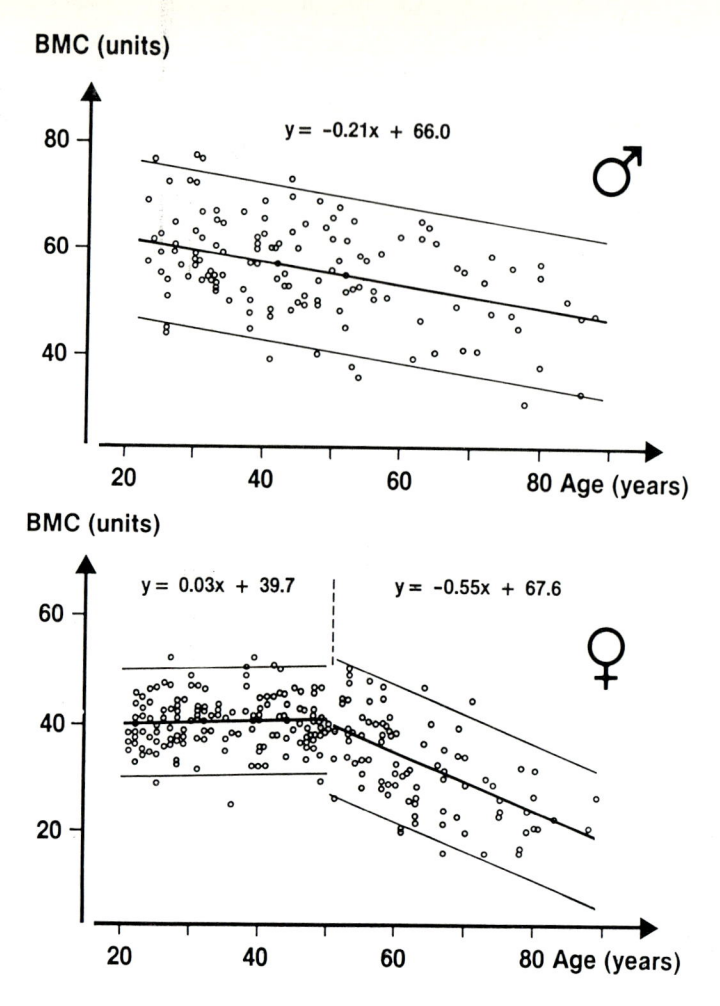

Figure 5
Bone mineral content as a function of age in normal men and women (Mean±2SD).
(Copyright C Christiansen, used with permission).

Conclusion
It is possible both to measure the peak bone mass and the rate of postmenopausal bone loss. The rate of bone loss may be determining for the future bone quality. Which role peak bone mass or bone quality play for development of osteoporosis will hopefully be clarified in future investigations.

REFERENCES

1. Finn Jensen, G.; Christiansen, C.; Boesen, J.; Hegedüs, V.; Transbøl, I.: Epidemiology of postmenopausal spinal and long bone fractures. Clin Orthop. 166: 75-81 (1982).

2. Cummings S.R., Kelsey J.L., Nevitt M.C., O'Dowd K.J. Epidemiology of osteoporosis and osteoporotic fractures. Epidemiol Reviews 7: 178-207 (1985).

3. Jensen, J.S.; Tøndevold, E.: Mortality after hip fractures. Acta Orthop Scand. 50: 161-167 (1979).

4. Johnston, Jr., C.C.; Hui, S.L.; Christian, J.C.: Some determinants of peak bone mass and subsequent rates of bone loss; in Christiansen et

al., Copenhagen International Symposium on Osteoporosis, Copenhagen 1984. No. 1, pp. 263-268 (Aalborg Stiftsbogtrykkeri, Aalborg 1984).

5. Heaney, R.P.: Nutritional factors and estrogen in age-related bone loss. Clin Invest Med. 5: 147-155 (1982).

6. Drinkwater, B.L.: Maximizing bone mass in the premenopausal years: Positive and negative factors. In Christiansen et al., International Symposium on Osteoporosis, Aalborg 1987. No. 1, pp. 484-488 (Osteopress Aps., Copenhagen 1987).

7. Thomsen, K.; Gotfredsen, A.; Christiansen, C.: Is postmenopausal bone loss an age-related phenomenon? Calcif Tissue Int. 39: 123-127 (1986).

8. Krølner, B.; Pors Nielsen, S.: Bone mineral content of the lumbar spine in normal and osteoporotic women: Cross-sectional and longitudinal studies. Clin Sci. 62: 329-336 (1982).

9. Geusens, P; Dequeker, J.; Verstraeten, A.; Nijs, J.: Age-, sex-, and menopause-related changes of vertebral and peripheral bone: Population study using dual and single photon absorptiometry and radiogrammetry. J Nucl Med. 27: 1540-1549 (1986).

10. Nilas, L.; Christiansen, C.: Bone mass and its relationship to age and the menopause. J Clin Endocrinol Metab. 65: 697-702 (1987).

11. Hui, S.L.; Slemenda, C.W.; Johnston, C.C.; Appledorn, C.R.: Effects of age and menopause on vertebral bone density. Bone and Mineral. 2: 141-146 (1987).

12. Christiansen, C.; Riis, B.J.; Rødbro, P.: Prediction of rapid bone loss in postmenopausal women. Lancet. i: 1105-1108 (1987).

13. Johnston, Jr., C.C.; Norton, Jr., J.A.; Khairi, R.A.; Longcope, C.: Age-related bone loss; in Barzel, Osteoporosis II, pp. 91-100 (Grüne & Stratton, New York 1979).

14. Ernst, M.; Schmid, Ch.; Froesch, E.R.: 17β-estradiol stimulated proliferation and type I procollagen gene expression in primary osteoblasts, in Christiansen et al., International Symposium on Osteoporosis, Aalborg 1987. No. 1, pp. 198-201 (Osteopress Aps., Copenhagen 1987).

15. Eriksen, E.F.; Berg, N.J.; Graham M.L.; Colvard, D.S.; Mann, K.G.; Spelsberg, T.C.; Riggs, B.L.: Multiple sex steroid receptors in cultured human osteoblast-like cells, in Abstract book of International Symposium on Osteoporosis, Aalborg 1987. Abstract No. 67 (1987).

16. Christiansen, C.; Christensen, M.S.; Transbøl, I.: Bone mass in postmenopausal women after withdrawal of oestrogen/gestagen replacement therapy. Lancet. i: 459-461 (1981).

17. Lindsay, R.; Aitken, J.M.; Anderson, J.B.; Hart, D.M.M; MacDonald, E.B.; Clarke, A.C.: Long-term prevention of postmenopausal osteoporosis by oestrogen. Lancet. i: 1038-1040 (1976).

18. Reginster J.Y., Albert A., Lecart M.P., Lambelin P., Denis D., Deroisy R., Fontaine M.A., Franchimont P. 1-year controlled randomised trial of prevention of early postmenopausal bone loss by intranasal calcitonin. Lancet ii: 1481-1483 (1987).

19. Christiansen C., Riis B., Rødbro P. Prediction of rapid bone loss in postmenopausal women. Lancet $\underline{i}$: 1105-1108 (1987).

20. Wasnich R.D., Ross P.D., Heilbrun L.K., Vogel J.M. Prediction of postmenopausal fracture risk with use of bone mineral measurements. Am J Obstet Gynecol $\underline{153}$: 745-751 (1985).

21. Nordin B.E.C. How can we prevent osteoporosis. In Christiansen et al., International Symposium on Osteoporosis, Aalborg 1987. No. 2, pp. 1204-1210 (Osteopress Aps., Copenhagen 1987).

22. Ott S.M., Kilcoyne R.F., Chesnut C.H. Ability of four different techniques of measuring bone mass to diagnose vertebral fractures in postmenopausal women. J Bone Min Res $\underline{2}$: 201-210 (1987).

23. Heaney R.P. Qualitative factors in osteoporotic fracture: The state of the question. In Christiansen et al., International Symposium on Osteoporosis, Aalborg 1987. No. 1, pp. 281-287 (Osteopress Aps., Copenhagen 1987).

Discussion:

DR. RIGGS (Rochester, MN): Just so there won't be misunderstanding for the audience, the slide that you showed of our data was cross-sectional and it was fit with a linear plot. But when we look at longitudinal data, we will follow these women up for five years, we do see an acceleration at the time of the menopause of about four to five-fold. So, that while we do still find a substantial premenopausal bone loss, there's no question that it has accelerated at the menopause.

DR. KOLB (San Francisco): Claus, what dose of transdermal estradiol is osteoprotective in most women?

DR. CHRISTIANSEN (Denmark): The estrogen we used was percutaneous 17B estradiol. We have no experience with the patch. I don't think that anybody in this auditorium has data which can tell which dose of the patch is enough to prevent bone loss.

DR. REEVE (England): I wasn't quite clear in your new study, whether you'd measured a lot more than one skeletal site. In which case, can you tell us whether using a different skeletal site, such as the spine, you get the same women in your various groups or whether they cross over into different groups?

DR. CHRISTIANSEN: If you use the biochemical data, to estimate the bone loss in the spine or total body or other areas of interest, you find highly significant correlations, but not as high as in the forearm. In my opinion, it is caused by the fact that we can measure the bone loss more precisely in the forearm than in any other place.

DR. REEVE: Then, do you get correlations between rates of loss in the spine and in the forearm that go along with that conclusion?

DR. CHRISTIANSEN: Yes.

DR. REEVE: You're implying that you get correlations between the two rates of loss in different sites?

DR. CHRISTIANSEN: Yes, in the order of 0.4 to 0.65

DR. BERGMANN (Belgium): Do you have still a predictive value for biological measurements if they are normalized for the skeletal size? Did you try to normalize hydroxyproline, for instance, for the skeletal size, and does it increase or decrease the predictive value?

DR. CHRISTIANSEN: We haven't done that. But I would actually expect that it would decrease the correlation.

DR. ETTINGER (San Francisco): I'd just like to mention that calcium seems to increase the effectiveness of suboptimal doses of estrogen. In a poster session at this meeting, we show that .5 of micronized estradiol is sufficient if it's used with additional calcium supplementation. This adds to the experience that we've had with .3 mg/day of conjugated estrogen with calcium and that Gallagher has also had with .3 mg/day.

It's also interesting to look at the effects of additional exercise on estrogen's effectiveness. And Notelovitz has some unpublished data showing that weightbearing exercise increases the effectiveness of estrogen.

DR. CHRISTIANSEN: I agree and we have also data to show that.

Optimizing Bone Mass in the Perimenopause: Calcitonin and Diphosphonates

CHARLES H. CHESNUT III

Osteoporosis Research Center
University of Washington School of Medicine
Seattle, WA

In the elderly female, the major determinants of postmenopausal osteoporosis, and osteoporotic fracture, are hypothetically the peak bone mass attained at adolescence, the maintenance of such peak bone mass during the premenopausal period, and the rate of bone loss after the menopause (1). The relative contributions of these determinants to postmenopausal osteoporosis and fracture are unclear; certainly an accelerated rate of bone loss postmenopausally can be expected to be a major factor in the occurrence of subsequent fractures. Therapies aimed at preventing such an accelerated bone loss after the menopause should theoretically be of value, by stabilizing that attained and maintained peak bone mass above an individual's hypothetical fracture threshold.

Therapeutic agents known to prevent bone loss are estrogen, calcitonin, and the bisphosphonates (diphosphonates); these agents work primarily by an inhibition of bone resorption, without a direct stimulatory effect on bone formation. An increase in bone mass has been noted for agents from each group, due to an inhibition of bone resorption without a corresponding inhibition of bone formation, allowing a transient net accrual of bone mass until normal coupling mechanisms are restored and bone formation is correspondingly decreased (2).

The ideal prophylactic agent for preventing bone loss immediately after the menopause has the qualities of therapeutic efficacy, safety, ease of administration (to assure compliance in a population at risk for, but as yet without, a disease), and a reasonable cost. Estrogens satisfy each of these criteria, except safety. How about calcitonin and the bisphosphonates?

Synthetic salmon calcitonin has been shown to be efficacious in osteoporotic individuals (3, 4, 5), with a 2 - year stabilization of bone mass at multiple skeletal sites, presumably by an inhibition of osteoclastic bone resorption. This therapeutic agent is quite safe, but its expense, route of administration (intramuscularly or subcutaneously), and as yet unproven prophylactic efficacy are less acceptable for the currently available calcitonin moities. However, a suitable route of administration by nasal spray is under evaluation in a number of laboratories, and at least one preliminary study (6) suggests maintenance of bone mass over 1 year in a group of immediately postmenopausal women treated with nasal spray calcitonin, compared to a similar group of women treated only with calcium; such a route of administration seems to be associated with few side effects and to be acceptable to women at risk for, but as yet without, osteoporosis. If proven effective, such an agent, with essentially no side effects, may have definite value as an alternative to estrogen for prevention of bone loss immediately after the menopause. Expense remains a problem with calcitonin, but if nasal spray calcitonin proves to be an effective prophylactic agent, an increased volume of usage could hopefully result in an overall cost reduction.

The bisphosphonates, also called diphosphonates, also possess a therapeutic rationale for usage in the prevention, and treatment, of postmenopausal bone loss (7). Both a physicochemical effect (inhibition of crystal dissolution of calcium phosphate in vitro) and a cellular effect (a change in the morphological aspect of osteoclasts, as well as a possible decrease in the number of osteoclasts, in vivo) are postulated, resulting in an overall decrease in bone resorption in vivo, an end result similar to that seen with estrogens and calcitonin (but achieved presumably through different pathways). As with calcitonin, studies are available noting a potential beneficial effect on bone mass in <u>osteoporotic</u> patients; Chesnut (2) noted a stabilization (and actually an increase) in bone mass over 2 years in osteoporotic patients intermittently treated with the bisphosphonate clodronate. Preliminary results from other studies are however conflicting. Storm et al (8) has shown an average 6% gain in spinal bone mineral content as assessed by dual photon absorptiometry techniques in 17 osteoporotic women receiving the bisphosphonate etidronate (EHDP) in a modified coherent therapy regiment (2 weeks of treatment with etidronate 400 mgm/day followed by a 13-week rest period with repetitive cycles over 150 weeks). Fifteen placebo patients lost an average 5.2% at the same site over the same period. Pacifici et al (9) on the other hand noted a mean loss of 8% at the spine as assessed by QCT methods in 30 osteoporotic women followed for 2 years on a coherent therapy regimen consisting of intermittent phosphate and etidronate. A similar group receiving hormonal (estrogen) replacement and calcium experienced no change in spine bone mass, while a 3.8% decrease was noted in a group treated with calcium alone. At this time therefore it appears that clodronate, and questionably etidronate may be effective in the osteoporotic individual. Whether these agents would be equally effective in the prevention of bone loss in individuals immediately postmenopausal is unproven. The bisphosphonates as a group, when administered intermittently, have few apparent side effects (although if administered continuously over a prolonged period a mineralization defect and potential osteomalacia may occur). The route of administration for bisphosphonates is quite acceptable in terms of prophylactic compliance (an oral medication), and they are associated with a reasonable expense. It remains to be seen however as to whether or not prophlactic efficacy comparable to that obtained with estrogens will be available from these agents; if bone loss can be prevented for 4 - 5 years it would certainly be an alternative to estrogen therapy in terms of relative safety, an equal cost, and a similar simplicity of administration.

It should also be noted that the majority of studies that have been completed with both calcitonin and the bisphosphonates utilize measurements of bone mass throughout the entire skeleton, or at the spine or wrist, as their primary parameters for establishing efficacy. Whether such therapy will be of value in preventing bone mass loss at the hip (4), and subsequent fractures at that site, is unclear. It should also be noted that the usage of these medications in such secondary osteoporoses as corticosteroid-induced bone loss, athletic amenorrhea, medically treated hyperparathyroidism, etc., is, while theoretically attractive, unproven at the present time.

Therefore, in 1988, a number of medications, calcitonin and the bisphosphonates, are under evaluation, or are being considered for evaluation, for usage as alternatives to estrogen in the prevention of bone mass loss immediately after the menopause. The prime attribute of these two potentially prophylactic therapies is their putative safety; such safety is a significant asset compared to estrogens, a medication which can prevent bone loss over an extended period of time, but occasionally at a high cost in terms of side effects.

<u>References</u>

1. Chesnut CH: Osteoporosis: the young, the athletic, the anorexic, and the old. In: Osteoporosis 1987. International Symposium on Osteoporosis Denmark 1987. Ed: Christiansen C, et al. Osteopress ApS, 49 - 51, 1987.
2. Chesnut CH: Synthetic salmon calcitonin, diphosphonates, and anabolic steroids in the treatment of postmenopausal osteoporosis. In: Osteoporosis. Copenhagen International Symposium on Osteoporosis 1984. Ed: Christiansen C et al. Aalborg, Stiftsbogtrykkeri, 549-555, 1984.
3. Gruber HE, Ivey JL, Baylink DJ, Matthews M, Nelp WB, Sisom K, Chesnut CH: Long-term calcitonin therapy in postmenopausal osteoporosis. Metab 33: 295-302, 1984.

4. Gennari C, Chierichetti SM, Bigazzi S, Fusi L, Gonnelli S, Ferrara R, Zacchei F: Comparative effects on bone mineral content of calcium and calcium plus calcitonin given in two different regimens in postmenopausal osteoporosis. Curr Ther Research 38:455-464, 1985.
5. Mazzuoli GF, Passeri M, Gennari C, Minisola S, Antonelli R, Valtorta C, Palummeri E, Cervellin GF, Gonnelli S, Francini G: Effects of salmon calcitonin in postmenopausal osteoporosis: a controlled double-blind clinical study. Calcif Tissue Intl 38:3-8, 1986.
6. Reginster JY, Denis D, Albert A, Deroisy R, Lecart MP, Fontaine MA, Lambelin P, Franchimont P: 1 year controlled randomised trial of prevention of early postmenopausal bone loss by intranasal calcitonin. Lancet, 1481-1483, Dec 26, 1987.
7. Fleisch H: Bisphosphonates - an introduction. In: Osteoporosis 1987. International Symposium on Osteoporosis Denmark 1987. Ed: Christiansen C, et al. Osteopress ApS, 1159-1164, 1987.
8. Storm T, Thamsburg G, Sorenson OH, Lund B: The effects of etidronate therapy in postmenopausal osteoporotic women: preliminary results. In: Osteoporosis 1987. International Symposium on Osteoporosis Denmark 1987. Ed: Christiansen C, et al. Osteopress Aps, 1172-1176, 1987.
9. Pacifici R, McMurtry C, Vered I, Rupich R, Avioli LV: Coherence therapy does not prevent axial bone loss in osteoporotic women: a preliminary comparative study. J Clin Endocrinol Metab 66: 747-753, 1988.

Discussion:

DR. RIGGS (Rochester, MN): You may want to correct yourself on one point, Charles. I think you mispoke when you indicated that the diphosphonates, in general, have the problem with a mineralization defect. You mean, just EHDP. I don't think there's any major mineralization defect with the other diphosphonates.

DR. CHESNUT (Seattle): I'm not sure that some of the others do not, but I'll accept your correction that it's predominantly EHDP.

DR. HARRIS (San Francisco): I just wanted to comment that, as you know, we're participating in ongoing studies of Didronel therapy with and without the addition of phosphorus. In the preliminary results that we're showing in a poster at this conference, it appears that our post Didronel results are very similar to those that you showed from the European experience.

There was an increase in spinal density, whether by DPA or QCT, of 5 to 10 percent, primarily within the first year of therapy. I really can't explain why our results are at variance with those observed in St. Louis. However, I'd be interested in remarks from the St. Louis group about that difference.

DR. CHESNUT: Good point. I think that the data will be very interesting when it is finally completed.

DR. ORTOLANI (Italy): Two questions: Can you define how many units of calcitonin are absorbed or the percentage of the absorbed calcitonin by nasal spray? And the second, you suggest that lower dosage of calcitonin can be more effective than the 100 you used in the '84 study. Will you note the dose you suggest for parenteral administration in this sense?

DR. CHESNUT: The question is, is for parenteral use, what dosage of calcitonin would we recommend, presumably for individuals with established disease. There's no definitive data, but I do feel that 100 units daily is an excessive dose. Our bias is that this is due to a down regulation of receptor sites. Other possible explanations would be counter-regulatory mechanisms.

For that reason, we would feel that 50 units every other day might be a more reasonable dosage in established osteoporosis. I think that probably 100 units every day is too much. In addition, by using 50 units every other day in the osteoporotic woman, you drop the cost down to a more acceptable level in our country, from about $200 to about $50 to $60 per month.

In terms of nasal spray, I think for prevention it's still questionable as to whether 50 units daily intranasally is going to be effective in preventing bone loss. The data from the Brussels groups would raise questions regarding that, so, I can't comment on that specifically.

I would think that 200 to 400 units daily may be needed for nasal spray calcitonin prevention of bone mass loss.

About the absorption of the nasal spray, I think that the data that is presented does show absorption of nasal spray calcitonin. Even without an activator, studies do show reasonable blood levels. One can put an activator into the nasal spray and probably get better absorption. On the other hand, in that situation, one pays the price of possible nasal irritation by putting in an activator such as taurocholic acid which can be irritating to the nasal mucosa.

So, you balance side effects against bioavailability. It appears currently that the nasal spray without the activator does achieve relative bioavailability.

DR. ZIEGLER (Germany): If you use calcitonin in osteoporosis, you don't have a biochemical marker for response. Using, for instance, salmon calcitonin nasal spray in Paget's disease of bone, we think that the development of antibody is a reasonably high predictor of non-response.

Do you have suggestions how to watch this phenomenon in studies using calcitonin in osteoporosis?

DR. CHESNUT: I'm afraid we're still left with bone mass measurements as the only way of monitoring therapeutic response. Our feeling is that antibody level does not correlate with lack of effectiveness, at least in osteoporosis. That's been our bias for years, and we still maintain it. So, I really don't have an answer to your question, other than to simply follow the clinical history and measurements of bone mass, to say that we have stabilization of the disease process or, perhaps, a slight improvement over a period of time.

Use of Vitamin D Metabolites in Osteoporosis

J.C. GALLAGHER

*Creighton University School of Medicine
Omaha, NE*

INTRODUCTION:
The use of Vitamin D in Osteoporosis treatment has been wide-spread for many years. This was because of the finding that osteoporotic patients have malabsorption of calcium. Over the years the most common preparation used in osteoporosis therapy has been Vitamin D2. It has never been clearly established what dose of Vitamin D should be used in the treatment of osteoporosis since measurement of calcium absorption is not readily available. However, an increase in the 24 hour urine calcium is usually a good indication that there has been an increase in calcium absorption. One of the problems in the management of patients using Vitamin D2 compounds is the limited number of therapeutic options open. Ideally, there should be doses of Vitamin D ranging in 1000 unit doses up to a level of 5000 units, however, the most commonly available preparation of Vitamin D2 is the 50,000 unit tablet which is most often given weekly. Some of the problems of Vitamin D2 compounds is their relative instability over time and in light. Also Vitamin D2 is stored in body fat and therefore may be released during episodes of weight loss into the active forms of Vitamin D, namely 25 hydroxy D and 1,25 dihydroxyvitamin D. In the last few years the synthesis of these active forms of Vitamin D have given us more alternatives. Although 25 hydroxy D is quite widely used in Europe, it is uncommonly used in the USA. There has been a trend recently toward using the final active metabolite of Vitamin D namely 1,25 dihydroxyvitamin D3 (calcitriol) or the analogue 1 α hydroxy D3 which must be converted in the liver to form 1,25 dihydroxyvitamin D3. A considerable amount of work has been carried out on these metabolites in the last few years because these metabolites are stable in capsule form and because of the ease and speed at which they increase calcium absorption.

RESULTS:
The therapeutic dose of 1 α hydroxy D3 has been evaluated with calcium absorption studies and calcium balance studies

(1-5). 1 microgram of 1 α hydroxy D3 did not always improve calcium absorption whereas 2 micrograms invariably did so. 5 micrograms caused hypercalcuria. Calcium balance improved on 2 micrograms/day compared to 1 microgram/day, but was less positive on 5 micrograms/day because of hypercalcuria. Some studies have shown an increase in radial density on 1 α hydroxy D3, and recent reports have shown a reduction in the vertebral fracture, rate on 1 hydroxy D3 (6-7).

In our own studies we have used 1,25 dihydroxy Vitamin D3 (8). We found a significant improvement in calcium balance on 0.5 micrograms/day. Calcium balance was more positive at 6 months than at 2 years. At the time we were uncertain as to whether this was due to the well known transient effect of therapeutic agents on bone or whether this could be do to an analytical difficulties with calcium balances repeated after two to three years. Our recent work with total body calcium measured by dual photon absorptiomery has shown no significant loss of bone over a period of two years. This implies that the patient has been in calcium balance during the period of observation. (Total Body Calcium measured by DPA has been cross calibrated against total body calcium measured by neutron activation.) Since urine calcium increased in all patients in our most recent study, the results suggest that there has been an increase in calcium absorption. Measurements of urinary hydroxyproline showed a significant reduction at the end of two years. Thus, it is likely that there was a decrease in bone turnover on calcitriol. Another study by Aloia, et al (9), has shown results very similar to those reported by us. However, in another study by Ott et al (10) no significant difference between calcitriol or placebo treated patients was detected at the end of two years. In the study by Ott et al, the average dose of calcitriol was 0.4 micrograms/day and the average number of fractures was 1.5/patient. In our study and that by Aloia et al, the dose of calcitriol used was 0.67 and 0.75 micrograms/daily respectively. The number of fractures, 4.5 fractures/patient, were similar in both studies. Thus, there may be a threshold dose response for calcitriol, also, it is possible that severe osteoporosis may be more responsive to treatment than milder disease. Vitamin D metabolites may have different actions depending upon the dose used. With relatively small doses of calcitriol,< 0.75 micrograms/day, the major effect of calcitriol is to increase calcium absorption, improve calcium balance and reduce bone turnover. On higher doses, 1.5 - 2 micrograms/daily, there is evidence of a direct action of calcitriol on bone. In a study of 10 patients treated with high doses of calcitriol, we found evidence of increased activation frequency measured by tetracycline labeling and increases in the measured bone formation rates (11). These preliminary results suggest that more work needs to be done on the potential impact of higher doses of Vitamin D metabolites on bone, given either as intermittent or as continuous therapy.

There has been concern about the safety of Vitamin D metabolites on renal function, because of the possibility that increased calcium absorption may lead to hypercalcuria and calcification within the kidney. On a free calcium intake (average 800 mg/day) we found that the incidence of hypercalcuria was less than 1% on 0.5 microgram/day, about 15% on 0.67 micrograms/day and 30% in patients on 0.75 micrograms/daily. However, when the calcium intake is restricted to 500 mg/day, patients can tolerate 1.5 - 2.0 micrograms/daily without developing hypercalcuria. In our most recent study we measured creatinine clearance in a placebo controlled study where the average dose of calcitriol was 0.67 micrograms/day. Patients collected 24 hour urines at regular monthly intervals over 2 years. At the end of the study the decline in creatinine clearance was identical in both groups. Thus, to date neither us or others have found any obvious difference in renal function in calcitriol treated osteoporotic patients. However, because of the potential toxicity, more sophisticated analysis such as ultrasound or computerized tomography of the kidneys to look for evidence of nephrocalcinosis probably should be performed in long term treated patients.

CONCLUSIONS:
Most of the published reports appear to show a beneficial effect of Vitamin D metabolites in osteoporotic patients, and nearly all studies show an advantage in calcitriol treatment compared to placebo in preventing bone loss. It is also clear that changes in bone density are relatively small and similar to those reported for example on Calcitonin. Unfortunately, there are no randomized studies of the use of calcium therapy or estrogen therapy for comparison in osteoporosis patients. It is likely that calcitriol reduces bone turnover and leads to a small transient increase in bone density. Larger increases in bone density, (5-8%) which imply significant deposition of bone and an increase in bone formation, have not been seen with small doses of calcitriol. Whether higher doses of calcitriol have a role to play in the treatment of osteoporosis remains to be seen. At the present time only small doses of calcitriol, 0.5 micrograms/daily, should be used to improve calcium balance. The calcium intake should be restricted to less than 800 mg/day in order to avoid the problem of hypercalcuria, which should be monitored with 24 hour urine calcium measurements.

REFERENCES
1. Lund B., Holm, P., Egsmose, C. Sorensen, H.,B., Mosekilde, L., Egsmose, C., Strom, T.L.,and Nielsen, S.P. 1985:Long-term treatment of senile osteopenia with 1 di-hydroxycholecalciferol. In: Vitamin D. A Chemical, Biochemical and Clinical Update, edited by A.W. Norman. K. Schaefer, H.- G. Grigoleit, and D.V. Herrath, pp. 1039-1040. Walter de Gruyter & Co., Berlin-New York.
2. Sorensen, O.H., Anderson, R.B., Christensen, M.S., Friis, T., Hjorth, L., Jorgensen, F.S., Lund, B., and Melsen, F. 1977: Treatment of senile osteoporosis with 1 di-hydroxyvitamin D3. Clin. Endocrinol., 7:169S-175S.
3. Lindholm, T.S., Nilsson, O.S., Kyhle, B.R., Elmstedt, E., Lindholm, T.C., and Eriksson, S.A. 1981: Failures and complications in treatment of osteoporotic patients treated with 1 di-hydroxyvitamin D3 supplemented by calcium. In: Osteoporotics, edited by C.Christiansen, C.D. Arnaud, B.E.C. Nordin, A.M. Parfitt, W.A. Peck, and B.L. Riggs, pp. 351-357. Aalborg Stiftsbogtrykkeri, Glostrup, Denmark.

4. Crilly, R.G., Marshall, D.H., Horsman, A., and Nordin, B.E.C. 1980: 1 alpha hydroxy D3 with and without estrogen in the treatment of osteoporosis. In: Osteoporosis: Recent Advances in Pathogenesis and Treatment, edited by H.F. DeLluca, H.M. Frost, W.S.S. Jee, and C.C. Johnston. University Park Press, Baltimore.
5. Marshall, D.H., Gallagher, J.C., Guha, P., Hanes, F., Oldfield, W., and Nordin, B.E.C. 1977: The effect of 1 alpha-hydroxycholecaliciferol and hormone therapy on the calcium balance of post-menopausal osteoporosis. Calcif. Tissue Res., 225:78-84.
6. Shiraki, M., Orimo, H., Ito, H. Akiguchi, I., Nakao, J., and Takahashi, R. 1985: Long-term treatment of postmenopausal osteoporosis with active vitamin D3, 1-alpha-hydroxycolecaliciferol (1OHD3) and 1,24 dihydroxycholecaliciferol (1,24(OH)2D3). Endocrinol. Jpn., 32:305--315.
7. Orimo H. Shiraki M., Hayashi T., Nakamura T. Reduced occurrence of vertebral crush fractures in senile osteoporosis treated with 1 (OH) Vitamin D3. Bone & Mineral. 3.(1) 4.7, 1987.
8. Gallagher, J.C., Jerpbak, C.M., Jee, W.S.S., Johnson, K.A., DeLuca, H.F., and Riggs, B.L. 1982: 1,25-Dihydroxyvitamin D3: Short-and long-term effects on bone and calcium metabolism in patients with postmenopausal osteoporosis. Proc. Natl. Acad. Sci., 79:3325-3329.
9. Aloia, John F., Vaswani, Ashok., Yeh, James K., Mineola, New York., Ellis, Kenneth., Yasumura, Seiichi., Cohn, Stanton H., Upton, New York., Am. J. Med., Calcitriol in the Treatment of Postmenopausal Osteoporosis., 84:401, 1988.
10. Ott, S. and Chestnut C., Personal Communication., 1987
11. Gallagher, J.C., and Recker, R.R. 1985: A Comparision of the Effects of Calcitriol or Calcium Supplements. on Bone in Postmenopausal Osteroporosis In: Vitamin D, A Chemical, Biochemical and Clinical Update, edited by A.W. Norman, K.Schaefer, H.-.G. Grigoleit, and D.V. Herrath, pp. 971-975. Walter de Gruyter & Co., Berlin-New York.

Discussion:

DR. CUMMINGS (San Francisco): In Aalborg, as I remember, Dr. Ott and the group from Seattle reported negative results in what sounded like a very similar protocol of therapy. Is that still true and, if so, how would you explain the discrepancies?

DR. CHESNUT (Seattle): I think one explanation is that her data was basically with a very low dosage. As a nephrologist, she was concerned about renal side effects and our mean drug ingestion was about .45 micrograms/day. We had few side effects at that level, outside of hypercalciuria. But we, indeed, did not have any difference at any site being measured, between the treated group, 1-25 plus calcium, and calcium alone. Both postmenopausal osteoporotic groups maintained bone mass, interestingly, over two years.

Why our data is different from the Creighton group and the Aloia group, I think may be related to a certain extent to dosage.

DR. GALLAGHER (Omaha): I think John Aloia published last week in the American Journal of Medicine results almost identical to those that you've seen this morning.

And I think to bring back a point that Charles made, both Aloia and I had two quite striking differences from the Seattle study. First of all, we had on average four and a half fractures per patient. And I think in your group it was more like one and a half to two fractures.

DR. CHESNUT: That's correct.

DR. GALLAGHER: And the second, this is that the average dose in the Seattle study was about .4 micrograms. Whereas, both Aloia and I were nearer to .7, .75 micrograms. And I think that may be an important difference.

DR. CUMMINGS: I have one other point of confusion and that is, it seems as though from your descriptions of the vertebral fractures, the age of the patients, that most of them -- or, many of them would be classified as Type 1 osteoporotics. And pathophysiologically, as you described earlier, vitamin D (1,25) therapy would be more appropriate for what's being called Type 2 osteoporosis. Are you testing the drug in a sense, in the wrong group?

DR. GALLAGHER: No, I think we're treating Type 1's, and I think that's the group to treat. They're the ones who most obviously have a low 1,25 group. But on the other hand, let's emphasize that only about 60 to 70 percent of patients with Type 1 have low absorption and low 1,25 levels. When you go into a double blind study, you make the assumption that everybody has the same problem.

Now, obviously, we're also treating people with normal absorption and normal 1,25, so that the results are to a certain extent biased against you in any double blind study. And, of course, that applies to all the studies we've heard this morning in therapeutic terms.

DR. DEQUEKER (Belgium): Have you seen any differential effect on the peripheral bone mass and the actual bone mass? You only showed the spinal bone mass and then the total body. Because using 1 alpha vitamin D has been shown in many studies to increase bone loss at peripheral and cortical bone. And we saw in rheumatoid arthritis, also, an increase in the spine, but an increased loss at peripheral bone.

DR. GALLAGHER: I didn't show the slide to save time. But, in fact, there were no significant differences between treatment and placebo on mid-shaft radial.

DR. ORTOLANI (Italy): Comments about the rationale for the use of the 1,25 in Type 1 osteoporosis. From the PTH challenge test of Riggs, it seems that the 1 alpha hydroxylase in these patients are normal. So, probably the low levels of 1,25 are an adaptive response to the increased sensitivity of the skeleton to the PTH resorptive action. So, it seems rational to increase the resistance of the skeleton to the resorption, than to increase intestinal calcium absorption.

DR. GALLAGHER: I think that the logical thing, really, to do in this kind of case is to treat patients only who have low absorption and low 1,25 levels. And this is what, of course, Dr. Canniggia has done in Italy, and has consistently, I think, seen much greater responses in terms of bone density.

DR. REEVE (England): I was a little bit disturbed to find, if I'm interpreting your slide correctly, that your control group lost somewhere between 10 and 15 percent of their GFR over two years. That's much more than the old work of Schock would have predicted, about two percent. Have you any explanation for this?

DR. GALLAGHER: I don't think that I would be too put out by the results. I'm not sure that I would agree with those reports that you came up with. In fact, if you do calculate an age-related change in GFR, it's really a quadratic function. An it's around 5 mls per minute, per year in elderly people. Actually, that's very close to the data that I showed here. Ten percent sounds quite a lot, but the decrease is falling off very rapidly in the last few years. I don't think it's out of line at all.

DR. HARRIS (San Francisco): Do you think there's an abnormality in the relationship between dietary phosphorus and 1,25 levels, either in normal elderly subjects or in osteoporotics?

DR. GALLAGHER: That's an interesting question. I don't have the information on that, though.

DR. SANTORA (Detroit): To follow up on your conclusion that there is an effect of 1,25 in Type 1 osteoporosis. I just wondered if there was a little bit of information you could give us about the demographics? Ideally, you'd like to have no patients, say, over 60. As we know, having Type 1 osteoporosis doesn't prevent one from getting Type 2 osteoporosis farther down the road. What are the demographics of the patients in your study? Are they a mixture of women, say, shortly after menopause, or does it extend to women in their 60s and 70s?

DR. GALLAGHER: I think that our patient group is probably a mixed one. I think they're predominately Type 1's. But I think there are some Type 2's there, also. And I suspect that the ideal population to treat would probably be the Type 1's who selectively have low 1,25 levels, which is a fairly easy measurement to make this day. And I think that would be a logical way to proceed.

Steroids and Osteoporosis: An Unsolvable Problem?

LAWRENCE G. RAISZ

University of Connecticut Health Center
Farmington, CT

INTRODUCTION

For anyone who has experienced the revolution in bone biology that has occurred over the past 20 years, the answer to the question posed in my title must be a resounding "no". We will surely find solutions to the problem of glucocorticoid-induced osteoporosis as we learn more about the regulation of bone cells. On the other hand, the problem is unsolved at present. We can seek solutions by a number of different pathways. The most obvious is to stop using systemic glucocorticoids. This seems highly unlikely to occur but some decrease in systemic glucocorticoid use can be expected as topical agents become more effective and alternative therapies are developed. However, alternative therapies may produce new problems. We do not yet know how much damage to the skeleton may be produced by other non-steroidal immunosuppressive agents. A second route would be to find glucocorticoids which have diminished adverse effects on skeletal tissue but are still good anti-inflammatory agents. Deflazacort is currently being examined in this regard, and there is evidence for its selective advantage over other clinically used steroids. The third most attractive approach is to learn more about the pathogenesis of glucocorticoid-induced osteoporosis and provide specific therapy to reverse this process. There is evidence that this approach is already effective in preventing those adverse effects of glucocorticoids due to increased bone resorption. Reversal of the inhibitory effects of glucocorticoids on bone formation has not yet been accomplished and may represent a much more difficult task. It is this problem that is most "unsolvable" at the present time. One difficulty in developing either preventive or therapeutic approaches to glucocorticoid-induced osteoporosis is the complexity and inconsistency of our data on epidemiology and pathogenesis. Although the population at risk has been characterized to some extent, we cannot predict accurately who among glucocorticoid-treated patients will develop systematic osteoporosis with fractures.

EPIDEMIOLOGY

The usual risk factors for the development of osteoporotic fractures do not necessarily apply in patients treated with glucocorticoids (1-3). Bone disease can develop in men and premenopausal women but as might be expected, is more common in postmenopausal women. The high incidence in the last group is probably due to the combination of postmenopausal and glucocorticoid-induced osteoporosis. In fact in one study, the difference in bone mass between postmenopausal glucocorticoid-treated patient and controls was not significant, although in others, larger differences have been observed (3-5). Patients on glucocorticoids are often immobilized by musculoskeletal, gastrointestinal or pulmonary disease and many of them have poor nutrition. Despite these complicating risk factors, there is a clear association between the dose and duration of steroid therapy and the severity of bone loss in patients treated with systemic glucocorticoids whether it be for connective tissue disease or other allergic disorders (6-9).

PATHOGENESIS

It is clear that both increased bone resorption and decreased bone formation play a role in reducing bone mass and strength in glucocorticoid-treated patients. Morphologic studies comparing glucocorticoid-induced osteoporosis with other forms show a striking difference in the degree of inhibition of bone formation in the steroid group (10). Moreover, therapy which is aimed at inhibiting bone resorption often has only a limited effect in improving bone mass and skeletal function in glucocorticoid-treated patients, suggesting that decreased formation is the more important abnormality (11).

Most of the available data support the hypothesis that increased bone resorption is a secondary response in glucocorticoid-treated patients, due to impaired intestinal absorption of calcium and secondary hyperparathyroidism. Nevertheless, a direct stimulatory effect of glucocorticoids on osteoclasts has been suggested. Such an effect has been observed in one study on neonatal mouse calvaria (12), and we have recently found a transient increase in the release of previously incorporated ^{45}Ca in fetal rat calvaria treated with cortisol (13). On the other hand, glucocorticoids can inhibit bone resorption in vitro (14). This effect occurs particularly in control unstimulated bone organ cultures, and cultures stimulated by the osteoclast activating factors (interleukin-1 and tumor necrosis factor). Glucocorticoids cannot block the increased bone resorption that occurs in hyperparathyroidism in vivo or with PTH administration in vitro. Glucocorticoids actually enhance certain PTH effects on bone cells. It is possible that the effect of glucocorticoids on the osteoclastic cell line is biphasic in a manner similar to their effects on osteoblastic cells. Thus, physiologic concentrations of glucocorticoids may be necessary for the late stages of differentiation and function of osteoclasts while the generation of new osteoclasts which involves cell replication may be inhibited. The inhibitory effect could be mediated by a change in the production of local regulators, since glucocorticoids can inhibit the formation of both interleukin-1 and prostaglandins in bone and adjacent connective or hematopoietic tissues (15-16).

While there is current consensus that glucocorticoids increase bone resorption largely by producing secondary hyperparathyroidism, the mechanism of this secondary effect is not completely clear. Increased PTH levels have been described, but the values are usually within the normal range. Moreover, some studies have found no elevation of PTH. Hence, PTH sensitivity rather than production may be increased. New studies using the more precise immunoradiometric assays for PTH may resolve this question.

Hyperparathyroidism is probably not dependent on impaired vitamin D activation since 1,25-dihydroxyvitamin D levels are usually not decreased. However, studies on production and metabolic clearance of 1,25-dihydroxyvitamin D are limited. Glucocorticoids have a direct effect to decrease Ca absorption which probably involves both a diminution in the response to 1,25-dihydroxyvitamin D and a decrease in intestinal cell receptors for this hormone (17-18). Acute studies with short-term high dose prednisone show an increase in 1,25-dihydroxyvitamin D which is presumably secondary to increased PTH secretion, but could be due to an effect on renal production or peripheral metabolism. Although the intestine is resistant to the actions of vitamin D metabolites, high doses can overcome the block and increase calcium absorption. While the intestinal effect is most important, effects on the kidney and on the parathyroid gland may contribute to secondary hyperparathyroidism. Hypercalciuria is common in glucocorticoid-treated patients. Phosphaturia also occurs and may be greater than would be expected from any increase in PTH. An increase in PTH secretion has been observed with glucocorticoid treatment of parathyroid glands in vitro (19), but it is not known whether this occurs in vivo.

The major pathogenetic mechanism in glucocorticoid-induced osteoporosis is probably inhibition of bone formation. However, the effects of glucocorticoids on cells of the osteoblastic lineage are complex and include both stimulation and inhibition of specific cell functions. Glucocorticoids can increase collagen synthesis acutely in organ culture (20). This effect is not dose related but occurs at low, physiologic concentrations and is reversed at higher, pathologic concentrations (21). This initial response is associated with an increase in PTH stimulation of cyclic AMP production in bone cells, which probably includes both an increase in cell receptor number and postreceptor adenylate cyclase activity. Glucocorticoids can increase the differentiation of isolated bone cells as indicated by an increase in the formation of nodules containing a mineralized matrix (22). The number of 1,25-dihydroxyvitamin D receptors is increased in some culture systems and decreased in others (23). This may be related to differences in species and in the stage of cell differentiation.

Early inhibitory effects of glucocorticoids are also observed. Decreased DNA synthesis in bone organ cultures, inhibition of prostaglandin production and a decrease in the production of at least one noncollagen protein of bone, osteocalcin or the bone GLA protein, can be seen within 24 hours of glucocorticoid administration (21,24). Since bone formation depends on constant cell renewal as each succeeding layer of osteoblasts lays down its portion of bone and becomes buried as an osteocyte, the effect on cell replication is probably the primary cause of the progressive decrease in bone formation. Morphologically, bones from patients and animals treated with high doses of glucocorticoids show a marked loss of cellularity, with a diminution in the activity and number of osteoblasts on the bone surface.

The degree to which factors which stimulate bone formation can reverse inhibition by glucocorticoids has not been studied extensively. In organ culture, PGE_2 can stimulate both early cell replication and late osteoblastic collagen synthesis and reverse the glucocorticoid effect (25). Insulin-like growth factor 1 is also a potent stimulator of bone growth which not only can reverse the inhibition but appears to be more effective in the presence of the physiologic concentrations of glucocorticoids (26). The ability of fluoride to stimulate bone formation has not been studied systematically in the presence of glucocorticoids but anecdotal clinical observations indicate that it can be effective. Similarly, the effects of exercise and mechanical loading of the skeleton have not been studied systematically, but here again, there is a clinical impression that the patients who are able to maintain a vigorous exercise program while on glucocorticoid therapy lose bone less rapidly and may even gain bone mass.

ASSESSMENT

While long-term glucocorticoid therapy certainly predisposes to the development of clinical osteoporosis, not all patients will show substantial losses in bone mass or develop fractures. Since the usual epidemiologic factors which predispose to osteoporosis may not operate in glucocorticoid-treated patients, other means of assessment are important. Early and frequent measurements of bone mass should be helpful. In the past, single beam photon absorptiometry of the distal radius, where there is a substantial amount of trabecular bone, was considered a sensitive index, but measurements of lumbar bone mass with dual beam photon absorptiometry or computerized tomography show disproportionately greater losses and are probably even more useful (27). The urinary calcium and hydroxyproline excretion in glucocorticoid-treated patients may be useful parameters to assess bone resorption. However, calcium excretion may increase disproportionately with effective calcium and vitamin D supplementation. In any case, it should be monitored frequently. If calcium excretion is excessive, thiazides and/or amiloride may be indicated both to prevent calcium loss and to decrease the likelihood of renal store formation. The reduction in the serum concentration of osteocalcin which occurs rapidly after high dose glucocorticoids and is sustained, certainly indicates an effect on bone cells. Whether it has prognostic implications for the development of symptomatic osteoporosis has not yet been determined. Because bone can be lost rapidly during the first year of glucocorticoid-treated patients, frequent assessment and rigorous efforts at prevention should be instituted early, particularly in patients who already show a low bone mass.

MANAGEMENT

As indicated above, there are at least three potential solutions to the glucocorticoid problem. Reduction of dose and the use of topical steroids combined with other therapeutic agents which might diminish the need for steroid therapy, is certainly desirable. On the other hand, many patients on chronic glucocorticoid therapy are in fact alive because of this therapy and must be continued or full doses. If there is a glucocorticoid which can produce anti-inflammatory or immunosuppressive effects equal to prednisone but substantially less bone loss, this clearly would represent a major solution to the problem of glucocorticoid-induced osteoporosis. Deflazacort is probably as effective as prednisone in the treatment of rheumatic diseases (28). Short-term studies indicate that deflazacort causes less inhibition of intestinal absorption of calcium and less trabecular bone loss than prednisone (29). However, in vitro data suggest that the active desacetyl form of deflazacort is as inhibitory to osteoblasts as prednisolone (30). Long-term trials will be necessary before we can be certain that deflazacort produces less bone disease at therapeutically effective doses than prednisone.

While reversing the increase in bone resorption by glucocorticoids cannot restore lost bone or prevent the glucocorticoid-induced decrease in bone formation, it should slow the rate of bone loss. Resorption can be reduced by increasing calcium supply, decreasing urinary calcium loss or by using direct inhibitors of bone resorption. Calcium supplements and vitamin D, particularly in the form of calcifediol (11), can reverse calcium deficiency and secondary hyperparathyroidism in glucocorticoid-treated patients. Diuretics which decrease urinary calcium, such as thiazide and amiloride, may enhance these effects and will also reduce the danger of renal stone formation. Short-term studies indicate that salmon calcitonin (31) and aminohydroxypropylidene bisphosphonate (32), both potent inhibitors of bone resorption can increase bone mass in patients who are maintained on steroids. Biopsies in patients treated with APD showed that while osteoclastic activity was markedly increased, osteoblastic activity decreased even further. Moreover, both inhibitors are likely to increase secondary hyperparathyroidism and could result in a rebound acceleration of bone loss when therapy is discontinued.

Sex hormone deficiency is likely to complicate glucocorticoid-induced osteoporosis in patients who are postmenopausal and might also occur in premenopausal women and men because glucocorticoids can suppress gonadotropin production. Unfortunately, sex hormone replacement therapy can be disastrous in some glucocorticoid treated patients, particularly those with lupus or autoimmune hepatic disease. On the other hand, the incidence of rheumatoid arthritis appears to be diminished in postmenopausal women on hormone replacement therapy (33). Unless there is a contraindication, hypogonadal men and women should be treated with the appropriate sex hormones. Whether anabolic steroids which are weak androgens are generally useful in men and women on corticosteroids, even if they have normal gonadal function, requires further study. These steroids may improve muscle and bone mass (34) but have side-effects which could outweigh any benefits.

The most important solution to the problem of glucocorticoid-induced osteoporosis will be the development of methods for stimulating bone formation in these patients. At present, fluoride is the only available therapeutic agent which acts largely to stimulate bone formation, although anabolic steroids and intermittent PTH may have this effect as well. Some patients with glucocorticoid-induced osteoporosis show an increase in bone mass on fluoride, but the only published therapeutic trial shows that fluoride did not prevent prednisone-induced bone loss (34). Unfortunately, the dose and duration of fluoride therapy in this study were insufficient for an adequate evaluation. Fluoride can be used in patients with progressive vertebral crush fractures who are on glucocorticoids just as it is in other osteoporotics with this severe form of the disease.

In the laboratory, we have at least three classes of factors which can stimulate bone growth; bone morphogenetic proteins (including transforming growth factor-β), insulin-like growth factors and prostaglandins. Fibroblast growth factors may also stimulate bone formation in some experimental models. Whether any of these compounds can be administered in such a way as to reverse glucocorticoid-induced osteoporosis, or for that matter, to increase bone formation in any form of osteoporosis remains to be determined.

CONCLUSIONS

This brief review of the epidemiology, pathology and management of glucocorticoid-induced osteoporosis is intended to describe a problem which is unsolved, but potentially solvable. To develop a solution, we will have to learn more about the specific pathogenesis of both decreased bone formation and increased bone resorption in glucocorticoid-treated patients. With this information it may become easier to reverse the resorptive abnormality, but it is likely to be much more difficult to stimulate bone formation. Unfortunately, stimulation of bone formation is probably necessary for effective long-term prevention of glucocorticoid-induced osteoporosis and certainly is needed for treatment of established bone loss. Thus, it seems particularly attractive to look for alternative preventive approaches involving the use of steroids or other anti-inflammatory agents which do not cause as much bone loss as the drugs we currently employ.

References

1. Dykman, T.R., Gluck, O.S., Murphy, W.A., Hahn, T.J., Hahn, B.H. Evaluation of factors associated with glucocorticoid-induced osteopenia in patients with rheumatic disease. Arth. Rheum. 28:361-368, 1985.

2. Seeman, E., Melton, L.J. III, O'Fallon, W.M., Riggs, B.L. Risk factors for spinal osteoporosis in man. Amer. J. Med. 75:977-983, 1983.

3. Als, O.S., Gotfredsen, A., Christiansen, C. The effect of glucocorticoids on bone mass in rheumatoid arthritis patients. Influence of menopausal state. Arth. Rheum. 28:369-375, 1985.

4. De deuxchaisnes, C.N., Devogelaer, J.P., Huaux, J.P., Esselinckx, W. Influence of the menopausal state on the effect of low-dose glucocorticoid

on bone mass in rheumatoid arthritis patients. Arth. Rheum. 29:693-694, 1986.

5. Reid, D.M., Kennedy, N.S.J., Smith, M.A., Tothill, P., Nuki, G. Total body calcium in rheumatoid arthritis: Effects of disease activity and corticosteroid treatment. Brit. Med. J. 285:330-332, 1982.

6. Sambrook, P.N., Eisman, J.A., Yeates, M.G., Pocock, N.A., Eberl, S., Champion, G.D. Osteoporosis in rheumatoid arthritis: Safety of low dose corticosteroids. Ann. Rheum. Dis. 45:950-953, 1986.

7. Reid, D.M., Nicoll, J.J., Smith, M.A., Higgins, B., Tothill, P., Nuki, G. Corticosteroids and bone mass in asthma: Comparisons with rheumatoid arthritis and polymyalgia rheumatica. Brit. Med. J. 293:1463-1466, 1986.

8. Verstraeten, A., Dequecker, J. Vertebral and peripheral bone mineral content and fracture incidence in postmenopausal patients with rheumatoid arthritis: Effect of low dose corticosteroids. Ann. Rheum. Dis. 45:852-857, 1986.

9. Ruegsegger, P., Medici, T.C., Anliker, M. Corticosteroid-induced bone loss. A longitudinal study of alternate day therapy in patients with bronchial asthma using quantitative computed tomography. Eur. J. Clin. Pharmacol. 25:615-620, 1983.

10. Dempster, D.W., Arlot, M.A., Meunier, P.J. Mean wall thickness and formation periods of trabecular bone packets in corticosteroid-induced osteoporosis. Calcif. Tis. Int. 35:410-417, 1983.

11. Hahn, T.J., Halstead, L.R., Teitelbaum, S.L., Hahn, B.H. Altered mineral metabolism in glucocorticoid-induced osteopenia: Effect of 25-hydroxyvitamin D. J. Clin. Invest. 64:655-665, 1979.

12. Reid, I.R., Katz, J.M., Ibbertson, H.K., Gray, D.H. The effects of hydrocortisone, parathyroid hormone and the bisphosphonate, APD, bone resorption in neonatal mouse calvaria. Calcif. Tis. Int. 38:38-43, 1985.

13. Gronowicz, G., McCarthy, M.B., Woodiel, F., Raisz, L.G. Effects of corticosterone and parathyroid hormone on formation and resorption in cultured fetal rat parietal bones. Amer. Soc. Bone and Mineral Research - Annual Meeting, 1988.

14. Raisz, L.G., Trummel, C.L., Werner, J.A., Simmons, H. Effect of glucocorticoids on bone resorption in tissue culture. Endocrinol. 90:961-967, 1972.

15. Raisz, L.G., Simmons, H.A. Effects of parathyroid hormone and cortisol on prostaglandin production by neonatal rat calvaria in vitro. Endocrine Res. 11:59-74, 1985.

16. Knudsen, P.J., Dinarello, C.A., Strom, T.B. Glucocorticoids inhibit transcriptional and post-transcriptional expression of interleukin-1 in U937. J. Immunol. 139:4129-4134, 1987.

17. Findling, J.W., Adams, N.D., Lemann, J., Gray, R.W., Thomas, C.J., Tyrell, J.B. Vitamin D metabolites and parathyroid hormone in Cushing's syndrome - Relationship to calcium and phosphorus homeostasis. J. Clin. Endocrinol. Metab. 54:1039-1044, 1982.

18. Nielsen, H.K., Eriksen, E.F., Storm, T., Mosekilde, L. The effects of short-term high-dose treatment with prednisone on the nuclear uptake of

1,25-dihydroxyvitamin D3 in monocytes from normal human subjects. Metabolism. 37:109-114, 1988.

19. Au, W.Y.W. Cortisol stimulation of parathyroid hormone secretion by rat parathyroid glands in organ culture. Science 193:1015-1017, 1976.

20. Dietrich, J.W., Canalis, E.M., Maina, D.M., Raisz, L.G. Effects of glucocorticoids on fetal rat bone collagen synthesis in vitro. Endocrinol. 104:715-721, 1979.

21. Chyun, Y.S., Kream, B.E., Raisz, L.G. Cortisol decreases bone formation by inhibiting periosteal cell proliferation. Endocrinol. 114:477-480, 1984.

22. Bellows, C.G., Aubin, J.E., Heersche, J.N.M. Physiological concentrations of glucocorticoids stimulate formation of bone nodules from isolated rat calvaria cells in vitro. Endocrinol. 121:1985-1992, 1987.

23. Chen, T.L., Hauschka, P.V., Feldman, D. Dexamethasone increases 1,25-dihydroxyvitamin D3 receptor levels and augments bioresponses in rat osteoblast-like cells. Endocrinol. 118:1119-1126, 1986.

24. Ekestam, E., Stalenheim, G., Hallgren, R. The acute effect of high dose corticosteroid treatment on serum osteocalcin. Metabolism 37:141-144, 1988.

25. Chyun, Y.S., Raisz, L.G. Stimulation of bone formation by prostaglandin E2. Prostaglandins 27:97-103, 1984.

26. Raisz, L.G., Kream, B.E. Regulation of bone formation. New Eng. J. Med. 309:29-35, 83-89, 1983.

27. Seeman, E., Wagner, H.W., Offord, K.P., Kumar, R., Johnson, W.J., Riggs, B.L. Differential effects of endocrine dysfunction on the axial and the appendicular skeleton. J. Clin. Invest. 69:1302-1320, 1982.

28. Lund, B., Egsmose, C., Jorgensen, S., Krogsgaard, M.R. Establishment of the relative anti-inflammatory potency of deflazacort and prednisone in polymyalgia rheumatica. Calcif. Tis. Int. 41:316-320, 1987.

29. Gennari, C., Imbimbo, B., Montagnani, M., Bernini, M., Nardi, P., Avioli, L.V. Effects of prednisone and deflazacort on mineral metabolism and parathyroid hormone activity in humans. Calcif. Tis. Int. 36:245-252.

30. Guenther, H.L., Felix, R., Fleisch, H. Comparative study of deflazacort, a new synthetic corticosteroid, and dexamethasone on the synthesis of collagen in different rat bone cell populations and rabbit articular chondrocytes. Calcif. Tis. Int. 36:145-152, 1984.

31. Ringe, J.D., Welzel, D. Salmon calcitonin in the therapy of corticoid-induced osteoporosis. Eur. J. Clin. Pharm. 33:35-39, 1987.

32. Reid, I.R., King, A.R., Alexander, C.J., Ibbertson, H.K. Prevention of steroid-induced osteoporosis with (3-amino-1-hydroxypropylidene)-1, 1-bisphosphonate (APD). Lancet 8578:143-146, 1988.

33. VandenBroucke, J.P., Witteman, J.C.M., Valkenburg, H.A., Boersma, J.W., Cats, A., Festen, J.J.M., Hartman, A.P., Huber-Bruning, O., Rasker, J.J., Weber, J. Noncontraceptive hormones and rheumatoid arthritis in perimenopausal and postmenopausal women. J.A.M.A. 225:1299-1303, 1986.

34. Rickers, H., Deding, A., Christiansen, C., Rodbro, P. Mineral loss in cortical and trabecular bone during high-dose prednisone treatment. Calcif. Tis. Int. 36:269-273, 1984.

Discussion:

DR. PARFITT (Detroit): When we treat patients with proven osteomalacia with vitamin D or its metabolites and show a 30 to 40 percent increase in mineralized bone in the ilium, and we look at so-called metaphyseal bone mass in these patients measured by SPA, we show less than a 2 percent increase over the same time period. How do you reconcile that with your apparent endorsement of a study which claimed a 15 percent increase in metaphyseal bone mass with a vitamin D metabolite in a group of patients who almost surely had a much lesser degree of osteoid accumulation and secondary hyperparathyroidism than our osteomalacic subjects?

DR. RAISZ (Connecticut): I can't reconcile it. Certainly the mechanism for the 15 percent increase shown here was not the filling up of osteomalacic seams, because on biopsy, as you know, these patients - although they may have a mineralization defect, they also have a marked defect in synthesizing matrix - don't have such wide seams. They don't have a place to put the calcium.

I must tell you that I'm at a loss to explain both this effect of 25-D, and why 1,25 didn't work. Is it possible that 25 has some trophic effect in the glucocorticoid treated patient? I can tell you that attempting to look for that in the laboratory, we've been unable to find it. No, I can't explain it.

DR. BOUILLON (Belgium): Can you speculate what would be the origin of the difference of cortisone effects on trabecular bone and cortical bone?

DR. RAISZ: I think it simply relates to the rate of turnover. In other words, the more bone formation is required to maintain that particular bone mass, the more an inhibitor of bone formation is going to affect that mass. And the rate - the proportion of new bone that is formed at the trabecular part of the skeleton per year - is so much greater than the proportion formed in the cortical that you see this much greater effect.

I don't think there's any more to it than that, although there may be some selective localization.

DR. DEMPSTER (New York): You mentioned your distress that many postmenopausal women with steroid-induced osteoporosis don't seem to be being prescribed estrogens. Do you know of any formal studies where the effect of estrogens has been examined?

DR. RAISZ: Just before I got up to give this talk I asked Norm Bell, in desperation, if he had seen such a study. I have searched the literature for this, and I'm glad you brought it up because I was going to ask this audience, "Have I missed something? Why don't we have a study of the effect of estrogen on glucocorticoid-induced osteoporosis?" All we have is everybody's anecdotal experience here. Many of us have used it. But I don't know of a single study, and it's certainly important to do. Intuitively, it shouldn't have any less effect on the resorptive response, which is probably mediated by the same things in the glucocorticoid patient. But we need those data desperately.

DR. GENANT (San Francisco): My comment on the relative rates of loss in the sites of trabecular bone are based upon some data that were presented last fall at the International Workshop on Densitometry in England. This was data presented by Montage from Munster, representing approximately 60 patients that were placed on high-dose Prednisone, doses ranging from 20 to 60 milligrams a day for a period of one month. And following vertebral bone mass in that case with quantitative CT, they documented an average rate of loss of about 17 or 18 percent in four weeks.

So, this emphasizes the rapidity with which these changes can occur. And furthermore, they took a subset of their patients and did treat them with sodium fluoride and showed either stabilization or increase in bone mass in a substantial number. I don't believe that that was a controlled study, but at least it supports, perhaps, the use of sodium fluoride in this setting.

DR. RAISZ: I just want to comment that that massive loss of bone must be the result of increased resorption as well as decreased formation. And, therefore, I need to adjust what I said before to Jonathan Reeve, I guess it was. Clearly, rapid increases in resorption derived from, let's say, marrow osteoclasts might occur to a greater extent on trabecular bone than on cortical bone.

DR. NAGANT (Belgium): To answer the question of Professor Parfitt, we were unable, giving calcifidiol, 40 micrograms per day, to patients with rheumatoid arthritis treated with glucocorticoids to significantly increase metaphyseal bone mass. But we were able to prevent bone loss at the metaphysis.

Now, to answer the question of Dr. Dempster. Evidently, when following patients with rheumatoid arthritis treated with an average 7.5 milligrams per day of Prednisone, before the menopause we were unable to see any significant bone loss, whereas after the menopause bone loss was very obvious. That doesn't answer the question entirely, but indicates that estrogens may be effective preventive therapy against small doses of glucocorticoids, which remains to be proven.

DR. RAISZ: But it means that we need to prove that estrogen is worthwhile in these patients, because there's a great resistance to giving estrogen in autoimmune disease, which is probably rational in lupus, although perhaps not even there. But certainly it doesn't seem to be rational in rheumatoid arthritis.

DR. GAGEL (Houston): Earlier in this week we heard from Gideon Rodan that in an immobilization model of the rat, that there was increased prostaglandin E2 production associated with immobilization bone loss. And perhaps more importantly that there was decreased bone formation in that model system.

Given that evidence and the evidence that PGE2 is primarily a stimulator of bone resorption, I was a little concerned about your conclusions that it might be a way of reversing glucocorticoid-induced osteoporosis. And I wonder if you could expand your comments to address these points.

DR. RAISZ: Well, I thought I was clearer than that. I said that I don't see how you could possibly use it to reverse glucocorticoid osteopenia because you could only use it if you could give it to the defective preosteoblasts and not to any other cells in the body. Because what you said is absolutely true. It does increase bone resorption. And an excess of PGE2 could be an adverse factor after menopause and other times in causing bone loss.

I might say that we don't have any evidence one way or the other about the relative effect of nonsteroidals on bone loss in rheumatoid arthritis patients. But the problem there is that when you look at these patients, they're receiving nonsteroidals in an intermittent fashion. And so, their net prostaglandin production may not be greatly affected anyway.

DR. PRICE (Maryland): When you are talking about using estrogen in people on steroids, are you talking about it in people who are recently postmenopausal, or people who are ten years or more out?

DR. RAISZ: I'm talking about anyone. I don't know when one would stop starting estrogen. If a patient came to you with rheumatoid arthritis on glucocorticoids and low bone mass and was 65 and hadn't received estrogen, I can't, at the moment, give you any reason why they shouldn't be considered for estrogen therapy. And we certainly do that.

DR. PRICE: I'm just curious, in people who are not on glucocorticoids, do you have the same approach if they have low bone mass and they're more than ten years after you use estrogens?

DR. RAISZ: I do. But that's other people's topic.

General Discussion

DR. ETTINGER (San Francisco): I have a comment and a caveat about 1,25 treatment for osteoporosis. In our hands, in San Francisco, using CT of the spine as well as the other measurements we found it quite ineffective in restoring bone mass to osteoporotic women. But beyond that, I'm really concerned about practitioners using 1,25. It's a drug that has to be handled extremely carefully.

Those of us who were involved in this multi-center study were seeing patients monthly, monitoring urinary and serum calciums frequently and finding unexpected rises in either serum or urine calcium at rather odd times during this study. Perhaps, it really might look fine for three months or four months and then suddenly the patient becomes hypercalcemic.

So, I don't think anyone should come away from here with the thought that this is something that can be applied to the treatment of osteoporotic women.

DR. GALLAGHER (Omaha): I think the point that Dr. Ettinger makes is quite correct. And I think that's something we need to point out to everybody, since you were involved in these studies, is that the way the study was designed, it was designed to take us to the point of toxicity. I mean, there was no doubt about that. But we produced hypercalcemia in every single patient as a deliberate maneuver, and then backed down a dose.

And I think that our experience, and Larry Riggs might make a comment here, is that generally on doses of half a microgram and an average calcium intake in this country, you do not, in fact, get hypercalcemia and hypercalciuria. I think we made some calculations out of 2,500 observations on urine calcium and serum calcium over a two-year period. I think we saw two episodes of mild hypercalciuria on half a microgram. It is unusual. But, of course, it would be a potential problem if you had calcium supplements.

And I think if you just want to make people aware that there's a potential toxicity problem there, yes, I think that's fine. But I think in half a microgram it's unusual. But above that, I think that it would be quite common. So, I think it's just a matter of laying down what the guidelines should be.

DR. CHESNUT (Seattle): I think in our study, Dr. Ott was concerned about side effects. And for that reason we never got the dose up very high.

Would you agree, Chris, that if we go up to .75 or a microgram of 1,25, even at that level are we going to have benefit on bone mass?

DR. GALLAGHER: I think there are two issues involved. At half a microgram of 1,25, we're dealing probably with a purely calcium absorption effect. That's my feeling. I think there is some evidence that once you get above one microgram there is a separate and independent effect in terms of stimulating bone. And then, of course, we would really have significant problems in terms of hypercalcemia and hypercalciuria, unless we control the calcium intake to less than 500 milligrams.

We've done that successfully for six months without any problems. But, nevertheless, I wouldn't advise that as a general maneuver at the present time. And I think, at our present state of knowledge, we should use half a microgram, or even slightly less, probably, as a calcium-absorbing hormone, until further information comes along.

DR. CHESNUT: In other words, we may still be able to say that there is a beneficial effect of 1,25 on bone formation mineralization or whatever, but we're unable to achieve that particular level due to side effects.

DR. GALLAGHER: Very nicely put.

DR. KHAIRI (Indianapolis): I'd like the experts to comment on the use of estrogen in women age 65 to 70. Is it too late to use it, or should we still consider using in that kind of a situation.

DR. RIGGS (Rochester, MN): I'd like to say this is, again, an area where there really is not good data. The older idea was that after you go through the period of accelerated bone loss following the menopause, which is probably no more than six or eight years at the most. Then you go into a stage of low bone turnover where depressed bone formation is the dominant process. That has never been explicitly looked at. And our more recent data suggests that, in fact, bone turnover does stay high in the older person.

So, I think if bone turnover is high, it's possible that estrogen could have a favorable effect. And we just don't have objective data. But I think from a practical standpoint that- particularly if you have a woman with vertebral fractures - that estrogen certainly could still be used.

DR. JOHNSTON (Indianapolis): There was a paper that appeared last summer from, I think, Los Angeles that demonstrated that at least until age 70 estrogen would inhibit bone loss compared to controls that were not on estrogen. So, we know that it is effective, certainly up until that age, at inhibiting loss.

DR. DUNCAN (Detroit): There are two points that Larry Raisz was speaking to on steroid-induced osteoporosis in the rheumatic diseases patients. Rheumatoid arthritis in particular is probably the worst example of rheumatic diseases we could use because of concurrent therapy, and that they already have a low bone turnover distant to affected joints.

In addition, the steroids are further reducing the bone turnover of our patients and if you add estrogen, how much do you expect estrogens to further suppress the turnover?

DR. RAISZ: I think that the issue is when you would give the estrogen in that case. And, maybe, in answering an earlier question, I should have been more conservative about how late we would use estrogen.

The problem is that among our glucocorticoid-induced osteoporosis patients, we don't know how great the contribution of increased bone resorption is, and how great the contribution of decreased bone formation is. And we certainly would expect that estrogen would have some positive effects to block further bone resorption.

DR. DUNCAN: Steroids' effects are very, very depressing.

DR. RAISZ: The other problem is that there's evidence from Larry Riggs and others that there is some anabolic effect of estrogen on bone cells. And if that pans out to be true for humans, then that will be an additional reason for using the estrogen.

DR. DUNCAN: I'd like to submit that there's a difference in the long-term low dose and the pulsing patterns that are going on at the present. We need to look at those particular situations.

DR. RAISZ: Yes, the possibility of giving an anti-resorptive agent during the pulse is something that I would love to see explored. And this might be calcitonin or a diphosphonate or estrogen.

DR. GALLAGHER: The point is not that bone resorption is increased, but that net bone resorption has increased. Your level of bone resorption can stay the same, but if your bone formation declines, then net bone resorption increases. And, therefore, to give any agent which slows down turnover further, such as estrogen, would reduce the amount of negative calcium balance coming out of bone. So there would be a benefit.

DR. GENANT: In the very short-term, perhaps the first six months of exposure to the corticosteroids, there is very accelerated bone loss. This almost certainly has to be accelerated bone resorption. And perhaps estrogen's role might be of greater importance. We have ourselves been following pulmonary patients over periods up to six months, observed 20 to 30 percent declines in vertebral mass over that period of time.

DR. DUNCAN: Wouldn't calcitonin be better? It's a much more specific osteoblast suppressant.

DR. GENANT: We have a prospective study just underway looking at that, in both treatment and prevention, actually.

DR. RIGGS: I might also comment that perhaps we should be careful in extrapolating the Hahn study from the bone changes at the metaphysis to the entire skeleton, since their patients had rheumatoid arthritis and undoubtedly, in many of them the wrist joint was involved. So, that these large increases in bone mass that they found may, indeed, not be representative of the entire skeleton.

DR. GENANT: I think that's an important point, and I'd like to comment on that also in that we studied approximately 30 patients with either corticosteroid-induced osteoporosis or Cushing's disease, and analyzed measurement sites including radial cortex, metaphysis, metacarpal cortical thickness, and spine.

In fact, in this group we were not able to find a disproportionate loss of the metaphyseal bone relative to the radial shaft. Now, that was not the ultra distal site, but was the traditional three centimeter distal site. And at that site, disproportionate loss was not observed.

DR. RAISZ: These really weren't enormous increases that Hahn showed, because there's a law of initial values. The levels of metaphyseal bone in these rheumatoid patients were down around 20, 30, 40 percent of normal. And so, an increase of 15 percent may have represented a relatively small amount of bone that was actually formed. And I think that's perhaps why those data will have been misleading in terms of the effectiveness of this therapy.

DR. LAFFERTY (Cleveland): This is a question to Dr. Raisz. Since patients who have fractures who are on large doses of corticosteroids have an exuberant callus formation, presumably chondroblastic activity, do you postulate that corticosteroids have a different effect on chondroblast than they do on osteoblast?

DR. RAISZ: I think that has to do with the remarkable fact that there is a tremendous amount of growth factor in the bone, in everyone, all the time. And if you can get that out as you do when you fracture the bone, or when you can add both factors from the circulation such as PDGF or IGF1 when coming from macrophages, all the things that move into that site, you can, in fact, overcome this inhibition of the normal preosteoblast/osteoblast system. Cartilage formation is slowed overall in glucocorticoid-treated patients.

But I think that this response to injury shows us that enough growth factors can overcome the glucocorticoid effect. And this is where the problem is, therefore, not unsolvable.

DR. DEQUEKER (Belgium): There is another argument to say that estrogen treatment in postmenopausal women with rheumatoid arthritis under corticosteroid therapy would have some benefit, and this has not been mentioned yet, namely, the negative feedback to the ACTH. The secretion of androstenedione, which is the only estrogen source in the postmenopause, will be suppressed by the cortocosteroids. So, they have a double disadvantage: direct negative effect of corticosteroids and the lower estrogen level compared to the other postmenopausal women.

DR. RAISZ: That's an excellent point. And I was remarking to someone earlier that we've not talked about androgens in the female at all so far, have we? Has anybody talked about them in this conference? There's quite a lot of reason to believe that the relatively low, but real levels of androgen, be they testosterone androstenedione, and DHEA's are related to bone mass in all kinds of osteoporosis. I don't have any specific evidence on that though. Do you? What happens? When you give the estrogen, can you make a little androgen from that? That doesn't work, does it?

VI
Metabolic Bone Disease and the Hip

Overview:
Metabolic Bone Disease and the Hip

ROBERT LINDSAY

Regional Bone Center
Helen Hayes Hospital
West Haverstraw, NY
and Department of Clinical Medicine
Columbia University
New York, NY

It is clear that fracture of the hip is the most serious of the fractures of the aging population. However the relationship between osteoporosis and fracture presentation has been questioned. Riggs and his colleagues have postulated that the aging bone loss that precedes fracture of the hip is consequent upon the gradual decline in the supply of 1,25-dihydroxy-cholecalciferol probably consequent upon reduction in renal function (1). This section of the symposium set out to examine some of these issues about hip fractures including its epidemiology, its relationship to bone disease and particularly to 1,25(OH)2-D supply, as well as current approaches to treatment of patients with hip fracture from both medical and surgical viewpoints.

In the initial presentation the epidemiology of falls and hip fractures was reviewed (2). It is well known that the risk of hip fracture increases with age in both males and females, as does the risk of falls. However only a small percentage of falls result in hip fracture (~1%).

A variety of factors are thought to influence this relationship, but the final conclusion seems inescapable. The energy from the fall that is transmitted to the femoral neck must exceed its strength, which is closely related to its mineral "density". Thus, there are larger differences in bone mass between those who have suffered a hip fracture and those who have fallen but did not fracture, than between the former group and "normals". Presumably, therefore, if bone mass did not fall with age then injury to the femoral neck would be significantly less likely, although clearly further study of the relationship is required. The conclusion might be, however, that hip fracture is a phenomenon of aging and consequently if everyone were to live long enough, all would fracture a hip. In the second presentation the techniques for measurement of bone in the femoral neck were evaluated (3). At present two techniques DPA and DEXA, the x-ray equivalent of DPA, are the only available methods. Unlike measurements of the spine, DEXA does not appear, on preliminary data, to provide significant improvements in precision over DPA, although the shorter scanning time will allow more intensive quality control. Curiously part of the overlap noted between normals and fracture patients could be attributed to the effect of variable distance between source and object (i.e. the femoral neck) and not due to true difference in bone mass.

Since the hip is not an easy site to measure the question of the inter-relationships between sites was examined (4). Using bone biopsy as the standard it was noted that while there were significant relationships between spine and iliac crest cancellous bone volume, the values obtained in the spine were always lower, with thinner trabeculae and different spatial configuration. Few data are available comparing femoral neck with biopsy, and clearly further study of this issue is required. Clarification of the relationship between spinal measurements and hip measurements was not examined, but clearly is also an issue, the importance of disproportionate loss of trabecular bone at each of these sites, being an issue that was raised during the discussion. Wide variability in turnover between sites has been observed in the few data available. This is clearly important since turnover data from the standard biopsy site are increasingly being used in deciding the therapeutic approach to the patient.

In the modeling approach to the assessment of risk, Dr Horsman presented information demonstrating how a model system might be used to determine the degree of risk of fracture of the hip for any individual (5). It is clear that to allow such a model to be put into clinical use more detailed information about the epidemiology of falls and their relationship to fracture is required. However predictability is important to the clinician since many patients will present either at menopause, or at the time of first fracture, usually of distal radius or spine, and treatments should probably be initiated at one of those time markers.

The second half of the session examined the potential role of vitamin D metabolism in the pathogenesis of the disorder. In the first of these two presentations Clemens reviewed the evidence for declining plasma levels of 1,25-(OH)2D with age (6). In the second Peacock noted the decline in 25-(OH)D seen most obviously in Great Britain, and suggested that insufficiency of this metabolite was a causative factor in bone loss and hip fracture. However both presentations stressed the importance of impaired conversion of 25-(OH)D to its 1-hydroxylated metabolite as part of the aging process. This was demonstrated by two different approaches, but the biological consequences have yet to be confirmed. Reduced calcium absorption does appear to result in hip fracture patients, in whom it appears not reversible with precursor administration, unlike healthy elderly (7).

As was evident from the detailed and wide ranging discussion, further work is clearly required in this area, particularly in determining the clinical consequences of these alterations in vitamin D metabolism, and subsequently in establishing treatment protocols to reverse them.

In the final section of this session attention was turned toward treatment aspects. Lane et al (8) emphasized the

Epidemiology of Hip Fractures and Falls

S.R. CUMMINGS and M.C. NEVITT

*Division of General Internal Medicine
and Department of Epidemiology and International Health
University of California
San Francisco, CA*

The incidence of fractures increases exponentially with age. White women have about a 15% lifetime risk of hip fracture compared to 2-5% for men and blacks (1). In 1985, 247,000 hip fractures occurred in the United States among women and men over age 45 (2). The age-specific incidence of hip fractures appears to be increasing in Northern Europe, but not in the United States (3). Since the number of elderly is steadily increasing, the annual number of hip fractures among women and men over age 50 in the United States will more than double by the year 2040, even if the age-specific incidence of hip fractures remains constant.

Those who suffer a hip fracture have about a 5-20% greater risk of dying within the first year than expected for age (4). Much of this mortality, however, might be due to concomitant disabling illnesses. Fewer than half of elderly patients who suffer a hip fracture fully recover their functional abilities one year later. Hip fractures cost over 7 billion dollars in 1984 in the United States alone. Assuming only a 3% rate of inflation, the annual cost of hip fractures would exceed $30 billion by the year 2020.

Falls

Among the elderly, the risk of falling increases with age. In the United States, the annual risk of falling increases from 19% among women who are 60-64 years old to 33% among those who are 80-84 (Figure 1). The number of falls per year actually increases more rapidly with age because more of the very elderly suffer several falls per year. Most studies indicate that the risk of falling is somewhat greater for women than men.

About half of all falls in the elderly cause injury, but most of these injuries are minor. Among community-dwelling elderly, about 4-6% of falls result in fractures (5); the rate is higher in nursing homes. Syncopal falls are several times more likely than nonsyncopal falls to cause fractures (Cummings SR and Nevitt MC, unpublished), suggesting that loss of protective responses during a fall substantially increases the risk of fracture. A very large number of risk factors for falls have been proposed, but few have been tested in prospective studies. We have recently found that past history of multiple falls or injurious falls, Caucasian race, Parkinson's disease, arthritis, difficulty standing up from a chair or performing a tandem-walk, and impaired depth perception were

Figure 1
Annual Risk of Falling Among Older Women*

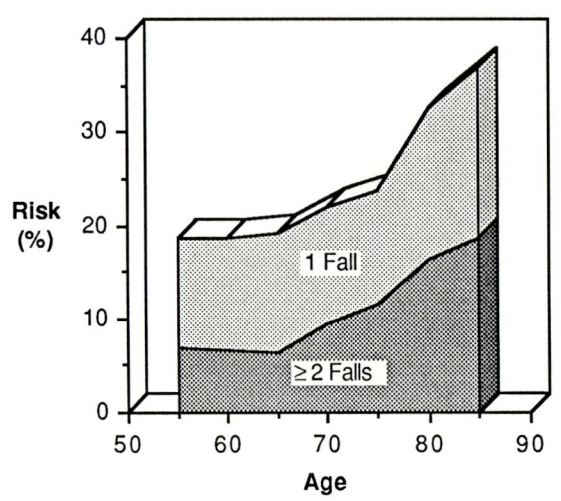

*Unpublished data from the 1984 United States Health Interview Survey, Supplement on Aging (National Center for Health Services Research)

independent predictors of multiple falls (unpublished). Other studies have found that regular use of sedative hypnotics also increases the risk of both falling and hip fracture.

Falls and the Pathogenesis of Hip Fracture

About 90% of hip fractures are due to moderate trauma, usually falls directly onto the hip (1,6,7). A fall from standing height has several times the potential energy necessary to fracture even a normal hip (8). But only 1% of falls result in hip fractures (Cummings and Nevitt, unpublished). Thus, in 99% of falls, most of the potential energy of the fall is diverted away from the hip or absorbed by other tissues before it is transmitted to the proximal femur.

We hypothesize that in order for the fall to cause a hip fracture, several conditions must be satisfied (Table 1): First, the fall must be oriented so as to land on or near the hip. This type of orientation is more likely when the faller has little or no forward momentum, such as when falls occur at slow gait speeds, during syncope, "drop attacks," transfers from bed to chair, or while descending stairs or curbs. Additionally, we hypothesize that some elderly have an abnormal reaction to losing their balance--a sudden loss of extensor muscle tone ("collapse reaction")-- that predisposes them to land on a hip or buttocks when they fall.

Second, normal protective responses, such as grabbing objects or landing on outstretched hands, must fail. The effectiveness of these responses may depend on reaction time and muscle strength. Third, local shock absorbers, such as fat and muscles around the hip, must fail to absorb enough energy to protect the proximal femur from breaking (7).

Finally, the *residual energy* of the fall transmitted to the proximal femur must exceed the strength of the bone. Since the mineral "density" (BMD) of the proximal femur is highly correlated with its strength, it is the best available index of bone strength. But other factors, such as the geometry and quality of bone are also important (9,10).

This hypothesis suggests that the risk of hip fractures will increase with increased risk of falling, decreased gait speed, slowed reaction time,

Table 1
The Pathogenesis of Hip Fractures due to Falls

Defenses against hip fracture	Factors that may impair defenses
1. Orientation of fall (away from hip)	Slow gait Fall during bed-chair transfer Fall while descending stairs or curbs Syncope, "drop attacks" "Collapse" reaction to loss of balance

2. Protective responses
  - Grabbing objects
  - Landing on extended arm
	Slowed reaction time
	Decreased strength

3. Local shock absorbers
  - Muscles surrounding hip
  - Peri-trochanteric fat and skin
	Muscle atrophy, weakness
	Thin body build
	Skin atrophy

4. Strength of proximal femur
  - Mass
  - Architecture
	Osteopenia
	Qualitative abnormalities

decreased strength, decreased fat and muscle around the hip, and decreased strength of the proximal femur. All of these factors change substantially with aging (Table 2) and may contribute to the exponential increase in incidence of hip fracture with aging.

Melton (11) has observed that the annual risk of hip fracture among women very low BMD in the proximal femur (< 0.6 g/cm^2), is only about 2%. This may be because the other 98% do not fall or, if they fall, they divert or absorb enough potential energy to avoid breaking their hip. Since osteopenia is only one of several causal factors, more rigorous studies have found that cases with hip fracture have only somewhat lower bone density than controls of similar age (12). But, as this hypothesis would predict, there are much larger

Table 2
Age-related Changes that May Contribute to Hip Fracture

Factor	Relative change from ages 60-65 to 80-85*
Risk of hip fracture	10 X increase
Number of falls [1]	≥2 X increase
Gait speed [2]	34% decrease
Muscle strength [2]	20-30% decrease
Reaction time [2]	16 - 22% decrease
Hip BMD [3]	29% decrease

* All estimates in this table are based on cross-sectional studies.
1. Unpublished data from the 1984 U.S. Health Interview Survey, Supplement on Aging.
2. Cummings SR, unpublished data.
3. Melton LJ, personal communication.

differences between the bone mass of women who have fractured their hip and women of similar age who have fallen on the hip but sustained no fracture (13).

Risk Factors for Hip Fracture

Most studies of risk factors for hip fracture have focused only on factors that might affect bone mass. There has been little research about factors that may increase the risk of falling or decrease the effectiveness of protective responses. There are several risk factors for hip fractures that appear to increase the risk of fracture because of an increased risk of falling: use of long-acting sedative-hypnotics, disabling rheumatoid arthritis, and impaired vision. Alcoholism may increase the risk of fracture by increasing the risk of falling, impairing protective responses to falls, and decreasing bone strength. Other factors that presumably influence the risk of hip fractures by their effects on bone mass, such as race, corticosteroid therapy, smoking, and estrogen therapy, could also affect neuromuscular function and the risk of falling. These possibilities need further study.

The best established risk and protective factors for hip fracture are age, sex, race, estrogen use, body build, and oopherectomy before natural menopause (Table 3). A recent study (14) suggests that the incidence of hip

Table 3
Risk Factors for Hip Fracture in Women*
(Increased risk: +, Protective: -)

STRONG EVIDENCE

Advanced age (+)	Female (+)
Caucasian (+)	Obesity (-)
Black, Mexican-American (-)	Thinness (+)
Bilateral oopherectomy before natural menopause (+)	Estrogen use (≥ 5 years) (-)

LIMITED EVIDENCE

Previous hip fracture (+)	Long-acting sedatives (+)
Heavy use of alcohol (+)	Cigarette smoking (+)
Chronic use of corticosteroids (+)	Disabling rheumatoid arthritis (+)
History of falling (+)	Asian race (+)
Impaired visual acuity (+)	

PROBABLY NO INCREASED RISK

Type II diabetes	Age at natural menopause,
Child-bearing	Breast feeding
Thyroid hormone (replacement doses)	Rheumatoid arthritis without disability

LITTLE OR NO EVIDENCE

Family history of osteoporosis	Caffeine
Calcium intake	Antacids
Moderate alcohol use (< 2 drinks/day)	Physical activity

* See references 1 & 15.

fractures among Asian women in the United States is similar to that of Caucasian women. Many factors commonly mentioned as risk factors, such as family history of osteoporosis, sedentary life-style and low calcium diet, have not yet been established as risk factors for hip fracture (1,15).

Prospects for Prevention

Long-term use of estrogen is the only well-substantiated method for preventing hip fractures. Estrogen protects against bone loss and reduces the risk of hip and other types of fractures by about 50% (1,14,16). Much of this protection may be lost within about five years after estrogens are discontinued (16). Less than 15% of white women over age 65 in the United States are currently using estrogen (see J. Cauley, this volume). Increased use of estrogen among postmenopausal women would slow but not prevent the steady increase in hip fractures. Because most hip fractures occur after age 75, it may take one or two decades before an increased long-term use of estrogen among 50-60 year old women would have a noticeable effect on the incidence of hip fractures.

Prevention of hip fractures among the very elderly could produce more immediate results. Since most elderly women are already osteopenic and rates of bone loss in this age group are relatively slow, efforts to prevent fractures in the very elderly must focus on preventing falls. The most efficient strategies would focus on preventing falls among those with the greatest risk of multiple falls and preventing the types of falls that are most likely to cause hip fractures. Pharmacologic treatments that strengthen the proximal femur or protective padding that absorbs much of the energy of a direct impact near the hip could also decrease the risk of hip fractures. Such interventions may be most beneficial for those who are prone to recurrent falls, have poor defenses against hip fracture, and have severe osteopenia. These types of preventive measures, however, remain to be developed and tested.

References

1. Cummings SR, Kelsey JL, Nevitt MC, O Dowd KJ. Epidemiology of osteoporosis and osteoporotic fractures. Epidemiol Rev 1985;7:178-208.

2. National Center for Health Statistics. 1985 Summary: National Hospital Discharge Survey. Advance Data from Vital and Health Statistics. No. 127, DHHS Pub. No. (PHS) 86-1250. Public Health Service. Hyattsville, MD. Sept. 25, 1986.

3. Melton LJ, O'Fallon WM, Riggs BL. Secular trends in the incidence of hip fractures. Calcif Tissue Int 1987;41:57-64.

4. Cummings SR. Osteoporotic fractures: the magnitude of the problem. In Christiansen C, Johansen JS, Riis BJ (eds). Osteoporosis 1987 (volume 2). Copenhagen. Osteopress, 1987:1193-6.

5. Gryfe CI, Amies A, Ashley MJ. A longitudinal study of falls in an elderly population: I. Incidence and morbidity. Age ageing 1977;6:201-10.

6. Clark ANG. Factors in fracture of the female femur: A clinical study of the environmental, physical, medical and preventative aspects of the injury. Geront Clin 1968;10:257-70.

7. Melton LJ, Riggs Bl. Risk factors for injury after a fall. Clin Geriatr Med 1985;1:1-15.

8. Frankel VH, Pugh JW. Biomechanics of the hip. In Frankel VE (ed). Basic Biomechanics of the skeletal system. Philadelphia: Lea and Febiger, 1980: 115-131.

9. Parfitt AM. Trabecular architecture in the pathogenesis and prevention of fracture. Am J Med 1987;82:68-71.

10. Hayes WC, Gerhart TN. Biomechanics of bone: applications for assessment of bone strength. In Peck WA (ed). Bone and Mineral Research/3. Amsterdam: Elsevier, 1985:259-94.

11. Melton LJ, Wahner HW, Richelson LS, O'Fallon WM, Riggs BL. Osteoporosis and the risk of hip fracture. Am J Epidemiol 1986;124:254-61.

12. Cummings SR. Are patients with hip fractures more osteoporotic? Review of the evidence. Am J Med 1985;78:487-94.

13. Cooper C, Barker DJP, Morris J, Briggs RSJ. Osteoporosis, risk of falling and neuromuscular protective responses in fracture of the proximal femur. In Christiansen C, Johansen JS, Riis BJ (eds). Osteoporosis 1987 (volume 1). Copenhagen. Osteopress, 1987:141-3.

14. Haber R, Hodgkins M, Black D. Racial differences in hip fracture incidence. Clin Res 1988;37: (in press).

15. Kelsey JL. Epidemiology of osteoporosis and associated fractures. In Peck WA, (ed). Bone and Mineral Research / 5. New York, Elsevier Science Publishers B.V.; 1987, 409-44.

16. Weiss NS, Ure CL, Ballard JH, et al. Decreased risk of fractures of the hip and lower forearm with postmenopausal use of estrogen. N Engl J Med 1980;303:1195-8.

Noninvasive Measurement of Bone Loss in the Femoral Neck

HEINZ W. WAHNER

Department of Diagnostic Radiology
Mayo Clinic and Foundation
Rochester, MN

INTRODUCTION

Until recently, information on bone loss in the hip was based mainly on changes in trabecular structure and cortical thickness, and measurements of bone mass were restricted to studies on excised bones. Technical developments in dual-photon absorptiometry (DPA) and more recently in quantitative computed tomography (QCT) make it possible to quantify, with acceptable accuracy and precision, bone mineral in the hip in vivo. These new developments stimulated new efforts in the understanding of bone loss and fracture in the hip.

This report reviews the presently available techniques for measuring in vivo bone loss in the hip. Because they are new, DPA and dual-energy X-ray absorptiometry (DEXA) are compared and described in more detail. As an introduction to the complexity of bone structure in the hips, the anatomy of the proximal femur and changes in bone structure and mass that occur during life are briefly described. The objective is to develop a test procedure that would allow the prediction of fracture risk in the hips of patients with osteoporosis.

DEVELOPMENTAL CHANGES IN THE PROXIMAL FEMUR

The shaft of the femur of the newborn human baby is ossified, whereas the femoral head and neck, the intertrochanteric crest, and the trochanters consist of a continuous mass of epiphyseal cartilage. At 3 years of age, bony lamellae are present in the region of the base of the lesser trochanter, the earliest signs of the calcar femorale. Bony lamellae become more abundant, and the trochanters and the intertrochanteric crest develop by budding out from the original oval diaphysis. The trabecular structure and the calcar femorale reach maximal size and density at early adulthood. With old age, there is progressive thinning of the trabeculae, and the space resulting from the reduction in trabecular bone mass is filled with fat. In addition, there is a change from red bone marrow to yellow marrow. These alterations result in a significant change in intraosseous fat content of the proximal femur during life. In 60% of the 110 persons 75 years old or older, Harty (1) found that Ward's triangle contained no trabecular bone but was occupied entirely by yellow marrow.

The medial angle between the shaft and the neck decreases during active growth and ranges between 110° and 145° in adulthood. After adulthood is reached, the angle remains constant into old age.

The medial and backward deviation of the femoral neck produces maximal pressure stresses on the inner posterior surfaces of the upper-fourth of the shaft. The calcar femorale reinforces the bone in this region. The trabecular structure and the cortical bone thickness in the proximal femur reflect the mechanical forces.

AGE-RELATED BONE REMODELING IN THE FEMUR

The internal architecture of the proximal femur is composed of two major trabecular systems that are arranged along the lines of compressive and tensile stresses produced during weight-bearing. A central region defines a neutral axis where tensile and compressive forces balance each other. Secondary compressive and tensile groups of trabeculae can be identified (see Fig. 1).

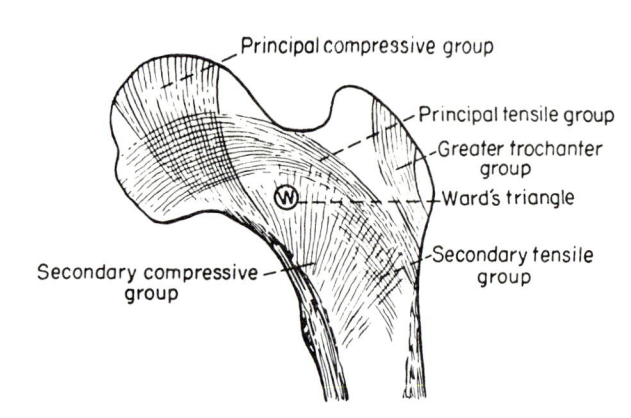

Fig. 1. Trabecular structure of proximal femur as used in trabecular grading pattern proposed by Singh (2).

Adaptive alterations of these patterns occur by bone remodeling as a result of changes in the vector of stress forces. This is seen in variations in the external configuration of the proximal femur, and alterations of the normal trabecular pattern are seen with weight-bearing changes.

With age, bone loss in the proximal femur is different from that in the spinal column (3). In the latter, bone loss starts with a loss of horizontal trabeculae, which results in pressure increase and hypertrophy of the remaining vertical trabeculae. In time, this leads to a decrease in the specific surface of trabecular bone (trabecular bone surface per volume of trabeculae) (4). Microfractures, repair, and hypertrophy constitute a chronic process that ultimately results in end-plate deformities and compression fractures. In the proximal femur, bone loss follows a definite pattern that reflects a hierarchy of function of the trabecular group in meeting the mechanical demands of weight-bearing. Secondary trabeculae are resorbed first, and Ward's triangle enlarges. Next there is a loss of tensile trabeculae starting centrally, the primary tensile group being the last to be absorbed (2). Trabecular hypertrophy is not observed. The decreasing mean trabecular diameter leads to an increase in the specific surface (4). This sequence of events is illustrated by the patterns of the Singh Index (Fig. 2).

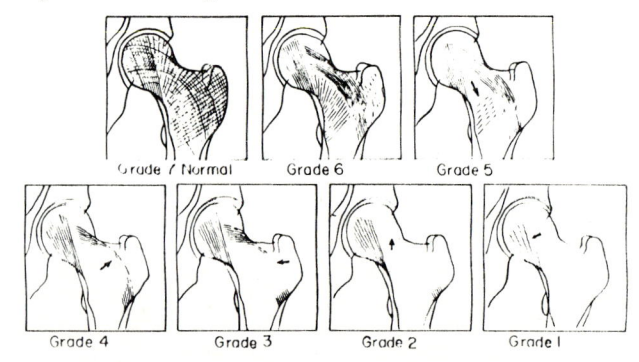

Fig. 2. Singh Index patterns. All subjects start with pattern 7 or 6. With progressing age, lower grades are observed in most but not all subjects.

In cancellous bone of excised specimens of proximal femur, there is a significant correlation between mechanical properties and bone mineral (5). Removal of the central trabecular bone portion from a specimen of proximal femur reduces the strength for impact loading by about 50%. This reduction suggests not only that trabecular bone has a major part in the strength of the bone but also that cortical bone has structural importance. Variations in compressive strength and modules of elasticity are large within and between femoral bone samples, larger than seen in the spinal column. This observation suggests that age-related bone loss in the hip is modulated more effectively by certain factors (exercise, life-style, nutrition) than is bone loss in the spinal column. Density alone does not fully account for the wide variation in mechanical properties, and microstructure must have a prominent role in mechanical behavior. The importance of the latter is also suggested by the relatively low correlation between appendicular cortical bone mass (radius) or distant trabecular bone mass (spine) and the trabecular pattern in the femur (6, 7).

MEASUREMENT TECHNIQUES

Several in vivo procedures have been used to study bone changes in the hip. Measurements on cadaver bones are the reference standard. The principal procedures are summarized in Table 1.

Table 1: Methods Used for Noninvasive Estimation of Bone Loss at the Hip

Principal approach	Information available	Technique
Imaging procedures (descriptive)	Description of trabecular structure and/or cortical bone thickness	Radiography; computed x-ray tomography; magnetic resonance imaging
Semi-quantitative procedures	Grading of trabecular bone pattern in proximal femur (Singh Index);	Radiographs of hips; inward rotation
	Thickness of calcar femorale; cortical Index	Frog lateral view
Quantitative procedures	Bone density at different sites of the proximal femur; integral bone area density (g/cm^2)	DPA and DEXA
	Trabecular and/or integral bone density (mg/mm^3)	Quantitative computed tomography; Transverse slice technique; histogram analysis technique; three-dimensional reconstruction technique

Earlier tests based on radiographs of the hips concentrated on structural information. Attempts to quantify trabecular bone changes in the hip resulted in the Singh Index (2), assessment of the calcar femorale, and the cortical index of the femoral neck and shaft (8, 9). Of interest are newer experimental imaging and image-processing techniques based on axial tomograms obtained with CT (10-12). These techniques image the cross-sectional distribution of trabeculae, including the femoral head and acetabulum, which are not readily accessible for detailed trabecular studies by other techniques. Thus far, this approach has been more important for the diagnosis of focal bone disease in the femur, such as avascular necrosis. Early observations on cross-sectional trabecular bone patterns in osteoporosis show an increase in spacing of the trabeculae and changes in spatial distribution of trabeculae (10). In general, morphology-based procedures had limited success in the prediction of fracture risk.

In studies on excised bone, bone density and bone mass are important determinants of bone strength (5). This makes bone mass measurements important for fracture risk prediction. Before direct noninvasive measurements of the femur were available, efforts were made to predict bone mass or density in the hip from measurements of appendicular bones (13). These also met with limited success. The introduction of DPA and QCT for the spinal column now opens possibilities for the direct measurements of hip density.

In osteoporosis, where fracture risk assessment is a major objective, measurements need to consider the complex bone structure of the hip, the region-specific relationship between trabecular and cortical bone, and the region-specific rate of bone loss. The same diagnostic strategies used at the spinal column or appendicular skeleton probably will not be successful at the hip.

Bone density measurements by DPA and DEXA are currently taken at the femoral neck, the Ward triangle, and the trochanter area. The femoral neck is the site of subcapital, rare midcervical, and uncommon basicervical fractures (63% of all proximal femur fractures). The trochanter is another site of fracture (37% of all proximal femur fractures). Ward's triangle at the base of the neck is a site of early trabecular bone loss.

Measurements at Ward's triangle give information on early bone loss and in some studies discriminate best between subjects with and without fractures (14).

DPA or DEXA measures integral bone as area density (bone mass per unit of area scanned) at different sites in the proximal femur. Details on both procedures are given later. Quantitative CT measurements on the hip are being developed for estimation of trabecular bone density (bone mass per unit of volume of trabecular bone, the latter including marrow and fat), as well as density of cortical bone. Technical requirements differ from those used in QCT of the spinal column. The geometrical complexity of the proximal femur prohibits the single-section approach used for measurement of cancellous bone in the spinal column. CT number determinations between contiguous 1-cm sections may vary up to 100% (11). Capability to select irregular regions of interest is required. The standard oval or circular regions of interest are not usable. Separation of cortical and trabecular bone (particularly the calcar femorale) is more difficult and time-consuming. Technical limitations inherent in QCT application in the hip are variable beam hardening and substantial partial volume artifacts. High x-ray dose techniques are required (500-1000 mrem).

NONINVASIVE BONE MINERAL MEASUREMENTS ON THE PROXIMAL FEMUR BY DPA AND DEXA

DPA and DEXA are of great interest as clinical and investigative procedures because of their success in measuring bone density in the spinal column and of the advanced state of technology. Commercial instruments are available. The study compared hip measurements made with an instrument based on DPA (Lunar, Inc. DP3) and those made with a DEXA-based instrument (Hologic, Inc. QDR-1000) and evaluated the limits within which accurate and precise measurements can be expected. Relevant features of the instruments are compared in Table 2.

METHOD

Several experiments were conducted to analyze the accuracy and precision of bone mineral results at three regions of interest in the hip. The effect of variation in body and bone marrow composition, femur positioning, and patient thickness on measurements of bone mineral density was evaluated. The experiments are summarized in Table 3.

Table 2: Comparison of DPA and DEXA Instruments

Method	Transmission scan	
	DPA	DEXA
Source	153-Gd	X-ray
Energy	44, 100 keV	70, 104 kVp
Source collimation (mm)	3	2
Detector collimation (mm)	8	None
Scan speed (m/sec)	2.5	60
Line increment (mm)	2.5	1
Scan time (min)	35	6-8
Processing time (min)	5	5
Table-detector distance (cm)	30	40
Daily calibration	3-bone phantom	Spine phantom

Accuracy was measured on a spine phantom and with ashed bones in 20 cm of water. The three regions of interest in the proximal femur are difficult to isolate and to ash with sufficient accuracy for comparison. The 8-mm collimator was used for all measurements with the DP3. With the DP3, software version 2.4 was used. The DEXA hip software was a prototype version not yet approved for clinical use. Data on body composition, patient thickness, and femur distance from the table were obtained by measurements on women being referred to the laboratory for bone mineral studies. Their ages ranged from 33 to 85 years. These results are given in the last column of Table 3.

Table 3: Experimental Procedures Used in the Evaluation of Bone Mineral Measurements in the Hip

Parameter	Experimental method	Remarks
Accuracy	Measured on a block and spine phantom and on ashed bones in 20 cm of water	Other than hip phantoms had to be used
Precision Short-term	Spine, hip phantom, ashed bones	DP3 instrument observed over 3 yrs
Long-term	Spine, hip phantom, ashed bones	QDR instrument over 8 mo
Effect of absorber (patient) thickness	Human proximal femur measured in water ranging from 10 to 30 cm in depth	Body thickness range in patients 12-30 cm at hip
Effect of femur distance from imaging table	Human proximal femur measured in 20 cm of water 0-15 cm distance from table top	Femur distance range in patients 10-15 cm
Effect of fat in media surrounding bone (body composition)	Human proximal femur measured in 20 cm of oil-water mixture with 0 to 75% oil	Bone marrow fat range in patients 20-80% (V/V)
Effect of fat in bone (marrow)	Human proximal femur with layers of margarine on top of bone	Range in patients 20-60%
Effect of rotation of femur (positioning) and side differences	Human proximal femur in different positions	Patient scanned with internal-rotation positioning device used

DPA   **DEXA**

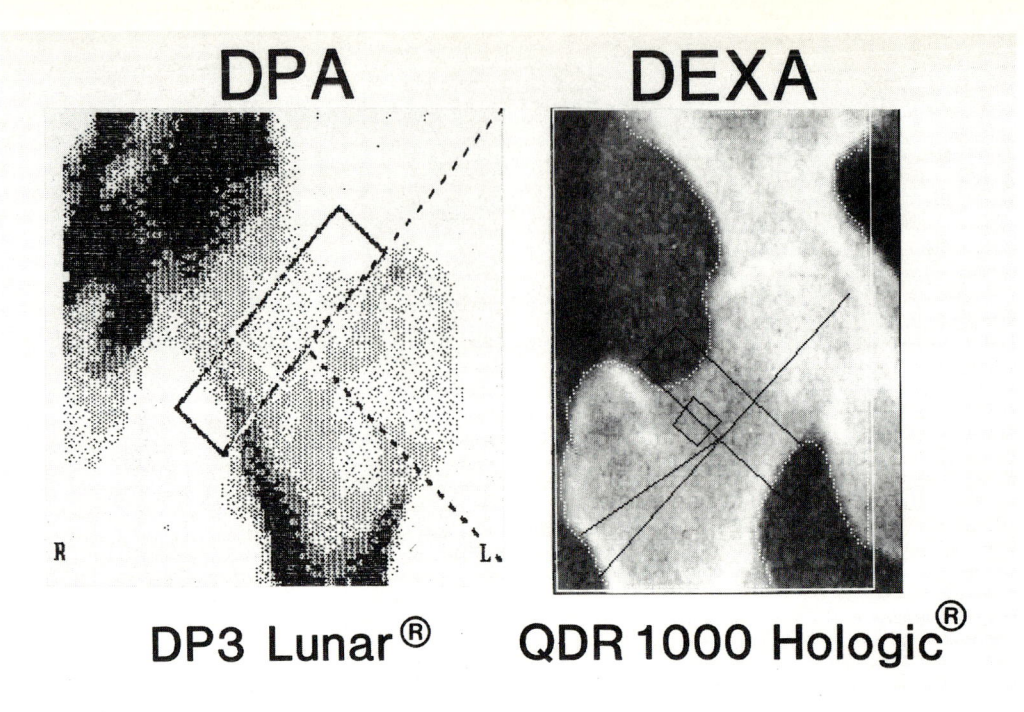

DP3 Lunar®   **QDR 1000 Hologic®**

Fig. 3. Data output from DPA and DEXA instruments.

RESULTS

(1) <u>Accuracy and Precision</u>.--Accuracy measured with a hydroxyapatite block phantom, ashed bones, and a spine phantom has previously been described for both instruments as part of a comparison of performance for measurements on the spinal column (15). In short, both instruments showed a linear response to increasing bone mineral content. For the DP3 instrument: bone mass (g) = - 0.117 + .953 x (measured mass), r = 0.999. For the QDR 1000 instrument: bone mass (g) = 1.085 + 0.925 x (measured mass), r = 0.999.

Long-term precision (6 months) simultaneously measured on both instruments with the Hologic spine phantom yielded a coefficient of variation (CV) of 1.5% (bone mineral density) for DPA and of 0.4% for DEXA. There was no significant slope of the linear regression bone mineral density on time in either instrument (15). Short-term precision in phantoms and patients is summarized in Table 4. Data on long-term precision of hip measurements are not available for the DPA instrument. Results from the DEXA instrument show that the high precision seen in the lumbar spine cannot be matched in the hip.

Table 4: Precision of Two Instruments for Bone Mineral Measurements in the Femur

Bone mineral density (g/cm^2)	DPA			DEXA		
	Neck	Ward's triangle	Trochanter	Neck	Ward's triangle	Trochanter
Patient mean				0.602	0.465	0.556
n	12 patients, duplicate			1 patient, triplicate		
CV%	5.0	8.8	5.1	2.2	1.4	0.5
Femur phantom (Hologic) mean	0.686	0.646	0.977	0.732	0.612	0.905
n	3 measurements			4 measurements		
CV%	0.58	1.16	0.58	1.9	1.2	1.6
Femur cadaver mean	0.693	0.565	0.680	0.684	0.498	0.569
n	5 measurements			5 measurements		
CV%	2.5	2.9	1.3	1.7	1.0	1.3
Long-term precision (8 mo) DPA (1 mo) DEXA	Available only for spine phantom 1.0% CV			0.730 17 2.2	0.605 17 1.9	0.907 17 1.3

242

(2) <u>Effect of Changing Absorber Thickness</u>.--In 23 consecutive women with suspected osteoporosis, body thickness at the hip are (table surface to anterior iliac crest) varied from 13 to 19 cm (median, 18 cm). The results of the experiments using a cadaver hip bone and changing water levels are summarized in Fig. 4. Data are expressed as percent of bone mineral density (g/cm^2) at the reference site (R)--that is, 15 cm of water. The shaded area encloses two standard deviations of the density value at the reference point. Within a range of 15 to 20 cm of water, both instruments performed well.

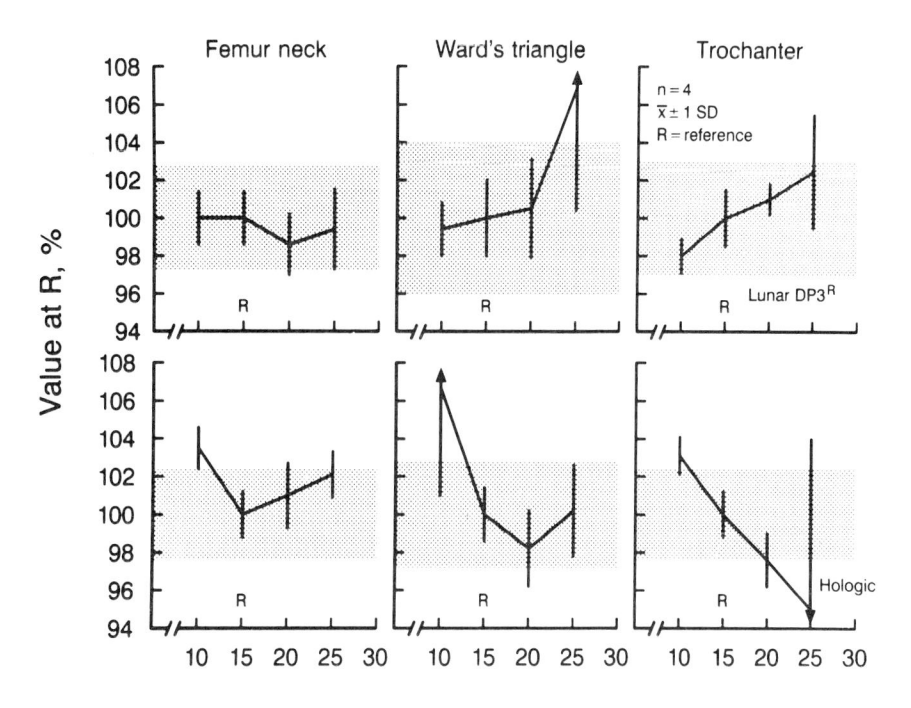

Fig. 4. Effect of absorber thickness on bone mineral values (g/cm^2) of femur. The shaded area encloses two standard deviations of the bone mineral values at R.

(3) <u>Effect of Bone Distance from Table Surface</u>.-- In the same 23 women, the table-to-trochanter distance varied between 9 and 14 cm (median, 10 cm). When the cadaver bone was moved within this range, bone mineral density was reproducible within 2 to 3%, except for Ward's triangle on the DPA and the trochanter region on the DEXA, where at 15 cm an 8% decrease in density was noted in both instruments (Fig. 5). The shaded area encloses two standard deviations of the bone mineral density at 10-cm table distance (R)

(4) <u>Effect of Fat in Absorber Surrounding Bone</u>.-- From RST measurements made with DPA, the fat content in tissue surrounding the hips of the 23 women ranged from 5 to 50% (median, <25%). RST is a number reflecting the absorption coefficient of tissue around the bone, available only on the DPA instrument. Within this RST range, there was little effect on fat changes with either instrument. However, further increases in fat content led to a false increase in bone mineral density (Fig. 6).

(5) <u>Effect of Fat in Bone</u>.--The possible effect of changing bone marrow fat over the lifetime of a subject was studied. On the DEXA instrument, a 1.5 cm-thick-fat (margarine) layer was put over the cadaver femur. Scanning in 20 cm of water produced no measurable effect. When the fat layer was 3.0 cm (diameter of femoral neck was 2 cm); bone mineral density in all three regions of interest was reduced by 8 to 10%. This reduction is

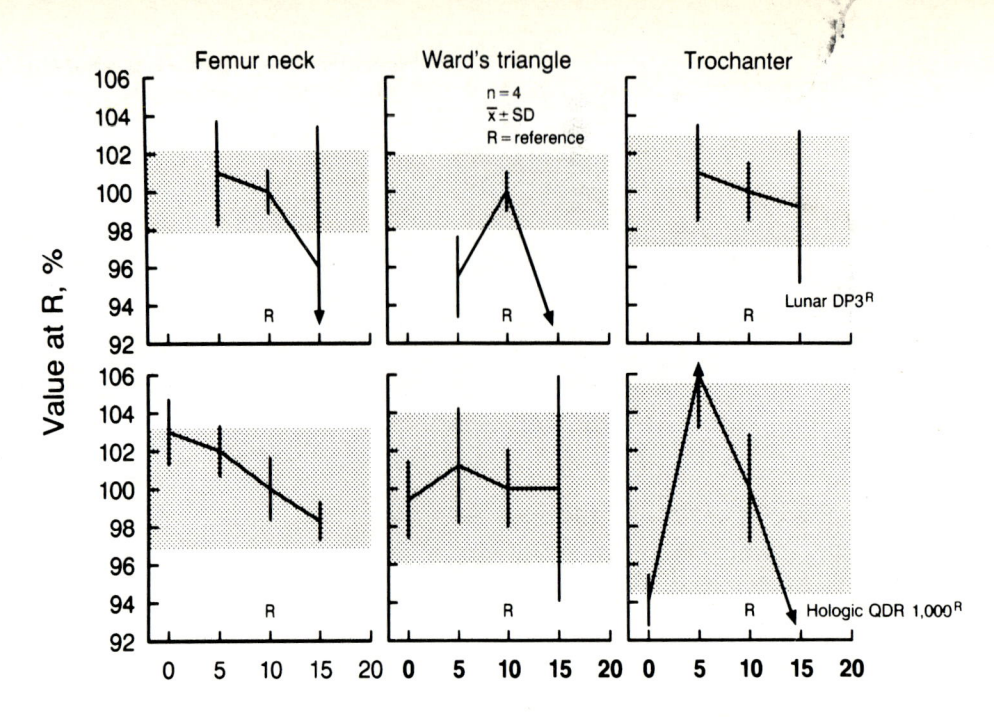

Fig. 5. Effect of distance from table surface on bone mineral values of femur.

similar to reductions reported by us earlier with a slightly different experimental set up for the DPA instrument (16).

(6) <u>Effect of Fat Around the Femoral Neck Only</u>.--To study the effect of variation in fat content along the bone surface, a 2-cm layer of margarine was wrapped around the neck of the cadaver femur and scanning was performed

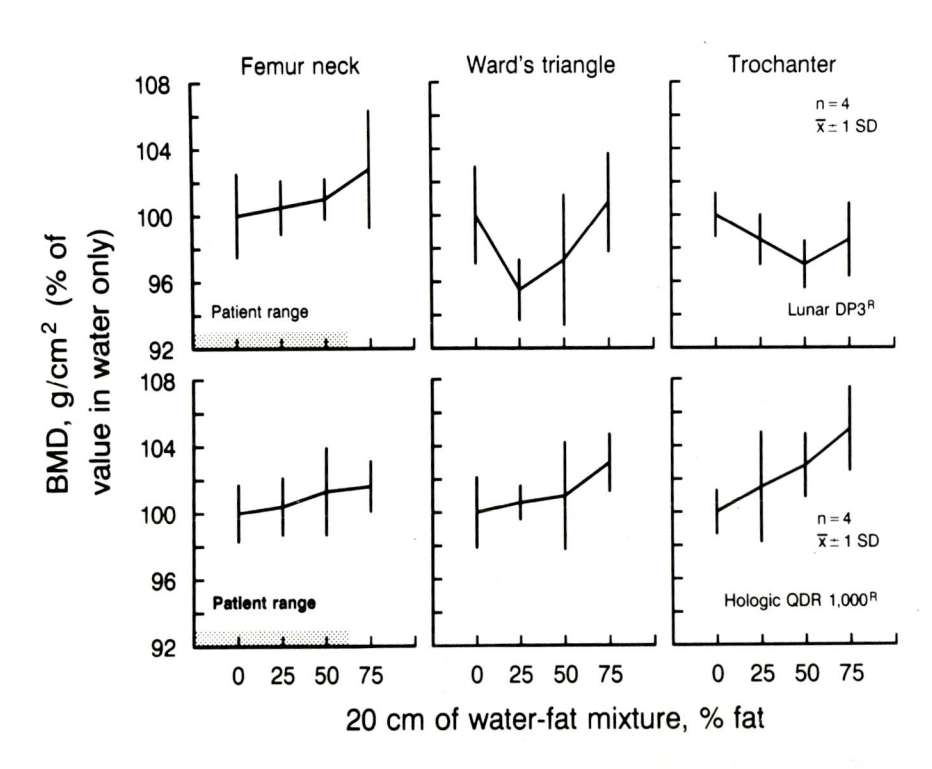

Fig. 6. Effect of fat surrounding bone on bone mineral measurements. The shaded area at the left-hand side along the abscissa shows the range of fat content seen in patients.

in 20 cm of water. DPA showed the predictable effect (from experiment 4) on all three regions of interest, even in those not near the fat. DEXA showed that fat affects only the femur neck and Ward's triangle, not the trochanter, which was not covered with fat.

(7) <u>Effect of Femur Positioning</u>.--The effect on bone mineral density in three regions of interest was evaluated: during rotation around the femur shaft axis, the angle of the femur shaft, and during scanning of the femur specimen in left (beam passes anteroposterior) or right position (beam passes posteroanterior). As previously shown (17), the algorithm of the DPA instrument is tolerant to changes in femur angle and rotation, although manual positioning of the regions of interest becomes necessary. Bone mineral density values are essentially unchanged at angle changes of less than 15°. Further changes lead to significant errors in measurement. The DEXA instrument would not process data obtained when the femur was angled in either axis by about 10°. No change was noted when the femur was scanned with the head pointing right or left on either instrument.

SUMMARY

DPA and DEXA can measure with acceptable accuracy and precision, regional bone mineral in vivo as area density. In contrast to the results obtained on the lumbar spine, where DEXA clearly shows better precision, results in the femur were about equal in both instruments. A series of studies with phantoms was performed to evaluate the tolerance limits of the techniques to changes in fat content around the bone, to fat changes in the bone itself, and to changes in body thickness. Because these experiments are incomplete models of actual changes in patients, they do not allow evaluation of the additive effect of multiple variations as they may occur in patients. The results are meant to stimulate further improvements in the technique and to serve as a caveat for data interpretation. Studies on more complex models are under way. Because a prototype version of the hip software was used on the DEXA instrument, there were restrictions on measuring bone mineral in patients. The data do not allow an assessment of how this instrument will perform in patient studies. The experiments on phantoms, however, show that the software is now ready for testing in patients.

With these restrictions, DPA and DEXA techniques for hip studies should be used with caution in patients whose body composition is outside a given range. Bone density in children or obese persons should not be measured without prior instrument calibration. Significant weight change during a study may affect longitudinal data. When populations are compared, significant differences in average weight may obscure true differences in bone density. It is suggested that RST (on DPA instruments), body thickness at the scanning site, height of the trochanter above the table, and patient's height and weight be recorded and inspected when the data are interpreted. DEXA and DPA show similar results and problems. DEXA requires less time to perform, which results in more efficient quality control (faster scans of phantoms), greater convenience for the patient, and faster patient turnover in the laboratory.

REFERENCES

1. Harty M: The calcar femorale and the femoral neck. J Bone Joint Surg (AM) 29:625-630, 1957.

2. Singh M, Nagrath AR, Maini PS: Changes in trabecular pattern of the upper end of the femur as an index of osteoporosis. J Bone Joint Surg (AM) 54:457-467, 1970.

3. Riggs BL, Wahner HW, Seeman E, Offord KP, Dunn WL, Mazess RB, Johnson KA, Melton JL: Changes in bone mineral density of the proximal femur

and spine with aging: differences between the postmenopausal and senile osteoporosis syndrome. J Clin Invest 70:716-723, 1982.

4. Pesch HJ, Henschke F, Siebold H: Einfluss von Mechanik und Alter auf den Spongiosaumbau in Lendenwirbelkorpern und im Schenkelhals. Virchows Arch A Path Anat and Histol 377:27-42, 1977.

5. Martens M, van Audekercke R, Delport P, Demeester P, Mulier JC: The mechanical characteristics of cancellous bone at the upper femoral region. J Biomech 16:971-983, 1983.

6. Khairi MRA, Cronin JH, Robb JA, Smith DM, Yu PL, Johnston CC: Femoral trabecular pattern index and bone mineral content measurement by photon absorption in senile osteoporosis. J Bone Joint Surg (AM) 58:221-226, 1976.

7. Kranendonk DH, Jurist JM, Lee HG: Femoral trabecular patterns and bone mineral content. J Bone Joint Surg (AM) 54:1472-1478, 1972.

8. Barnett E, Nordin BEC: The radiological diagnosis of osteoporosis: a new apprroach. Clin Radiol 11:166-174, 1960.

9. Fredensborg N, Nilsson BE: Cortical index of the femoral neck. Acta Radiol Diag 18:492-496, 1977 (Fasc 4 July).

10. Kerr R, Resnick D, Sartoris DJ, Kursunaglu S, Pineda C, Haghighi P, Greenway G, Guerra J Jr: Computerized tomography of proximal femoral trabecular patterns. J Orthop Res 4:45-56, 1986.

11. Sartoris DJ, Andre M, Resnick C, Resnick D: Trabecular bone density in the proximal femur: quantitative CT assessment. (Work in Progress) Radiology 160:707-712, 1986.

12. Gluer CC, Genant HK: Quantitative computed tomography of the hip. IN: Osteoporosis Update 1987. HK Genant ed., Radiology Research Education and Foundation, San Francisco, CA, pg 187-195, 1987.

13. Leichter I, Margulies JY, Weinrieb A, et al: The relationship between bone density, mineral content and mechanical strength in the femoral neck. Clin Orthop 163:272-281, 1982.

14. Mazess RB, Barden H, Ettinger M, Shultz E: Bone density of the radius, spine, and proximal femur in osteoporosis. J Bone Min Res 3:13-18, 1988.

15. Wahner HW, Dunn WL, Brown ML, Morin R: Comparison of quantitative digital radiography (QDR) and dual-photon absorptiometry (DPA) for bone mineral measurements on the L-spine. Proceedings Intern Workshop: Noninvasive Bone Measurements, Leuven, Belgium, September 24-25, 1987 (to be published).

16. Wahner HW, Dunn WL, Mazess RB, Towsley M, Lindsay R, Markhard L, Dempster D: Dual-photon Gd-153 absorptiometry of bone. Radiology 156:203-206, 1985.

17. Wahner HW, Dunn WL, DiMagno M: Bone mineral (BM) measurements of the hip by dual-photon absorptiometry (DPA): precision and performance evaluation. Proceedings Intern Workshop: Noninvasive Bone Measurements, Leuven, Belgium, September 24-25, 1987 (to be published).

Relationship Between the Iliac Crest Bone Biopsy and Other Skeletal Sites

DAVID W. DEMPSTER

Regional Bone Center
Helen Hayes Hospital
New York State Department of Health
West Haverstraw, NY
and Department of Pathology
Columbia University
New York, NY

The iliac crest biopsy is widely acknowledged as being one of the most powerful clinical and research tools available for the study of metabolic bone disease. However, although a large body of data has been accumulated for the standard iliac biopsy site, there is still relatively little information on how this site relates to other, more clinically relevant, skeletal sites, such as the vertebrae and the proximal femur. This paper will review the available data on this topic in terms of bone structure, strength and remodeling activity. The histomorphometric terms and abbreviations used will be consistent with recommendations of the American Society for Bone and Mineral Research.[1]

Bone mass and structure

Meunier and Courpron[2] compared cancellous bone volume (Cn-BV/TV) in the iliac crest with that in the third lumbar vertebra in 45 control subjects. They found the vertebral Cn-BV/TV to be lower in all cases than the iliac values and that there was a significant positive correlation between the two sites with a correlation coefficient of 0.78. Similar results were obtained by Podenphant et al.[3] in a detailed study of 14 cadavers in which they compared the sites histomorphometrically and also measured bone mass in the lumbar spine by dual photon absorptiometry (DPA). They found that the iliac biopsy provides a better estimate of the amount of cancellous bone in the lumbar vertebrae than DPA. The lower Cn-BV/TV in vertebral bodies is due to the fact that the trabecular plates are both thinner and more widely separated than in the ilium[3,4] (Figure 1). Podenphant et al.[3] also showed that iliac Cn-BV/TV was significantly correlated with the cancellous bone density in the distal radius and ulna. However, the cortical thickness (Ct.Th) and cortical porosity in the iliac crest were not significantly correlated with those in the lumbar spine, nor with cortical bone density in the forearm. In addition to a reasonably good concordance between Cn-BV/TV in the iliac crest and the spine, the compressive strength of vertebral cancellous bone and whole vertebral bodies can be reliably predicted from that of cancellous bone from the standard biopsy site.[5,6]

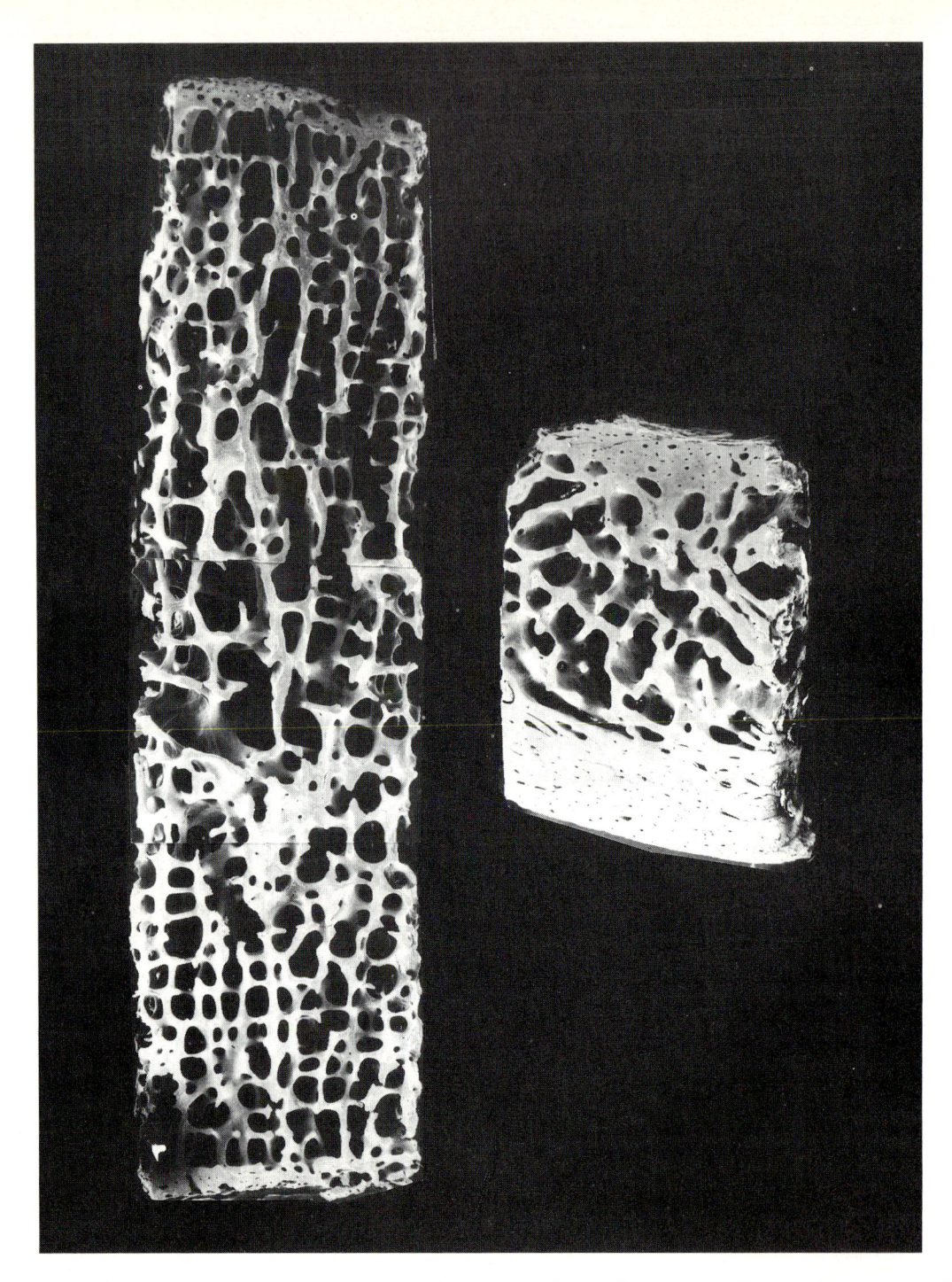

Figure 1: Scanning electron micrographs of cores from the second lumbar vertebra (left) and the standard iliac biopsy site (right). Samples were obtained at autopsy from a 45 year-old man who had suffered sudden death without evidence of bone disease. Note the significantly thicker cortices in the iliac sample. Structural parameters of cancellous bone, determined on thin, undecalcified sections of the iliac and vertebral samples, respectively, were as follows: bone volume: 29.6 vs. 15.2%; trabecular number: 1.66 vs. 1.50 per mm; trabecular separation: 414 vs. 542 μm; and trabecular thickness: 170 vs. 85 μm. The specimens were prepared according to Dempster et al.[7] Field height = 25 mm.

There are few studies that have been performed with the specific aim of comparing bone structure in the ilium and the proximal femur. Krempien et al[8] compared the two sites in eight control subjects and found the Cn-BV/TV in the iliac crest to be to be approximately 2/3 of that in the proximal femur, with the same ratio being maintained in patients with either chronic renal failure or malignant tumors. In a comparative study of these two regions in patients with intracapsular femoral neck fractures, Frisch and Eventov[9] evaluated the degree of hematopoiesis, osteopenia and osseous remodeling. Unfortunately, neither raw data nor definitions of these parameters were provided, making it extremely difficult to interpret the results. The authors' conclusion was that osteopenia in the iliac crest is of the "high turnover type" while that in the femoral neck is of the "low turnover type". Although it was not a comparative inter-site study as such, Johnston et al.[10] published an important paper, which indicated that different patterns of bone loss in the iliac crest were associated with different fracture syndromes in postmenopausal women. Specifically, those patients with femoral neck fractures had a higher Cn-BV/TV and a lower Ct.Th than those with vertebral crush fractures. Lips et al.[11] compared histomorphometric parameters with the Singh index of cancellous bone architecture in the upper end of the femur. There was a statistically significant correlation between iliac Ct.Th and the Singh index, but the correlation coefficient was very low (0.27). Iliac Cn-BV/TV and the Singh index were not significantly correlated.

Several authors have compared biopsy indices of bone mass with results obtained by other, non-invasive techniques. Bydder et al.[12] reported a highly significant correlation (r=0.75) between iliac Cn-BV/TV and spinal cancellous bone density, determined by computed tomography, in 18 patients with idiopathic vertebral osteoporosis. But, in a more recent study[13] of 122 postmenopausal women with osteoporosis, Cn-BV/TV correlated only weakly (r values: 0.20-0.26) with total body calcium (by neutron activation analysis), cancellous and total vertebral bone mass (by quantitative computed tomography), height loss, and a vertebral fracture index. In agreement with the study mentioned above,[3] there was no significant relationship with vertebral bone mass by DPA, nor with radial bone mass by single photon absorptiometry (SPA). The correlations between Cn-BV/TV and the non-invasive measures were much weaker than those among the non-invasive techniques themselves.

Thus, in general, the amount of cancellous bone in the iliac crest biopsy site appears to be reasonably predictive of that in the spine with, not surprisingly, much better correlations being obtained when the same assessment technique, i.e., histomorphometry, is used at each site. Insufficient data of this type are available to comment on the representativeness of the ilium with regard to the appendicular skeleton, in general, and the neck of femur, in particular. Correlations between histomorphometric and other, non-invasive measures of bone mass are weaker. This is probably due, at least in part, to the fact that different parameters are being measured and, specifically, that the absorptiometric techniques (DPA and SPA) include variable amounts of cortical bone, depending upon the site of measurement.

Bone turnover
The turnover rate in cortical bone is roughly 1/10 of that in cancellous bone and there is considerable site to site variation

in turnover rates throughout the skeleton in both types of bone. According to Parfitt,[14] the turnover rate of cancellous bone in the ilium is higher than in other bones with an estimated value of 40% per year compared to approximately 20% in the vertebrae. Despite this high value for iliac cancellous bone, his histomorphometric estimate of whole-body bone turnover (cancellous + cortical) is some 2/3 of the value obtained by radiokinetic methods. A formal comparison of histomorphometric and whole body ^{85}Sr kinetic data on bone resorption and formation rates has recently been conducted in patients with vertebral osteoporosis.[15] Reasonable correlations were found between the two methods for both parameters. The relationship between the histomorphometric and kinetic indices of bone formation were better when based on the extent of double tetracycline labels than on measurements of osteoid parameters. When both treated and untreated patients were considered, the best estimate of an exchange-corrected kinetic index of total body bone formation rate was given by double-labeled osteoid volume, that is, (dLS/OS) x OV. Eroded surface (ES) was fairly well correlated with exchange-corrected kinetic indices of resorption and, again, better relationships were obtained when a volume referent was employed (ES x $\sqrt{\text{Cn-BV/TV}}$). Osteoid volume was also found to be an independent predictor of kinetically determined bone resorption, with a stronger association than might be expected simply from the coupling between resorption and formation. Osteoclast number was only rather weakly correlated with kinetic estimates of resorption and formation. The authors concluded that, although they have the advantage of being atraumatic, the best kinetic techniques of assessing bone turnover require a prolonged period of study (up to 5 months) and that similar data can be obtained much more rapidly by histomorphometry. This study also allowed another important conclusion to be drawn, which is that in osteoporosis, bone formation and resorption rates throughout the skeleton can be reliably estimated by histomorphometric analysis of the iliac crest biopsy. However, while this may be true in groups of patients, a recent paper[16] indicates that it may not necessarily be the case in a single patient. In this study, the sudden death of an osteoporotic patient, while participating in a therapeutic trial involving bone biopsy, afforded the authors the opportunity to compare tetracycline uptake in 24 different skeletal sites. There was considerable regional variation in the dynamic parameters. In cancellous bone, the mineral apposition rate ranged from <0.2 to 1.2 µm/day. The extent of tetracycline uptake was even more variable with the result that the bone formation rate (BFR) ranged from 1.7% per year (in the tenth thoracic vertebra) to 37.1% per year (in the standard iliac biopsy site). BFR was not uniformly low in the spine, however, with values of up to 21.1% per year being recorded in other vertebral bodies. Significantly, the BFR determined in the left iliac biopsy was almost four times higher than that in the right, with obvious implications for investigations involving repeat biopsies. Inter-site discrepancies of similar magnitude were also present in cortical bone. Therefore, with the caveat that this observation is based on a sample of one, it would appear that in the management of individual patients with osteoporosis the iliac biopsy should not be solely relied upon to predict the overall rate of bone formation.

The question of the representativeness of the iliac sample in various other types of bone disease has also been addressed. Krempien et al.[8] compared static remodeling parameters among four sites in control subjects and in patients with chronic renal failure or malignant tumors with skeletal metastases. Marked disparity among the different skeletal sites in osteoid surface and osteoblast surface implied significant differences in local remodeling rates (iliac crest > lumbar vertebra > femoral head > distal femur). Nevertheless, in uremia, systematic changes in the parameters at all four sites were generally observed. As would be expected, those sites with higher turnover (ilium and vertebra) displayed a greater accumulation of inactive osteoid than in the femoral sites. Villanueva et al.[17] compared Haversian remodeling in iliac crest and the 11th rib in six patients, three of whom had osteomalacia and the others, osteoporosis. Highly significant correlations were found for ten of 11 parameters measured with the exception being the number of resorption spaces. Moreover, there were no significant differences between the mean value for each site in any of the measures. Close correlations have also been observed between histomorphometric and calcium kinetic or biochemical indices of bone turnover in Paget's disease,[18] and in thyroid and parathyroid hormone excess or deficiency.[14,19,20]

In conclusion, there is clearly considerable variation in remodeling activity throughout the skeleton. However, in metabolic bone disease, systemic factors override local factors and the iliac crest biopsy provides a reasonably accurate reflection of overall skeletal status. As a consequence of the higher turnover rate in the ilium, the biopsy is a very sensitive indicator of skeletal disturbances. Although this is distinctly preferable to low sensitivity, it should be borne in mind when the biopsy is used to assess the overall severity of bone disease.

Acknowledgements

This work was partly supported by National Institutes of Health grants AR35647 and AR39191. The author is grateful to Ms. Wendy Horbert for expert technical assistance in the preparation of the scanning electron micrographs.

REFERENCES

1. Parfitt AM, Drezner MK, Glorieux FH, Kanis JA, Malluche H, Meunier PJ, Ott SM, Recker RR 1987 Bone histomorphometry: Standardization of nomenclature, symbols, and units. J Bone Min Res **2**:595-610.
2. Meunier PJ, Courpron P 1976 Iliac trabecular bone volume in 236 controls: Representativeness of iliac samples. In: Jaworski ZFG (ed) Proceedings of the First Workshop on Bone Morphometry, University of Ottowa Press, pp 100-105.
3. Podenphant J, Gotfredsen A, Nilas L, Norgaard H, Braendstrup O 1986 Iliac crest biopsy: Representativity for the amount of mineralized bone. Bone **7**:427-430.
4. Dempster DW, Fey C, Horbert W, Parisien MV 1988 A comparison of structural parameters of cancellous bone in the ilium and the second lumbar vertebra. In: Proceedings of the Fifth International Congress on Bone Morphometry, Niigata, Japan, July 24-29.
5. Mosekilde L, Viidik A, Mosekilde L 1985 Correlation between the compressive strength of iliac and vertebral trabecular bone in normal individuals. Bone **6**:291-295.
6. Mosekilde L, Mosekilde L 1986 Normal vertebral body size and compressive strength: Relations to age and to vertebral and iliac trabecular bone compressive strength. Bone **7**:207-212.

7. Dempster DW, Shane E, Horbert W, Lindsay R 1986 A simple method for correlative light and scanning electron microscopy of human iliac crest bone biopsies: Qualitative observations in normal and osteoporotic subjects. J Bone Min Res 1:15-21.
8. Krempien B, Lemminger F-M, Ritz E, Weber E 1978 The reaction of different skeletal sites to metabolic bone disease - a micromorphometric study. Klin Wschr 56:755-759.
9. Frisch B, Eventov I 1986 Hematopoiesis in osteoporosis-preliminary report comparing biopsies of the femoral neck and iliac crest. Isr J Med Sci 22:380-384.
10. Johnston CC, Norton J, Khairi MRA, Kernek C, Edouard C, Arlot M, Meunier PJ 1985 Heterogeneity of fracture syndromes in postmenopausal women. J Clin Endocrinol Metab **61**:551-556.
11. Lips P, Taconis WK, Van Ginkel FC, Netelenbos JC 1984 Radiologic morphometry in patients with femoral neck fractures and elderly control subjects. Clin Orthop Rel Res **183**:64-70.
12. Bydder GM, Elsasser U, Hesp R, Kreel L, Reeve J, Charhon S, Edouard C, Meunier PJ 1983 Peripheral and axial measurements of trabecular bone density in patients suspected of idiopathic vertebral osteoporosis. J Comp Tomography **7**:357-361.
13. Ott SM, Kilcoyne RF, Chesnut, III CH 1988 Comparisons among methods of measuring bone mass and relationship to severity of vertebral fractures in osteoporosis. J Clin Endocrinol Metab **66**:501-507.
14. Parfitt AM 1983 The physiologic and clinical significance of bone histomorphometric data. In: Recker RR (ed) Bone Histomorphometry: Techniques and Interpretation, Boca Raton, Florida, CRC Press, pp 143-223.
15. Reeve J, Arlot ME, Chavassieux PM, Edouard C, Green JR, Hesp R, Tellez M, Meunier PJ 1987 The assessment of bone formation and bone resorption in osteoporosis: A comparison between tetracycline based iliac histomorphometry and whole body ^{85}Sr Kinetics. J Bone Min Res **2**:479-489.
16. Podenphant J, Engel U 1987 Regional variations in histomorphometric bone dynamics from the skeleton of an osteoporotic woman. Calcif Tissue Int **40**:184-188.
17. Villanueva AR, Parfitt AM, Duncan H 1977 Comparison of Haversian bone dynamics between 11th rib and iliac trephine biopsies. In: Meunier PJ (ed) Bone Histomorphometry: Second International Workshop, Societe de la Nouvelle Imprimerie Fournie, Toulouse, France, pp 75-77.
18. Lauffenburger T, Olah AJ, Dambacher MA, Guncaga, J, Lentner C, Haas HG 1977 Bone remodeling and calcium metabolism: a correlated histomorphometric, calcium kinetic, and biochemical study in patients with osteoporosis and Paget's disease. Metabolism **26**:589-605.
19. Delmas PD, Meunier PJ, Faysse E, Saubier EC 1986 Bone histomorphometry and serum bone Gla-protein in the diagnosis of primary hyperparathyroidism. World J Surg **10**:572-578.
20. Charles P, Eriksen EF, Mosekilde L, Melsen F, Jensen FT 1987 Bone turnover and balance evaluated by a combined calcium balance and ^{47}calcium kinetic study and dynamic histomorphometry. Metabolism **36**:1118-1124.

Stochastic Models of Femoral Bone Loss and Hip Fracture Risk

A. HORSMAN[1] and L. BURKINSHAW[2]

[1]MRC Bone Mineralisation Group
[2]MRC Body Composition Group
Department of Medical Physics
University of Leeds
Leeds, UK

Introduction

Dual photon absorptiometry of the lumbar spine and femoral neck is now widely performed with the expectation that the resulting measurement at each site predicts the risk that the person measured will later suffer an osteoporotic fracture there [1]. Research effort and screening procedures using this technique usually concentrate on postmenopausal women, who are collectively at greater risk of osteoporotic fractures than young adults and elderly men [2]. Screening is intended to identify women most likely to benefit (in terms of reduced fracture risk) from prophylaxis given to reduce subsequent bone loss [3,4].

We therefore chose to explore numerical consequences of the hypothesis that in women the amount of bone mineral in the femoral neck is a determinant of the risk of hip fracture following a fall, using Monte Carlo techniques to implement two similar stochastic models. Evaluations were carried out using a linear descriptor of age-related mineral loss [5] and also a descriptor which more closely resembles real data now available on the femoral neck in females [6]. In the latter case an additional aim was to compare the predicted mean mineral deficit in groups of elderly fracture cases (relative to age-matched non-fracture cases) with the observed value [7].

Stochastic models of bone loss, falls and fracture risk

Two similar models ('linear' and 'non-linear') were investigated, the non-linear model being an extension of (but not a replacement for) the linear case and more relevant in the context of currently available measurements on the femoral neck. Monte Carlo methods were applied in both models to simulate mineral loss, falls and fractures in an ageing cohort, using techniques set out in full elsewhere [5]. Fractures were assumed to occur only as a consequence of falling; hip fractures which are the cause of falls are thought to be rare. The frequency of falls, which increases with age, was described by the same function in both models.

The linear model was so-called because a linear function was used to describe the age-related decrease in a hypothetical bone mineral measurement on the femoral neck. Denoting the risk that an individual will fracture following a fall by Q, and the bone mineral measurement in the femoral neck <u>at the time of the fall</u> by BM then, by definition, Q = F(BM) where F(BM) is an unknown function to be determined. F was defined to be a smooth function of BM only (not age).

The second model used a non-linear function to describe the age-related decrease in a real, measurable property of the femoral neck, the bone mineral density. An important difference between this and the linear model is inclusion in the calculation of fracture risk of an extra age-dependent function, S(a) (a is age), which can in part be regarded as describing how the severity of falls increases with age; its inclusion was <u>necessitated</u> by the form used for the descriptor for age-related bone loss. For the non-linear model, by definition the risk Q = S(a).G(BMD) where the fall occurs at age a and BMD is the current bone mineral density (dimensions ML^{-2}). Both S(a) and G(BMD) were unknown functions to be determined. G was defined to be a smooth function of BMD.

The linear model

Fig. 1 outlines the approach used to simulate events in a cohort of women ageing from maturity to extreme old age. Each woman was first allocated values for BM at maturity and its subsequent rate of decrease. Each was then allocated falls on the basis of the known incidence of falls as a function of age. Next all falls were examined and a decision made whether or not to associate a fracture with each fall; BM at the time of fall was noted and the risk of fracture interpolated from the function relating BM and fracture risk. This function was initially given arbitrary values so that the following iteration could start.

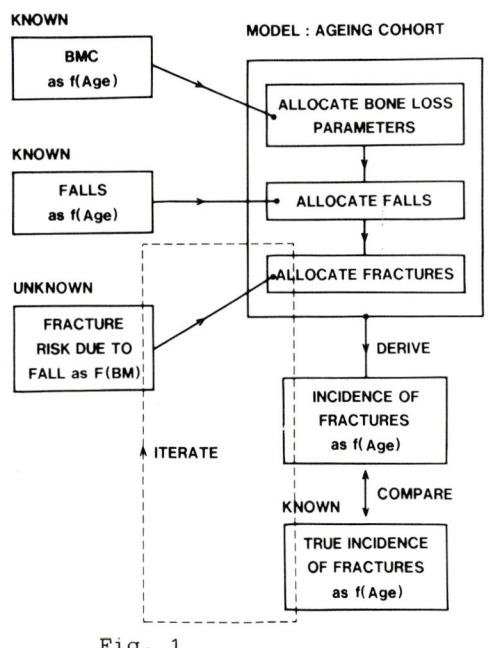

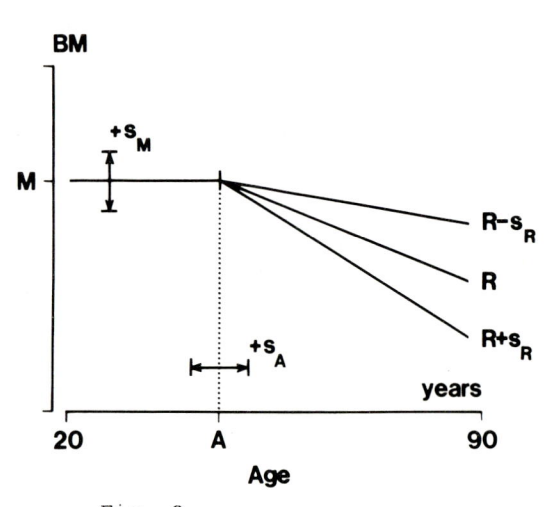

Fig. 1
Schematic representation of the implementation of the linear model.

Fig. 2
Parameters of the linear model defining age-related changes in BM.

The age-specific incidence of fractures was computed by counting the number of fractures occurring in 5-year intervals. That was then compared with the known true (idealised) incidence of hip fractures in women. Any mismatch was attributed to errors in the specification of the unknown function relating fracture risk to BM. That specification was then modified to reduce the difference between predicted and true incidences. Iteration continued until the two incidences matched.

Practical implementation

Simulations were performed using a program written in compiled BASIC on an IBM compatible personal computer. The curvilinear relationships between incidence of falls and age and between fracture risk due to a fall and BM were represented by low-pass filtered piecewise-linear approximations (annual samples). Using a 20 megabyte hard disc to store the data for retrospective analysis, cohorts of 20,000 women were simulated without difficulty.

Values of parameters

Parameters describing BM as a function of age are illustrated in Fig. 2. It was assumed that in young women the skeleton is in dynamic equilibrium. An individual's BM value (BM(i)) during the equilibrium phase was held constant. BM values in the young were assumed to be Gaussianly distributed with standard deviation (SD) s_M. In practice s_M/M (M is the mean) was taken to be 0.11, with BM values scaled so that M=90. The equilibrium phase continued in the ith individual until age A(i), where the distribution was Gaussian with mean A and SD s_A. A was taken to be 50 years and s_A 2 years [8]. At the end of the equilibrium phase, each woman was assumed to lose mineral indefinitely at a constant rate R(i) units/year which was independent of her young adult value BM(i) (with R(i) and BM(i) in consistent units). R(i) values were assumed to be Gaussianly distributed with mean R and SD s_R. R was taken to be 1.0 units/year [9]; no data were available from which s_R could be determined. It was assumed that $s_R/R=0.10$; arguments for this choice are given in reference [5]. Values of BM(i), A(i) and R(i) were statistically independent of one another.

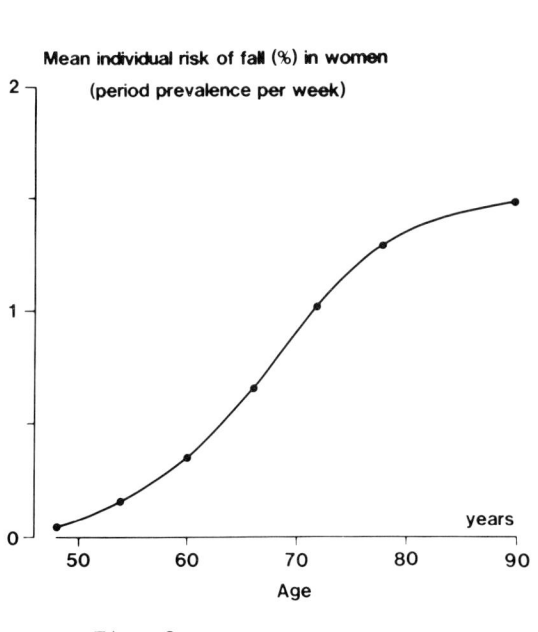

Fig. 3
Age-specific period prevalence (per week) of falls in women

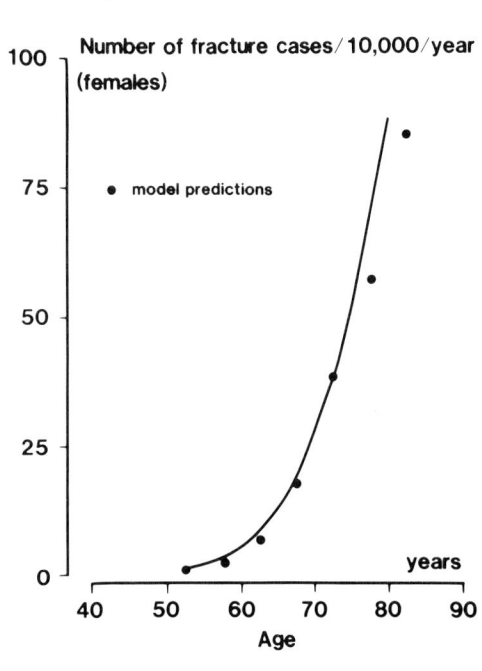

Fig. 4
Comparison of predicted (points) and idealised true hip fracture incidence.

Two sources were used to derive the age-specific period prevalence (per week) of falls in women shown in Fig. 3. Relative values in the range 50-70 years were derived from reference [10]; absolute values from 60 onwards were obtained from a DHSS survey in the UK analysed by the MRC Epidemiology Unit in Southampton. Underlying the randomness of falls in the individual there might be systematic differences between individuals in the frequency of falling; each individual was therefore allocated a multiplier which acted as a personalised scaling factor for the general curve shown in Fig. 3. The multiplier was arbitrarily assumed to have a mean of 1 and SD 0.3; the value of the SD did not affect the conclusions drawn.

Initial estimates of hip fracture risk over the whole range of BM values were made from the known age-specific incidence of fractures, the mean frequencies of falls and the mean values of BM at ages 60 and 80. Initial estimates were forced rapidly to zero for values of BM above the highest present in the population and to 100% as BM tended to zero.

Because sets of real data on age-specific incidence of hip fracture vary due to sampling artefacts and systematic differences between populations studied, real data were idealised as an exponential rising to 50 cases/10,000/year at age 75 and doubling every 5 years. The idealised curve is shown in Fig. 4.

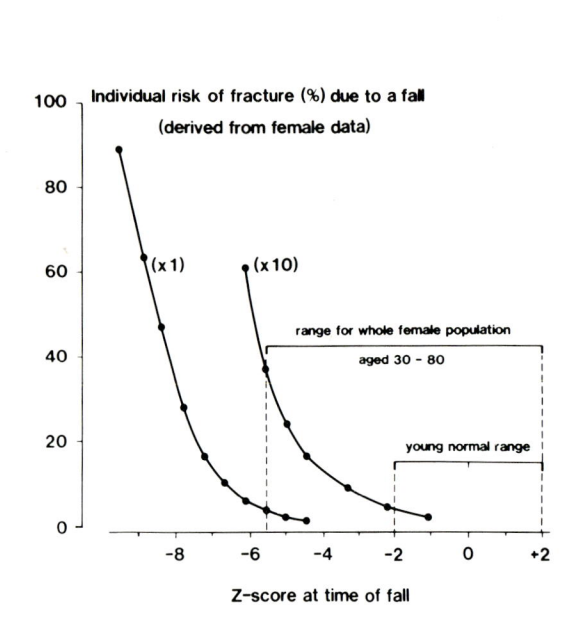

Fig. 5
Relationship between risk of fracture due to a fall and BM expressed as a Z-score at the time of the fall (linear model).

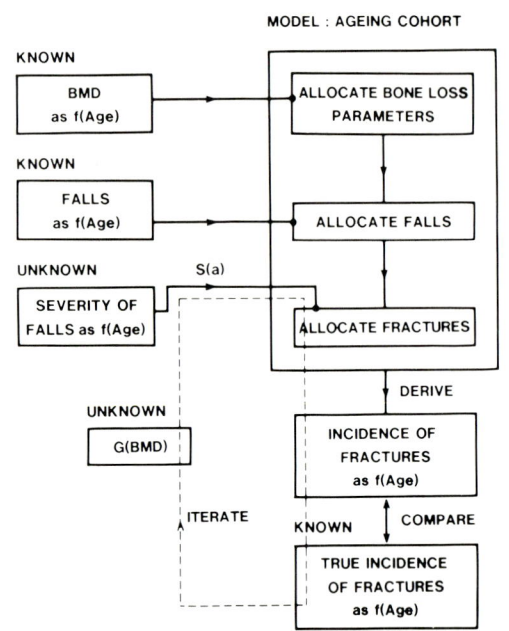

Fig. 6
Schematic representation of the implementation of the non-linear model.

Results

Fig. 4 also shows the match achieved after 5 iterations between the age-specific incidence of fractures predicted by the linear model and the idealised incidence of hip fractures in women. Because real incidence curves are probably sigmoidal rather than exponential, greater importance was attached during iteration to matching model predictions with the idealised incidence in the lower age-groups. The fact that at high ages the model generated values below the exponential curve was anticipated.

Fig. 5 shows the previously unknown function relating the individual's risk of fracture due to a fall to BM (expressed as a Z-score) at the time of the fall. Z was derived by linear transformation of BM in such a way that Z=0 corresponded to the young mean and Z=-1 to 1SD below that value. That particular function, coupled with the function describing the incidence of falls in relation to age (Fig. 3), generated the predicted fracture incidence data shown in Fig. 4. By definition, that function (Fig. 5) applied whenever members of the simulated cohort fell; it quantified the relationship between the bone mineral measurement (BM) on the femoral neck and the risk that the hip would fracture when loaded during a fall.

The function (Fig. 5) tended to 100% at low Z values (below -5.5) that rarely occurred in the simulated cohort. As the magnified (x10) curve shows, the risk at the lowest values reached in the cohort (-2SD limit at age 80) was just under 4%. The risk was so low because there were many more falls than fractures. Furthermore the curve was highly non-linear within the range of values observed in the population, and for positive Z approached zero asymptotically.

Because all individual data were stored by the simulation program, it was possible retrospectively to pose complex questions in the form of database queries. One such question was 'If a woman age 70 has a BM value in the femoral neck equivalent to Z=-2.5, what is the chance that she will fracture her hip if she survives to age 80?' The answer resulting from analysis of the database was 4.0%. If Z had been -2.0, the answer would have been 2.8%. If the woman had not been measured, then the risk estimate (based solely on the known fracture prevalences at age 70 and age 80) would have been 5%.

The non-linear model

Fig. 6 outlines the approach used to simulate events in the ageing female cohort. Each woman was first allocated parameters describing her lifelong changes in BMD, then falls were allocated as before. The function $S(a)$ was initialised to 1 for all ages a. Because the curve in Fig. 5 closely approximated an exponential function (see below, Fig. 9), G(BMD) was represented as $G(BMD)=\exp(k_1-k_2 \cdot BMD)$ and initialised using $k_1=6$ and $k_2=0.1$. The numerical value of k_2 is dependent on the scale of BMD. Values of G(BMD) were limited to 100 (% risk). Next every fall was examined and a fracture associated with it, conditional upon the current fracture risk which was by definition $S(a) \cdot G(BMD)$, where BMD here denotes the value of BMD at the age of the fall a.

Fracture incidence was assessed as before and compared with the idealised true incidence shown in Fig. 4. Mismatch in the age range 40-70 years was attributed to errors in the specified values of k_1 and k_2. These were then changed so that in successive iterations predicted and true incidences in that age range converged. The age constraint had to be applied because (with $S(a)=1$ for all a) it proved impossible in practice to find any values of k_1 and k_2 which generated a match over the whole range up to age 90.

After iteration, new point values for $S(a)$ (ages over 70) were estimated as the ratio of the true to predicted incidences in 5-year groups. Because in practice the point values of $S(a)$ for ages in the range 70 to 85 appeared to rise exponentially, $S(a)$ was subsequently evaluated analytically: i.e. $S(a)=1$ for ages below 68; $S(a)=\exp(k_3 \cdot a - k_4)$ for ages over 67, where $k_3=0.0650$ and $k_4=4.388$. Using the resulting values for $S(a)$ and unaltered values for k_1 and k_2, the association between the falls and fractures was reworked and the predicted fracture incidence recomputed. No iteration was necessary.

Practical implementation

Simulations of cohorts of 20,000 women were performed using extended versions of the programs which implemented the linear model.

Values of parameters

Parameters describing how BMD changed with age in individuals are illustrated in Fig. 7. Growth occurred at mean rate R0 with SD s_{R0} until mean age of maturity A1 with SD s_{A1}. Thereafter the equilibrium phase (R1=0 in everyone) continued until mean age A2 with SD s_{A2}, when bone loss started with mean rate of change R2 and SD s_{R2}. Later in life at mean age A3 with SD s_{A3} bone loss slowed down to a mean rate of change R3 with SD s_{R3}. Individual values of all variables were statistically independent of one-another.

Values of those parameters were chosen so that age-related changes in the whole cohort would mimic results of cross-sectional absorptiometric studies of the femoral neck published recently [6]. Mean values used (SD in brackets) were R0=4.5(0.405)/year, A1=20(1) years, R1=0(0), A2=35(2), R2=-0.864(0.063), A3=60(2), R3=-0.18 (0.018). The period prevalence of falls used was as before (Fig. 3), with the same distribution of falls frequency multiplier (mean 1, SD 0.3). Initial values of k_1 and k_2 have been given above.

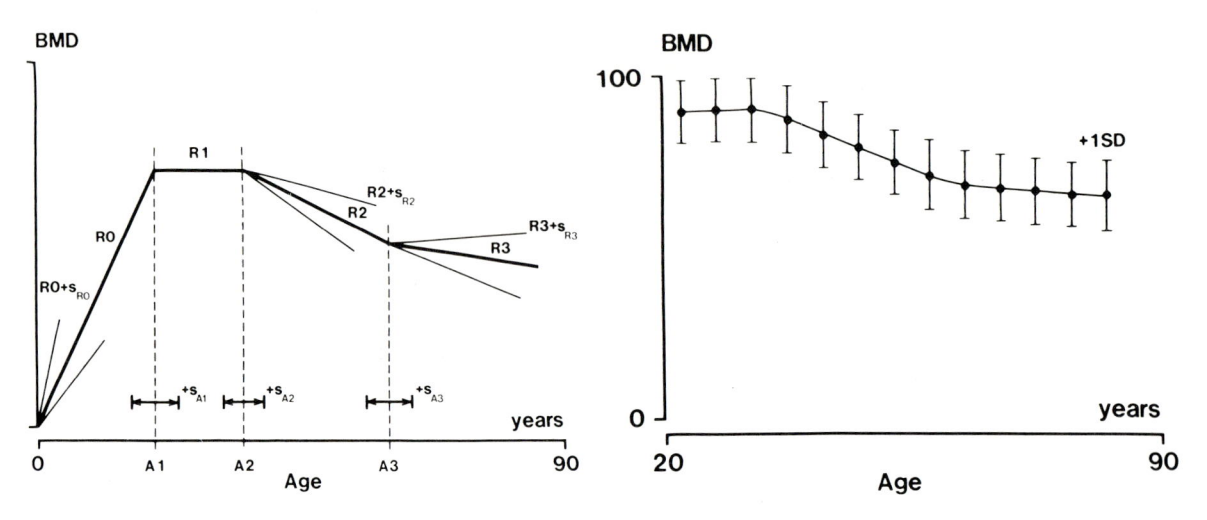

Fig. 7
Parameters of the non-linear model defining age-related changes in BMD.

Fig. 8
Changes in BMD in the ageing cohort.

Results

Fig. 8 illustrates how the distribution of BMD changed as the cohort aged from 20 to 85 years. The young mean value of BMD was 90.1 with SD 9.3 (coefficient of variation 10.3%); by age 60 the mean was 77% and by age 80 was 70% of the young mean value. The SD at age 80 was 10.5.

Final values of k_1 and k_2 after iterating to match the incidence curve in Fig. 4 in the age range 40-70 years were 6.32 and 0.1128 respectively. Fig. 9 shows the relationship between $\log_{10}(G(BMD))$ and BMD expressed as Z-score. This is effectively the relationship between log(% risk) and Z which applies up to age 67. The slope of the straight line in Fig. 9 is such that the risk increases by a factor of 2.84 for a decrease in Z of 1 unit. The same figure illustrates the relationship between log(% risk) and Z for the linear model which applies in that case at all ages. As previously stated, that curve approximates an exponential; the risk increases by a factor of about 2 for 1 unit decrease in Z.

Fig. 10 illustrates the match achieved between the predicted and true incidence at the end of the iteration when S(a)=1 for all a, and after S(a) had been adjusted as described above. Values of S(a) at ages 70,75, and 80 were then respectively 1.18, 1.63 and 2.25.

Retrospective analysis of the database permitted fracture cases who had their first fracture in specified age-groups to be identified. For 5-year groups centred on ages 62.5, 67.5, 72.5 and 77.5 the group mean values of BMD were 57.6(8.0), 57.0(8.3), 57.5(8.6) and 55.9(8.0) respectively (SDs in brackets). These mean values were equivalent to Z-scores about 1.1 units below the mean values in age-matched non-fracture cases.

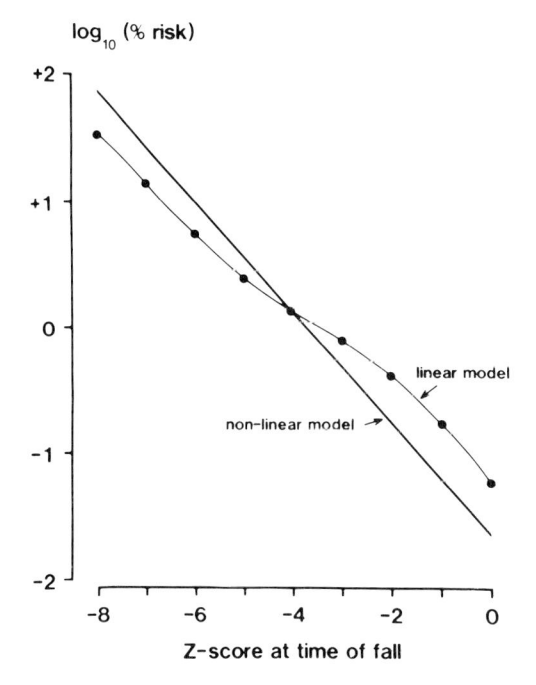

Fig. 9
Log(% risk) in relation to
Z-score. For the non-linear
model this applies only for
ages below 68.

Fig. 10
Comparison of predicted
(points) and idealised true
hip fracture incidence for
the non-linear model.

Discussion

Linear model

Although in the linear model BM was treated as a measurable risk factor for fracture, it is not implied that BM must be the only relevant variable. It is highly likely that other properties of bone (and body build and musculature) in reality also control whether or not a woman fractures her femur when she falls. Those properties must include the spatial distribution of mineral within and amongst trabeculae, the spatial organisation of trabeculae in the metaphyses, the cortical porosity and organisation of the Haversian systems and the integrity of the organic matrix including micro-structure and cross-linking of collagen fibrils. In the context of these microscopic properties, any non-invasive bone measurement is a large-scale and relatively crude property of the bone.

It is possible that some real absorptiometric measurement on the femoral neck (but not BMD) in reality changes in the way formulated for BM in the linear model. If so, the fact that the linear model can accurately predict hip fracture incidence over the whole age span implies that age-related changes in these other quantities which are co-determinants of risk must on the whole parallel the changes in bone.

Non-linear model

This model was designed to simulate observations which more closely describe real data [6]. Initial exploratory work immediately revealed the necessity of introducing an extra age-related variable, S(a), regarded above as a measure of the severity of falls. This is a helpful conceptual simplification only; S(a) is better regarded as a function which ascribes to age multiplicative risk factors which cannot be estimated from BMD at the time of the fall. It is important to realise that the final numerical values of

S(a) were dependent on three other functions: the idealised true age-specific incidence of fractures, which probably becomes increasingly unrealistic at ages over 80; the age-dependent frequency of falls, which might not be relevant to the population on whom BMD was measured; and the function describing how BMD changes with age in individuals (no data were available to verify some of the parameter values used). It is conceivable, but in our view unlikely, that if all these limitations were overcome it would be possible to predict accurately the incidence of hip fracture over the whole age span with S(a)=1 for all a (i.e. with S(a) becoming redundant).

Reductions in BMD in fracture cases aged 60-79 predicted by the model were slightly lower than observed reductions equivalent to about 1.4 standard deviation units [7]; the small residual difference (about 0.3 units) is most likely another manifestation of some of the limitations mentioned above.

At present, photon absorptiometry is in practice the only technique which can provide non-invasively and with very small radiation exposure a bone measurement that is an indirect estimator of fracture risk. Photon absorptiometry is therefore currently the method of choice as a screening procedure. The approaches described above provide mechanisms for computing the numerical value of risk from the resulting measurements. This does not exclude the possibility that observations of body weight and height (which jointly determine the potential energy to be dissipated in a fall from the standing position) or of muscle function can usefully supplement absorptiometric observations. Future extensions of the model will attempt to take these variables into account.

Acknowledgement

This work was carried out while both authors were supported by MRC External Scientific Staff programme grants.

References

1. Wasnich R D, Ross P D, Heilbrun L K and Vogel J M 1985 Prediction of postmenopausal fracture risk with use of bone mineral measurements Am J Obstet Gynecol 153 745-751
2. Knowelden J, Buhr A J and Dunbar O 1964 Incidence of fractures in persons over 35 years of age. A report to the MRC working party on fractures in the elderly Brit J Prev Soc Med 18 130-141
3. Nordin B E C, Horsman A, Marshall D H, Simpson M and Waterhouse G M 1979 Calcium requirement and calcium therapy Clin Orthop Rel Res 140 216-239
4. Horsman A, Jones M, Francis R and Nordin B E C 1983 The effect of oestrogen dose on postmenopausal bone loss New England Journal of Medicine 309 1405-1407
5. Horsman A, Marshall D H and Peacock M 1985 A stochastic model of age-related bone loss and fractures Clin Orthop Rel Res 195 207-215
6. Mazess R B, Barden H S and Green G 1987 Bone mineral density of the spine in normal white women Presented at Am. Soc. Bone Mineral Research (Indianapolis), Abstract #330.
7. Mazess R B, Barden H, Ettinger M and Schultz E 1988 Bone density of the radius, spine and proximal femur in osteoporosis J Bone and Mineral Research 3, 13-18
8. Jaszmann L 1973 Epidemiology of climacteric and postclimacteric complaints Front Hormone Res 2 22-30
9. Riggs B L, Wahner H W, Seeman E, Offord K P, Dunn W L, Mazess R B, Johnson K A and Melton L J 1982 Changes in bone mineral density of the proximal femur and spine with aging. Differences between postmenopausal and senile osteoporosis syndromes J Clin Invest 70 716-723
10. Aitken M 1984 Osteoporosis in Clinical Practice (Wright, Bristol)

Discussion:

DR. GENANT (San Francisco): Dr. Wahner, you have demonstrated, in one of the examples you showed a histogram across the femoral neck showing the density tracing of a normal versus an osteoporotic fracture. In that osteoporotic fracture, you show a disproportionate loss of trabecular bone while the cortical bone showed smaller losses.

Secondly, the last slide that you really did not have time to explain showed relatively good separation between fracture/non-fracture patients based upon measurements at Ward's triangle, again suggesting, perhaps, a greater discriminatory capability in the region of trabecular bone within the femoral neck, perhaps also consistent with the Singh approach.

What I'm questioning is whether this type of information might not question the concept of the Type 1 and Type 2 osteoporosis, wherein one thinks of Type 2 osteoporosis as a proportionate loss of trabecular and cortical bone contribution to hip fracture in the very elderly. We have some indirect evidence now, and perhaps also some direct evidence, suggesting that it is not a proportionate loss but a disproportionate loss of trabecular bone even in the femoral neck region that may be, in part, accounting for the fracture susceptibility.

DR. WAHNER (Rochester, MN): That is an interesting interpretation of the data. We certainly have now the tools to settle this issue. I'm aware of the fact that, for example, the trabecular bone, which is only 30 percent or so in the neck, accounts for half of the compressive strength in the specimen. But I have no facts to add.

DR. SINGH (Chicago): You know, it was very nice to see my work being presented by Dr. Wahner here. And when he first presented this paper at the meeting in 1973 in Washington, Dr. Riggs was sitting next to me. And after the presentation I told Larry, "If I had a machine to sell along with this observation, it would be considered very significant." But now we have the machine. And the thing which I wanted to say was that, we are not using the machine for comparing different areas of the proximal femur within the same bone but are focusing our attention on one or other part of the bone. We know that, because of the unusual structure of the femoral neck, the trabecular bone in the proximal femur behaves differently in different parts.

If you look at the greater trochanter, the part which does not take part in direct weightbearing, that bone behaves more like the cancellous bone in the vertebrae, and changes in the cancellous bone of the trochanter, follow the vertebral density changes more closely. On the other hand, the compressive trabeculae in the femur behave more like cortical bone, and changes in the compressive trabeculae follow more closely the changes in the cortical bone of the middle radius.

My question, then, is do we have any data on the comparative values of density in the proximal femur? Have you compared any density changes to the Singh index?

DR. WAHNER: I fully agree that bone loss in itself is not the real end point we want. I think we want to have the location which best predicts fracture. We should not look for the area in the spine which shows the lowest bone mineral or even the highest loss, but rather the area which will ultimately show the best fracture prediction.

DR. SINGH: I would say that the geometry is equally as important as density of bone in predicting fractures and we should be looking at comparing different areas within the proximal femur to get an idea about the hip fracture risk.

DR. WAHNER: I believe the histogram display of bone mineral is probably the closest thing we have right now to work on.

DR. JOHNSTON (Indianapolis): Tony Horsman's model, I think, is very interesting and provocative and very important. Some of the assumptions, particularly about falls, I would question. How solid is the evidence that falls actually level off with age? For example, Iskrantz published a graph of death-related falls from the public health service here, and that's an exponential increase, which would somewhat alter your second model. But it's still a very interesting and important model. And I'd also be interested in Steve Cumming's comments on it as well.

DR. HORSMAN (England): First of all, let me say that I accept the limitations of the input data as far as the prevalence of falls is concerned. At the time I set the model up, that was the only set of figures available to me, and it was based on some data analyzed by the MRC unit in Southampton using results of a Department of Health survey carried out in 1973. Changing that input function would certainly affect the function that I call S, the severity of falls.

DR. CUMMINGS (San Francisco): I agree. I think that it's a very nice model. And I also agree that not all studies, including the data I showed earlier about the incidence of falls with age in the United States, which I think is the best population-based data. If one takes account, not only of the risk of falling but of the number of falls that occur with age, one tends to see a more exponential rise because the number of falls per person that fall increases with age. Now, that makes some sense.

It might be very interesting to use the United States data in the Horsman model to see how that changes the assumptions. But, otherwise, I think that to some degree the model that he proposes fits very nicely with the hypothesis of hip fractures that were presented earlier. And so, I think it's an exciting convergence.

DR. RIGGS (Rochester, MN): I know Dr. Genant is too good a scientist to try to develop general conclusions from measurements in two single individuals. I think when you look at the measurements made in a large number of individuals, looking at a measurement of the spine, for example, that contains mostly trabecular bone, and the mid-radius, entirely cortical bone, that you will see that in older people the loss of trabecular and cortical bone is approximately proportionate.

Now, of course, the process of Type 1 osteoporosis is the accelerated disproportionate loss of trabecular bone. And those individuals will lose the trabecular bone from their hip as well, during that 15 to 20 year period after menopause, as Dr. Mazess has shown in his paper in the JBMR. But if you make those measurements later in life, at the time when hip fractures usually occur, you don't see the good discrimination on separation.

DR. PARFITT (Detroit): The available published data indicate that the hip fracture risk is very much smaller in Blacks in South Africa than in Blacks in the United States. I would ask each member of the panel to say how they account for that, whether in terms of personal observations or any of the theoretical models relating fracture risk to bone measurements that have been put forward.

DR. CUMMINGS: I wish I knew more about Blacks in South Africa. But the models it proposed suggested it's either falling-protection against fracture during falls - or something to do with bone strength that may not be measured by measurements that were made in that study. And beyond speculation, the author of that paper speculated that it was a more careful mode of walking. I've never seen people walk there and I can't imagine that that accounts for the entirety of the difference. But I'm intrigued that there may be other structural or bone-strength-related parameters that might account for at least part of that difference.

One other thing. It's also interesting that within the same countries, for example, there are strong urban/rural differences that some have speculated may be due to both physical activity and isolation, that is, people in urban areas living alone and being, therefore, more prone to falling badly.

DR. MAZESS (Madison, WI): With regard to the question of compact bone and trabecular bone in the proximal femur, there's very definite excess loss of the trabecular bone. That is evidenced by the decreased values in the Ward's triangle area in virtually any osteoporotic with a hip fracture that one examines.

I think there may well be a Type 1 and Type 2 osteoporosis, but that hip fracture is a case where there is preferential loss at the hip rather than in the spine, and that is perhaps more of a distinction.

A second distinction that is not made here, because we all tend to normalize our bone values in terms of density, is that people with hip fracture almost invariably are smaller and have a lower bone mineral content than their age-matched controls. They actually have smaller bones. So that, if we look at the difference in the BMC rather than the BMD, it's much larger. But the variance of the BMC is so large that the diagnostic sensitivity is not enhanced by using BMC.

Those who are investigating hip fracture, however, should really look at the absolute values of BMC rather than the density itself, because I think there may be some information that we get from doing so that is not achieved or is obscured by looking at density.

DR. MALLUCHE (Lexington, KY): I have a question and comment to Dr. Dempster's interesting presentation. When one addresses the predictive value of bone histology for assessing bone mass, one needs to take into consideration the way the iliac crest bone biopsy is being performed. We did studies on the variability of bone mass within iliac bone and could show that the variability exists from superior to inferior, and there is very little, if any, variability from anterior to posterior.

If you take your bone sample in a vertical manner, you will cover that variability within your specimen if it is of sufficient size and doesn't stop right under the cortex. Whereas, when you take your biopsy in a horizontal manner, you're subject to the superior/inferior variability and, therefore, the bone biopsy is not as predictive as when taken in a vertical manner. How were your bone samples obtained?

DR. DEMPSTER (New York): Our samples were taken in a horizontal manner.

DR. SCHNITZLER (Johannesburg): I should like to comment on Dr. Parfitt's reference to the femoral neck fractures in Blacks in South Africa. We do see femoral neck fractures in the Black population. But the epidemiological pattern is different. We see as many men with femoral neck fractures as women. They are somewhat younger than in Whites; the average age, roughly, is about 60. They are usually in individuals who have abused alcohol. And it is in the periurban and urban areas that we begin to see these fractures now, where hard liquor is being consumed.

One other comment relates to the agility of the aging Black population. These people live in a much less protected environment than we do. Their coordination and perhaps, also, their reaction times may be better and protect them against falls.

Lastly, there is evidence that trabecular bone mass is greater, trabecular thickness is greater, trabecular number is greater, and trabecular separation is lower.

Femoral Fracture: The Role of Vitamin D

MUNRO PEACOCK[1] and LESLIE HORDON[2]

[1]Indiana University School of Medicine
Indiana University Hospital
General Clinical Research Center
Indianapolis, IN
[2]Department of Rheumatology
The General Infirmary
Leeds, England

Introduction

Aging does not spare the skeleton. On average 30% of the bone mass of the young adult is lost between the age of 50 and 80. This loss is associated with an age-related increase in osteoporotic fractures the commonest of which, in people over the age of 65, is fracture of the proximal femur. In populations in North Europe and America about 1% of women and 0.2% of men aged 80 sustain a femoral fracture every year.[1] Because of the high rates of morbidity and mortality arising from this fracture, the expense incurred by its treatment and the increasing number of people living beyond the age of 65, prevention of the fracture is now a major goal in health care.

The injury causing the fracture is usually minor and precipitated by a number of physical and environmental disabilities common in people over the age of 65. However, the fact that minor trauma results in fracture implicates the quantity and/or quality of bone as a major risk factor. The lower bone mass and higher incidence of fracture in women than men also suggests that the quantity of bone is a major determinant of the fracture.

Age-related bone loss is accompanied by changes in the architecture of bone in the hip.[2] At its simplest level this involves the relative distribution of bone between cortex, trabeculae and medulla. At a more complex level the thickness, number and alignment of individual trabecula are involved. With age there is an outward expansion of the cortex due to subperiostial growth and endostial resorption and a thinning and loss of trabeculae. In healthy males, thinning is the more prominent feature whereas trabecular loss is more prominent in women.

Unlike quantity and distribution of bone, there is little to suggest that aging per se alters bone quality. On the other hand, osteomalacia is reported in some studies to affect up to 20% of patients with femoral fracture.[3]

A number of disabilities and diseases affecting both the quantity and quality of bone become increasingly common with age. Of particular concern in this article is the decrease with age in calcium absorption since calcium malabsorption is a common risk factor in both primary and secondary osteoporosis and in plasma 25OHD and 1,25(OH)$_2$D, since they have a primary role in regulating both calcium absorption and bone mineralization.

The theme of this article is to describe and collate a number of studies aimed at defining abnormalities in vitamin D and calcium metabolism in relation to the pathogenesis of the abnormalities in bone in patients with hip fracture.

Results

Effect of Age on Plasma 25OHD, Creatinine Clearance and Radiocalcium Absorption in Women.[4] (Fig 1)

In healthy women with no evidence of bone disease there is a steady decline in plasma 25OHD with age. After the age of 70 the mean value is less than the lower limit of the range in young women and continues to decrease into the 10th decade. The absorption of calcium, measured by radiocalcium, and glomerular filtration rate, measured by creatinine clearance from 24 hour urine collections, show little change until the age of 70. Thereafter however they decrease with age and the mean values are less than the lower limit of the ranges in young healthy women.

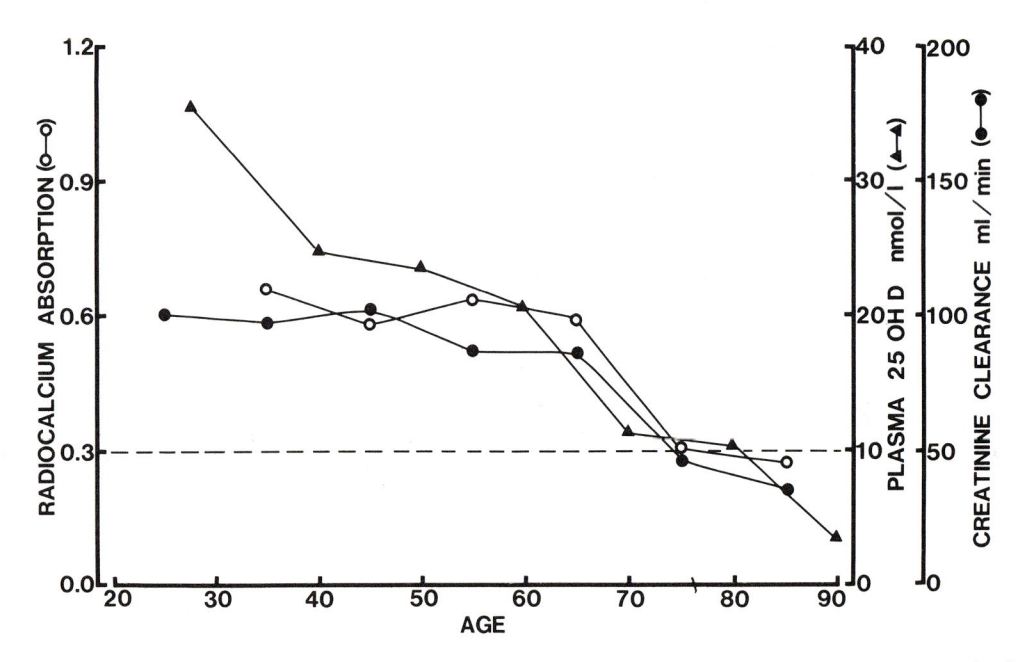

Fig. 1 The relationship between mean plasma 25OHD, creatinine clearance and radiocalcium absorption and age in three separate groups of healthy women. The lower limits in women aged 20 to 60 are indicated by the interrupted line.

Effect of Age on Plasma 1,25(OH)$_2$D and PTH. (Fig 2)

In healthy women there is a steady decline in plasma 1,25(OH)$_2$D with age. By the ninth decade the mean plasma 1,25(OH)$_2$D is below the lower limit of normal of young adult women. In contrast the plasma PTH rises steadily with age and by

NORMAL WOMEN

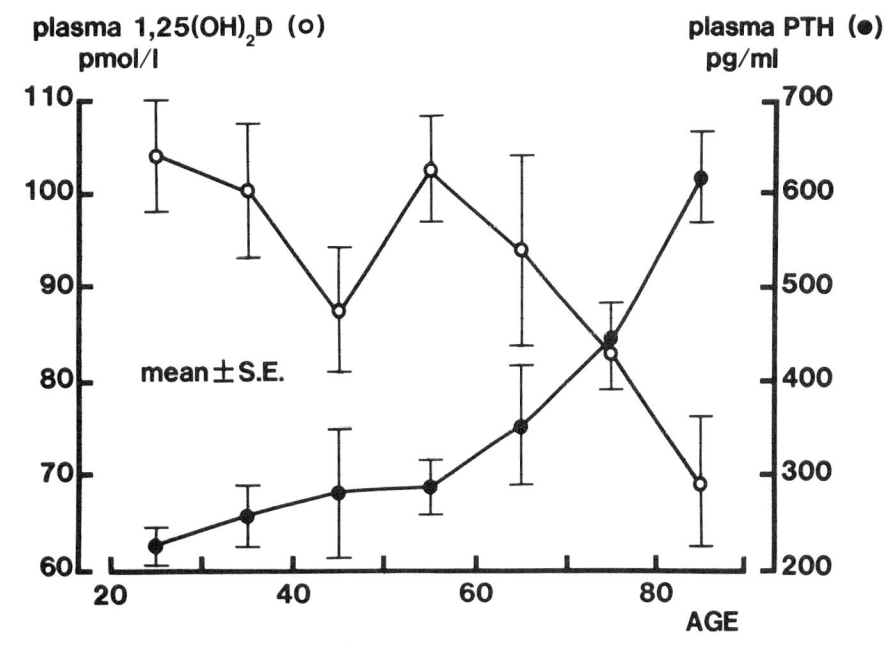

Fig. 2   The relationship between mean plasma 1,25(OH)$_2$D and PTH and age in two separate groups of healthy women.

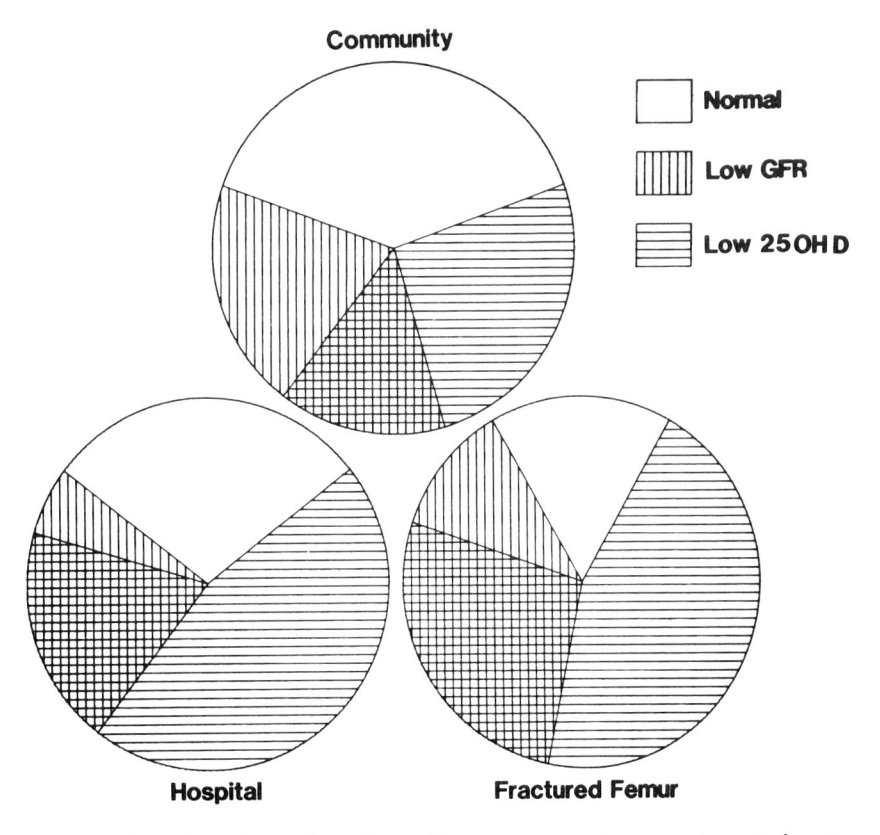

Fig. 3   Pie charts showing the percentage of subjects with a reduced GFR (assessed by plasma creatinine), reduced plasma 25OHD and with both abnormalities in a population of hospitalized patients with femoral fracture, age-matched hospital controls and age-matched controls in the community from which the hospital populations were drawn.

the ninth decade the mean plasma PTH is above the upper limit of normal young women.

Biochemical Abnormalities in Femoral Fracture Patients and their Age-Matched Hospital and Non-Hospital Controls (Fig 3)

All groups of elderly subjects show biochemical abnormalities in plasma vitamin D metabolites and renal function. However, as compared to their age-matched controls hospitalized for minor intercurrent illnesses, femoral fracture patients show a higher prevalence of biochemical abnormalities. Both groups are, however, more often affected than healthy age-matched controls in the community from which they are drawn.

Biochemistry in Femoral Fracture Patients and Controls and the Change induced by 40 ug/day of oral 25(OH)D$_3$ for 7 days[5] (Table 1 & Fig 4)

Table 1. Biochemistry in 23 patients with femoral fracture and their controls before (basal) and after 7 days treatment with 40 ug of 25(OH)D$_3$ given orally; results are shown as mean and SEM.

		Control			Fracture		Normal (Young Adult)
Plasma							
25(OH)D (nmol/l)	Basal	13.5	1.2		13.3	0.9	9-90
	Treated	49.3	2.7		46.3	2.2	
Creatinine (umol/l)	Basal	97	6		83	5	80-120
	Treated	96	7		83	6	
RadioCa absorption (fr/h)	Basal	(n=21) 0.42	0.05	(n=18)	0.29	0.04	0.4-1.2
	Treated	0.51	0.05		0.32	0.03	
PTH (pg/ml)	Basal	(n=22) 374.3	28.9		237.4	1.5	125-375
	Treated	345.8	34.3		203.8	17.0	
1,25(OH)$_2$D (pmol/l)	Basal	93.8	5.8		81.4	8.4	75-165
	Treated	140.6	8.7		89.1	5.6	

Patients with femoral fracture studied at the time of fracture do not differ substantially in their biochemical variables as compared with age-matched control women admitted to a geriatric ward for assessment of minor disabilities. But they tend to have lower plasma 1,25(OH)$_2$D and PTH levels and radiocalcium absorption. However, the response in biochemistry to oral 25OHD is markedly different. Unlike their controls the fracture patients fail to increase plasma 1,25(OH)$_2$D and radiocalcium absorption. These defects are shown in relation to the slopes of the change in plasma 1,25(OH)$_2$D and calcium absorption and the basal plasma 25OHD concentration established from the responses in various diagnostic groups[6] (Fig 4).

Bone Histology in Patients with Femoral Fracture (Fig 4).

Histomorphometry of bone biopsied from the iliac crest at the time of fracture showed that out of 72 patients only 31% were completely normal. Osteoporosis (bone volume <15%) was present

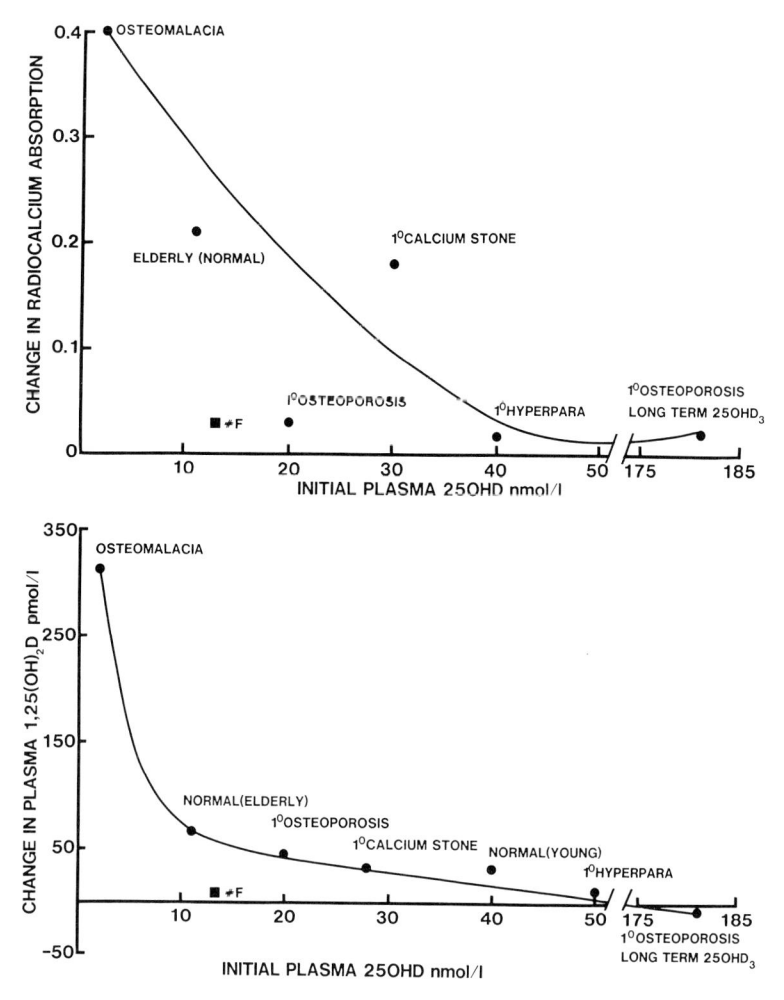

Fig. 4   The relationship between the change in radiocalcium (top panel) and plasma 1,25(OH)$_2$D and the basal plasma 25OHD induced by 7 days of 40ug 25OHD$_3$ orally in groups of patients with various diseases. The arbitrary line of relationship is shown and the data from the femoral fracture patients is indicated, #F ■.

in 47%. In 32% osteoporosis was the sole abnormality, but in 5% there was also osteomalacia (osteoid surfaces >24% and calcification fronts <60%) and in 10% there was an abnormally low calcification front. The overall prevalence of osteomalacia was 15% but 5% also had osteoporosis.

The prevalence of osteoporosis increased with age. However, the relationship between osteomalacia and age was much steeper and 62% of the patients with osteomalacia were over the age of 80.

Biochemically there was no distinguishing features which separated patients with osteoporosis. However, the osteomalacic patients showed biochemical evidence of renal failure, hyperparathyroidism and reduced plasma levels of vitamin D metabolites.

Discussion

The general phenomenon of age-related loss of bone in healthy people over the age of 65 is accompanied by decreases in plasma

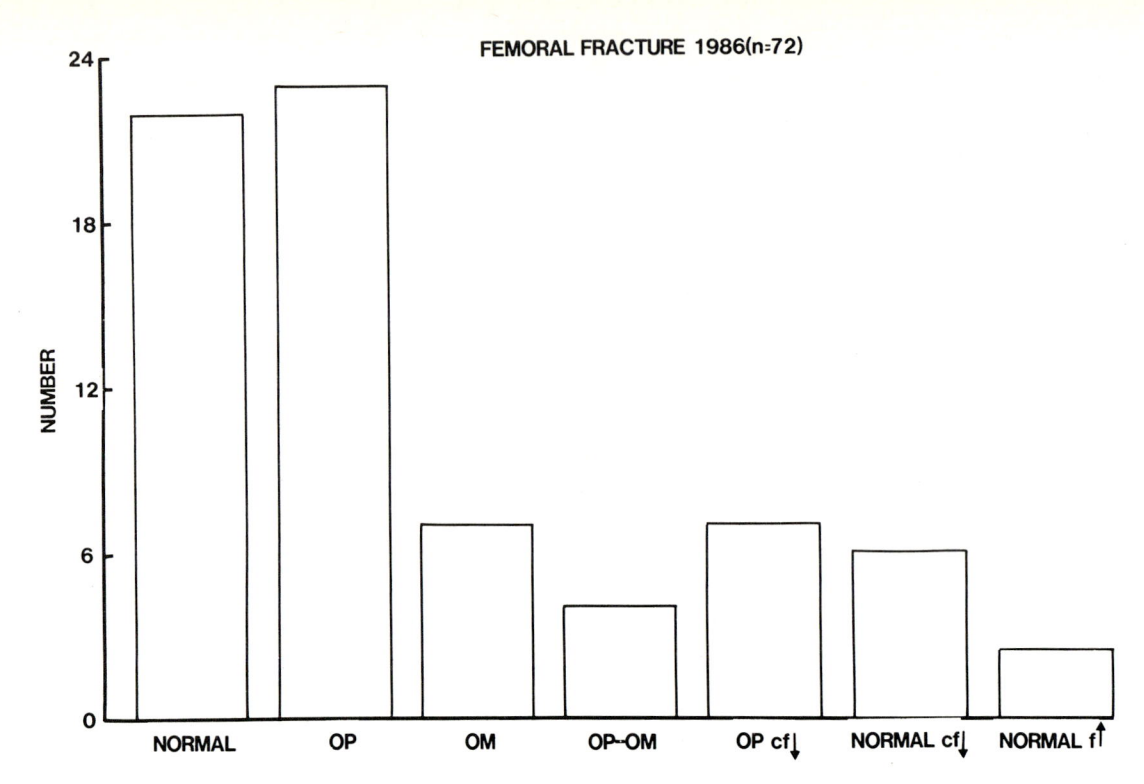

Fig. 5 Histomorphometry in femoral fracture patients (OP = osteoporosis, OM = osteomalacia, OP-OM = both osteomalacia and osteoporosis, cf = % calcification front, f = % osteoid surfaces).

25OH and 1,25(OH)$_2$D which by virtue of their effect on calcium absorption, plasma PTH levels and on mineralization are important in determining both the amount of bone lost and the quality of bone remaining. Impaired calcium absorption leads to generalized osteopenia; increased plasma PTH levels to bone loss, particularly in the cortex and low plasma levels of 1,25(OH)$_2$D and 25OHD to an increased prevalence of calcification defects.

We have argued that as the vitamin D stores are chronically depleted the individual passes from a state of vitamin D sufficiency to one of insufficiency and finally to one of deficiency which can be defined by the response in plasma 1,25(OH)$_2$D to a standard oral dose of 25OHD$_3$ (Fig. 4). Insufficiency causes impaired absorption which leads to osteoporosis. Insufficiency, however, readily progresses to deficiency and causes, in addition, secondary hyperparathyroidism and osteomalacia. This sequence of events is supported by the prevalences of osteoporosis and osteomalacia in patients with femoral fracture and their relationship to age. As the plasma levels of 25OHD and 1,25(OH)$_2$D become progressively lower with age the prevalences of osteoporosis and osteomalacia in biopsies from femoral fracture patients increase. However the osteomalacia is confined to the oldest patients and "osteoporotic-osteomalacic" is common suggesting that osteoporosis itself is a risk factor for the development of osteomalacia.

Since these decreases in vitamin D will tend to alter both the quantity and quality of bone and therefore promote fracture, it would be expected that the abnormalities are more common in patients with femoral fracture. In general this is true if the fracture patients are compared with healthy people in the community (Fig. 3). It is less obvious when they are compared with elderly people hospitalized for minor illnesses (Fig. 3). Like bone mass itself, there is a large overlap in these variables between people with and without femoral fracture.

When small numbers of patients are compared (table 1), only calcium absorption is significantly lower in the fracture patients as compared to elderly control subjects in hospital. Plasma 25OHD and 1,25(OH)$_2$D are low in both groups and PTH is not increased. A clear difference however is apparent between femoral fracture patients and their controls when both groups are given a daily oral dose of 25OHD$_3$ for a week. The control subjects and the fracture patients show a normal and equivalent rise in plasma 25OHD levels. However, the normal rise in plasma 1,25(OH)$_2$D and calcium absorption does not occur in the femoral fracture patients (table 1, Fig. 4). The cause of this failure is not obvious. It is not due to impaired renal function since plasma creatinine in the fracture patients is lower than the controls. Whether it is an intrinsic or transitory abnormality induced by the fracture episode is not clear. In six patients followed for six months after the fracture there was partial recovery of the responses to oral 25OHD$_3$ suggesting that it may be transitory. Whatever the cause it is clear that biochemistry taken at the time of fracture is unable to differentiate between patients with and without osteomalacia and except in the severest cases histological diagnosis remains at present necessary for diagnosis.

REFERENCES

1. Hedlund, R., Lindgren, V., Ahlborn, A. (1987) Age and sex-specific incidence of femoral neck and trochanteric fractures. Clin Orthop **222**,132-139

2. Singh, M., Nagrath, A.R., Marni, P.S. (1970) Changes in trabecular pattern of the upper end of the femur as an index of osteoporosis. J Bone Joint Surg **52A**,457-4

3. Aaron, J.E., Gallagher, J.C., Anderson, J., Stasiack, L., Longton, E.B., Nordin, B.E.C., Nicholson, M. (1974) Frequency of osteomalacia and osteoporosis in fractures of the proximal femur. Lancet **1**:229-233

4. Peacock, M., Francis, R.M., Selby, P.L. (1983) Vitamin D and osteoporosis. In: Dixon A STJ et al eds. Osteoporosis, A Multi-Disciplinary Problem. Roy Soc Med Internat Congress & Symposium, Series No. 55, Academic Press & Roy Soc Med; London, p 245-254

5. Hordon, L.D., Peacock, M. (1987) Vitamin D metabolism in women with femoral neck fracture. Bone and Mineral **2**:413-426

6. Peacock, M., Selby, P.L, Francis, R.M., Brown, W.B., Hordon, L.D. 1985) Vitamin D deficiency, insufficiency, sufficiency and intoxication. What do they mean? In: Norman AW et al eds. Sixth Workshop on Vitamin D. Berlin, New York: Walter de Gruyter, p 569-570

Vitamin D Nutrition and Metabolism in Aging and Osteoporosis

THOMAS L. CLEMENS

Regional Bone Center
Helen Hayes Hospital
West Haverstraw, NY
and Department of Pathology
Columbia University
New York, NY

Introduction

Vitamin D is a principal determinant of intestinal calcium absorption and has important actions on skeletal remodeling. It has been proposed that age-related disturbances in the calcium-vitamin D endocrine system contribute to the bone loss associated with aging. In this chapter, recent work on the nutrition, metabolism and action of vitamin D will be reviewed with specific reference to age-related bone loss in humans.

Theoretical considerations

Vitamin D is available to man from two sources. The principal source is the skin where it is produced by a photochemical process. Provitamin D_3 (7-dehydrocholesterol) present in the epidermis is photolyzed to pre-vitamin D_3, which, in turn, undergoes thermal rearrangement to form vitamin D_3 (1). Vitamin D is also available in the diet, mainly in foods fortified with it. Vitamin D from either source is converted in the liver to the most abundant circulating metabolite, 25-hydroxyvitamin D_3 (25-(OH)D). In the kidney, 25-(OH)D is converted to the active, hormonal form, 1,25-dihydroxyvitamin D (1,25-$(OH)_2$D). This step is normally tightly regulated according to the prevailing requirement for calcium. The major regulating factors are parathyroid hormone, calcium and phosphate and also the amount of substrate 25-(OH)D available for conversion. 1,25-$(OH)_2$D acts through specific intracellular receptors in the intestine where it enhances calcium and phosphate absorption, and in bone where it causes bone mineral mobilization and alters osteoblast function (2).

Theoretically, deficiency in vitamin D with aging could cause at least two different disorders. Chronic, severe vitamin D deficiency causes intestinal hypoabsorption of calcium and phosphorus leading to osteomalacia. This disorder has been reported to be relatively common among elderly subjects in Great Britain, but is now rarely seen in the U.S.

Increasing evidence suggests that alterations in vitamin D metabolism with age contribute to the genesis of osteoporosis. The mechanisms by which this occurs are probably different from those that produce osteomalacia. Age-related defects could arise at several levels along the vitamin D metabolic pathway (Fig.1). Each of these possible disturbances will now be considered.

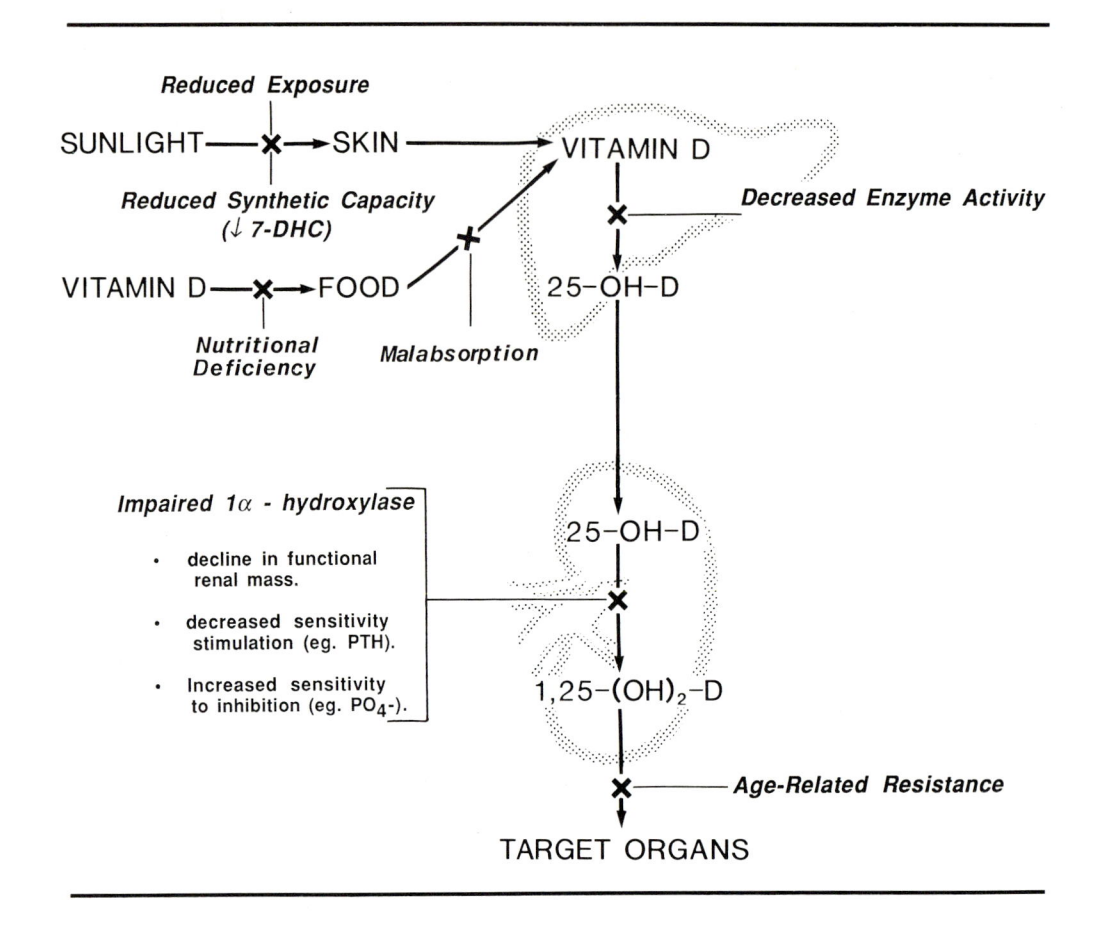

Figure 1: Possible sites for age-related disturbances in vitamin D production, metabolism and action.

Vitamin D supply in the elderly

The vitamin D status and nutritional requirements among elderly U.S. citizens are still not well understood. It is likely that the elderly have a reduced total intake of vitamin D. Recent evidence suggests that aging decreases the skin's capacity to synthesize vitamin D_3 in response to sunlight exposure. Pro-vitamin D_3 content is reduced in skin of elderly individuals compared with young people (3). The physiological relevance of this difference has not yet been determined, because ultraviolet irradiation can raise serum 25-(OH)D concentrations in elderly subjects to levels comparable to those achieved in young subjects (4). Most elderly, however, habitually get less exposure to sunlight than do young people. This is obviously true in people who are institutionalized or house-bound. Our recent studies in New York nursing homes suggest that most residents get no sunlight exposure (5).

Vitamin D status in the elderly could also be reduced because of inadequate dietary intake. A popular notion is that the elderly avoid dairy products because of the associated intestinal discomfort. Dietary intake data of a healthy elderly population in New Mexico indicate that 60 percent of subjects who were not taking supplements had a vitamin D intake of below 100 IU per day (6). This value is not much different from that obtained for a group of young adult women when the contribution from vitamin supplements was subtracted (7). Elderly subjects in nursing homes might be expected to ingest less vitamin D than non-institutionalized subjects, but our recent surveys in New York suggest the opposite. In these subjects, the mean intake was 350 IU. While vitamin D supplements were the major determinant of intake, the ingestion of milk accounted for as much as one-third of the supply (5). Based on interview information, there was no evidence that these individuals declined dairy products because of gastrointestinal discomfort. Obviously, this finding may not hold true for all nursing homes.

It has also been proposed that the elderly malabsorb vitamin D, and some experimental support for this concept exists (8). We have used an oral absorption test, which was originally developed to detect severe vitamin D malabsorption in inflammatory bowel disease, to evaluate the effect of age on vitamin D absorption. In these studies, elderly subjects given a single oral dose of 50,000 IU vitamin D_2 had increments in serum vitamin D_2 comparable to those of young adults (Fig 2). Thus, aging apparently is not associated with severe intestinal malabsorption of vitamin D.

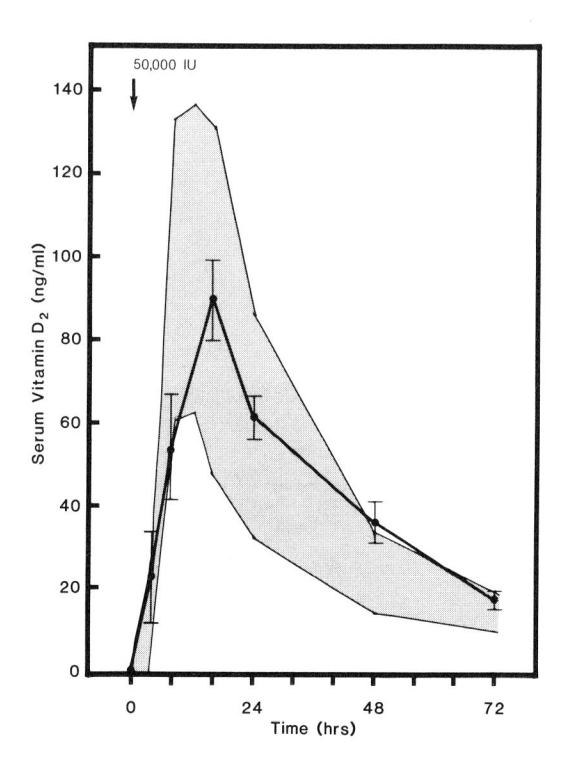

Figure 2: Mean serum vitamin D_2 concentrations in seven elderly subjects before and after a single dose of 50,000 IU vitamin D_2. The shaded area represents the range of levels achieved in eight young healthy subjects. Reproduced with permission (9).

It is also possible to evoke a mechanism whereby hepatic 25-hydroxylation declines with age. Attempts to investigate this possibility by determining the influence of large doses of vitamin D on circulating 25-(OH)D concentrations (10) are difficult to interpret and inconclusive.

Circulating vitamin D metabolite concentrations in elderly individuals

Measurement of serum vitamin D metabolite levels in elderly populations has been revealing with regard to understanding their vitamin D status. It is not surprising, given the evidence discussed above, that most studies have disclosed lowered 25-(OH)D levels in elderly subjects compared with younger control groups (11). In general, however, reported values were not grossly low and were well above the threshold that would be associated with osteomalacia. Even in chronically institutionalized subjects, serum 25-(OH)D concentrations can be maintained at a normal level by dietary ingestion of adequate amounts of dairy products and supplements (5,9). These findings are in contrast to those from Great Britain and France where serum 25-(OH)D levels in elderly subjects have been reported to be at or below the limit of normal (11). A clue to the difference between these populations is found in a study of 25-(OH)D levels of patients in a long-stay mental hospital in England (12). These subjects had normal 25-(OH)D levels because they were receiving vitamin D supplements. Taken together, these data suggest that reduced sunlight exposure is the main reason for a lowered 25-(OH)D status among elderly, and that vitamin D supplementation is important in the maintenance of normal 25-(OH)D levels.

Serum $1,25-(OH)_2D$ concentrations, however, clearly fall with age (Fig.3) and can reach abnormally low levels (13,14). We have now surveyed individuals from three separate nursing homes as well as a population of ambulatory elderly in the New York area. Our data suggest that approximately 15 to 30 percent of individuals within the age range from 60 to 100 years have serum concentrations below 20 pg/ml despite having a normal 25-(OH)D (5,9).

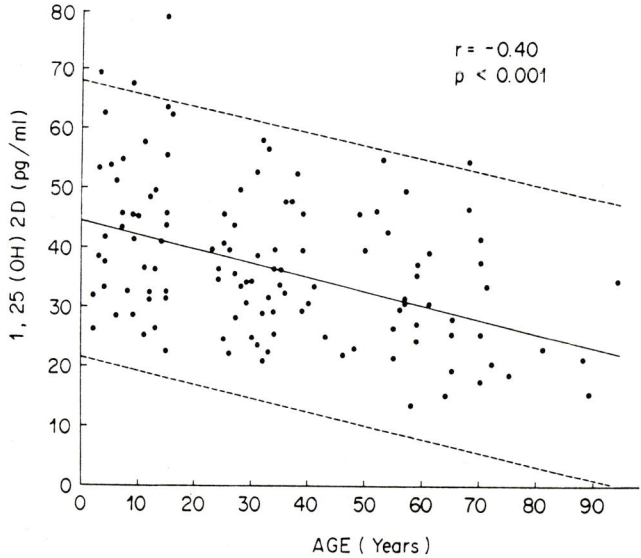

Figure 3: Influence of age on plasma concentration of $1,25-(OH)_2D$ in normal humans. Reproduced with permission (13).

Mechanism for the age-related decline in 1,25-(OH)$_2$D production

It is not yet clear what mechanism is responsible for the reduction in serum 1,25-(OH)$_2$D level with age. A decline in GFR probably plays a role but does not completely explain the fall in serum 1,25-(OH)$_2$D concentration. For example, in patients with chronic renal disease, serum levels of 1,25-(OH)$_2$D appear not to decline significantly until GFR reaches 40-50 ml/min. We have found that elderly subjects with relatively normal renal function can have abnormally low serum levels of 1,25-(OH)$_2$D (5,9). A more likely possibility is that aging disturbs the regulation of the renal 1-hydroxylase. Therefore, the enzyme might be resistant to the hormones and factors that normally stimulate its activity, such as parathyroid hormone, and be more sensitive to factors that suppress its activity, such as blood phosphate and calcium.

Dynamic testing of the parathyroid-renal 1-hydroxylase axis has recently been applied to the study of the mechanism for age-related decline in 1,25-(OH)$_2$D production. Infusions or bolus injections of human parathyroid hormone cause a transient rise in blood metabolite levels. Young people demonstrate a greater increase in serum 1,25-(OH)$_2$D in response to parathyroid hormone than do older subjects (15,16). In one study, the increment in serum 1,25-(OH)$_2$D was correlated with the GFR, but parathyroid hormone infusion produced a similar rise in cAMP in old and young women. This further suggests that renal impairment is not the sole cause for the impaired 1,25-(OH)$_2$D production. In a group of younger osteoporotic women (within 20 years of menopause), there was no evidence for a blunted 1,25-(OH)$_2$D production (16). Therefore, the defect is probably a function of aging rather than osteoporosis *per se*.

Oral phosphate administration can be used to evaluate the sensitivity of renal 1-hydroxylase to inhibition in aging and osteoporosis (17,18). Administration of one gram of neutral phosphate acutely lowers serum ionized calcium, which stimulates parathyroid hormone secretion. If phosphate dosing is repeated daily, serum 1,25-(OH)$_2$D levels fall after three to five days in elderly osteoporotic subjects by as much as 50 percent that of baseline (Fig.4).

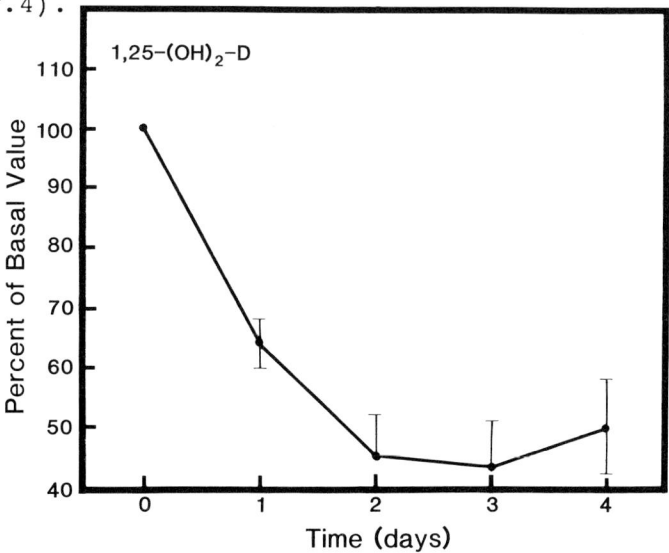

Figure 4: Effect of oral phosphate administration on circulating 1,25-(OH)$_2$D concentrations in elderly osteoporotic subjects. Reproduced with permission (17).

Phosphate administration to young people results in comparable changes in calcium and parathyroid hormone but does not significantly reduce serum 1,25-(OH)$_2$D levels (18). This observation suggests that aging might also be associated with an enhanced sensitivity to suppression of renal 1-hydroxylase activity by phosphate.

Age-related resistance to 1,25-(OH)$_2$D

Aging could also result in a decreased sensitivity of the intestine and possibly bone to the action of 1,25-(OH)$_2$D, which would further predispose to bone loss. This phenomenon appears to occur in aging rats and is supported by a study of human subjects (19). Nevertheless, oral administration of 1,25-(OH)$_2$D$_3$ can increase intestinal calcium absorption in elderly subjects (20) which demonstrates that any intestinal resistance is not absolute.

It is also possible to assess skeletal response to 1,25-(OH)$_2$D in aging. The production of bone Gla (BGP) protein or osteocalcin, which is produced by the osteoblast, is known to be stimulated by 1,25-(OH)$_2$D and appears in serum following dosing with the hormone. This has been used as a marker for the responsiveness of bone to 1,25-(OH)$_2$D. Patients with postmenopausal osteoporosis have an even greater BGP after oral 1,25-(OH)$_2$D$_3$ than do age-matched control women (21). This test has yet to be applied to evaluate the influence of age on skeletal response to 1,25-(OH)$_2$D.

Consequences of reduced 1,25-(OH)$_2$D in the elderly

The impact of a chronically reduced serum level of 1,25-(OH)$_2$D is not fully appreciated. Whether this represents the primary defect in the genesis of senile osteoporosis is still open to debate. In this scenario, a reduced 1,25-(OH)$_2$D serum level would be followed by a decline in intestinal calcium absorption and a state of mild secondary hyperparathyroidism with bone resorption surpassing formation. Recent measurements of serum parathyroid hormone using new assays for the biologically active hormone have shown that levels do rise with age. There remain, however, many unanswered questions that deserve attention in the coming years. Do elderly subjects with a chronically reduced level of 1,25-(OH)$_2$D have a reduced bone mass? If so, would these individuals benefit from treatment with 1,25-(OH)$_2$D$_3$? Although serum 25-(OH)D levels are not grossly low in most elderly individuals, they might be inappropriately low given the less efficient conversion to the active metabolite. If this were true, then it may be feasible to supplement these individuals with vitamin D to increase the substrate levels and thereby raise their serum 1,25-(OH)$_2$D levels to normal. Clearly, given the established importance of 1,25-(OH)$_2$D to mineral homeostasis and its possible involvement in cell differentiation and immune function, further study of age-related perturbations in vitamin D metabolism and action is warranted.

References

1. Holick, M.F. (1981) J. Invest. Dermatol. 76,651-657.
2. Deluca, H.F. (1988) FASEB. J. 2, 224-236.
3. MacLaughlin, J.A. and Holick, M.F. (1985) J. Clin. Invest. 76, 1536-1538.
4. Davie, M., and Lawson, D.E.M. (1980) Clin. Sci. 58, 235-242.

5. O'Dowd, K.J., Clemens, T.L., Lindsay, R. and Kelsey, J.L. (1988) J. Bone. Min. Res. (abstract in press).
6. Omdahl, J.L., Garry, P.J., Hunzaker, L.A., Hunt, M.A. and Goodwin, J.S. (1982) Am. J. Clin. Nutr. 36, 1225-1233.
7. Sowers, M., Wallace, R.B., Hollis, B.W. and Lemke, J.H. (1986) Am. J. Clin. Nutr. 43, 621-628.
8. Barragry, J.M., France, M.W., Corless, D., Gupta, S.P., Switala, S., Boucher, B.J. and Cohen, R.D. (1978) Clin. Sci. Mol. Med. 32, 213-220.
9. Clemens, T.L., Zhou, X-Y., Myles, M., Endres, D. and Lindsay,R. (1986) J. Clin. Endocrinol. Metab. 63, 656-660.
10. Skinner, R.K. (1979) in "Vitamin D. Basic Research and its Clinical Application", ed. A.W. Norman, De Gruyter, New York, p.1001.
11. Parfitt, M.A., Gallagher, J.C., Heany, R.P., Johnston, C.C., Neer, R. and Whedon, G.D. (1982) Am. J. Clin. Nutr. 36, 1014-1031.
12. Sheltawy, M., Newton, H., Hay, A. Morgan, D.B. and Hullin, R.P. (1984) Hum. Nutr: Clin. Nutr. 38C, 191-194.
13. Manolagas, S.C., Culler, F.L., Howard, J.E., Brinkman, A.S. and Deftos, L.J. (1983) J. Clin. Endocrinol. Metab. 56, 751-756.
14. Gallagher, J.C., Riggs, B.L., Eisman, J., Hamstra, A., Arnaud, S.B. and DeLuca, H.F. (1979) J. Clin. Invest. 64, 729-736.
15. Slovik, D.M. Adams, J.S., Neer, R.M., Holick, M.F. and Potts, J.T.,Jr. (1981) N. Eng. J. Med. 305, 372-374.
16. Tsai, K-S., Heath, H., Kumar, R. and Riggs, B.L. (1984) J. Clin. Invest. 73, 1668-1670.
17. Clemens, T.L., Silverberg, S.J., Dempster, D.W., Shane, E., Segre, G.V., Williams, S., Lindsay, R. and Bilezikian, J.P. (1985) In: "Vitamin D. Chemical, Biochemical and Clinical Update" ed A.W. Norman, DeGruyter, New york, pp. 1010-1011.
18. Silverberg, S.J., Shane, E., Clemens, T.L., Dempster, D.W., Segre, G.V., Lindsay, R. and Bilezikian, J.P. (1987) J. Bone. Min. Res. 1, 383-388.
19. Francis, R.M., Peacock, M, Taylor, G.A., Storer, J.H. and Nordin, B.E.C. (1984) Clin. Sci. 66, 103-107.
20. Gallagher, J.C., Jerpbak, C.M., Jee, W.S.S., Johnson, K.A. DeLuca, H.F. and Riggs, B.L. (1982) Proc. Natl. Acad. Sci. 79, 3325-3329.
21. Duda, R.J., Kumar, R., Nelson, K.I., Zinsmeister, A.R., Mann, K.G. and Riggs, B.L. (1987) J. Clin. Invest. 79, 1249-1253.

Discussion:

DR. MARCUS (Stanford): We've had recent experience touching on both of these fascinating presentations that I wish to share with the audience. One has to do with the question of how much of the apparent defect in 1-alpha-hydroxylase in elderly women is due to age, per se, or what might be a component of estrogen deficiency.

The way we approached this problem was to study these women with provocative stimulation of calcitriol production before and after a 30-day trial of 1.25 milligrams a day of conjugated estrogen. The experimental model that we used was EDTA-induced hypocalcemia, with a rise in spontaneous parathyroid hormone secretion.

Although estrogen treatment led to significant increases in plasma 1,25 D static levels in this group of women, average age 70, there was no change in the response to the rise in PTH that was induced by hypocalcemia. So, we have been unable to show any evidence that this 1-alpha-hydroxylase defect is reversible by estrogen.

The second point I wanted to raise confirms the hypothesis that Munro Peacock just presented that the level of sufficiency for vitamin D is considerably higher than traditional values which we associate with osteomalacia.

We have studied 150 normal, ambulatory volunteers from the Palo Alto community and assessed the relationship between circulating 25-hydroxy D and immunoreactive parathyroid hormone. There is a statistically significant negative correlation between circulating PTH and 25-hydroxy D, and that relationship holds up in a multiple regression analysis when the effects of glomerular filtration rate and age are cancelled.

However, if one limits the analysis of PTH versus 25-hydroxy D only to subjects whose values of 25-hydroxy D are greater than 25 nanograms per milliliter, there is no significant relationship between 25-hydroxy and PTH.

As we start to include more subjects at the lower end of 25 OHD, that is, to levels about 20 nanograms per milliliter, the inverse relationship between 25-hydroxy D and PTH becomes statistically significant. No further significance is obtained by going down to our very lowest values.

Therefore, it appears that something happens at 25 OHD of about 20 nanograms per milliliter that leads to an increase in PTH. There's ample literature confirmation for the idea of a threshold effect for 25-hydroxy D on PTH. Your study certainly suggests that. Your data, I think, were expressed as nanomols per liter. Multiplying by .4 is the proper correction to ng/ml. Therefore, a level around 20 nanograms per milliliter is where you might define vitamin D sufficiency from your study. Thus, I'm happy to report that our data appear to confirm your hypothesis.

DR. PEACOCK (Indianapolis): The values of 20 ng/ml is close to what I would call sufficiency.

DR. BOUILLON (Belgium): I think that there is a basic problem because the interpretation for the etiology of Type 2 osteoporosis is being discussed here. We have looked at vitamin D, 1,25 and 25-hydroxy vitamin D levels in an elderly population in Belgium, which is at the latitude of Canada, and in south of Spain, Cordoba, which is at the latitude of the middle of the United States. Indeed, concentrations of both are frequently low in these population, but they are totally correctible with oral 25-hydroxy vitamin D. So, I would share the opinion of Munro Peacock, that it is not a primary deficiency of the renal 1-alpha hydroxylase activity, but substrate deficiency which causes the low 1,25 dihydroxy vitamin D levels.

I would like to ask Dr. Clemens if you looked at the effects of serum phosphate, serum creatinine, and calcium intake in your population to look for an alternative explanation for the low 1,25 dihydroxy vitamin D levels in some of your subjects?

DR. CLEMENS (New York): Yes, they were all normal. I think there is a difference between these two populations and that one of the differences is, I think, that in Europe, and I believe in Leeds, you're looking at people who just have lower 25-hydroxy vitamin D concentrations. So, you're going to see the normalization in 1,25. Whereas, the nursing home group we looked at had a relatively normal vitamin D intake and a much higher 25-hydroxy vitamin D concentration.

DR. BOUILLON: But a relationship with serum creatinine was not found?

DR. CLEMENS: No.

DR. BAYLINK (Loma Linda, CA): I agree that calcium absorption decreases with aging, and in some geographic areas that plasma 25 OHD also decreases. But there are a large number of patients who malabsorb calcium, who are aged, who have normal levels of serum 1,25 vitamin D. I'm just wondering if Dr. Clemens could comment on the mechanism for this. Does this involve some aspect of vitamin D utilization, or are there other factors that might be involved?

DR. CLEMENS: One of the points I tried to make is that I think reliance on a static measurement of plasma 1,25 D in a given population, especially in cross-sectional studies, is dangerous. And I think the use of a dynamic stimulation test along the lines which I just showed may be helpful. I agree, you can't explain some of these observations.

DR. BAYLINK: Not terribly practical, though.

DR. CLEMENS: That's correct.

DR. PEACOCK: I think, by definition, you would call that resistance.

DR. BAYLINK: Well, they respond quite well to 1,25 vitamin D in low dose, but they have normal levels.

DR. PEACOCK: Yes, but that is likely to be a direct action of oral 1,25 D in the gut. When you give half a microgram of 1,25 D the response in absorption doesn't correlate with the blood 1,25 D level which hardly changes.

DR. BAYLINK: Have you evaluated whether that might be resistance?

DR. PEACOCK: Yes. In our osteoporotic population up to the age of 75, we found a subgroup who had malabsorption of calcium, normal plasma 1,25 D concentrations and who did not respond to changes in plasma 1,25 D induced by oral 25 OHD. We called that resistance. It's very easily overcome by giving oral 1,25 D. But I don't think that's a true test of resistance because of its local action in the gut.

DR. HEANEY (Omaha): I have questions for both Drs. Peacock and Clemens. As you know, Dr. Peacock, your work in this regard has been fascinating for years and it was nice to see it again today. Where would you put the boundary line between insufficiency and sufficiency, as far as 25 hydroxy D levels are concerned?

DR. PEACOCK: It would be in that area about 50 nanomols per liter.

DR. HEANEY: So, it would be in the range of 50 to 60 nanomols per liter?

DR. PEACOCK: Yes.

DR. HEANEY: Which would translate to be something very close to Bob Marcus' figure of 20 to 25 nanograms per mil, right?

DR. PEACOCK: Yes.

DR. HEANEY: Then I guess I would ask, in view of the general consensus from several groups that this kind of a phenomenon is going on, why are we waltzing around the term deficiency and calling this simply insufficiency and putting deficiency somewhere farther down the scale?

DR. PEACOCK: I think, historically, vitamin D deficiency has been synonymous with osteomalacia. I would recommend using insufficiency when there is only calcium malabsorption, which of course produces osteopenia.

DR. HEANEY: Dr. Clemens, you spoke about the response of the serum 25 hydroxy D levels to D intake as an evidence that absorption was at least qualitatively okay. But that is not satisfactory evidence of that because, of course, you would want to know what the slope was. And we didn't have any data on the slope of that response in young versus older individuals.

DR. CLEMENS: No, and I think, in fact, the relationship between plasma 25 OHD and dietary D intake that I showed was a line which, in fact, dissected the ordinate at about ten nanograms per mil but I don't think it is a simple relationship. I think it's curvilinear, but we have not done any more assessment of that.

DR. HEANEY: But is it the same relationship in the young as in the elderly?

DR. CLEMENS: We haven't looked at that.

DR. HEANEY: Okay. So, we know there is some absorption, but we don't know whether it's normal or not?

DR. CLEMENS: That's correct.

DR. PARFITT (Detroit): Just a comment on the definition of osteomalacia and its relationship to vitamin D. Without tetracycline labeling, it is impossible to differentiate osteomalacia from so called preosteomalacia, which is a state of increased bone turnover due to secondary hyperparathyroidism with osteoid accumulation. And that state is undoubtedly a manifestation of mild vitamin D deficiency, whereas osteomalacia, in the strict sense, is a manifestation of more severe vitamin D deficiency.

The prevalences you have shown for osteomalacia are almost certainly much higher than reality. For example, I would not accept any of the cases put forth by Dr. Sokoloff as having osteomalacia. In a rather extensive study of iliac histology in hip fracture patients in Detroit some years ago, we found not a single case which I would accept as having osteomalacia.

We did, however, find a substantial proportion of cases who had an increased extent of osteoclasts on the cancellous bone surface which inversely correlated with the serum level of calcidiol. I think PTH-mediated bone loss due to subclinical vitamin D deficiency may be a very important contributory mechanism in a small subset of patients with hip fracture. But the prevalence of that cannot be identified by using osteomalacia as the hallmark of vitamin D deficiency.

DR. PEACOCK: I agree with all these comments and I pointed out the great difficulties we have in the static histomorphometry taken at the time of fracture. This is an area that needs further studies.

To define osteomalacia, we have used two criteria: the increase in formation surfaces and the decrease in the calcification fronts. In well documented D deficiency these give good separation from normals and hyperparathyroid biopsies, and the lesions are completely reversible with vitamin D treatment.

DR. REEVE: Carrying on a little bit on that theme, I'm very

interested in the extended but normal thickness osteoid seams that you've shown in Leeds. Paul Lips has recently quantified about 40 of our biopsies and found the same sort of distribution of osteoid extent without very many biopsies showing thick osteoid seams.

The interesting point was that in Paul's own Dutch series he found a correlation, and a very strong inverse correlation, between the thickness of the cortices and the extent of the osteoid seams.

And in osteoporotic patients, who had bone density measurements made at the mid shaft of the radius, there was this same inverse correlation. So, it does look as though extended thin osteoid seams are correlated with bad indices of cortical bone density elsewhere. And I was very interested to hear Michael Parfitt's comments that this may be a high bone turnover state which, of course, might predispose to loss of cortical bone.

I wonder if you have any comparable data in your own series, Munro. Have you looked at indices of bone mass at any other site or in the biopsy itself, in your larger series?

DR. PEACOCK: We have done neither. We would agree with the observation of very thin cortices in osteomalacia or high turnover states in the elderly. It's very striking.

DR. RIGGS (Rochester, MN): Just two brief comments. First, with respect to Dr. Bouillon's comments, in the study that Dr. Clemens showed from the Mayo Clinic, we selected those patients so that they all had normal 25 hydroxy vitamin D. So, the young individuals and the elderly individuals had the same level of 25 hydroxy vitamin D. Yet, when we infused PTH, they had a clear blunting of the response.

I don't think that 25 hydroxy vitamin D deficiency, which certainly may be important in some patients, particularly in northern Europe, can explain all of the problems, and there clearly is a hydroxylase defect in the elderly.

On the other hand, I would agree with Munro Peacock. Our most recent data suggests that there is also a problem of resistance to 1,25 dihydroxy vitamin D action, in that, in the larger series of patients, we now find that serum 1,25 dihydroxy vitamin D increases, and then plateaus or decreases as a hydroxylase defect comes in.

DR. BELL (Charleston): We have found that obese Caucasian subjects have vitamin D insufficiency. Serum vitamin D values are strikingly low and serum 25 OHD values are about half of those of non-obese individuals. These individuals also had elevated serum immunoreactive PTH, 1,25-dihydroxy vitamin D urinary cyclic AMP and low urinary calcium. These changes are reversed by administration of 25-hydroxyvitamin D.

The point to be made is that 25-hydroxyvitamin D has biologic activity, even when serum values are within the normal physiologic range. The subjects who have low serum 25-hydroxyvitamin D values with normal serum values of 1,25-dihydroxyvitamin D calcium that are malabsorbing calcium may be malabsorbing because of the lack of 25-hydroxyvitamin D. Would you care to comment on these observations?

DR. PEACOCK: I agree with that but it acts through 1,25 dihydroxy vitamin D. This morning, we were talking about calcium having a threshold. Vitamin D doesn't have a threshold. When we're considering calcium intake, we must consider its intake in relation to plasma 25-hydroxyvitamin D level. They cannot be considered separately.

DR. PECK (St. Louis): I'd like to ask Dr. Parfitt a question that stems from his comment. Do you find a continuum of osteoid seam thickness or extent of osteoid coverage that correlates inversely with vitamin D levels? Or are we talking about different effects on bone altogether, at different levels of vitamin D?

DR. PARFITT: The histologic findings certainly constitute a spectrum reflecting histologic evolution. If one looks at a large number of patients with vitamin D deficiency, whether nutritional or due to malabsorption, in general, the osteoid surface increases in extent first, at which time bone formation rate and osteoclasts are increased and PTH nephrogenous cyclic AMP and alkaline phosphatase are high, and calcidiol levels are low and the calcitriol levels are normal. Later, the formation rates gradually fall and the osteoid seam gets thicker and eventually the mineralization defect evolves and culminates in a state in which there is complete absence of tetracycline double labeling. In those patients whom everyone would say, even without tetracycline labeling, that they have severe osteomalacia, the calcitriol levels are low.

DR. PECK: I'm just trying to extend the concept that Bob Heaney was proposing, that at mild states of vitamin D deficiency, one sees both osteoidosis and increased bone resorption?

DR. PARFITT: Correct.

DR. RAISZ (Connecticut): We looked at a series of biopsies of osteoporotics and compared the extent of osteoid seams, which were not wide, with everything we could think of. There was no correlation at all with 25-hydroxyvitamin D. The only correlation we got was with albumin levels.

We ended up wondering whether or not these extended osteoid seams have something to do with the ability to make proteins. These extended osteoid seams are not a function of a mineralization defect. They're a function of some defect in this finishing off of bone, a phenomenon which we don't understand very well, laying down that last bit, of whatever it is, that gives us a finished bone surface as opposed to a slightly osteoidal bone surface. Have you looked at your albumin levels?

DR. PEACOCK: Albumin is interesting. Jonathan Reeve, from his studies, suggested that it is a useful biochemical test as a risk factor for hip fracture. Certainly, hip fracture patients have low plasma albumin. It also correlates with calcium malabsorption. The malabsorbers have the lowest plasma albumin. I think what you're seeing is that section of the population who are either very ill or most deprived nutritionally. We have not found a correlation with osteoid.

DR. MALLUCHE (Lexington, KY): When you address vitamin D deficiency and talk about osteomalacia in the elderly, I think there's a caveat in place. That is, you need to rule out that you are not talking about early renal osteodystrophy.

If glomerular filtration rate falls to levels of 70 milliliters per minute, you don't have significant changes in serum creatinine, but bone changes occur that are very similar to what you showed. Could you address that problem, please?

DR. PEACOCK: I think I would need to ask what your criteria are for early renal osteodystrophy and how these differ from osteomalacia.

DR. MALLUCHE: Well, I can't go into a detailed discussion of what is osteomalacia. I think that there is some need to clarify the nomenclature. One thing is sure, that the data that you presented would go along with what we see in patients with renal osteodystrophy, that is, an increase in PTH, and a somewhat low 1,25 dihydroxyvitamin D level but still in the normal range. It was shown that the 1,25 dihydroxyvitamin D levels, even though still in the normal range, correlate with GFR. In addition, you see an increase in the fraction of trabecular surface covered by osteoid, without an increase in osteoid seam thickness, and signs of hyperparathyroid bone disease.

DR. PEACOCK: I think that's a difficult one. I certainly agree with you that renal failure is a risk factor for osteomalacia. If you examine the osteomalacic group, there will be one or two patients with high plasma creatinines. However, the major factor correlating with plasma 25-hydroxyvitamin D is 1,25 dihydroxyvitamin D and not plasma creatinine.

DR. SERRANO (Spain): We have studied 100 biopsies from elderly patients with hip fractures and no case of osteomalacia has been found in this 100 cases. The criteria used were static increased osteoid seam width and decreased osteoblastic osteoid rate. And with these two static criteria, we can't find any case of osteomalacia.

The Orthopaedist and Hip Fractures

J.M. LANE, C.N. CORNELL, M. BANSAL,
S.B. SCHWARTZ, and R. SCHNEIDER

Metabolic Bone Disease Unit
The Hospital for Special Surgery
Cornell University Medical College
New York, NY

Mechanism of Fracture

Bone is organized into both a cortical and trabecular structure with different mechanical roles for each of the two bone types[7]. Areas with large multidirectional impact stress have trabecular patterns while cortical bone is predominant in regions of high torque and bending. Trabecular bone has a high surface to volume ratio and appears more metabolically active. The skeletal areas rich in trabecular bone such as the vertebral spine sustain an early onset of postmenopausal bone loss and diminution of structural integrity. Cortical bone with a low surface to volume ratio is only slowly resorbed and consequently there is a late rise in the intertrochanteric fracture of the hip.

The mechanical strength of bone is related to its mass and structure[3]. A gross loss of bone mass increases the fracture rate in an exponential manner, and the hip fracture incidence is related to the bone density squared. This clinical observation is supported by laboratory studies. Structurally, the further the osseous mass is situated from the central axis of the bone, the greater the resistance is to bending and torque loads. Although, the fracture rate is indirectly proportional to an exponential of the bone mass and structure, other factors including extent and nature of trauma, potential for healing microfractures, bone quality, structural considerations, general health of the individual and age all significantly affect fracture incidence and risk.

Management of Osteoporotic Fractures

The impact of skeletal bone loss becomes evident as the skeleton begins to fail in its ability to withstand required loads. When fractures appear, osteoporosis becomes a disorder which alters the quality of life and adversely affects survival[7,6]. One patient in twenty past the age of 65 currently occupying a hospital bed is recovering from a hip fracture. In the most optimal environment, 40% of patients sustaining a hip fracture will not survive two years following this injury. Of the patients originating from a nursing home, 70% will not survive one year. Only one-third of patients following a hip fracture will return to a life-style and level of independence comparable to that prior to the injury.

A reasonable return of function following hip fracture in elderly patients can only be achieved by early, definitive stabilization of the injured extremities[7]. Immobilization of the patient as a whole rather than definitive operative treatment positions the patient at risk of venoembolic disease, pulmonary decompensation, decubitus formation, and further musculoskeletal deterioration from which recovery becomes difficult. In recent years, the treatment of osteoporotic fractures has improved considerably as a result of an understanding of the biology and mechanics of fracture healing in osteoporotic bone and improvements in the design of internal fixation devices. Based upon a large experience of treating osteoporotic fractures at The Hospital for Special Surgery and The New York Hospital Cornell Medical Center, the following therapeutic principles have been conceived:

1. Elderly patients are best served by rapid, definitive fracture care aimed at early restoration of mobility and function.

2. The aim of the intervention should be to achieve stable fracture fixation that allows early return of function.

3. The primary mode of failure of internal fixation results from bone failure rather than implant failure.

4. The underlying metabolic bone disease must be defined and treated.

A study at New York Hospital of 75 consecutive hip fracture patients compared their bone density and iliac bone histomorphometry with age matched controls and osteoporotic patients with spinal fractures[4]. Hip fracture patients did not differ from the age-matched non hip fracture population bone density of the lumbar spine (DBA). Both osteoporotic patients with either spinal or hip fractures had comparable bone histomorphometry. Both groups demonstrated 8% of the patients with hyperosteoidosis and similarly equal percentages of patients with slightly enhanced resorption. Within the hip fracture population, total bone volume, cortical bone volume, and cancellous bone volume as assessed by quantitative iliac crest histomorphometry did not differ with respect to hip fracture type (femoral neck versus intertrochanteric). See Table I below. From

TABLE I

	Bone Volume Total Bone Volume	Cortical Bone Volume	Cancellous Bone Volume
Fracture Pts. (total)	28.7+/-10.1	18.1+/-9.1	10.6+/4.3
Femoral Neck Fracture Patients	27.8+/- 9.9	17.2+/-9.0	10.6+/-4.7
Intertrochanteric Fracture Patients	29.6+/-10.8	18.9+/-9.7	10.7+/-4.2
All Matched Control	30.6+/-10.5	17.0+/-8.1	13.6+/-7.6

the patients studied, those older than 60 were sufficiently osteopenic with femoral bone densities below the hip fracture threshold. The mechanism of injury, rather than selective loss of either cortical or trabecular bone or metabolic dynamics of the bone disease, determines whether the patient sustains a subcapital fracture or a intertrochanteric fracture.

Femoral Neck Fractures

Femoral neck fractures nevertheless present a problem because of a high incidence of nonunion and avascular necrosis that occurs in spite of adequate treatment[7]. Closed reduction and pin or screw fixation using a variety of implants is consistently associated with a 14% incidence of nonunion, and a 15% incidence of symptomatic segmental collapse following avascular necrosis. Although these complications can be minimized by accurate reduction and fixation, patients with severe osteopenia (<15% trabecular bone volume) had a higher incidence of failure secondary to loss of bony fixation at New York Hospital[10].

The treatment options for femoral neck fractures are reduction and internal fixation versus hemiarthroplasty. Although the complications of fracture healing would be eliminated by hemiarthroplasty, it also has its own unique problems. Hemiarthroplasty is unable to provide hip function equal to an intact hip joint and long-term complications include dislocation, loosening and breakage of the implant and late infection. In spite of prior reports, modern techniques have resulted in perioperative morbidity rates nearly comparable to that of closed reduction and pinning[7].

Our current protocol for treatment of displaced femoral neck fractures utilizes closed reduction and internal fixation with Knowles pins or compression screws as the primary form of treatment. In our most recent review of 251 patients at New York Hospital who underwent closed reduction and Knowles pinning for femoral neck fractures between 1979 and 1981, 80% of patients with Garden III or IV fractures in whom good reductions were obtained, had good to excellent results at six months[1]. This study clearly emphasized the importance of good reduction. Primary hemiarthroplasty using a cemented bipolar prosthesis is selected for patients who are physiologically 70 years of age and who are active household or community ambulators. Nonambulatory patients unless due to metastatic disease are always pinned. Other indications for primary hemiarthroplasty include severe osteopenia (<15% trabecular bone volume or DBA <.75 gm/cm^2)[2] and neuromuscular disease precluding partial weight bearing. In a recent review of 120 cemented bipolar hemiarthroplasties performed for displaced femoral neck fractures at New York Hospital, the six month mortality rate was 5%. The survival rate at six months was not improved by treating the acute fracture by closed reduction and pinning followed by delayed hemiarthroplasty if the primary Knowles pinning failed. Complications included 1% early and 2% late dislocation, 2% loosening and 1% revision surgery. These encouraging results have prompted us to utilize primary hemiarthroplasty in patients over 70 with displaced femoral neck fractures.

Intertrochanteric Fractures

Intertrochanteric fractures primarily affect elderly women and men with osteopenic metabolic bone disease. Unlike femoral neck fractures in which nonunion and avascular necrosis are common, intertrochanteric fractures rarely have those complications. Instead, the incidence of malunion and resulting varus, shortening and external rotation deformity is significant and can be disabling [8]. Formerly treatment of intertrochanteric fractures utilized fixed nail/side plate devices such as the Jewett Nail. Because of poor bone quality and quantity, these devices were beset with problems of high rates of loss of fixation and pin penetration into the hip joint and neck cut out [8]. A fixed nail plate device is a load-bearing device. It does not allow impaction of the fracture into a stable position and, hence, requires stable reduction of the fracture fragments to be successful. In the absence of stable reduction, high loads are generated at the interface between the trabecular bone of the femoral head and the nail. This inevitably predisposes to loss of fixation when osteopenia is significant. Consequently, fixed nail plate devices violate our principles of design of internal fixation devices for osteoporotic fracture [7].

The medial displacement osteotomy was developed to rectify this situation by creating bony stability, but the osteotomy, itself, is technically demanding and results in a shortened limb with weakened abductor power and a gluteus lurch [5]. In addition, failure of fixation following medial displacement osteotomy is reported to vary from 10 to 30% [9].

Sliding hip screws represent an improvement over fixed nail plate devices in that they allow controlled impaction of the fracture until a stable fracture complex is achieved. The great advantage of this device is that it has load-sharing properties that reduce the stresses between implant and bone. In spite of significantly improved functional results with such devices, there still occurs a finite incidence of malunion and loss of fixation. Medial displacement osteotomy does not appear to significantly improve results when a sliding nail plate is used.

Intramedullary condylocephalic nails provide the advantages of intramedullary fixation with less intraoperative blood loss and fewer wound infections. They achieve results comparable to sliding nail plates and give rise to a new set of complications. At New York Hospital Ender's nails were used for treatment of stable and unstable intertrochanteric fractures from 1979-1983. Although operative time and surgical blood loss were less, the complication rates related to nail penetration, back out and loss of fixation were to such a degree, the fracture service reverted back to anatomic reduction and internal fixation using the sliding nail plate devices. To this date we continue to use this latter method as our treatment of choice for both stable and unstable intertrochanteric hip fractures.

The essential to success in using sliding nail plate devices is attention to detail and a thorough understanding of the principles of design. To achieve optimal bony purchase, the screw must be placed in the center of the femoral head and must engage subchondral bone. New screw designs with extra large thread intended to improve "the bite" in soft osteopenic bone have been introduced and, when necessary, methyl methacrylate can be used to provide adjunctive fixation [2]. Large greater and lesser trochanteric fragments should be incorporated into the fracture implant composite by utilizing interfragmentary compression screws. Lastly, the amount of impaction by the fracture should be anticipated. Grossly unstable fractures are best treated with short barrels which allow maximal slide. It is not uncommon for the screw to slide completely down a long barrel side plate converting the device into a fixed device with resultant loss of fixation.

Summary

We have discussed the biomechanical and biomaterial properties of bone and emphasized the microenvironment. The microdensity of bone tissues determines the resistance to compressive forces. The structural orientation of bone critically determines its ability to withstand torsion and bending forces. Highly remodeled bone is brittle and fractures easily due to the multiple reversal planes within the bony plates.

Hip fractures have been discussed in terms of their pathophysiology and treatment options. The most important concept in reviewing osteoporotic fractures is prevention, that is, falls must be prevented and bone loss must be prevented starting in young adulthood. The basic principles in the management of osteoporotic fractures are to recognize and address the underlying metabolic bone disease when fracture occurs. Elderly patients are best served by rapid, definitive fracture care directed at early restoration of mobility and function, Remember, the aim of intervention should be to achieve stable fracture fixation that allows early return of function. The primary mode of failure of internal fixation results from osteopenic bone failure rather than implant failure. The hallmark of osteoporosis fracture treatment must be its prevention.

Bibliography

1. Arnold, W.D.: The effect of early weight-bearing on the stability of femoral neck fractures treated with Knowles pins. J. Bone Joint Surgery 66-A: 847-852, 1984.

2. Bartucci, E.J., Gonzalez, M.H., Cooperman, D.R., Freedberg, H.I., Barmada, R., and Laros, G.S.: The effect of adjunctive methylmethacrylate on failures of fixation and function in patients with intertrochanteric fractures and osteoporosis. J. Bone Joint Surgery 67-A: 1094-1107, 1985.

3. Carter, D.R. and Hayes, W.C.: The compressive behavior of bone as a two-phase porous structure. J. Bone Joint Surgery 59-A: 954-962, 1977.

4. Cornell, CN., Schwartz, S., Bansal, M., Lane, J.M., and Bullough, P.B.: Quantification of Osteopenia in hip fracture patients. Bone in press.

5. Dimon, J.H., III, and Hughston, J.C.: Unstable intertrochanteric fractures of the hip. J. Bone Joint Surgery 49-A:440-450, 1967.

6. Holbrook, T.L., Grazier, K.L., Kelsey, J.L., and Stauffer, R.N.: Human and Economic Impact of Injuries and Crippling Disorders of the Musculoskeletal System. American Academy of Orthopaedic Surgeons, Chicago, 1984.

7. Lane, J.M., Cornell, C.N., and Healey, J.H.: Orthopaedic consequences of osteoporosis. In Osteoporosis: Etiology,

Diagnosis, and Management, edited by B.L. Riggs and L.J. Melton III, pp.433-455. Raven Press, New York, 1988.

8. Moller, B.N., Lucht, U., Grymer, F,, and Bartholdy, N.J.: Instability of trochanteric hip fractures following internal fixation. Acta Orthop. Scand 55:517-520, 1984.

9. Rao, J.P., Banzon, M.T., Weiss, A.B., and Rayhack, J.: Treatment of unstable intertrochanteric fractures with anatomic reduction and compression hip screw fixation. Clin. Orthop. 175: 65-71, 1983.

10. Scileppi, K.P., Stulberg,B., Vigorita, V.J., Lane, J.M., Vossburgh, R., Bullough, P.G., and Arnold, W.D.: Bone histomorphometry in femoral neck fractures. Surg Forum 32: 543-545, 1981.

Medical Management of Osteoporosis of the Hip

M.E. KRAENZLIN, E.E. SCHULZ, C.R. LIBANATI, L.A. TUDTUD-HANS,
M.R. MARIANO-MENEZ, and D.J. BAYLINK

Departments of Medicine and Radiology
Loma Linda University
and Jerry L. Pettis VA Hospital
Loma Linda, CA

INTRODUCTION:

Osteoporosis and associated fractures represent a major health problem for the aging population. In particular fractures of the hip are associated with more morbidity, mortality and medical costs than all other osteoporotic fractures combined (1). In the past 2 decades several drugs have been shown to have osteotropic effects on the osteoporotic skeleton including estrogen, anabolic agents, calcium, 1,25-vitamin D, calcitonin, didronel, parathyroid hormone (PTH), and fluoride (2-5). Of these the only agent tested on the hip is estrogen, which has been shown to decrease hip fracture incidence (6). Apart from this one drug there is paucity of information regarding the effect of therapeutic agents on the hip. Moreover if we extrapolate from the effect of estrogen treatment on the spine to the hip we would conclude that estrogen does not increase hip density; rather it only prevents hip bone loss. One reason for the lack of information on the medical treatment of hip osteoporosis has been the lack of instruments to measure hip bone density. In the past few years such technology has become available. We selected fluoride as the therapeutic agent for treatment of osteoporosis of the hip because only fluoride and PTH have been shown to actually increase bone density in the osteoporotic skeleton, in this case the spine (7,8)

METHODS:

Fifty-five ambulatory female patients treated for at least 1 year with fluoride were included in the study. All subjects were referred for treatment of axial osteoporosis as evidenced by one or more atraumatic vertebral compression fractures. The mean age was 69 years with a range from 35 to 92 years. Forty-seven patients had primary osteoporosis, and 8 patients had secondary osteoporosis, 5 due to glucocorticoid therapy and 3 due to malabsorption. The dose of elemental fluoride for individual subjects ranged from 24 to 44 mg/d in divided doses after meals. The mean dose of sodium fluoride for the group was 38 mg/d.

Bone mineral content of the hip was measured by dual-photon absorptiometry (Lunar Radiation, Wisconsin) at three specific regions of the proximal femur: the femoral neck, the Ward's triangle, and the trochanteric region. Measurements were performed on both hips. In view of the good correlation between the left and right site, as well as between the three measurement sites the data from the 3 sites and from the left and right sides were pooled to improve our precision (see results). Bone mineral density of the spine and the femoral condyle was measured by quantitative computer tomography (9).

Statistics: Data are expressed as mean±SEM. Quantitative data were compared by paired Student's two tailed t-test. Correlation studies were done by linear regression analysis.

RESULTS:

Table 1 summarizes the correlations between the measurements of the right and left hip, and the correlation between the individual measurement sites in the hip. By pooling the data obtained from the left and right hip, as well as from the three measurement sites the coefficient of variation decreased from 18-21% to 16%.

Table 1: Correlation of the bone mineral content of the right(R) and the left(L) hip, and the correlations between the measurement sites-femoral neck (Neck), Ward's triangle (Ward) and trochanteric (Troch) region.

	r-value:	p-value:
Neck-R vs Neck-L	0.834	<0.001
Ward-R vs Ward-L	0.849	<0.001
Troch-R vs Troch-L	0.841	<0.001
Neck vs Ward	0.939	<0.001
Neck vs Troch	0.765	<0.001
Ward vs Troch	0.712	<0.001

The bone density of the hip increased by 0.0121±0.005 g/cm^2 (p<0.05) after 12 months and by 0.0261±0.01 g/cm^2 (p<0.025) after 24 months of fluoride treatment (Fig.1). The spinal bone density increased by 23.2±3 mg/cm^3 (p<0.001) and by 29.1±5 g/cm^3 (p<0.001) after 12 and 24 months of fluoride treatment, respectievely (Fig.1). The femoral bone density increased by 13.4±2.6 g/cm3 (p<0.001) and 20.0±3.1 g/cm^3 (p<0.001) after 12 and 24 months respectively (Fig.1).

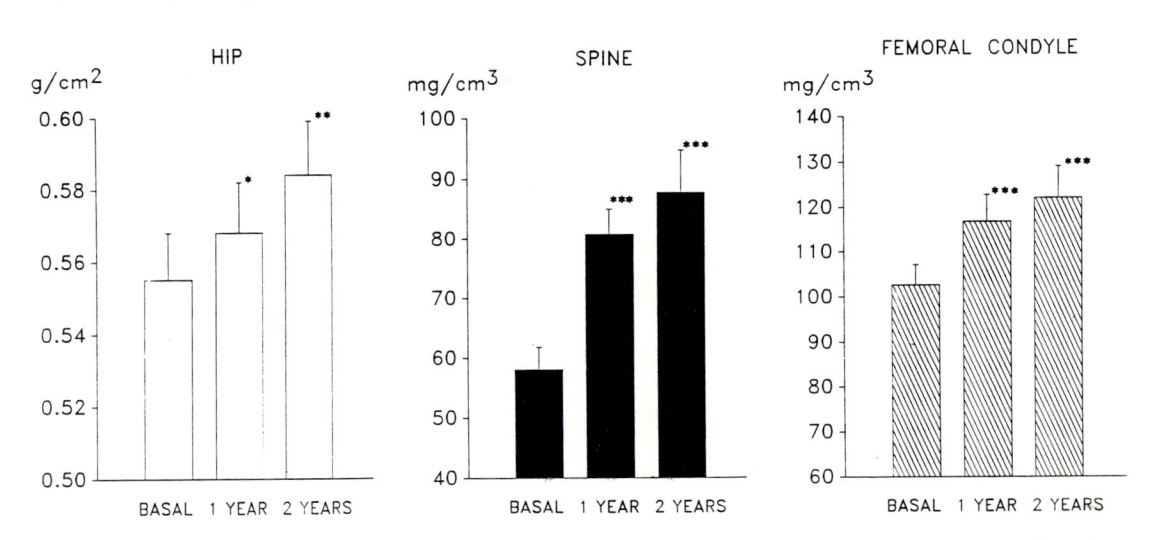

Fig.1 Effect of fluoride treatment on bone density of the hip (open box), spine(solid box) and femoral condyle (shaded box), (mean±SEM), 1 year n = 55, 2 year = 18 .

* p <0.05, ** p<0.025, *** P<0.001

The increase in hip bone density was negatively correlated at 24 months with the pretreatment values, r=-0.682, p<0.001. The increases in hip, spine and femoral condyle were not correlated with one another.

DISCUSSION:

This study demonstrates for the first time that fluoride treatment of osteoporotic patients results not only in an increase in spinal bone density but also in density of the hip. Thus fluoride treatment resulted in a significant increase in hip bone density by 2-3% at 12 months and by 5-6% at 24 months. It also significantly increased spinal bone density, 38 and 50% respectively, and femoral condyle bone density by 13 and 20% respectively. Thus fluoride action was site preferential being more effective at restoring bone in the spine than in the femoral condyle and hip. Because fluoride increases bone density by increasing bone formation, it follows that bone formation during fluoride treatment proceeds at different rates in different skeletal sites. This may be related to local differences in bone surface area between the spine, hip, and femoral condyle, since an increase in bone mass is achieved by deposition of bone on surfaces. Furthermore, the net gain of bone density at the different distant sites did not correlate with one another, e.g. a gain in spinal bone density is not necessarily accompanied by a gain in hip bone density. This is the first demonstration of a dissociation of the effects of fluoride on bone mineral density.

The increase in hip bone density negatively correlated with the pretreatment hip bone density, indicating that the lower the initial (pretreatment) hip bone density, the greater the response to fluoride treatment. This relationship was not seen in the spine or femoral condyle.

In summary, the present investigation demonstrates that in osteoporotic subjects, fluoride treatment not only increases bone density in the spine and femoral condyle, but also in the hip. The response to fluoride treatment occurred in the following decreasing order: spine, femoral condyle, and hip. The increase in hip bone density was negatively correlated with the pretreatment hip bone density. We conclude that fluoride treatment has a positive effect on bone density at the hip and that those patients most at risk for hip fracture show the greatest response to treatment.

REFERENCES:

1. Cummings SR, Kelsey JL, Nevitt MC and O'Dowd KJ: Epidemiology of osteoporosis and osteoporotic fractures. Epidemiol.Review 1985;7:178.

2. Lindsay R, Aitkin JM, Anderson JB, Hart DM, MacDonald EB and Clarke AC: Long-term prevention of postmenopausal osteoporosis by estrogen. Lancet 1976;1:1038.

3. Geusens P, and Dequeker J: Long-term effect of nandrolone decanoate, 1a-hydroxyvitamin D3 or intermittent calcium infusion therapy on bone mineral content, bone remodelling and fracture rate in symptomatic osteoporosis: a double-blind controlled study. Bone and Mineral 1986;1:347.

4. Briancon D, Meunier PJ: Treatment of osteoporosis with fluoride, calcium, and vitamin D. Orthop.Clin.North.Am. 1981;12:629.

5. Riggs BL, Seeman E, Hodgson SF, Taves DR and O'Fallon WM: Effect of fluoride/calcium regimen on vertebral fracture occurrence in postmenopausal osteoporosis. N.Engl.J.Med.1982;306:446.

6. Kiel PK, Felson DT, Anderson JJ, Wilson PWF and Moskowitz MA: Hip fracture and the use of estrogens in postmenopausal women. N.Engl.J.Med. 1987;317:1169.

7. Chesnut CH, Gruber HE, Ivey JL, Matthews M, Sisom K, Nelp WB, Taggart HM, Roos BA and Baylink DJ: Synthetic salmon calcitonin in the treatment of postmenopausal osteoporosis. In: Proceedings, International Workshop on Human Calcitonin. A.Caniggia (ed), Italy, Elli and Pagani Ciba-Geigy), 1983, p119.

8. Farley SM, Schulz EE, Libanati CR and Baylink DJ: A successfull strategy for the use of fluoride therapy in osteoporosis in terms of efficacy and side effects. J.Bone and Min. Res. 1986;1(suppl.1):263.

9. Cann CF, and Genant HK: Precise measurement of vertebral mineral content using computed tomography. J.Comput.Assist. Tomogr. 1980;4:493.

Discussion:

DR. GENANT (San Francisco): Dr. Baylink, I have a question in regard to the differential response that you have presented. You have measured, in the spine, purely trabecular bone with quantitative CT. You've measured purely trabecular bone in the femoral condyle with CT. In both cases, you observed substantial increases in response to sodium fluoride, but a differential of, perhaps, two to three-fold between the spine and the condyle. It is conceivable that this differential could be related to the relative amounts of active marrow, red marrow, in the spine and essentially, yellow marrow in the femoral condyle. On the other hand, the changes that you saw in the proximal femur, where an integral of trabecular and compact bone was measured, probably the majority was cortical bone. Thus it is possible that the differential response that you observed is more related to trabecular versus cortical measurements and red versus yellow marrow or active versus inactive marrow, than it is in relationship to local factors that you have suggested in the second portion of your presentation.

DR. BAYLINK (Loma Linda, CA): I think those are good points. I'd like to comment on them briefly. We're measuring change, and I don't think the marrow changes that much in the 24 months.

As far as the different types of parameters being measured, there is at least 50 percent cortical bone in the neck, whereas, we're measuring 100 percent trabecular bone in the spine. We basically multiplied our values in the hip to try to equate them with what we might have gotten had we measured only trabecular bone in the hip, and still end up with a much lower response.

As far as the condyle comparison is concerned, that's total condyle, not just trabecular condyle. The condyle in the hip doesn't contain 50 percent cortical bone, but only about 20 percent. If you make the calculations, trying to adjust all the values or all the responses to similar amounts of trabecular cortical bone, you still get a higher response in the spine and a mid response in the condyle and the lowest response in the hip.

DR. GENANT: The point I was making about the marrow was not that it would have changed or affected the accuracy or precision of your measure, but that perhaps the relative amount of active marrow may have something to do with the trabecular bone turnover in the spine versus the femoral condyle where the marrow surrounding the trabecular bone is, essentially, inactive fatty marrow.

DR. BAYLINK: I think that's an excellent point. I'm sure that there's a lot of cooperation between red marrow and bone.

DR. CODY (Detroit): Dr. Lane, you stated early in your talk that you felt that cortical bone had a bigger effect on fracture risk of the hip than trabecular bone. Can you follow up on why you feel that way?

DR. LANE (New York): Well, it really depends on which bone you're basically looking at. For instance, if you look at the spine, Toby Hayes sanded off the cortical bone of the spine. And in that he found that only decreased the strength by seven percent. If you look at the metaphysis of the knee, there again, almost all the strength is basically within trabecular bone.

If you follow through the same kind of experiments into the hip, the calcar is very critical for the strength of the femoral neck. Now, this has been tested in vitro, and I'm not sure if the loading is exactly the same as in vivo where there may be more torque. I think there is a much greater role for cortical bone in that particular location, but I can't exclude some importance to trabecular bone.

If you look at the strength of bone, the mass is out at the periphery of the cylinder. If you add a lot of material on the inner part, it provides very little biomechanical strength. It's the distribution of the bone from the periphery that is important in a torque-loaded injury. If it's a tensile or compressive injury, then the trabecular bone is very important.

DR. CODY: Where in the hip would you look for the cortical bone if you were going to measure it, specifically?

DR. LANE: Well, you'd have to look where the fractures occurred, take anatomical specimens and look at those locations and define exactly the alignment of the fractures (it's never exactly vertical), and then do a distribution.

For instance, if you get a femoral head that's been cut off after a fracture, you'd be able to look at it yourself and you can get a chance to do the distribution.

DR. CODY: You had mentioned bone structure. Do you feel that there is a need for more descriptive system for looking at bone structure in the hip, or is the Singh index all we need?

DR. LANE: Toby Hayes has a formula for this in terms of doing distribution of the bone in terms of torque testing, and its distribution can be determined.

The next step will be based on methodology like Dr. Genant's. He will have to work out a CAT scan looking at the structural distribution and put that into the formula.

DR. RIGGS (Rochester, MN): David, I certainly enjoyed seeing your new data and I like your hypothesis. I think, for example, that the two conditions where stress fractures occur relatively commonly are runners and fluoride therapy. I would like to make one caveat. I think that before we project the value of fluoride therapy in terms of changing bone mass, I think it is important to establish that fluoridic bone has the same strength as normal bone, and, as you know, studies are underway to look at that.

DR. BAYLINK: I think that's a good point. But I think there is also a misconception about the extent to which fluoride might modify bone strength. Now, it's been claimed for many years that fluoride caused a woven bone kind of matrix and that's entirely incorrect. It does not cause woven bone matrix. It causes a normal lamellar matrix. It does cause an increase in osteoid. But an increase in osteoid under no conditions that I know of will have any adverse affect on bone strength, everything else being equal.

Now, it certainly may not be as strong as young bone because, if one has large pillars instead of small pillars, which would be the effect of increasing bone density back to normal, with fluoride, one might not have the same strength despite the same density.

So, under those conditions you might not have the same strength. I agree that bone strength studies must be done, but I am not discouraged by claims that fluoride causes abnormal bone. I think we're going to see that the fluoride effect on bone strength is very substantial. This is borne out by at least a half dozen studies in the literature showing that fluoride decreases fracture frequency and, of course, your study is one of those.

DR. CONTE (Boston): Dr. Baylink, I was interested in your characterization of fluoride as a mitogen enhancer. In terms of your bone scans, could some of these positive uptakes be a result of synovitis in those joints, and do you know of any effect on fluoride in terms of synovial cells or IL1 enhancement, and isn't mitogen either in skeletal cells or synovial cells?

DR. BAYLINK: I can't answer your question about IL1. With

respect to why we see the uptake in these sites, on some occasions we've been able to see a new layer of periosteal bone formation, and I believe that the reason for the increased uptake is not a synovitis but actually an increase in bone formation, which is not limited to the periosteum. So, I think we're just seeing increases in the level of bone formation at the sites.

If it's an osteoarthritic site fluoride seems to accentuate that even more. The hot spot that you see on the basal scan will have enhanced activity after a few months of fluoride therapy and that can be associated with pain. Just as rapid growth rates are associated with pain in children, you see pain at these sites with rapid growth rates in these metaphyseal sites of the knee and ankle.

DR. PARFITT (Detroit): I have a brief comment and a question. The comment has to do with the difficulty of deciding exactly what is cortical and what is cancellous bone in the hip. The structure of the calcar femorale has been alluded to several times. This is a solid bar of bone, which is cortical in structure in the sense that it's solid, but it's cancellous in location, in that it runs through the marrow cavity. So, what are you going to call it?

Now, the question has to do with what to do once the patient has had a hip fracture. We've heard a lot about very promising ways of preventing hip fracture. But is there any intervention that can be applied to a patient who's had the first hip fracture that will help to prevent that person getting a second hip fracture?

DR. LANE: The fracture rate is relatively low. And I think the way to solve this would have to be a large cooperative study. Unfortunately, no institution clearly can have enough patients to make that judgment right now.

DR. KLEEREKOPER (Detroit): Dr. Lane, can I just verify that you said you've reduced your post-hip fracture mortality to five percent, and you've done that by just adding calcium?

DR. LANE: No, not by calcium. Using the approach of aggressive hemiarthroplasty. And we have a six-month survival rate of around 95 percent for hip fractures.

DR. KLEEREKOPER: Dr. Baylink, can I interpret from your data that there's more load bearing on the spine than there is on the hip?

DR. BAYLINK: That's a very good point. If you look carefully at the spine's response to fluoride, you'll find that the biggest response is seen in the lumbar area, next in the thoracic area, and least in the cervical area. But I think Dr. Genant has a good point here. I think there are other factors that will determine local levels of growth factor release than just mechanical stress. So, I'm not sure how much this hypothesis applies to the axial skeleton.

DR. RAISZ (Connecticut): I gather, Dr. Lane, that all your hip fracture patients are getting replacement of the hip now?

DR. LANE: If they're physiologically over 70 or if they have significant osteopenia. We're just getting a bone density instrumentation in the fracture service.

DR. RAISZ: You're going to do bone densities on the way to the O.R.?

DR. LANE: Absolutely.

DR. RAISZ: But you're not looking at anything about the bone itself? You're not doing the biopsy?

DR. LANE: Oh, yes. We biopsy all our hip fractures.

DR. RAISZ: You can't do an intraoperative microradiograph?

DR. LANE: No. I think the densitometry is probably the only method available at this time that has any potential.

DR. RAISZ: What proportion are you replacing hips on?

DR. LANE: I would say probably around 60 percent.

DR. SCHNITZLER (Johannesburg): I see Dr. Baylink smiling. I don't think he would want me to go away without putting on record that I don't entirely agree with his interpretation of the increased uptake in the metaphyseal regions. I am not saying that he's not correct. I'm sure you are, that there is increased turnover in these regions. But where you have asymmetrical uptake, particularly in areas with highly increased uptake and pain, it would be nice if one could have a few biopsies. You seem to see more of these lesions than we do.

And we actually had the opportunity of biopsying one such area in the calcaneum which has definitely shown that there are microfractures with callus and a RAP phenomenon in that region. I personally continue to believe that these are stress fractures and that the periosteal reaction is, in fact, a feature of a healing fracture. Radiologically, scintigraphically and chronologically, these lesions behave like stress fractures.

DR. BAYLINK: I think it's difficult, from a standpoint of giving a patient optimum care, to biopsy the fracture sites. So, I dismiss that as a means to pursue this issue. But, as I've mentioned, we've looked at some of these sites very carefully with x-ray and also with CT. And by this means, one can see increased periosteal bone formation not stress fracture. And certainly CT is the best method that I know of to see a stress fracture.

Most of the cases that we've examined do not show stress fractures. Basically, I think we're in conflict here because you think that the hot spots are due to stress fractures and I totally disagree with that concept. I am certain that these hot spots are due to sites of increased bone formation without stress fractures. But I know that there are other people who will agree with you in that position.

I would like just to mention, in defense of my own position, that we see these hot spots in patients who are good responders. We don't see them in patients who are poor responders. It should be the other way around if the hot spots were due to stress fractures.

I have seen stress fractures in patients treated with fluoride. But you must remember that every patient that comes into my clinic and probably the clinic of most of the others in this audience are put on an exercise program as soon as they walk in. And that could induce stress fractures.

DR. SCHNITZLER: I don't deny that these may be due to increased activity because generally these patients do feel better. Whether that is due to fluoride therapy or the calcium and the D we give with it, I'm not sure, but what we have observed is one must not x-ray these patients within two or three weeks of the onset of pain. One doesn't see any change. In some cases, especially those who have had non-steroidal anti-inflammatories for their pain, especially Indocid, it may take months for the healing callus to appear radiologically.

We have also examined, in a number of patients, iliac crest biopsies at the time of the stress fracture and compared these with pre-treatment and biopsies. And the details of that I shall present at the Toronto meeting. But suffice it to say at the moment, that there is a significant increase in bone resorption surfaces at the time of the stress fracture.

DR. DEMPSTER (New York): This is really a follow-up question to Dr. Lane. Please correct me if I picked you up wrongly, but I think you said you didn't see any specific changes in the biopsies of patients with hip fracture. I wondered if you'd looked specifically in the cortical bone given the findings reported by Drs. Johnston and Meunier a few years ago, where they saw a selective reduction in cortical thickness in patients with hip fracture and, conversely, a greater decrease in cancellous bone volume in patients with vertebral fracture?

DR. LANE: We are aware of that study, and we had difficulty seeing that. Now we're going to try and do some cluster analysis. But we are impressed by the relative similarity of all osteoporotic patients.

DR. TEOTIA (India): We have been studying the problem of endemic fluorosis since 1964, and have a series of more than 2,200 patients we have investigated. We have biopsy data from the iliac crest on a large number of these cases. I must say, invariably these biopsies have shown disordered, granular orientation of the bone, with poorly formed lamellar systems. Ruined bone, immature bone, partially malacic bone is a constant feature in these biopsies. These patients show excessive production of the osteoid tissue, which resembles osteomalacia, with poor uptake of tetracycline labels. These patients go into secondary hyperparathyroidism not only seen on histology, but also confirmed by high levels of PTH in plasma. This has been well documented by many workers in this country and also in my country.

Recently, we have shown that, if I were to give three slides to the best histomorphometrist in the country, of a patient of endemic fluorosis or osteomalacia, one cannot differentiate.

Periosteal bone formation is a constant feature of fluorosis and, therefore, I confirm that ruined bone is a constant feature in patients with fluorosis.

DR. BAYLINK: I think what you're implying is that the bone has a disordered structure in fluorosis. And I'd like to emphasize that we shouldn't equate the changes you're finding in endemic fluorosis with those that we see in patients who are treated with much lower levels of fluoride.

Many years ago, Dr. Singh sent me a sample of bone from an endemic fluorotic area, and in that bone I definitely did see disordered collagen structure. On the other hand, I've examined more than 100 biopsies from patients treated with fluoride, and I believe that Dr. Meunier's data are identical to mine. Neither of us have ever seen any woven bone in these patients.

I think what you're trying to do is similar to saying that sunlight is bad. I mean, we need sunlight for vitamin D, but if you take too much of it, you'll have disordered skin. And I think if you take fluoride, you'll increase your bone formation and increase bone strength. But if you take too much of it, it will disorder the bone as well.

DR. KLEEREKOPER: I'd like to buy into the stress factor argument, only to tell you that you see the same hot spots in patients treated with placebo as you do with fluoride. I can't tell you the rates because the trial is still double-blinded. But you have to look at controls as well as everything else when you're doing these studies.

VII
PTH-Related Disorders

Overview: Parathyroid Hormone-Related Disorders

JOHN P. BILEZIKIAN[1] and T.J. MARTIN[2]

[1]College of Physicians and Surgeons
New York, NY
[2]Department of Medicine
Repatriation General Hospital
Heidelberg West, Victoria, Australia

PATHOGENESIS OF PARATHYROID HYPERSECRETION

The pathogenesis of primary hyperparathyroidism is the subject of several different experimental approaches which are summarized in this first part of the overview. Genetic control of the hyperparathyroid secretory state could be due to a single lesion in a single cell giving rise to a monoclonal origin of the hyperparathyroidism. Alternatively, the hyperparathyroid gland could have its genetic roots in a multicellular process in which the tissue responds to a variety of more pervasive external influences such as humoral factors, circulating antibodies, or cell-to-cell spread of a tumorigenic virus. Molecular genetics have helped to begin to test further the hypothesis that the single adenomatous parathyroid gland is a monoclonal neoplasm whereas the form of hyperparathyroidism due to four-gland hyperplasia is a polyclonal disorder. Arnold and Kronenberg have applied the technique of restriction fragment length polymorphism (RFLP) to examine this issue. Eight of 43 adenomas and 5 of 23 hyperplastic glands were found to be heterozygous for the BamHI/HPRT polymorphism and thus available for study by this technique. Six of 8 adenomas showed clear loss of one allele, consistent with monoclonality, while all 5 hyperplastic parathyroids showed relative nonpreferential HpaII cleavage consistent with polyclonality. Certain technical limitations of this approach require that these results be confirmed by other molecular tests as well as by more classical genetic approaches. The data however do indicate that a majority of parathyroid adenomas are monoclonal neoplasms and suggest a fundamental difference in their pathogenesis as compared to the multiglandular form of primary hyperparathyroidism.

The parathyroid cell is an unusual secretory cell in terms of its relationship to calcium. Whereas most secretory cells are stimulated by cellular calcium (classical stimulus-secretion coupling), the parathyroid cell is inhibited by cellular calcium. In normal parathyroid tissue, the relationship between parathyroid hormone secretion and extracellular calcium is steep with the major element of control by calcium being exerted over the physiological range of calcium (1-1.25 mM). In primary hyperparathyroidism, sensitivity to control by calcium is reduced both by virtue of the increased number of parathyroid cells and by an increase in the "set-point" for calcium-regulated parathyroid hormone release. The work presented by Brown, Chen and Leboff has begun to provide a conceptual framework within which altered regulation by calcium in primary hyperparathyroidism can be understood. The studies have emphasized the physiological regulation of normal parathyroid cells. As previously shown by Fitzpatrick and Aurbach, pertussis toxin blocks the inhibitory effects of high extracellular calcium on parathyroid hormone release, suggesting a role for a guanine nucleotide binding protein in transducing the signal generated by calcium. However, the rise in inositol phosphates and cellular calcium induced by extracellular calcium is not inhibited by pertussis toxin suggesting that at this step at least the putative G protein is not a pertussis toxin substrate. A number of other potentially important physiologically relevant agonists besides calcium have been shown to regulate parathyroid hormone secretion. Biogenic amines such as dopamine, stimulators of protein kinase C such as phorbol esters, and guanine nucleotides are all potential secretagogues that may not be mediated by changes in cellular calcium or cyclic AMP. In hyperparathyroidism the abnormal regulation by calcium of parathyroid hormone can be best described by pathophysiological changes in the maximal secretory rate at low calcium concentrations, the set-point itself, the slope of the curve at its midpoint, and the minimal secretory rate at high calcium concentration.

Insight into the pathophysiological disturbance of the primary hyperparathyroidism associated with Multiple Endocrine Neoplasia, Type I (FMENI) has been made by Brandi, Zimering, Marx, DeGrange, Goldsmith, Sakaguchi and Aurbach. They hypothesized that a substance stimulating parathyroid cell proliferation is involved in the pathophysiology of the disorder. Plasma from FMENI was shown to be selectively mitogenic for parathyroid cells. Plasma from other hyperparathyroid syndromes was considerably less mitogenic. Characterization of the factor shows it to have an apparent molecular weight of 50 kilodaltons and to share certain properties of the fibroblast growth factor-related proteins. Evidence has recently been obtained to suggest that the target cell of this growth factor appears to be the endothelial cell of the parathyroid vasculature. The parathyroid epithelial cell and other endothelial cells do not show reactivity to the parathyroid growth factor. How this factor is released into the circulation, its exact relationship to FGF-like proteins and/or ongogene products related to the FGF family as well as its source are all questions for further intense investigation.

PSEUDOHYPOPARATHYROIDISM

This classic genetic disorder of calcium metabolism has distinctive characteristics: short stature, round facies, short neck, foreshortened metacarpal and metatarsal bones, a tendency to mental retardation and calcifications in the basal ganglia (Albright's Hereditary Osteodystrophy or Pseudohypoparathyroidism, Type Ia). In contrast to true hypoparathyroidism, the hypocalcemia is accompanied by elevated immunoreactive parathyroid hormone levels; hence the designation, pseudohypoparathyroidism. The salient biochemical feature of pseudohypoparathyroidism, Ia, resistance to the actions of parathyroid hormone, is seen by the lack of a phosphaturic and cyclic AMP response to parathyroid hormone. Pseudohypoparathyroidism, Type Ib, is identical to Type Ia except for the fact that Albright's Hereditary Osteodystrophy is not present and other hormone resistant states, typical of the Ia phenotype, are not seen. Patients do have the biochemical abnormalities. After Albright described pseudohypoparathyroidism, he observed a patient with the typical body habitus of pseudohypoparathyroidism but without evidence for hypocalcemia or target organ resistance. In his attempt to distinguish this variant from classical pseudohypoparathyroidism, Albright dubbed it pseudopseudohypoparathyroidism. Pseudo- and pseudopseudohypoparathyroidism clearly belong to the same genetic family as evidenced by family trees that contain both forms of the disorder, by selected patients whose biochemical profile has been known to crossover to the other, and by the molecular basis of the disorder.

Important clues to the defect in pseudohypoparathyroidism were gained by observations of Levine and his collaborators as well as by several other groups. The constellation of hormone resistant states included in the syndrome involves the adenylate cyclase messenger system. A site common to all hormones that utilize adenylate cyclase is the guanine nucleotide binding protein, Gs, that links their different receptors to the catalytic unit of adenylate cyclase. Patients with Albright's Hereditary Osteodystrophy (Pseudohypoparathyroidism, Type Ia) demonstrate a 50% reduction in the alpha subunit of Gs. There does not appear to be any gross gene deletions or rearrangements of the gene encoding Gsalpha. Levels of the alpha subunit of the inhibitory guanine nucleotide binding protein, Gi, are normal. Despite the enthusiasm generated by this observation, reduced Gsalpha levels do not entirely account for the syndrome. Patients with pseudopseudohypoparathyroidism in which the typical physiognomy is not accompanied by hormone resistance, nevertheless, do have reduced Gsalpha levels. Only patients with the classical disorder, but not all, have the reduction in Gsalpha. Patients with type Ib and parathyroid resistance in the absence of any other hormone resistance, have normal levels of Gs, implicating that this isolated hormone resistant state might be due to a defect in the parathyroid hormone receptor *per se*. Even within the group of patients who show reductions in Gsalpha, there is heterogeneity. Most, but not all, patients manifesting a reduction in Gsalpha activity show a decrease in messenger RNA by Northern blot analysis.

In view of the fact that the G protein abnormality does not appear to account entirely for the syndrome, Goltzman, Mitchell and Hendy as well as others have examined the possibility that characteristics of parathyroid hormone *per se* might contribute to the manifestations of functional hypoparathyroidism in pseudohypoparathyroidism. Characteristics of circulating PTH were examined in three patients with the classical syndrome. In the plasma of these patients were elevations in immunoreactive PTH but reductions in biologically active PTH as determined by cytochemical bioassay. In addition, the plasma of these patients appeared to contain an inhibitor of exogenous, biologically active

PTH by two _in vitro_ bioassays. The biochemical profile of immunoreactive PTH in patient plasma showed differences from normal plasma in that the bulk of the circulating immunoreactivity in pseudohypoparathyroidism consisted of more hydrophobic moieties. These results are consistent with the presence of an alteration in parathyroid hormone metabolism within the parathyroid gland in pseudohypoparathyroidism. The defect in Gsalpha might accommodate such an hypothesis because the parathyroid cell presumably also is impaired in this regard. Goltzman et al, have pursued this possibility further by investigating an experimental model of parathyroid hormone resistance in the vitamin D deficient rat. Elevated levels of parathyroid hormone in this syndrome are associated with post PTH receptor reductions in Gsalpha that extend to other hormones that utilize the adenylate cyclase system. When these observations are viewed together, they suggest that reduced levels of Gs are not necessarily causally related to hormone resistance in pseudohypoparathyroidism and also that the underlying mechanisms for the various forms of pseudohypoparathyroidism are likely to be heterogeneous.

PRIMARY HYPERPARATHYROIDISM

Primary hyperparathyroidism has become a relatively common endocrine disorder due to the widespread use of multichannel autoanalyzers in medicine. The increased incidence has been accompanied by a marked reduction in the presence of obvious signs and symptoms related to the hyperparathyroid state. These observations have led to a change in the therapeutic approach to primary hyperparathyroidism. Patients are not always subjected to parathyroidectomy because many are asymptomatic and do not appear to be suffering adverse consequences of the disease. In an effort to gain greater insight into the modern-day presentation of primary hyperparathyroidism, Ljunghall and his associates have reviewed an experience of 570 patients who underwent parathyroid exploration between 1965 and 1984. The average postoperative follow-up period was 7 years. The average age was 59 with women predominating over men by 3:1. Adenomas were found in 80%. The overwhelming majority of patients with adenomatous disease became normocalcemic (93%). Recurrences, however, tended to increase with time for both adenomatous and hyperplastic disease. Postoperative results focused on the relatively non-specific aspects of primary hyperparathyroidism because classical bone and stone disease have become relatively infrequent. A fair number of patients, however, did report postoperative improvement in complaints such as easy fatigability, memory, concentrating ability, depression, and several neuro-psychiatric complaints. Ljunghall et al, have also assessed other disorders believed to be associated with primary hyperparathyroidism such as hypertension and diabetes mellitus. They found little evidence for a pathophysiological association between either disease and primary hyperparathyroidism in that successful parathyroid surgery does not appear to alter the hypertension or the diabetes. They have also addressed the epidemiological evidence for increased mortality from cardiovascular and malignant disease in primary hyperparathyroidism.

Bilezikian and his associates are examining the asymptomatic patient with primary hyperparathyroidism in a prospective long-term study. They are addressing two key questions: in mild, asymptomatic primary hyperparathyroidism, can other evidence for parathyroid bone disease be discovered upon more detailed evaluation? which asymptomatic patients are at risk for developing complications of primary hyperparathyroidism? Among the 67 patients evaluated so far, the average age is 55 with women predominating over men by 2.5:1. The biochemical indices are typical with mild hypercalcemia (11.1 ± 0.1 mg/dl) and elevations in parathyroid hormone by radioimmunoassay. 'Mid-molecule' radioimmunoassay and 'intact' immunoradiometric assays show frankly elevated values in well over 90% of patients. No patient has radiologically overt parathyroid bone disease; 19% of patients had nephrolithiasis. Only one patient showed classical neuromuscular disease of primary hyperparathyroidism.

By bone densitometry, patients showed reductions in bone mineral density that was preferential to cortical bone. The distal radius, consisting of predominantly cortical bone, showed a reduction in bone mineral density to less than 80% of expected in 58% of the patients. In contrast, trabecular bone appeared to be relatively preserved. Only 13% of patients showed a reduction in trabecular bone mineral density to less than 80% of expected. These results were confirmed by results of the percutaneous bone biopsy in which the vast majority of patients (84%) had mean cortical width determinations below expected whereas an equivalently large number of patients (85%) showed trabecular bone volume greater than average. These early results indicate that the routine assignment of patient with primary hyperparathyroidism to an asymptomatic cohort, if they don't show clinically apparent complications, should be tempered by the likely possibility of skeletal involvement after more detailed testing. The results raise questions about the definition of asymptomatic primary hyperparathyroidism and call for additional long-term studies in order to define better the risk factors for complications of this disease.

Approaches to the Clonality of Human Tumors and Their Application to Parathyroid Adenomas

ANDREW ARNOLD and HENRY M. KRONENBERG

*Endocrine Unit, Massachusetts General Hospital
and Harvard Medical School
Boston, MA*

The finding that most cancers are monoclonal, i.e. derived from a single cell, constituted crucial early evidence in favor of the somatic mutation theories of carcinogenesis. Monoclonality in a tumor implies that the complete series of cellular events needed for neoplastic transformation and tumor progression to a clinically evident state occurs only rarely. Genetic lesions appear to be the most important of these cellular "hits", and in various tumor types studied to date have been demonstrated to include interchromosomal translocations, chromosome deletions, point mutations, insertion of viral DNA, and other DNA rearrangements. Even patients with certain familial tumor syndromes (eg. retinoblastoma/osteosarcoma), who inherit one key predisposing mutation (and which is thus present in all their somatic cells), generally develop monoclonal tumors, attesting to the rarity at the cellular level of the additional changes required for tumor emergence. Monoclonality, however, need not imply malignancy. Benign tumors can be monoclonal, and genetic changes conferring properties of tissue invasion and metastasis are not necessarily central to an initial transformation event but may represent steps in clonal progression or evolution. Benign monoclonal gammopathy, for example, is a clonal expansion that remains subject to normal regulatory controls over many years in most patients.

Polyclonality in a tumor, however, implies a different type of pathogenesis. Hyperplastic responses of normal tissues to humoral factors or circulating antibodies, as in the thyroid enlargement of Graves' disease, are polyclonal expansions. The multicellular origin suggested by a tumor's polyclonality could also be consistent with local cell-to-cell spread of a tumorigenic virus or other such field effects.

Prior to the 1980's, only three experimental approaches were available for the assessment of clonality in human tumors. Cytogenetic analysis provided evidence of clonal chromosomal abnormalities, for example, the reciprocal translocation between chromosomes 9 and 22 (Philadelphia chromosome) in chronic myelogenous leukemia. The requirement for actively dividing cells and a number of other technical considerations have in large part limited application of this method to hematopoietic tumors, although recent advances in solid tumor cytogenetics have greatly heightened its potential utility. Lymphomas containing B-cells that expressed surface immunoglobulin could be assessed for clonality by staining for surface kappa and lambda light chain protein; since allelic exclusion limits an individual B-cell to expression of kappa or lambda, but not both, the finding of a single light chain type on all cells of a lymphoid proliferation served as evidence for its monoclonality, while both types were expected in a polyclonal proliferation. Another way to take advantage of naturally occurring cellular mosaicism in humans for the study of clonality was widely applied by Fialkow and colleagues, to lymphoid and nonlymphoid tumors (1). Tumors from women heterozygous for electrophoretically distinguishable isoforms of the X-chromosome encoded enzyme glucose-6-phosphate dehydrogenase (G6PD) were analyzed. Because random inactivation of either the maternally-derived or paternally-derived X-chromosome occurs early in female embryogenesis, and because the particular "choice" of an inactive X in a cell is transmitted to its progeny, a polyclonal tumor in such a heterozygous patient is expected to contain both of her G6PD isoforms, while only a single enzyme phenotype is expected in a monoclonal tumor. G6PD analysis proved extremely valuable, and provided the first indication of the monoclonality of many human tumors. A few tumor types, however, appeared to be polyclonal with the G6PD method; they included hereditary neurofibromas, multiple trichoepitheliomas, intestinal polyps in Gardner's syndrome, certain colon and cervical carcinomas, and parathyroid adenomas (to be discussed below).

The development of recombinant DNA technology in the 1970's paved the way for several novel approaches to the study of clonality in the 1980's. The availability of cloned DNA probes, restriction endonucleases, and the Southern blotting procedure enabled investigators to exploit the physiologic rearrangements of the immunoglobulin genes in B-lymphocytes; the detection of unique non-germline immunoglobulin restriction fragments in a tumor provided a sensitive marker of its clonality and B-lymphoid nature (2). More recently, the cloning of the genes encoding the antigen-specific T-cell receptor permitted an analogous approach to the clonality of T-cell proliferations. Under usual conditions, the identical nongermline immunoglobulin or T-cell receptor restriction fragment need be contained in only 1-5% of the tumor cells in order to be detected by Southern blotting, so even minority clonal populations are detectable in this fashion.

In another molecular study, leukemias in patients with HTLV-I infection were shown to be monoclonal by the demonstration that the HTLV-I integration site in the host genome was identical in all leukemic cells from a given patient, while the integration sites varied from patient to patient. Other abnormal, tumor-specific restriction fragments, whose detection reflects the presence of a clonal population of cells in which all members possess the identical DNA sequence alteration, have been described, emphasizing the powerful nature of molecular genetic approaches in determining the clonal status of neoplastic proliferations (3).

The use of restriction fragment length polymorphisms (RFLPs) has provided independent, equally powerful molecular alternatives for clonal assessment. RFLPs permit one to distinguish the two alleles of a given gene in somatic cells by virtue of neutral variation in their DNA sequences or the sequences of nearby flanking DNA. In a number of cancers recently studied, it was found that a patient could be constitutionally heterozygous for a certain RFLP, but homozygous (or hemizygous) at that locus in his tumor DNA (4). This tumor-specific loss of heterozygosity, seen as loss of a band on a Southern blot, constitutes evidence of clonality because all such tumor cells likely contain the identical chromosomal loss or nucleotide change necessary for the elimination of at least one normally present restriction enzyme site. Another method based on the use of RFLPs, but, like the G6PD method, dependent on X-chromosome inactivation patterns, has been applied to the problem of parathyroid tumor clonality and is described below.

Jackson, Fialkow, and colleagues first recognized the importance of assessing the clonality of parathyroid adenomas as a clue to their underlying mechanism of tumorigenesis (5,6). This issue is crucial in the context of the longstanding controversy regarding the origins of parathyroid adenomas versus primary parathyroid hyperplasia. In a majority of cases of primary hyperparathyroidism, only one hypercellular gland is found, and its removal cures the patient. The usual clinicopathologic characteristics of such "adenomas" implies that they are the result of abnormalities intrinsic to the single tumorous gland only. In primary hyperplasia, the underlying abnormality apparently affects all 4 glands, and more than one gland may be removed to cure the patient; this pattern suggests that all parathyroid tissue may be responding together to an extrinsic stimulus. The difference between adenoma and hyperplasia, however, is not always clear-cut. Glandular enlargement in primary hyperplasia can be asymmetric, and the existence of "double adenomas" is thought by some to be not uncommon, while others believe them to exist extremely rarely if at all. Importantly, histopathologic examination is unable to distinguish adenoma from hyperplasia. The existence of these ambiguities led to the emergence of the hypothesis that parathyroid adenomatous and hyperplastic disease were really variants of the same fundamental disorder. Study of the clonality of apparently single parathyroid adenomas with the G6PD method in fact supported this view, since adenomas from a total of 10 heterozygous women displayed a double enzyme phenotype; this polyclonality would be expected in generalized hyperplasia, and suggested that adenomas and hyperplastic glands shared a pathogenesis consistent with multicellular origin (5,6).

Because of certain limitations inherent in the G6PD methodology (discussed below), we decided to re-examine the issue of clonality in parathyroid adenomas with newly available molecular genetic methods. One method, like G6PD, relies on the Lyon hypothesis of X-chromosome inactivation, but directly examines X-chromosome DNA instead of a polymorphic gene product (7). To apply this technique, the two X-chromosomes of a woman must be distinguishable by a restriction fragment length polymorphism, and "epigenetic" differences, in this case cytosine methylation patterns, serve to distinguish alleles on the active versus inactive X-chromosome. Vogelstein initially determined that the hypoxanthine phosphoribosyltransferase (HPRT) gene would be useful for such clonal analysis; subsequently the phosphoglycerate kinase (PGK) gene was found to complement HPRT analysis for this purpose. Intron I of the HPRT gene contains the stretch of DNA from BamHI sites B1 to B2 shown below:

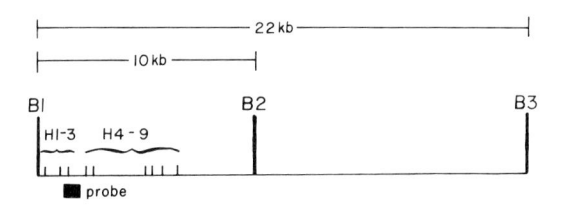

Figure 1

B2 is polymorphic, however, and is present on about 16% of X-chromosomes; B1 and B3 are always present, so roughly 1 of 4 women is expected to be heterozygous with respect to this BamHI polymorphism. Such heterozygosity is detectable by digestion of a woman's normal (or tumor) DNA with endonuclease BamHI, separation of resulting fragments by agarose gel electrophoresis, Southern transfer to nitrocellulose or nylon, and hybridization with a radioactively labelled cloned HPRT DNA fragment ("probe" in Figure 1). The probe will bind to a 10 kilobase (kb) BamHI fragment within the patient's genomic DNA when B2 is present, and to a 22 kb fragment when B2 is absent. Both bands are visible on a Southern blot of DNA from a heterozygous woman, and distinctively mark her two X-chromosomes.

Next, the differing methylation patterns of inactive versus active X-chromosome DNA in this region is exploited with the use of another restriction endonuclease, HpaII. HpaII cleaves DNA at the sequence CCGG, but only if the internal cytosine is not methylated. HpaII sites in the relevant part of the HPRT gene are marked by small vertical lines in Figure 1; at least one of HpaII sites H4-9 is unmethylated on virtually all inactive X-chromosomes, while all of these 6 sites are methylated in a substantial fraction of active X-chromosomes.

Therefore, cleavage of BamHI-digested DNA with HpaII can reflect whether one X-chromosome in tumor DNA uniformly contains inactive (or active) HPRT DNA. A polyclonal proliferation is expected to demonstrate relatively nonpreferential cleavage of the two BamHI bands by HpaII in a heterozygous woman, since about 50% of each X-chromosome complement contains inactive (cleavable) HPRT DNA; this is seen on a Southern blot as a decreased intensity of close to 50% for both the 22 kb and 10 kb BamHI bands after HpaII digestion (Figure 2). In contrast, a monoclonal tumor is characterized by the activity (or inactivity) of <u>all</u> the tumor's X-chromosomes marked by a particular BamHI polymorphism (either the 22 or 10 kb allele). Therefore, when both BamHI and HpaII are used to cleave monoclonal tumor DNA, the band representing the inactive X will be obliterated from the Southern blot, since all the individual HPRT genes contributing to its intensity will have been cleaved by HpaII; occasionally the smaller HpaII digestion products will be visible on such blots. Figure 2 summarizes the Southern blot patterns that can distinguish monoclonal from polyclonal tumors with this method.

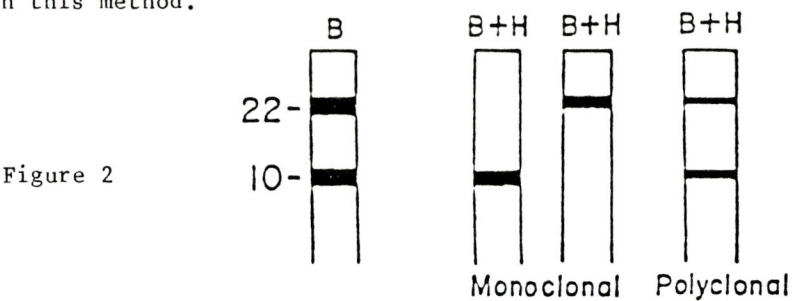

Figure 2

We began by screening 43 parathyroid adenoma DNA samples from women; 8 of these were found to be heterozygous for the BamHI/HPRT polymorphism and therefore applicable for study of clonality with the X-inactivation method. Similarly, 5 of 23 hyperplastic glands were heterozygous. The BamHI plus HpaII patterns for 6 of the 8 adenomas showed a clear preferential loss of one allele, consistent with monoclonality, while 2 adenomas plus all 5 parathyroid hyperplasia controls exhibited relatively nonpreferential HpaII cleavage consistent with polyclonality (8). A quantitative plot of the data is shown in Figure 3. "X-inactivation ratios" were calculated from densitometrically determined band intensities on the above Southern blots. The ratio was defined (to be >1) as the HpaII-induced loss of intensity for one BamHI band divided by the HpaII-induced loss for the other, and therefore indicated the degree to which HpaII cleavage of a particular allele was preferential.

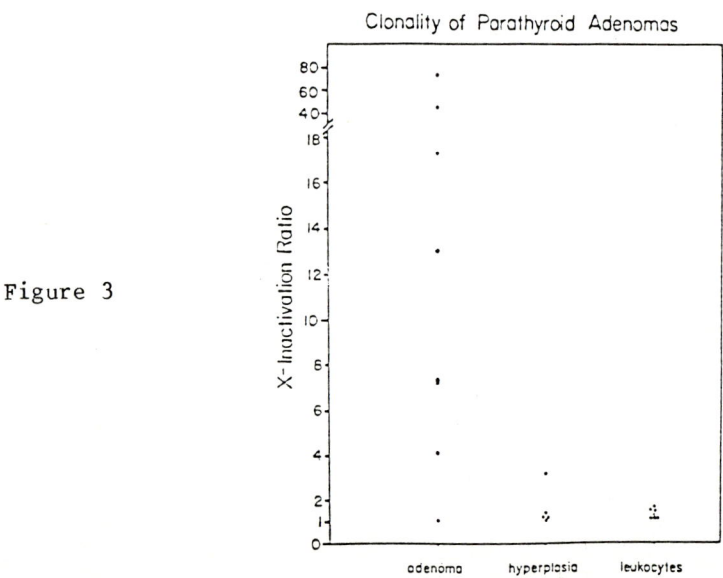

Figure 3

In interpreting this data, it must be recognized that polyclonality is a less definitive finding with this technique than is monoclonality. Admixture of normal stromal components or other "contaminants" has the potential to obscure the detection of a truly monoclonal population; it is also possible that aberrant DNA methylation of a monoclonal tumor's inactive X-chromosome could give the false appearance of polyclonality. Therefore, while it is certainly possible that the two "polyclonal" adenomas were indeed polyclonal, the possibility that they were monoclonal remains prominent. The RFLP X-inactivation method is much more reliable when it indicates monoclonality, although confounding circumstances can be envisioned. For example, 50% of biclonal tumors would appear monoclonal with this method. Also, if the "patch size" of normal parathyroid glands were large, i.e. if a large portion of a gland was derived from a single embryonic progenitor whose offspring (after X-inactivation) remained physically near one another, a polyclonal tumor could falsely appear to be monoclonal with any method based on X-inactivation. This possibility is unlikely, however, given our parathyroid hyperplasia control data; in none of these samples was a monoclonal pattern observed, suggesting that the "patch size" of parathyroid tissue is quite small relative to the amount of tissue we used for extraction of DNA.

While the RFLP-based X-inactivation method shares certain limitations with the G6PD method, it has several potentially important advantages. First, it is much more widely applicable; given the recent availability of the PGK polymorphism for this purpose, approximately 50% of women will be able to be studied fruitfully. Second, the method is not dependent on gene expression, protein synthesis, etc., which may function aberrantly in tumor tissue. It is possible, for example, that neoplastic parathyroid cells synthesize less G6PD than does "contaminating" mesenchymal tissue; such a situation could greatly decrease the sensitivity of the G6PD method for detecting a monoclonal subpopulation. Third, because it assays DNA directly, the RFLP-based method may detect monoclonal cells with amplified efficiency, taking advantage of the hyperdiploidy found in many neoplasms. Some parathyroid adenomas do in fact appear to be hyperdiploid on the basis of nuclear DNA staining, and to the extent this occurs the DNA-based method will preferentially "see" the clonal cells compared with mesenchymal contaminants. It is possible that one or both of the latter two factors explains the difference between the G6PD results and our RFLP-based X-inactivation results, and that most parathyroid adenomas are in fact clonal neoplasms. It is also possible that the tumors studied by G6PD analysis were truly polyclonal, and that differences related to the distinct patient populations examined or other factors result in a fundamental pathogenetic heterogeneity for apparently single parathyroid adenomas. To help resolve this issue, doubly heterozygous parathyroid adenomas could be examined for clonality by both methods. It may be relevant to this discussion that with the RFLP-based approach, Vogelstein and colleagues recently demonstrated the monoclonality of the benign adenomas in familial intestinal polyposis syndromes (9), entities previously found to be polyclonal with the G6PD method. Efforts to explain these discrepancies may well yield interesting data relevant to parathyroid cell and tumor biology.

Because of the potential difficulties inherent in the use of any X-inactivation approach to study clonality, it is desirable that data from an independent method be brought to bear on the question. We have found abnormal, tumor-specific restriction fragments, detectable with PTH gene probes, in DNA from 2 otherwise typical parathyroid adenomas. These abnormalities were clonal (a major population of cells from a tumor contained the precisely identical DNA alteration) and appeared to affect one of each tumor's two PTH alleles (8). Further investigation revealed that these somatic restriction fragment abnormalities resulted from major chromosomal rearrangements involving the PTH locus. We are currently examining the possible functional relevance of such rearrangements to parathyroid tumorigenesis, but regardless of function they serve to provide independent evidence of the monoclonality of the tumors in which they occur.

One would predict that if most parathyroid adenomas are indeed monoclonal neoplasms, then additional clonal genetic changes will be identified, as has been the case in other tumor models. For example, molecular evidence of a major, specific chromosomal deletion was recently found in two MEN I-related insulinomas (10) and a similar phenomenon has also been seen in some types of nonfamilial tumors. Demonstration of nonrandom chromosomal deletion in parathyroid adenomas would provide additional evidence for their monoclonality, and would of course raise other interesting issues relevant to tumor pathogenesis.

Our data, therefore, indicates that at least some and perhaps many parathyroid adenomas are monoclonal neoplasms, and implies that there is a fundamental difference in their pathogenesis compared with that of multigland hyperplasia. This difference could prove relevant clinically, and should contribute to the conceptual basis for future investigation of the molecular mechanisms underlying these disorders.

REFERENCES

1. Fialkow PJ. Clonal origin of human tumors. Biochim Biophys Acta 1976; 458:283-321.

2. Arnold A, Cossman J, Bakhshi A, Jafee ES, Waldmann TA, Korsmeyer SJ. Immunoglobulin-gene rearrangements as unique clonal markers in human lymphoid neoplasms. N Engl J Med 1983; 309:1593-9.

3. Masuda H, Miller C, Koeffler HP, Battifora H, Cline MJ. Rearrangement of the p53 gene in human osteogenic sarcomas. Proc Natl Acad Sci USA 1987; 84:7716-9.

4. Friend SH, Dryja TP, Weinberg RA. Oncogenes and tumor-suppressing genes. N Engl J Med 1988; 318:618-22.

5. Fialkow PJ, Jackson CE, Block MA, Greenawald KA. Multicellular origin of parathyroid "adenomas." N Engl J Med 1977; 297:696-8.

6. Jackson CE, Cerny JC, Block MA, Fialkow PJ. Probable clonal origin of aldosteronomas versus multicellular origin of parathyroid "adenomas." Surgery 1982; 92:875-9.

7. Vogelstein B, Fearon ER, Hamilton Sr, Feinberg AP. Use of restriction fragment length polymorphisms to determine the clonal origin of human tumors. Science 1985; 227:642-5.

8. Arnold A, Staunton CE, Kim HG, Gaz RD, Kronenberg HM. Monoclonality and abnormal parathyroid hormone genes in parathyroid adenomas. N Engl J Med 1988; 318:658-62.

9. Fearon ER, Hamilton SR, Vogelstein B. Clonal analysis of human colorectal tumors. Science 1987; 238:193-7.

10. Larsson C, Skogseid B, Oberg K, Nakamura Y, Nordenskjold M. Multiple endocrine neoplasia type I gene maps to chromosome 11 and is lost in insulinoma. Nature 1988; 332:85-7.

Physiology and Pathophysiology of Ca^{++}-Regulated PTH Release

EDWARD M. BROWN, CHU J. CHEN, and MERYL S. LEBOFF

*Endocrine-Hypertension Unit and Department of Medicine
Brigham and Women's Hospital and Harvard Medical School
Boston, MA*

The parathyroid cell is unusual for its inverse relationship between parathyroid hormone (PTH) release and the extracellular Ca^{++} concentration (1,2). In contrast to most secretory cells showing more classical stimulus-secretion coupling, increases in both the extracellular and intracellular Ca^{++} concentrations are associated with inhibition of PTH release (3). In normal parathyroid tissue, there is a steep inverse sigmoidal relationship between PTH secretion and the extracellular Ca^{++} concentration, with most of the modulation in hormone secretion occurring over a physiologic range of Ca^{++} concentrations (1-1.25 mM) in vivo (4). In most cases of hyperparathyroidism, on the other hand, there is reduced sensitivity to the effects of extracellular Ca^{++}, which is manifested both by cellular hyperplasia and an increase in the "set-point" for Ca^{++}-regulated PTH release (the Ca^{++} concentration required for half-maximal inhibition of PTH secretion)(4,5). The mechanisms underlying the normal and abnormal control of PTH release by Ca^{++} have remained elusive. Recent evidence, which will be reviewed below, have begun to provide a conceptual framework within which to understand normal and deranged Ca^{++}-regulated PTH secretion.

The relationship between PTH release and Ca^{++} in intact and permeabilized parathyroid cells. Raising the extracellular Ca^{++} concentration promotes an increase in the cytosolic Ca^{++} in quin-2-loaded parathyroid cells from about 200 to 600-700 nM (3). Although there is a very close, inverse relationship between the cytosolic Ca^{++} cocentration and PTH release, these parameters may be dissociated, suggesting that there may not be a causal linkage between increases in cytosolic Ca^{++} concentration and inhibition of PTH release (3,6). Nevertheless, the parathyroid cell secretes at near maximal rates at levels of extracellular and cytosolic Ca^{++} concentrations of 100 nM or less, suggesting an unusual relationship between Ca^{++} and PTH release in this cell type(3).

In contrast to results in the intact cell, PTH release from electrically permeabilized cells, in which Ca^{++} equilibrates rapidly between the outside and inside of the cell, is low at low Ca^{++} and is either not affected by (7) or, in our hands, stimulated by increases in Ca^{++} (8). We have interpreted this latter result to indicate that the underlying, Ca^{++}-stimulated secretory mechanism in the parathyroid cell is not dissimilar from that of other secretory cells. What differentiates the parathyroid cell from other cells, therefore, may not be the underlying secretory mechanism but rather the superimposition of additional control mechanisms which invert the usual relationship between the intra- and extracellular Ca^{++} concentrations, on the one hand, and hormonal secretion, on the other. At least two mechanisms might be required to effect this change: (1) A factor or factors which stimulate PTH release at low Ca^{++} concentrations: (2) mechanisms which inhibit PTH release in association with increases in the extracellular Ca^{++} concentration.

Mediators stimulating PTH release at resting or low cytosolic Ca^{++} concentrations. At least three physiologically relevant intracellular mediators stimulate PTH secretion at levels of Ca^{++} equivalent to or lower than those present in the intact cell at low extracellular Ca^{++} concentrations. First, agents increasing intracellular cAMP, such as dopamine, stimulate PTH release in the absence of any measurable increase in cytosolic Ca^{++} (3). Moreover, dopamine also enhances PTH secretion in the absence of extracellular Ca^{++}, when intracellular Ca^{++} is less than 100 nM (3,9). Since cAMP rises in parathyroid cells at low extracellular Ca^{++}, this cyclic nucleotide is a candidate for contributing to low Ca^{++}-stimulated PTH release. On a quantitative basis, however, it appears unlikely that cAMP alone can account for the stimulatory effects of low extracellular Ca^{++}.

Second, agents stimulating protein kinase C, such as phorbol esters and synthetic diacyglycerols, stimulate PTH release from both intact and permeabilized parathyroid cells (8,10,11). In intact cells, the stimulation of secretion takes place with either no change (11) or a decrease (6) in the cytosolic Ca^{++} concentration, while in permeabilized cells both TPA and dioctanoylglycerol enhance PTH secretion at Ca^{++} concentrations of 10^{-8} M or less (8). Endogenous levels of diacylglycerol have been reported to be higher at low than at high extracellular Ca^{++} and might contribute to the elevated secretory rates for PTH at low Ca^{++} (12). Finally, non-hydrolyzable analogues of GTP, such as GppNHp and GTPγS, are potent secretagogues in permeabilized parathyroid cells (13). It is not known whether the G-protein presumed to mediate this effect is active in parathyroid cells at low extracellular Ca^{++}.

Evidence for receptor-mediated regulation of parathyroid function by Ca^{++}. An increasing body of information supports the concept that high extracellular concentrations of Ca^{++} and other polyvalent cations regulate parathyroid function by a receptor-like mechanism which is coupled to intracellular effector systems by one or more G-proteins (14). This concept was initially suggested by the electrophysiologic studies of Lopez-Barneo and Armstrong, who hypothesized that the depolarization of rat parathyroid cells by various divalent cations was most readily explained by a cell surface receptor which was likely coupled to inhibition of potassium channels (15). Fitzpatrick and Aurbach subsequently found that pertussis toxin blocks the inhibitory effects of high extracellular Ca^{++} on PTH release, suggesting that a G-protein may be interposed between the recognition of changes in extracellular Ca^{++} and the subsequent control of PTH release (16). Additional, recent data extend the analogy between Ca^{++}-regulated PTH release and regulation of other cells by more classical hormone-receptor systems.

In contrast to results in quin-2-loaded cells, in which high extracellular Ca^{++} promotes only a sustained rise in cytosolic Ca^{++}, high Ca^{++} also evokes an initial, transient spike in cytosolic Ca^{++} in fura-2-loaded bovine parathyroid cells (17). This pattern of an "agonist"-evoked spike in cytosolic Ca^{++}, arising from intracellular stores, followed by a sustained increase, resulting from uptake of extracellular Ca^{++}, bears a distinct resemblance to the changes in intracellular Ca^{++} dynamics produced by more classical Ca^{++}-mobilizing hormones, such as TRH. The latter act, at least in part, by promoting hydrolysis of phosphoinositides, with attendant generation of IP_3 and IP_4. For this reason, we measured the effects of various polyvalent cations on inositol phosphate metabolism. High extracellular Ca^{++} and Mg^{++} promote the accumulation of IP_3 (18) and IP_4 (D.Hawkins and E.M.Brown, submitted for publication), with a relative potency similar to their relative effectiveness in inhibiting PTH release. IP_3 may mediate the Ca^{++}-induced spikes in cytosolic Ca^{++}, while IP_4 may contribute to the subsequent enhanced uptake of extracellular Ca^{++}. Finally, we recently found that a variety of divalent cations (i.e.

Ca^{++}, Mg^{++}, Ba^{++}) potently inhibit agonist-stimulated cAMP generation. Moreover, this inhibitory effect is totally blocked by preincubation with pertussis toxin, suggesting that it may be mediated through a receptor-like mechanism, coupled in an inhibitory fashion to adenylate cyclase via G_i (C.Chen and E.M. Brown, submitted for publication). Pertussis toxin does not, however, prevent the Ca^{++}-induced rise in cytosolic Ca^{++} or inositol phosphate accumulation, suggesting that the putative G-protein(s) involved in these changes are not pertussis toxin-sensitive. In addition, it is unlikely that pertussis toxin blocks the effects of divalent cations on agonist-stimulated cAMP accumulation simply as a secondary effect, acting on some other second messenger such as intracellular Ca^{++} and/or components of the phosphoinositide cycle.

Is there cooperativity in the regulation of parathyroid function by Ca^{++}? One of the most striking characteristics of the control of parathyroid function by a variety of divalent cations is the steepness of the dose-response relationships (3,4,18). For example, nearly all of the effects of high Ca^{++} in elevating cytosolic Ca^{++} and inhibiting PTH release takes place over a 4-5 fold range of Ca^{++} concentrations or less. Similarly, Ca^{++}-induced increases in inositol phosphates or lowering of agonist-stimulated cAMP occur over 5-10 fold ranges in extracellular Ca^{++}, and the curves relating divalent cations to membrane voltage in parathyroid cells are also very steep (15). In contrast, the effects of other agents, either stimulatory or inhibitory, which modulate parathyroid function take place over about two orders of magnitude, which is characteristic of non-cooperative, one-on-one interactions of a ligand with its binding site. Examples of agents acting in this latter fashion include stimulatory ligands, such as isoproterenol and dopamine, and inhibitory ones, such as prostaglandin F_{2alpha} (14). It is of interest that although both high Ca^{++} and PGF_{2alpha} (19) lower cAMP to a similar extent and the effects of both are are blocked by pertussis toxin (presumably by inactivation of G_i), the slopes of their respective dose-response curves for effects on cAMP differ markedly. It is possible, therefore, that this difference is the result of positive cooperativity at the level of the putative Ca^{++} receptor. Such cooperativity could be the result of multiple metal binding sites on one or more subunits and would be critical in ensuring that changes in parathyroid function take place over a narrow, physiologically relevant range of extracellular Ca^{++} concentrations in vivo.

The integrated control of parathyroid function. The evidence outlines above suggests that inverse control of PTH release by Ca^{++} may be accomplished by stimulation of PTH release at low extracellular and cytosolic Ca^{++} by one or more mediators such as cAMP, diacylglycerol, and/or GTP, as well as receptor-mediated inhibition of PTH release at high Ca^{++}. The linkage of Ca^{++}-regulated changes in second messengers to control of PTH secretion remains poorly understood. In most cells, agonist-stimulated increases in phosphoinositide turnover are accompanied by increases rather than decreases in secretion. Furthermore, it is unclear why an increase in the accumulation of inositol phosphates at high Ca^{++} is associated with a decrease rather than the expected increase in levels of diacylglycerol. Perhaps regulation of diacylglycerol production and metabolism by mechanisms other than phosphoinositide turnover play a dominant role in dtermining diacylglycerol levels. Moreover, it is possible that secretory control is exerted through pathways other than second messengers per se. For example, in addition to stimulatory effects of GTP on secretion at a site close to the exocytotic mechanism, some systems show inhibition of secretion by GTP analogues in permeabilized cells, which cannot be overcome by agents such diacylglycerol or Ca^{++} (20). Further progress in elucidating secretory control of PTH release would be greatly facilitated by the development of techniques for directly identifying and characterizing the putative parathyroid Ca^{++} receptor.

Derangements in the control of parathyroid function by Ca^{++} in states of parathyroid dysfunction. In states of parathyroid hyperfunction, there is frequently reduced sensitivity to the suppressive effects of high extracellular Ca^{++} on PTH release in vitro (5). Conversely, in hypoparathyroidism, circulating levels of

PTH are inappropriately low for the prevailing ionized calcium concentration in vivo. These derangements in the regulation of PTH secretion by Ca^{++} can be understood in pathophysiologic terms as alterations in the inverse sigmoidal curves relating PTH release to the extracellular Ca^{++} concentration. Such curves can be described by four parameters- (a) maximal secretory rate at low Ca^{++} concentrations, (b) the set-point, (c) the slope of the curve at its midpoint, and (d) the minimal secretory rate at high Ca^{++} (e.g. the nonsuppressible component of PTH release) (4). Hyperparathyroidism is related to changes in these parameters which increase the release of PTH at any given extracellular Ca^{++} concentration, such as an increase in the maximal secretory rate (i.e. an increase in parathyroid cell mass), an increase in set-point, and/or an increase in non-suppressible secretion. Conversely, hypoparathyroidism results from reduced PTH secretion at any given Ca^{++}, due to a decrease in maximal secretion and/or set-point. Although such analyses help to elucidate the pathophysiology of abnormal secretory control in hyper- and hypoparathyroidism, they contribute little to our understanding of the mechanisms of secretory dysfunction in these settings. If Ca^{++}-regulated PTH release is conceptualized as a receptor-mediated process, on the other hand, this provides a theoretical framework within which it is possible to understand potential sites of dysfunction in Ca^{++}-regulated PTH release encountered in states of abnormal parathyroid function.

Altered Ca^{++}-regulated PTH release related to perturbations of the cell surface. If recognition of changes in the extracellular Ca^{++} concentration is carried out by a cell-surface receptor, it should be possible to perturb this process through agents binding to the cell surface at or near the putative receptor. There are several examples of such effects. Monoclonal antibodies, for instance, can either inhibit PTH release (21) or block the inhibitory effects of Ca^{++} on secretion (22). In both cases, the change in secretory function is accompanied by the expected alteration in cytosolic Ca^{++} if the antibody were interacting at or near the Ca^{++}-"receptor"--elevation in cytosolic Ca^{++} in the first case and prevention of the Ca^{++}-induced increase in cytosolic Ca^{++} in the latter. The lectin concanavalin A can also block the effects of Ca^{++} on PTH release and cytosolic Ca^{++}, presumably by binding to the cell surface (23). Antibodies mimicking the effects of high extracellular Ca^{++} on PTH release and cytosolic Ca^{++} could conceivably contribute to the pathogenesis of autoimmune hypoparathyroidism by acting as Ca^{++}-agonists. Alternatively, a Ca^{++} receptor which was overly sensitive to extracellular Ca^{++} (i.e. with too low a set-point) could be the basis for congenital hypoparathyroidism.

In the case of parathyroid hypersecretion, a theoretical cause of primary hyperparathyroidism might be the presence of an antibody blocking the effects of Ca^{++} on the putative Ca^{++} receptor. Such an abnormality would be analogous to Grave's disease except that "autoimmune" hyperparathyroidism would be due to blockade of an inhibitory mechanism rather than activation of a stimulatory one. Abnormalities of the Ca^{++}-sensing mechanism reducing its sensitivity to Ca^{++} might also arise spontaneously, either as a primary abnormality leading to deranged control of secretion and cell growth or as a result of an initial derangement in cell growth control secondarily perturbing secretory regulation. The development of techniques for directly identifying the putative Ca^{++} receptor will be necessary to document such abnormalities.

Abnormal Ca^{++}-regulated PTH release due to changes in the coupling of the Ca^{++}-receptor to intracellular effector systems. The failure of pertussis toxin-intoxicated cells to respond to the inhibitory effects of high Ca^{++} on cAMP accumulation and PTH release (16) may be a model of naturally occurring states in which the Ca^{++} receptor is uncoupled from its intracellular actions. Phorbol esters may produce an analogous effect. We recently found, in preliminary experiments, that TPA reduces the stimulation of the accumulation of inositol phosphates at any given extracellular Ca^{++} concentration. In addition to disorders in which the receptor was uncoupled from its effectors, one could conceive of abnormalities in G-protein function enhancing this coupling (i.e. analogous to the effects of cholera toxin). Direct demonstration of such disorders would require identification of the G-protein presumed to mediate the effects of Ca^{++} on parathyroid function and assessing their activity in reconstituted systems.

"Distal" defects in the regulation of parathyroid function by Ca^{++}. In most pathologic parathyroid cells which we have studied, there are parallel decreases in sensitivity to the effects of extracellular Ca^{++} on PTH release (4,5) and cytosolic Ca^{++} (5). This type of response would be consistent with an abnormality at the level of the Ca^{++}-receptor and/or G-protein (i.e. a "proximal" defect residing at the plasma membrane). In one case, however, we encountered a gland in which severe resistance to the suppressive effects of Ca^{++} on PTH release was associated with relatively normal relationships between the extra- and intracellular Ca^{++} concentrations (5). This latter case could represent an example of a distal "post receptor" defect. The effects of Li^+ on parathyroid function, in turn, might be a model for such a distal defect. Li^+ reduces the sensitivity of bovine parathyroid cells to Ca^{++} in vitro (24), an observation which may be related to the development of hypercalcemia in some patients treated with lithium in vivo (25). We recently found that lithium markedly increases inositol phosphates in bovine parathyroid cells at high extracellular Ca^{++} (18). This effect results from the lithium-induced inhibition of the recycling of inositol into the phosphoinositide cycle through inhibition of the inositol monophosphate phosphatase. This pharmacologic effect of lithium might also raise diacylglycerol levels at any given level of extracellular Ca^{++}. Since TPA and diacylglycerol both stimulate PTH release, such a change in diacylglycerol metabolism might shift the set-point to the right in patients treated with lithium.

Summary. Recent studies provide increasing evidence that extracellular Ca^{++} and other divalent cations regulate parathyroid function through a receptor-like mechanism which is coupled to intracellular effector systems and PTH release via one or more G-proteins. This formulation provides a conceptual framework within which to understand possible defects in Ca^{++}-regulated parathyroid function. Both parathyroid hyper- and hypofunction might result from alterations in the sensitivity of the putative receptor to Ca^{++}, from changes in the coupling of receptor to its effector systems, and/or more distal defects in the generation of or response to these effectors. Further progress in elucidating normal and abnormal Ca^{++}-regulated PTH release will be greatly facilitated by the development of techniques for directly identifying the Ca^{++}-"receptor" as well as the G-proteins and effector systems to which it is coupled.

Acknowledgements. The author gratefully acknowledges the expert secretarial work of E.Brown, M.D. in preparing this manuscript. This work was supported by USPHS grants AM36796 and AM36801.

References.

1. Sherwood, L.M., Potts, J.T. Jr, Care, A.D., Mayer, G.P., and Aurbach, G.D. (1966) Nature 209, 52.
2. Habener, J.F. and Potts, J.T. (1976) Endocrinology 98, 197.
3. Shoback, D.M., Thatcher, J.G., Leombruno, R., and Brown, E.M. (1984) Proc. Natl. Acad. Sci. (USA) 81, 1984.
4. Brown, E.M. (1983) J. Clin. Endocrinol. Metab. 56, 572.
5. LeBoff, M.S., Shoback, D., Brown, E.M., Thatcher, J.G., Leombruno, R., Beaudoin, D., Henry, M., Wilson, R., Pallotta, J., Marynick, S., Stock, J., and Leight, G. (1985) J. Clin. Invest. 75, 49.
6. Nemeth, E.F., Wallace, J., and Scarpa, A. (1986) J. Biol. Chem. 261, 2668.
7. Muff, R., and Fischer, J.A. (1986) Bichem. Biophys. Res. Commun. 139, 1233.
8. Oetting, M., LeBoff, M.S., Levy, S., Swiston, L., Preston, J., Chen, C., and Brown, E.M. (1987) Endocrinology 121, 1571.
9. Brown, E.M., Watson, E.J., Leombruno, R., and Underwood, R. (1983) Metabolism 32, 1038.

10. Morrissey, J. (1984) Clin. Res. 32, 404A.
11. Brown, E.M., Redgrave, J., and Thatcher, J. (1984) FEBS Lett. 175, 72.
12. Morrissey, J. (1985) Clin. Res. 33, 440A.
13. Oetting, M., LeBoff, M., Swiston, L., Preston, J., and Brown, E. (1986) FEBS Lett. 208, 99.
14. Brown, E.M., LeBoff, M.S., Oetting, M., Posillico, J.T., and Chen, C. (1987) Recent Prog. Hormone Res. 43, 337.
15. Lopez-Barneo, J., and Armstrong, C.M. (1983) J. Gen. Physiol. 82, 269.
16. Fitzpatrick, L.A., Brandi, M.L., and Aurbach, G.D. (1986) Endocrinology 119, 2700.
17. Nemeth, E.F., and Scarpa, A., (1986) FEBS Lett. 203, 15.
18. Brown, E., Enyedi, P., LeBoff, M., Rotberg, J., Preston, J., and Chen, C. (1987) FEBS Lett. 218, 113.
19. Fitzpatrick, L.A., and Aurbach, G.D. (1986) Endocrinology 118, 2115.
20. Knight, D.E. and Baker, P.F. (1987) Ann. N.Y. Acad. Sci. 493, 504.
21. Posillico, J.T., Srikanta, S., Eisenbarth, G., Quaranta, V., Kajiji, S., and Brown, E.M. (1987) J. Clin. Endocrinol. Metab. 64, 43.
22. Juhlin, C., Holmdahl, R., Johansson, H., Rastad, J., Akerstrom, G., and Klareskog, T. (1987) Proc. Natl. Acad. Sci. (USA) 84, 2990.
23. Posillico, J.T., Burrowes, M., and Brown, E.M. (1986) Annu. Meet. Am. Soc. Bone Min. Res., 8th, Anaheim, Abstr. No. 311.
24. Brown, E.M. (1981) J. Clin. Endocrinol. Metab. 52, 1046.
25. Shen, F.H., and Sherard, D.J. (1982) Ann. Int. Med. 101, 63.

Multiple Endocrine Neoplasia Type I: Role of a Circulating Growth Factor in Parathyroid Cell Hyperplasia

M.L. BRANDI, M.B. ZIMERING, S.J. MARX, D. DeGRANGE,
P. GOLDSMITH, K. SAKAGUCHI, and G.D. AURBACH

*Metabolic Diseases Branch
National Institute of Diabetes and Digestive and Kidney Diseases
National Institutes of Health
Bethesda, MD*

Multiple endocrine neoplasia type I (MENI) includes hereditary and nonhereditary disorders displaying hyperfunction of at least two of the following endocrine tissues: parathyroid, anterior pituitary or pancreatic islet. The hereditary form, familial multiple endocrine neoplasia type I (FMENI), is an autosomal dominant disorder. Wermer in 1954 described (1) a family with "adenomatosis" of the endocrine glands, proposed that the syndrome was a genetic disorder, and prompted investigation of other such families. Although relatively rare, MENI is of general endocrine interest and a number of families have been studied. Knowledge gained from studies on multiple endocrine neoplasia syndromes would be important not only for patient care but for understanding of genetics of the disorder, embryological development of the endocrine system and mechanisms that control growth of endocrine tissues.

Clinical studies suggest that almost all gene carriers in FMENI can be detected by endocrine screening tests by age 40, whereas penetrance for the trait is pratically zero before age 15 (2). Hyperparathyroidism is generally the first and most common clinically evident lesion in FMENI, and autopsy findings have suggested that with increasing age, all three tissues (parathyroid, pancreatic islets, and anterior pituitary) inevitably show abnormality. Endocrine hyperfunction in FMENI is believed to reflect a multicellular origin in the parathyroid; either hyperplasia or clonal neoplasia may occur in the endocrine pancreas and pituitary.

A number of theories have been offered to account for the multiplicity of endocrine gland involvement in MENI (Table I); none is wholly satisfactory. Discovery of the true etiology must explain why tumors hypersecreting hormones develop in the pancreas and pituitary, whereas parathyroid hyperfunction in this syndrome reflects hyperplasia of all parathyroid glands. One popular theory invokes a genetic disturbance of the neuroectoderm, or more specifically, neural crest cell differentiation. This hypothesis is virtually untenable for MENI, since parathyroid and pancreatic endocrine tissues are not derived from the neuroectoderm. The nesidioblastosis theory wherein pancreatic endocrine tumors derived from duct cells would control parathyroid and pituitary gland

Table I

MENI - Theories

Intrinsic factors
    "Neural crest" hypothesis
    Nesidioblastosis
    Chromosomal defects
    Oncogene activation
    Suppressor gene inactivation
Extrinsic factors
    Humoral - Secretagogue
    Autoimmune
    Growth factors
    Other
Interaction among intrinsic and extrinsic factors
    "Two hit" hypothesis
    Positive feedback among 2 or more paracrine/endocrine mechanisms
    Multistage neoplasia development

involvement is improbable in that many patients with MENI syndrome express pituitary and parathyroid gland involvement, without showing any islet cell hyperfunction clinically. The recent localization of a mutant gene for FMENI to the long arm of chromosome 11 (3) should speed identification of the gene and of the biochemical disturbance. Oncogene activation is another potential mechanism. Oncogenes, implicated in the etiology of a number of tumors, activate proliferation by producing growth factors or their receptors or nuclear regulators. Humoral secretagogues as well as autoimmune mechanisms have been postulated but never proven to be causes of the syndrome. The cause of the syndrome may well involve more than one etiological factor acting in concert. In the "two hit" model of Knudson (4) the gene carrier inherits a genetic abnormality facilitating development of neoplasms; a second postnatal hit (somatic mutation) is necessary to transform the mutant cell to neoplastic. Another type of cooperative interaction might involve positive feedback among 2 or more paracrine/endocrine mechanisms. A valid hypothesis must account for the following observations: 1) the most common endocrinopathy in FMENI is hyperparathyroidism; 2) hyperplasia of all four parathyroid glands is virtually always found; 3) the rate of recurrence of hyperparathyroidism in FMENI after subtotal parathyroidectomy is particularly high. We explored the possibility that a substance stimulating parathyroid cell proliferation is involved in the pathophysiology of the disorder (5).

    Plasma from subjects with FMENI is highly mitogenic for bovine parathyroid cells in long-term culture (PT-b). The cells grow in a serum-free medium and maintain differentiated characteristics for many passages (6). Using this system and (^{3}H) thymidine incorporation as a test, we found that plasma from FMENI was remarkably mitogenic for parathyroid cells. Plasmas from primary hyperparathyroidism (caused by adenoma, cancer, or sporadic hyperplasia), multiple endocrine neoplasia type 2, sporadic primary hypergastrinemia, sporadic primary hyperpituitarism, or uremia were all considerably less mitogenic toward parathyroid cells. FMENI plasma produced no unusually high mitogenic activity toward other cell lines tested including rat pancreatic islet, pituitary, thyroid, or osteosarcoma cells, bovine aortic or pulmonary endothelial cells, human umbilical vein endothelial cells, and bovine or human fibroblasts from parathyroid. Plasma from FMENI showed higher mitogenic activity on parathyroid cells than other purified factors including epidermal growth factor, platelet-derived growth factor, nerve growth factor, acidic fibroblast growth factor, and multiplication-stimulating activity. The FMENI factor does not appear to be an autocrine product of the parathyroid, since we found no concentration gradient betwen peripheral and parathyroid venous blood. If the factor were cleared very slowly from blood, such a gradient might not be detected. The persistence of activity in plasma for up to four years after surgical induction of hypoparathyroidism, however, ruled out the parathyroid as source of the factor. Analyses of petrosal sinus samples or pancreatic venous samples from FMENI patients have not revealed the source of the factor. In gel-filtration studies, parathyroid mitogenic activity from the plasma of patients with FMENI eluted as a single peak with an apparent molecular weight of 50,000 to 55,000. In order to characterize better the parathyroid mitogenic activity, we have begun to develop methods to purify it from plasma of subjects with FMENI. Plasma was obtained from consenting subjects by plasmapheresis. The factor was precipitated from plasma with 50% ammonium sulphate. The concentrated material was submitted to chromatography on DEAE Affigel blue matrix and then to gel filtration on an S-200 column. This scheme produced a fifteen-fold purification, and provided material for further characterization. The active fractions from the S-200 column were pooled and applied to a DEAE column in high performance liquid chromatography. Activity eluted in a region separated from most of the protein. Good recovery of activity, however, was not obtained. The factor was acid labile and inactivated by reducing agents. We concluded that FMENI parathyroid growth factor appeared to be a protein of approximately 50 kilodaltons.

The identification and chemical characterization of molecular entities involved in FMENI have been the subject of intense investigation in the last two years in our laboratory. Progress on purification has been slow because of limited supplies of plasma and the low concentrations of substance in plasma. Recent observations, however, have provided further insight into the problem. Certain properties of the plasma factor are similar to those of the basic FGF-related proteins. Other observations indicated that our culture system contained not only secretory cells but endothelial cells as well. Indeed, bovine parathyroid glands, our source of cells, represent a highly vascularized endocrine organ, and approximately one third of the cell population is estimated to be endothelial in nature. Moreover, bovine parathyroid cells, although maintained in long-term culture for many passages, could not be cloned, suggesting the possibility of interactions among different cell types in the culture facilitating long-term growth. Favorable growth of the bovine parathyroid cells was fostered in a medium containing bovine pituitary and hypothalamic extracts. The latter contain fibroblast growth factors, which are potent mitogens for endothelial cells. Bovine parathyroid cells allowed to remain at confluence without transfer in a medium without growth factors produce networks. These branching strands varied in diameter and appeared randomly distributed throughout the culture dish (Fig. 1). These observations prompted us to clone selectively endothelial cells from bovine parathyroid tissue. This was particularly feasible since bovine endothelial cells seem to grow more readily than those of other animal species. The cells were cultured and cloned from parathyroid tissue using a very rich medium and low serum concentrations.

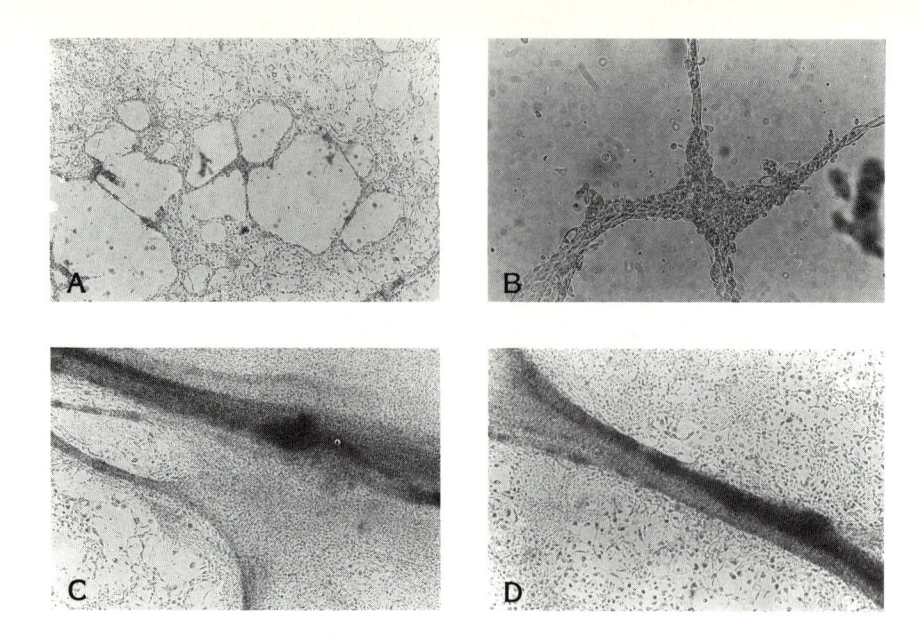

Figure 1: Phase-contrast micorgraphs showing a branching tubular network produced by Pt-b cells allowed to remain at confluence for 2 months (A and B) and 3 months (C and D). The networks array as branching strands that vary in diameter and appear randomly distributed throughout the culture dish. Note debris inside the macroscopic tubular forms (C and D, arrowheads).

The parathyroid endothelial cells grow rapidly on plastic surfaces, exhibit positive reaction for Factor VIII related antigen, and take up acetylated low density lipoproteins, markers of endothelial cell differentiation. These cells also take up parathyroid hormone itself. The ultrastructure of bovine parathyroid endothelial cells is consistent with the classical phenotype of endothelium (Brandi et al., unpublished).

Examination of our long-term culture of bovine parathyroid cells labelled with acetylated low density lipoproteins and analyzed by flow cytometry, showed that endothelial cells exist in primary culture and increase in number with each passage. Using this information we sought to identify the cell type representing the target of the FMENI factor. We examined cloned bovine parathyroid endothelial cells (BPE-1), cloned rat parathyroid epithelial cells (Pt-r) (7), and mixed bovine parathyroid cells in long-term culture (Pt-b) (6). Either BPE-1 or PT-b cells, showed extremely high mitogenic responses to the FMENI factor. PT-r cells did not differ in response to FMENI or normal plasma (Fig. 2). Moreover none of other groups of endothelial cells, bovine aortic, adrenal medullary or pulmunary arterial, or human umbilical vein cells responded to the FMENI factor. The lack of response with rat parathyroid epithelial cells or other bovine endothelial cells suggests that the actions of the FMENI factor are highly selective for parathyroid endothelium.

We now believe that the circulating factor in FMENI is related to basic fibroblast growth factor (bFGF), a substance known to stimulate growth of endothelial cells. Basic FGF also stimulates BPE-1 DNA synthesis but not to the extent of FMENI plasma. Properties apparently shared by bFGF and FMENI factor include: 1) affinity for immobilized heparin; 2) inhibition of the mitogenic effect of FMENI plasma on BPE-1 cells by a polyclonal antiserum against bFGF (1-24) (8). What is the pathophysiological significance of these findings? Angiogenesis, i.e. new blood vessel

MITOGENIC EFFECT OF MENI PLASMA FACTOR ON PARATHYROID CELL TYPES

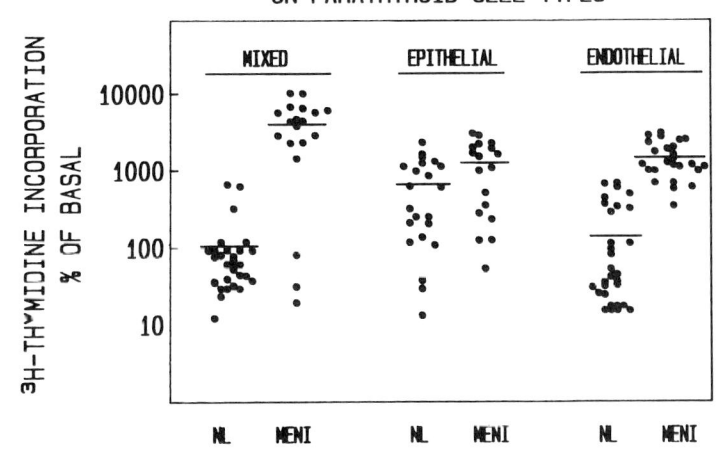

Figure 2: Effect of plasma (1:5 dilution) taken from subjects with FMENI and from normals on mitogenic activity of cultured PT-b, PT-r, and BPE-1 cells. Mitogenic activity is expressed as percent of control (no added plasma) of [^{3}H]-thymidine uptake.

formation, is required for growth of solid tumors. Immediately after fertilization vessels form and conditions favoring growth of endothelium promote also proliferation of surrounding tissues. Studies on the histogenesis of human parathyroid glands indicate that embryologic vascularization of the parathyroid glands is followed by a period of active hyperplasia, marked increase in cell number and a consequent increase in gland size. The relationship between parenchymal and vascular elements and cell polarity may be anatomic features of basic physiological significance. The importance of "angiogenesis" is emphasized by the fact that many of the known growth factors are angiogenic, TGFbeta, TGFalpha, and FGFs. The FGF family especially has been studied as an inducer of angiogenesis. Characteristic of acid and basic FGF is the lack of a secretory signal sequence and association mainly with cells and basement membrane; they are not released except locally in response to cell injury. Prevention of release could be a mechanism for regulation of FGFs activity or could be important for their intracellular function.

The FMENI factor appears in the circulation and hence a mechanism must exist accounting for its release from cells. We might speculate that in FMENI a bFGF-like growth factor with specificity for parathyroid and possibly other endocrine systems is released into the circulation. This possibility is made even more attractive by the recent findings of a new family of growth factors, likely oncogene products, related to the FGF family (Table II). The predicted products, based on cDNA sequences of these

Table II

FGF-Related Oncogenes

Oncogene		Origin
int-2	(9)	Virus-induced mouse mammary tumor
KS	(10)	Kaposi sarcoma
FGF3	(11)	Human bladder cancer

oncogenes, bear high degrees of homology to bFGF. The int-2 predicted product is larger than bFGF, with a short stretch of non-charged residues at the amino terminus, an extra central sequence, and a carboxy-terminal extension. The amino terminal extension might function as signal sequence, and the extra mid-or the extended carboxy-terminus might confer an unusual specificity on int-2, different from that displayed by other members of this family of mitogens. Perhaps the FMENI factor will prove similar to the int-2 product. We note in particular that, according to recent findings, the mutant gene in FMENI is localized to the pericentric region of chromosome 11, a region that is near int-2. Hence studies on int-2 may be of particular relevance to the genetics and pathophysiology of FMENI. Many questions remain to be answered. How could a mutation on chromosome 11 cause abnormal release of the FMENI factor into the circulation? What is the source of the factor? Does the same factor affect endothelial cells from pituitary and pancreatic islets? Is there indeed a relation between the int-2 gene and the disease?

Acknowledgements

We are grateful to Dr. A. Baird for the gift of the antiserum against bFGF (1-24) and to Mrs. Joan Glass for expert secretarial assistance.

References

1. Wermer, P. (1954) Am. J. Med. 16, 363
2. Marx, S.J., Vinik, A.I., Santen, R.J., Floyd, J.C., Mills, J.L., and Green J. III (1986) Medicine 65, 226
3. Larsson, C., Skogseid, B., Oberg, K., Nakamura, Y., and Nordenskjold, M. (1988) Nature 332, 85
4. Knudson, Jr., A.G. (1975) Genetics 79, 305
5. Brandi, M.L., Aurbach, G.D., Fitzpatrick, L.A., Quarto, R., Spiegel, A.M., Bliziotes, M.M., Norton, J.A., Doppman, J.L., and Marx, S.J. (1986) N. Eng. J. Med. 314, 1287
6. Brandi, M:.L., Fitzpatrick, L.A., Coon, H.G., and Aurbach, G.D (1986) Proc. Natl. Acad. Sci. USA 83: 1709
7. Sakaguchi, K., Santora, A., Zimering, M., Curcio, F., Aurbach, G.D., and Brandi, M.L. (1987) Proc. Natl. Acad. Sci. USA 84, 3269
8. Baird, A., Esch, F., Mormede, P., Ueno, N., Ling, N., Bohlen, P., Ying, S-Y., Wehrenberg, W.B., and Guillemin, R. (1986) Rec. Prog. Horm. Res. 42, 143
9. Peters, G., Brookes, S., Smith, R., and Dickson, C. (1983) Cell 33, 364
10. Delli Bovi, P., and Basilico, C. (1987) Proc. Natl. Acad. Sci. USA 84, 5660.
11. Zhan, X., Culpepper, A., Reddy, M., Loveless, J., and Goldfarb, M. (1987) Oncogene 1, 369

Discussion:

DR. OGATA (Tokyo): I'd like to make additional comment to the presentation of Dr. Brown by showing our new data in two slides. Drs. Michiko Yamamato and Tetsei Aloshi of my department measured blood calcium level by infusing a saline solution with or without calcium and with or without calcitonin and EGTA into rats. By that means, we could obtain the intended levels of serum calcium level for 48 hours.

Then we removed parathyroid glands from the rats, extracted RNA and measured PTH messenger RNA by means of primary extension method utilizing P30 to detect C DNA fragments of rat PTH gene.

Could I have the first slide, please?

On the top, this is representative data of a series of experiments. We also measured concurrently the messenger RNA for beta actin and used this as internal reference. The top panel shows the messenger RNA bands. We quantified messenger RNA by densitometric measurements as shown in the middle table. In the lower panel the amount of PTH messenger RNA is demonstrated along with the plasma calcium level.

When we infused medium with that calcium for 48 hours, these rats showed moderate hypercalcemia. If we infused these rats with medium containing 40 millimoles calcium, those rats exhibit moderate hypercalcemia. Now, the PTH messenger RNA. In the rats of mild hypercalcemia, PTH messenger RNA levels goes up dramatically. In sharp contrast, where the rat becomes hypocalcemic, PTH messenger RNA levels are depressed. We repeated this series of experiments under a variety of conditions.

The last slide please.

Here we plotted PTH messenger RNA level as a function of plasma calcium concentration when the parathyroid gland was removed. Here you see the quite beautiful and vast relationship between the PTH messenger RNA level in the PTH cells and plasma calcium levels. And this relationship just reminiscent of the data just shown by Dr. Brown between the rate of secretion of PTH and serum calcium levels.

So, I'd like to make three points. One, I believe this is the first experimental evidence that hypocalcemia of the near physiological range caused a definite increment in the PTH messenger RNA levels in parathyroid cells. Second, this kind of response occurred not before 24 hours, but after 48 hours. Therefore, this response belongs to the rate/onset type of response. Thirdly, I think there are three sets of processes where parathyroid cells respond to external calcium. Number one is an early response, correlated perhaps to secretion of stored parathyroid hormone and also a regulated degradation of the parathyroid molecule, or related molecule. Second, maybe the regulated synthesis of parathyroid hormone depends on the preexisting PTH messenger RNA. Third may be the regulation of messenger RNA itself. So, therefore, we should consider at least three elements of cellular machinery to interpret or elucidate the pathophysiology of parathyroid abnormalities.

DR. BROWN (Boston): Those are very beautiful studies, and I very much enjoyed your presentation. It looked as though the regulation of message follows very much the same curve as the regulation of secretion. I think I missed it, but what was the duration of the different periods of infusion?

DR. OGATA: At least more than 24 hours.

DR. BROWN: So, your time frame would be similar to what people have seen in other types of parathyroid cells, where it does take a matter of hours to several days to see these changes. You do differ, apparently, from the studies in the bovine system in seeing a quite potent increase in PTH or RNA in response to hypocalcemia, which is not seen in the bovine cells.

DR. OGATA: Yes. I believe no one could prove the incremental messenger RNA levels by lowering extracellular calcium. So, I think this is the first observation, I believe.

DR. BROWN: Right. Is there any change in the mass of the parathyroid glands or their mitotic index?

DR. OGATA: No. This is only 48 hours.

DR. BROWN: You also seem to see quite dramatic changes in the actin content. Is there any particular explanation for that?

DR. OGATA: The content of actin did not change.

DR. BROWN: I'm sorry, I may have misinterpreted the slide. It looked as though it went down in the later time points.

DR. OGATA: It depends on the exposure of the autography.

DR. RIGGS (Rochester, MN): I would like to congratulate Dr. Brandi again for continuing her very beautiful studies in this area. If basic FGF is intimately involved in the pathogenesis of the parathyroid hyperplasia one might expect that if you take MEN I serum and test the mitogenic effect on fibroblasts as compared to normal serum, if there would be increased mitotic activity. Have you done that experiment, and if so, what are the results?

DR. BRANDI (Bethesda, MD): Basic FGF, just like acidic FGF, are not released in the circulation. In fact, the basic FGF's lack the secretory signal sequence and you don't find them in the circulation even by radioimmunoassay.

So, if there is a mitotic effect of the plasma on fibroblasts, it is not due to fibroblast growth factors, at least to the known fibroblast growth factors.

DR. GAGEL (Houston): I have a question for Dr. Arnold. In hereditary and, I believe, also sporadic retinoblastoma, a deletion of 13 Q 14 has been shown to be the probably cause of the tumor. It is now known that for MEN I that there is linkage to a point near the centromere of chromosome 11 and MEN II is linked to a point near the centromere of chromosome 10. Because parathyroid disease is a component of each of these syndromes, I wondered whether you have looked for evidence of a deletion in your parathyroid adenomas?

DR. ARNOLD (Boston): Well, we're certainly interested in doing so, and have begun to look at those issues, as I mentioned near the end of my talk.

Whether the MEN I gene, when it's precisely characterized, will turn out to be relevant to parathyroid adenomatous disease in a non-familial setting is uncertain, but the same type of mechanism could be operative. In both familial and sporadic retinoblastoma, the same antioncogene locus on chromosome 13 appears to be involved. I don't know whether one could expect that to be the case in sporadic and familial parathyroid disease, because the presumably non-clonal parathyroid hyperplasia seen in MEN I appears to be a different process from the clonal neoplasia of sporadic adenomas.

DR. BELL (Charleston): I enjoyed your talk very much, Dr. Brandi. It's very exciting work. You indicated that you do not know the source of the factor. An obvious one would be the hyperplastic parathyroid glands. Have you determined whether there is increased activity in the hyperplastic parathyroid glands?

DR. BRANDI: As I explained during my talk, we do not think that parathyroid is the source of the factor, because in parathyroidectomized patients with surgical hypoparathyroidism we do find the factor. We are in the process, now, of looking to other neoplastic tissues in MEN I, just like pituitary as well as islet cells adenomas to evaluate if these might eventually be the source of the factor.

DR. JACKSON (Detroit): I'd like to congratulate Dr. Arnold on his presentation and the approach that his group has taken. About five years ago we presented at this meeting the work with G6PD, and I've talked to Dr. Fialkow and some of the other authors about that work. We cannot quite see where the discrepancy in the findings is, unless it is possibly in the selection of patients, or because in the 11 G6PD heterozygotes we studied, we found evidence of multicellular origin.

We think that these studies are very important. And I've talked to Hank Kronenberg about doing such studies on the same individuals. It's a little difficult to get a G6PD heterozygote who's also a heterozygote for HGPRT, but there may be the possibility of eventually finding those. And perhaps others in the audience, if they have black females who are G6PD heterozygotes, could study these cases using both techniques.

I would like to show a slide, if I may.

This is what we proposed as the mechanism of sporadic non-neoplastic hyperplasia, namely that one would see a multicellular origin in which both A and B G6PD cells were present. This could also apply to the HGPRT with two different types of cells. And one would see with the hyperplasia or, possibly with adenomas, in our studies, the multicellular origin or lack of clonality.

In hereditary hyperparathyroidism, because there's inactivation at a later point, both A and B cells would become multicellular with the first hit or first mutational event, and the second mutational event might produce a cancer.

We cited evidence that in MEN I there are, in the literature, several cases of parathyroid cancer within families of MEN I. Using radiation-induced hyperparathyroidism as an example, and this has never been studied, one would expect a clonal origin because the first hit would be a mutational event affecting one cell, in this instance shown as a G6PD B cell with the A inactivated, and in those instances parathyroid cancer could result. We think that this type of study is very important because it gets at the very pathogenesis of parathyroid tumors, whether they are neoplastic or hyperplastic-related, as Dr. Brandi said, to a substance which is circulating.

I would like to ask if any of the cases that Dr. Arnold has studied were hereditary hyperparathyroidism and if any were radiation-induced?

DR. ARNOLD: Two of the eight patients with adenomas had histories of neck irradiation. One of those was one of the two patients with an apparently polyclonal tumor pattern. Additionally, one of the six patients whose adenomas had monoclonal x-inactivation patterns had a history of neck irradiation.

None of the eight adenoma patients had hereditary hyperparathyroidism, or any family history of endocrine disease. They were quite typical sporadic single gland disease patients who have been followed postoperatively for many years, and have remained normocalcemic.

DR. JACKSON: It's now possible to study DNA on paraffin block formalin-fixed tissue. Have you been able to study that type of parathyroid adenoma?

DR. ARNOLD: That's an extremely good point. We haven't embarked on that yet, mostly because the DNA obtainable from paraffin blocks is somewhat degraded. The x-inactivation analysis

I've spoken about requires good quality, high molecular weight DNA in order to see a band as large as 22 kilobases. However, with some newer polymorphisms, like PGK, the relevant bands are of much smaller size. I think, therefore, that it's now very appropriate to try to obtain DNA from tissues stored in that fashion.

DR. JACKSON: It may be that we can dig out our parathyroid adenomas that have been studied and study them with your technique. Thank you.

DR. ARNOLD: Yes, I'd certainly agree that it's well worth doing these analyses on the same tumors. I would just add that in addition to the possibility that there's an important difference in the patient populations studied, another mechanism could possibly explain the discrepancy between the G6PD data and ours. Perhaps, on a per-cell basis, neoplastic parathyroid cells could be producing less G6PD than the contaminating normal cells. The presence of the monoclonal parathyroid cells would then be masked when total G6PD content is assayed.

G Proteins As Signal Transducers

MICHAEL A. LEVINE

The Johns Hopkins University School of Medicine
Baltimore, MD

The manner in which cell surface receptors transmit information to the rest of the cell is a question of fundamental biological importance. In some instances, receptor-effector coupling is a fairly straightforward affair. As an example, the binding of acetylcholine, glutamate, GABA and glycine to particular receptors directly leads to conformational changes in the structure of specific ion channels that result in activation of the channels. In other cases, however, the generation of intracellular signals in response to occupation of membrane receptors involves an additional component, a "transducing" element, that intervenes between the receptor recognition site and the effector molecule. For many signal-transduction systems, relevant receptors coupled to the effector by a member of a family of guanine nucleotide-binding proteins-the G proteins (1-4).

G PROTEINS

Through complementary approaches, molecular cloning and biochemistry have thus far identified at least eight members of the G protein family. In many instances, molecular cloning has revealed the existence of more than one protein that might subserve the role of a specific G protein that was first identified by function (e.g., three distinct forms of G_i have been cloned). Thus, adenylate cyclase is controlled by stimulatory (G_s) and inhibitory (G_i) G proteins; light-activation of cyclic GMP-phosphodiesterase in the retina is controlled by one form of transducin (G_{t1}) in photodetector rod cells and by another form (G_{t2}) in cones, the color detector cells; signal transduction in specialized olfactory cells is regulated by G_{olf}; hydrolysis of polyphosphoinositides by phospholipase C is controlled by the putative G protein G_{PLC} and inward-rectifying potassium channels are opened by activation of G_k. Activity of another G protein system is modulated by G_o - for "other"- because its function is at present not entirely clear. G_o is found in very high concentration in the nervous system, where one proposed role is as a regulator of voltage-sensitive calcium channels in neural cells. In addition to G_o, several other more mysterious entities including G_{ins}, G_e, and other as yet unnamed species have also been identified as candidate transducing proteins (1-4).

The G proteins share a common heterotrimeric structure, consisting of a major α-subunit (39-52, kDa), which binds guanyl nucleotides, and two smaller tightly coupled subunits designated β (35-36 kDa) and γ (8 kDa). The α-subunits clearly differ among the members of the G protein family, and appear to define the functional specificity and character. The β and γ subunits are more highly conserved, and although some heterogeneity may exist, are probably shared among some α chains to form the specific heterotrimers.

The G proteins also share a common mechanism by which the heterotrimeric protein activates its target effector system. G proteins cycle between an inactive GDP state and an active GTP state. When GDP is bound, α associates with $\beta\gamma$ complex to form the inactive holoprotein (G-GDP). Binding of GTP causes a change in the conformation of the G_α subunit that leads to its dissociation from the $\beta\gamma$ complex. Consequently, the free "activated" G_α-GTP subunit is capable of regulating the activity of the target effector system. The rate limiting step in the activation of G proteins appears to be dissociation of GDP. Indeed, a characteristic feature of G protein activation is that conversion from the GDP-bound state to the GTP-bound state is slow in the absence of an excited receptor. The interaction of G with an excited receptor catalyzes the activation of the G protein by markedly accelerating the rate of exchange of GTP for bound GDP.

The excitation of a receptor (R) by interaction with an appropriate agonist (e.g., hormone, neurotransmitter, photon, etc.) leads to a signal amplification cycle involving R,G, and effector system. The affinity of an excited R (R*) for G-GDP is sufficient to drive their interaction and lead to formation of a stable but transitory R*G-GDP intermediate. R* "opens" the guanine nucleotide-binding site on the G_α subunit and thereby permits GDP-GTP exchange. R*-stimulated exchange of guanine nucleotides requires the $\beta\gamma$ complex of the G protein. Once the holoprotein has interacted with R* it releases GDP and binds GTP. The activated G_α-GTP subunit then dissociates from the $\beta\gamma$ subunit and activates its effector. Binding of GTP causes R* to dissociate from the R*-G protein complex, and permits a single R* complex to activate many molecules of G. The catalytic action of R* and the relatively long lifetime of the activated G_α-GTP subunit provide considerable amplification of the incoming "signal".

The activation of G_α by its physiologic activator, GTP, is reversible, in that nucleotide hydrolysis is involved. The G_α subunit has an endogenous GTPase activity that converts bound GTP to GDP to terminate the regulatory effect of the G protein. Hydrolysis of GTP to GDP returns the G_α subunit to the G_α-GDP form, which has higher affinity for the $\beta\gamma$ subunit complex. The subsequent reassociation of G_α-GDP with the $\beta\gamma$ complex restores the G protein to its inactive state. The holoprotein then returns to its orientation with R and is ready to participate in another cycle of nucleotide exchange.

In solution, G proteins may also be activated by non-hydrolyzable analogs of GTP such as guanosine (3'-0-thio)-triphosphate (GTPγS), by aluminum fluoride (5), or by elevated concentrations of magnesium (6-8).

The members of the G protein family exhibit several additional structural and functional similarities. For example, exotoxins elaborated by the bacteria Vibrio cholerae and Bordetella pertussis catalyze the mono-ADP-ribosylation of many G proteins. These bacterial toxins transfer the ADP-ribose moiety from the cofactor nicotinamide adenine dinucleotide (NAD) to a specific amino acid on the α-subunit of G proteins, and thereby produce a distinctive alteration in the function of the G protein. G_s, G_t, and several other less well-characterized G proteins (9,10) are substrates for ADP-ribosylation by cholera toxin. ADP-ribosylation of $G_{s\alpha}$ by cholera toxin requires the presence of another protein, termed ADP-ribosylation factor (ARF) (11), that is a 21 kd GTP-binding protein. It is not clear whether ARF is required for ADP-ribosylation of $G_{t\alpha}$. An arginine residue in the midportion of $G_{s\alpha}$ and $G_{t\alpha}$ is the site of modification by cholera toxin. ADP-ribosylation of $G_{s\alpha}$ appears to decrease the affinity of $G_{s\alpha}$ for the $\beta\gamma$ complex and also to reduce the intrinsic GTPase activity of $G_{s\alpha}$. This is consistent with the observation that GTP activates G_s almost as well as non-hydrolyzable GTP analogs (e.g. GTPγS), and maintains $G_{s\alpha}$ in a state of persistant activation. The ultimate result of ADP-ribosylation of $G_{s\alpha}$ is <u>increased</u> signal transduction, which leads to enhanced activation of adenylate cyclase and increased formation of cyclic AMP.

Pertussis toxin catalyzes transfer of an ADP-ribose moiety from NAD to a cysteine residue four amino acids removed from the carboxy terminus of the α chains of G_i, G_o, and G_t. ADP-ribosylation by pertussis toxin appears to block interactions between G proteins and R. The "uncoupling" of R and G blocks R*-dependent stimulation of guanine nucleotide exchange, and thereby leads to reduced agonist-stimulated GTPase activity. The end result of pertussis toxin action is <u>reduced</u> signal transduction by the specific G protein substrate.

The effects of bacterial toxins on hormone-stimulated hydrolysis of phosphoinositides by phospholipase C suggest that several distinct G proteins may be "G_{PLC}". For example, pertussis toxin blocks agonist stimulation of phosphoinosite break-down in polymorphonuclear leukocytes (12) and mast cells (13). This suggests that a G protein that is a pertussis toxin substrate couples R to phospholipase C. In contrast, cholera toxin catalyzed ADP-ribosylation of a 41 kD protein in membranes of a macrophage (14) and T-cell line (15) is associated with reduced agonist stimulation of phospholipase C. Finally, neither pertussis toxin or cholera toxin alters receptor-stimulated activity of phospholipase C in hepatocytes (16), cardiac myocytes (17), astrocytoma cells (17), and fibroblasts (18). These observations are consistent with the participation of several distinct G proteins in regulation of phospholipase C in different cell types, including a novel G protein which is toxin-insensitive. One candidate for this latter G protein is $G_{x\alpha}$, a recently identified α chain which may be refractory to modification by pertussis toxin because the cysteine residue in the fourth position from the carboxy terminus is replaced by isoleucine (19,20).

ADENYLYL CYCLASE

The classic example of a G protein-regulated transmembrane signaling system is the adenylyl cyclase complex, the enzyme that catalyzes the synthesis of the second messenger cyclic AMP. It is well known that some agonists produce stimulation of the enzyme and some produce inhibition. This dual regulation is accomplished through the interaction of stimulatory receptors (R_s) with G_s and inhibitory receptors (R_i) with G_i. The molecular mechanisms involved in the G protein-coupled regulation of adenylyl cyclase have been recently reviewed in detail (1-4). The agonist-bound R_s is activated and associates with G_s, which leads to exchange of GDP for GTP and release of free $G_{s\alpha}$-GTP. $G_{s\alpha}$-GTP stimulates adenylyl cyclase activity and thereby increases synthesis of cyclic AMP. Two different forms of $G_{s\alpha}$ protein, 45 and 52 kDa, have been characterized. These multiple forms of $G_{s\alpha}$ protein arise from translation of at least four distinct $G_{s\alpha}$ mRNAs (two long and two short) that result from alternative RNA splicing of a primary transcript encoded by a single gene (21,22). Stimulatory receptors include those for β-adrenergic agonists, PTH, ACTH, gonadotropins, glucagon, TSH, and many other hormones and neurotransmitters. The intracellular accumulation of cyclic AMP produces a biochemical chain reaction that begins with activation of protein kinase A and phosphorylation of specific protein substrates, and ultimately concludes with expression of the physiologic response to agonist recognition by the cell.

Hormonal inhibition of adenylyl cyclase activity is mediated through activation of G_i by inhibitory receptors. These R_i's include those that recognize somatostatin, opioids, α_2-adrenergic agonists, and certain muscarinic cholinergic agents. The interaction of G_i with R_i* is similar to that of G_s

with R_s^*, with the exchange of GTP for GDP leading to dissociation of G_i and release of free $G_{i\alpha}$-GTP and $G_{\beta\gamma}$. The mechanism of inhibition of adenylyl cyclase by the resolved subunits of G_i is not straightforward, however. $G_{i\alpha}$-GTP has only a modest inhibitory effect on adenylyl cyclase, but enzyme activity is profoundly reduced by the free $G_{\beta\gamma}$ subunit complex (23). Moreover, whereas the inhibitory activity of $G_{i\alpha}$-GTP is due to a direct effect on the adenylyl cyclase catalyst, the inhibitory activity of $G_{\beta\gamma}$ is dependent on the presence of G_s. One current model to explain these observations proposes that G_β can mediate hormonal inhibition of adenylyl cyclase by interaction with $G_{s\alpha}$:

$$G_{s\alpha} + G_{\beta\gamma} \rightleftharpoons G_{s\alpha\beta\gamma}$$

Accordingly, activation of G_i through inhibitory receptor agonists should release sufficient $G_{\beta\gamma}$ complexes from G_i to either retard G_s dissociation or favor re-association of $G_{s\alpha}$ to form the inactive $G_{\alpha\beta\gamma}$ holoprotein.

The actions of numerous hormones and neurotransmitters in diverse tissues are mediated by cyclic AMP. One might well ask the question: How can cyclic AMP alone mediate so many different physiological effects through so many different agents? It appears that the specificity of the system does not reside in cyclic AMP itself but in the cell-surface receptors (i.e., TSH receptors are located primarily on thyroid follicular cells, whereas PTH receptors are located primarily on bone osteoblasts and renal tubular cells) and in the endogenous protein substrates for cyclic AMP-dependent phosphorylation. Other components of the system-the G proteins, the catalytic moiety of adenylyl cyclase, cyclic AMP phosphodiesterase and the cyclic AMP-dependent protein kinase-are all very similar, if not identical, from cell to cell.

DISEASES PRODUCED BY ALTERED G PROTEINS

One form of pseudohypoparathyroidism (PHP), the type Ia variant, provides an example of a clinical disorder caused by a dominantly inherited mutation affecting G_s. Albright's original description of PHP focused on PTH resistance in this disorder (24). Subjects with PHP type I excrete significantly less cyclic AMP in the urine in response to PTH infusion than do normal subjects or subjects with other forms of hypoparathyroidism (25). Resistance to PTH alone would be consistent with a defect in the receptor for PTH. However, some patients with PHP type I display resistance to multiple hormones that activate adenylyl cyclase, and express additional abnormalities, such as hypothyroidism (26), hypogonadism (26), mental retardation (27), impaired olfaction (28), and a peculiar phenotype characterized by subcutaneous ossifications, brachydactyly, obesity, round facies, and short stature (Albright's hereditary osteodystrophy) (24). The presence of these multiple defects is consistent with a generalized abnormality that impairs production of cyclic AMP in all tissues. By analogy with the cyc⁻ mutant cell line of S49 murine lymphoma, in which adenylyl cyclase is unresponsive to hormone stimulation because of a genetic deficiency of $G_{s\alpha}$ (29), patients with PHP Ia show an approximately 50% reduction in $G_{s\alpha}$ activity in plasma membranes from multiple cell types (30). In contrast, subjects with hormone resistance that is limited to PTH target tissues have normal $G_{s\alpha}$ activity and are considered to have PHP Ib.

The molecular basis for reduced $G_{s\alpha}$ activity has not been clearly defined. $G_{s\alpha}$ deficiency has been detected in PHP Ia both by functional "complementation assay" (restoration of adenylyl cyclase activity in membranes of $G_{s\alpha}$-deficient S49 cyc⁻ cells by detergent extracts of patient plasma membranes) and by cholera toxin-catalyzed labeling of plasma membrane $G_{s\alpha}$ protein with [^{32}P]ADP-ribose. Normal amounts of $G_{i\alpha}$ have been found.

Recent molecular studies using cDNA hybridization probes for $G_{s\alpha}$ and $G_{i\alpha}$

have extended these earlier observations. Thus cultured fibroblasts from most (but not all) patients with PHP Ia and decreased $G_{s\alpha}$ activity show an approximately 50% reduction in mRNA content for $G_{s\alpha}$ (31,32). As expected, normal amounts of $G_{i\alpha}$ mRNA are present (31). The decrease in total cellular $G_{s\alpha}$ mRNA represents a decrease in all four forms of $G_{s\alpha}$-specific message (32), and is consistent with equivalent decreases in both the 45-kDa and 52-kDa forms of $G_{s\alpha}$ protein in fibroblast membranes (33). The inheritance pattern of $G_{s\alpha}$ deficiency among these subjects is most consistent with autosomal dominant transmission of a defective $G_{s\alpha}$ allele. However, restriction endonuclease analysis of genomic DNA from these subjects reveals no evidence for large deletions or rearrangements of the $G_{s\alpha}$ gene itself that could account for altered gene expression (31,32).

Subjects with PHP Ia whose cultured fibroblasts contain reduced levels of $G_{s\alpha}$ mRNA also have decreased $G_{s\alpha}$ protein on immunoblots of erythrocyte membranes. It is thus conceivable that deficient $G_{s\alpha}$ activity in these patients is due to reduced synthesis of normal functional $G_{s\alpha}$ protein as a direct consequence of the lower level of $G_{s\alpha}$ mRNA. In contrast, the molecular basis for reduced $G_{s\alpha}$ activity in PHP Ia patients who have normal cellular levels of $G_{s\alpha}$-specific mRNA is more difficult to explain. A mutation within the gene for $G_{s\alpha}$ could lead to production of $G_{s\alpha}$ mRNAs that yield structurally abnormal or unstable $G_{s\alpha}$ proteins that are nonfunctional. Indeed, our recent identification of an $G_{s\alpha}$ protein of increased size (Mr≈90 kDa) in erythrocyte membranes of two subjects with reduced $G_{s\alpha}$ activity is consistent with this model. Stronger evidence that this $G_{s\alpha}$ protein is structurally abnormal comes from immunoblots with antisera raised against synthetic peptides derived from sequences common to all G protein α chains (562), or near the amino terminus (A572) or the carboxy terminus (C584) of $G_{s\alpha}$ (34). This unique $G_{s\alpha}$ protein shows normal immunoreactivity with antisera C584 and 562, but is not detected by antiserum A572. Moreover, in contrast to normal forms of $G_{s\alpha}$, the abnormal $G_{s\alpha}$ protein is not (^{32}P)ADP-ribosylated by cholera toxin. These results suggest that a variety of inherited defects and mutational mechanisms may produce the biochemical phenotype of $G_{s\alpha}$ deficiency.

Altered G proteins play a role in the pathophysiology of several other disorders. Other relevant endocrine diseases may possibly include insulin-dependent diabetes mellitus (rats rendered insulin deficient by treatment with streptozotocin have decreased hepatic G_i, a lesion that produces increased cyclic AMP and results in antagonism to the effects of insulin), certain human growth hormone-secreting pituitary adenomas (an abnormal form of G_s has been identified that appears to be persistently activated) (35), and hypothyroidism (in which increased levels of G_i may explain decreased heart rate and hypoglycemia).

Among other disorders linked to specific defects in G protein function are at least two infectious diseases. The severe and potentially fatal secretion of salt and water into the gut of patients with cholera results from cholera toxin-catalyzed ADP-ribosylation of G_s in intestinal mucosal cells. This modification keeps $G_{s\alpha}$ in a state of (relatively) persistant activation and leads to increased adenylyl cyclase activity. The resulting increase in intracellular cyclic AMP produces changes in water and ion transport across membranes of intestinal cells that result in severe watery diarrhea. A similar mechanism may explain traveler's diarrhea, often caused by strains of Escherichia coli that produce a heat-labile enterotoxin.

The toxin secreted by Bordetella pertussis plays a major role in the pathogenesis of whooping cough. The toxin ADP-ribosylates G_i in many cells, although the precise target cell(s) in the respiratory epithelium remains as yet unidentified. Many of the clinical manifestations of whooping cough result from toxin-catalyzed inactivation of G_i, with consequent increased cyclic AMP formation. In the pancreatic islets this results in increased insulin secretion due to blockade of the α-2-adrenergic response that inhibits insulin release.

Finally, given the ubiquitous distribution of G proteins and their importance in signal transduction, it is only reasonable to assume that as our understanding of G protein function increases so will our appreciation of how altered G proteins may contribute to the pathogenesis of many disorders not now linked to signaling processes.

ACKNOWLEDGEMENTS

This work was supported in part by grants from the March of Dimes (1-1065) and the National Institutes of Health (DK-34281).

REFERENCES

1. Gilman, A.G. (1987) Ann. Rev. Biochem. 56, 615-649.
2. Iyengar, R. and Birnbaumer, L. (1987) ISI Atlas Sci. Pharmacol. 1, 213-222.
3. Spiegel, A.M. (1987) Mol. Cell. Endocrinol. 49, 1-16.
4. Stryer, L. and Bourne, H.R. (1986) Ann. Rev. Cell. Biol. 2, 319-419.
5. Sternweis, P.C. and Gilman, A.G. (1982) Proc. Natl. Acad. Sci. U.S.A. 79, 4888-4891.
6. Iyengar, R. and Birnbaumer, L. (1982) Proc. Natl. Acad. Sci. U.S.A. 79, 5179-5183.
7. Katada, T., Northrup, J.K., Bokoch, G.M., Vi, M. and Gilman, A.G. (1984) J. Biol. Chem. 259, 3578-3585.
8. Deterre, P. Bigay, J., Pfister, C. and Chabre, M. (1984) FEBS Lett. 178, 228-232.
9. Lo, W.W.Y. and Hughes, J. (1987) FEBS Lett, 220, 327-331.
10. Xuan, Y.-T., Su, Y.-F., Chang, K.-J. and Watkins, W.D. (1987) Biochem. Biophys. Res. Commun. 146, 898-906.
11. Kahn, R.A. and Gilman, A.G. (1986) J. Biol. Chem. 261:7906-7911.
12. Ohta, H., Okajima, F., Ui, M. (1985) J. Biol. Chem. 260, 15771-15780.
13. Nakamura, T. and Ui, M. (1985) J. Biol. Chem. 260, 3584-3593.
14. Aksamit, R.R., Backlund, Jr., P.S. and Cantoni, G.L. (1985) Proc. Natl. Acad. Sci. U.S.A. 82, 7475-7479.
15. Imboden, J.B., Shoback, D.M., Pattison, G. and Stobo, J.D. (1986) Proc. Natl. Acad. Sci. U.S.A. 83, 5673-5677.
16. Uhing, R.J., Prpic, V., Jiang, H., Exton, J.H. (1986) J. Biol. Chem. 261, 2140-2146.
17. Masters, S.B., Martin, M.W., Harden, T.K., Brown, J.H. (1985) Biochem. J. 227, 933-937.
18. Murayama, T. and Ui, M. (1985) J. Biol. Chem. 260, 7226-7233.
19. Matsuoka, M., Itoh, H., Kozasa, T. and Kaziro, Y. (1988) Proc. Natl. Acad. Sci. U.S.A. 85, 5384-5388.
20. Fong, H.K.W., Yoshimoto, K.K., Eversole-Cire, P., and Simon, M.I. (1988) Proc. Natl. Acad. Sci. U.S.A. 85, 3066-3070.
21. Bray, P., Carter, A., Simons, C., Guo, V., Puckett, C., Kamholz, J., Spiegel, A.M. and Nirenberg, M. (1986) Proc. Natl. Acad. Sci. U.S.A. 83, 8893-8897.
22. Kozasa, T., Itoh, H., Tsukamoto, T. and Kaziro, Y. (1988) Proc. Natl. Acad. Sci. U.S.A. 85, 2081-2085.
23. Katada, T., Northrup, J.K., Bokoch, G.M., Ui, M. and Gilman, A.G. (1984) J. Biol. Chem. 259, 3578-3585.
24. Albright, F., Burnett, C.H. and Smith, P.H. (1942) Endocrinology 30, 922-932.
25. Chase, L.R., Melson, G.L. and Aurbach, G.D. (1969) J. Clin. Invest. 48, 1832-1844.

26. Levine, M.A., Downs, R.W., Jr., Moses, A.M., Breslau, N.A., Marx, S.J., Lasker, R.D., Rizzoli, R.E., Aurbach, G.D. and Spiegel, A.M. (1983) Am. J. Med. 74, 545-556.
27. Farfel, Z. and Friedman, E. (1986) Ann. Int. Med. 105(2), 197-199.
28. Weinstock, R.S., Wright, H.N., Spiegel, A.M., Levine, M.A. and Moses, A.M. (1986) Nature (London) 332, 635-636.
29. Harris, B.A., Robishaw, J.D., Mumby, S.M. and Gilman, A.G. (1985) Science 229, 1274-1276.
30. Levine, M.A. and Aurbach, G.D. (1988) Endocrinology, Ed. L.J. Degroot, Saunders, p. 1065-1079.
31. Levine, M.A., Ahn, T.G., Klupt, S.F., Kaufman, K.D., Smallwood, P.M., Bourne, H.R., Sullivan, K.A. and Van Dop, C. (1988) Proc. Natl. Acad. Sci. U.S.A. 85, 617-621.
32. Carter, A., Bardin, C., Collins, R., Simons, C., Bray, P. and Spiegel, A. (1987) Proc. Natl. Acad. Sci. U.S.A. 84, 7266-7269.
33. Levine, M.A., Eil, C., Downs, R.W., Jr. and Spiegel, A.M. (1983) J. Clin. Invest. 72, 316-324.
34. Mumby, S.M., Kahn, R.A., Manning, D.R. and Gilman, A.G. (1986) Proc. Natl. Acad. Sci. U.S.A. 83, 265-269.
35. Spiegel, A.M. (1988) Hospital Practice June 15, 71-88.

Pseudohypoparathyroidism: Studies of the Pathogenesis of Parathyroid Hormone Resistance

D. GOLTZMAN, J.A. MITCHELL, and G.N. HENDY

Departments of Medicine and Physiology
McGill University and Royal Victoria Hospital
Montreal, Canada

Pseudohypoparathyroidism [1] is a congenital disorder characterized by functional hypoparathyroidism in association with elevated levels of immunoreactive parathyroid hormone (PTH). Administration of exogenous bioactive PTH fails to augment both urinary cyclic AMP excretion and phosphate excretion, in the type I syndrome [2]. In the type II syndrome, exogenous bioactive PTH can increase urinary cyclic AMP excretion but the phosphaturic response is impaired [3]. The type I syndrome may be associated with a constellation of somatic abnormalities collectively referred to as Albright's hereditary osteodystrophy (AHO) and comprising short stature, round facies, brachydactyly, obesity, metastatic subcutaneous calcifications and a tendency toward mental retardation. Additionally, other endocrine deficiency states, such as hypothyroidism and gonadal failure, have been described in association with pseudohypoparathyroidism and AHO [4]. Consequently, this sub-group has been termed type Ia to distinguish it from the form (type Ib) without AHO and without multiple endocrine deficiency syndromes. Although pseudohypoparathyroid states may be familial, the genetics of these disorders have not as yet been well defined.

In the search for the mechanism of PTH resistance in pseudohypoparathyroidism, a reduction was found in the type Ia syndrome in levels of the alpha subunit of the stimulatory guanine nucleotide regulatory protein ($G_s\alpha$) [5] of the adenylate cyclase complex. This reduction [6,7] was described in a PTH target tissue (kidney) [8] as well as in a variety of non-target tissues and in cultured skin fibroblasts [9] and has been found only in association with individuals expressing AHO and other components of the type Ia phenotype. In most, but not all, patients manifesting a reduction in $G_s\alpha$ activity, a decrease in messenger RNA encoding $G_s\alpha$ has been found on Northern blot analysis, whereas Southern blotting has failed to identify any gross deletions or rearrangements of the gene encoding $G_s\alpha$ [10,11]. These studies have led to the concept that a genetic reduction in $G_s\alpha$ results in defective adenylate cyclase activity in tissues of affected individuals causing the pleiotropic somatic and endocrine manifestations of the type Ia syndrome. The major caveat, however, appears to be that not all patients with functional hypoparathyroidism and the type Ia syndrome display diminished $G_s\alpha$ activity whereas family members with AHO but without functional hypoparathyroidism (so called "pseudo-pseudohypoparathyroid" patients) may have reduced levels of $G_s\alpha$ [6,7,12]. Consequently, reductions in $G_s\alpha$ as measured in non-target tissues, do not necessarily correlate with the hypoparathyroid state and, even when

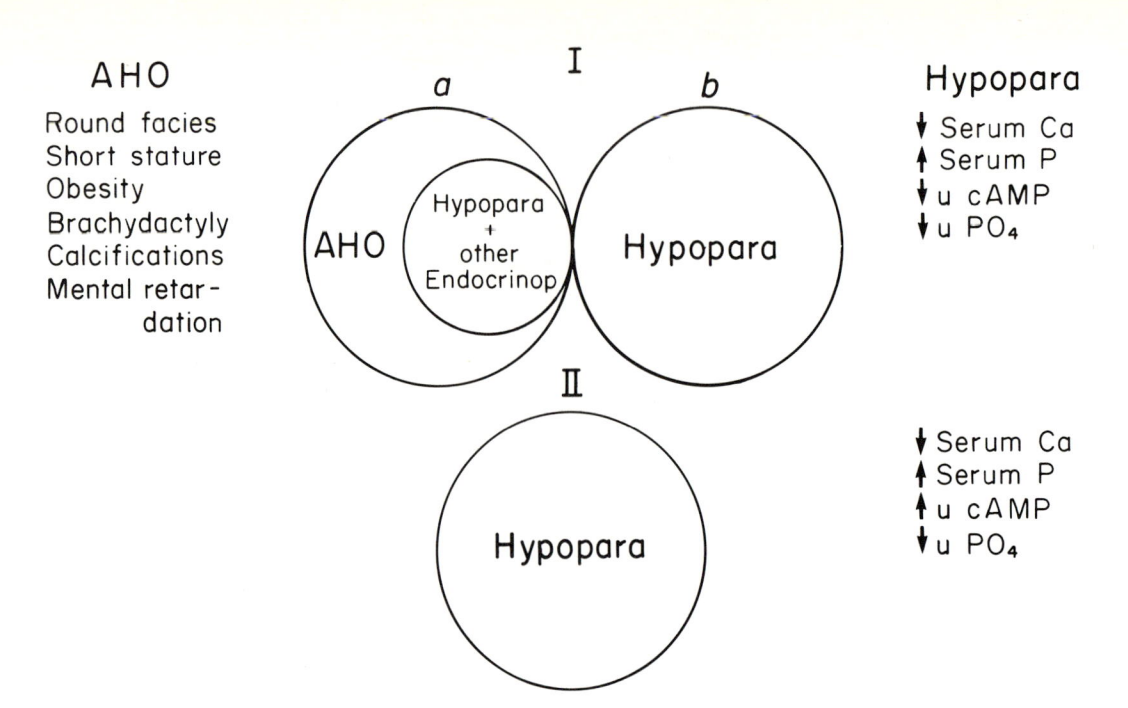

AHO
Round facies
Short stature
Obesity
Brachydactyly
Calcifications
Mental retardation

Hypopara
↓ Serum Ca
↑ Serum P
↓ u cAMP
↓ u PO₄

↓ Serum Ca
↑ Serum P
↑ u cAMP
↓ u PO₄

Figure 1. Classification of pseudohypoparathyroid states. Both type I and type II syndromes are characterized by resistance to exogenous PTH; however, in the former syndrome, the resistance is at the level of the receptor-adenylate cyclase complex; whereas, in the latter, resistance is distal to cyclic AMP generation. Type Ia is distinguished from type Ib by the presence of AHO (Albright's hereditary osteodystrophy) and other endocrinopathies in addition to hypoparathyroidism.

present, do not account for the observation that hypoparathyroidism is the predominant manifestation of endocrine deficiency.

Consequently, we and others have examined the possibility that characteristics of parathyroid hormone *per se* might contribute to the manifestations of functional hypoparathyroidism in this disorder.

I. "Pre-Receptor and Receptor" Resistance

Several studies initially reported a dissociation between the circulating levels of bioactivity and of immunoreactivity in untreated patients with pseudohypoparathyroidism type Ia [13,14] and indicated that a circulating inhibitor to the action of PTH might be present in this disorder. We examined the characteristics of circulating PTH in three patients with this syndrome [15], all of whom were being treated with oral vitamin D_2 and all of whom consequently had normal levels of serum calcium. The activity of the adenylate cyclase guanine nucleotide regulatory protein (G protein) was reduced in the one patient in whom it was measured. Despite normocalcemia, basal immunoreactive PTH levels (measured with a COOH-terminal or mid-region assay) were elevated in all three patients; nevertheless, bioactive PTH, when measured concomitantly with a renal cytochemical bioassay [16], was within the low normal range of the assay or below normal. The levels of PTH bioactivity, therefore, were consistent with the maintenance of normocalcemia by the vitamin D therapy. Associated with the absence of elevated levels of bioactivity in the plasma of our patients was the finding that patient plasma could diminish the stimulatory effect of exogenous biologically active PTH in two *in vitro* bioassays; thus, dose-dependent inhibition by patient plasma of PTH action was observed in a renal adenylate cyclase assay and in a renal cytochemical bioassay. No correlation was found between the initial level of total immunoreactive PTH and the capacity of each serum to shift the dose-response curves of stimulation in the in vitro assays by exogenous PTH. We then examined the effect of reducing the baseline level of immunoreactivity on the inhibitory capacity of patient plasma. Thus, baseline levels of immunoreactive PTH were reduced by short term calcium infusion and the plasma obtained during the peak of calcium elevation was tested. No reduction in the inhibitory capacity of plasma was observed despite the partial decrease in immunoreactive hormone levels which was achieved. Whether the inhibitory activity persisted in the basal non-suppressible component of immunoreactive PTH or whether the inhibitory moiety failed to react with PTH radioimmunoassays remains to be clarified. Studies of others have indicated that prolonged hypercalcemia can remove or reduce the level of inhibitory activity in the plasma of pseudohypoparathyroid patients [17].

To assess whether circulating plasma moieties in pseudohypoparathyroidism might directly interact with PTH, the capacity of patient plasma to bind bioactive iodinated hormone was tested. No significant plasma binding of iodinated PTH was observed. Consequently, the locus of in vitro PTH antagonism appeared to be at the level of the renal cell membrane receptor in the in vitro assays employed.

Finally, the profile of immunoreactive PTH in patient plasma was analyzed after fractionation by reversed-phase high performance liquid chromatography. Profiles were concomitantly analyzed in plasma from patients with primary or secondary hyperparathyroidism for comparison. Profiles of the latter indicated that circulating immunoreactivity was composed mainly of multiple early-eluting carboxyl-terminal fragments. In contrast, in the plasma of patients with pseudohypoparathyroidism, the concentration of early eluting carboxyl-terminal fragments was reduced and the bulk of the circulating immunoreactivity consisted of different, more hydrophobic moieties.

The overall interpretation of these studies, therefore, was consistent with the presence of an alteration in parathyroid hormone metabolism within the parathyroid gland in pseudohypoparathyroidism, such that aberrant immunoreactive moieties with reduced bioactivity were being released. Such entities were potentially the cause of the inhibitory activity observed in pseudohypoparathyroid plasma. Inasmuch as the defect in the stimulatory guanine nucleotide-regulatory protein in pseudohypoparathyroidism has been shown to be widespread in multiple tissues, such a defect would presumably also impair the adenylate cyclase system of the parathyroid cell. Therefore, the plasma abnormalities described in pseudohypoparathyroidism could be attributed to modification of the adenylate cyclase system in the processing, intracellular metabolism and/or release of parathyroid hormone.

II. "Post-Receptor" Resistance

Loveridge et al have reported that it is possible to distinguish inhibitory activity from bioactive PTH in the plasma of hypocalcemic patients with pseudohypoparathyroidism after fractionation of plasma by gel permeation chromatography [18]. Consequently, bioactive hormone may circulate in patients with this disorder, although concentrations of the bioactive moiety and, perhaps, of inhibitory activity may fluctuate. We, therefore, examined the influence of prolonged elevations of circulating PTH on target tissue function using a rat model of vitamin D deficiency [19].

Vitamin D deficient animals displayed elevated steady-state levels of circulating PTH with concomitant hypocalcemia, thereby fulfilling the criteria of parathyroid hormone resistance. Concentrations of 1,25-dihydroxyvitamin D were undetectable. This constellation of biochemical findings is, therefore, analogous to that seen in patients with pseudohypoparathyroidism prior to treatment. The characteristics of the PTH resistance were then examined in vitro in renal membranes prepared from the vitamin D deficient (D-) rats and compared to similarly prepared renal membranes from vitamin D sufficient (D+) animals.

PTH-stimulated adenylate cyclase activity was found to be reduced in the renal membranes of the D- animals when compared to activity in membranes of D+ animals. When receptor binding characteristics were then examined, PTH receptor binding was found to be reduced in the D- membranes and Scatchard analysis revealed that this reduction was due to a decrease in receptor capacity but not affinity. Consequently, the hyperparathyroid state had produced a characteristic hormonal down-regulation phenomenon. When the calcitonin-stimulated adenylate cyclase response was then examined in the same two groups of renal membranes, however, a reduction in calcitonin-stimulated activity was also seen in the D-membranes. This occurred despite the absence of hypercalcitoninemia and despite normal calcitonin receptor binding to the D- renal membranes. This observation suggested that the hyperparathyroidism might be causing a defect not only at the PTH receptor level, but at a more distal locus, i.e. at a component of the adenylate cyclase complex which might be shared by several hormones interacting on a common target cell. The reduced calcitonin bioactivity would, therefore, be a manifestation of such a post-receptor defect. Consequently, we next investigated the functional integrity of the G protein and of the catalytic moiety of the adenylate cyclase complex.

Effectors of the stimulatory G protein including the non-hydrolyzable GTP analog, guanylyl imidodiphosphate (Gpp(NH)p), and NaF were used to probe the functional capacity of $G_s\alpha$, and the diterpene forskolin was used as a direct activator of the catalytic moiety. In these studies, a reduced capacity of activators of $G_s\alpha$ to stimulate adenylate cyclase was found in renal membranes of D- animals, whereas the response to forskolin was unaltered in D- as compared to D+ membranes. Consequently, there appeared to be a post-receptor abnormality at the level of $G_s\alpha$. The catalytic unit was, however, unimpaired. Two

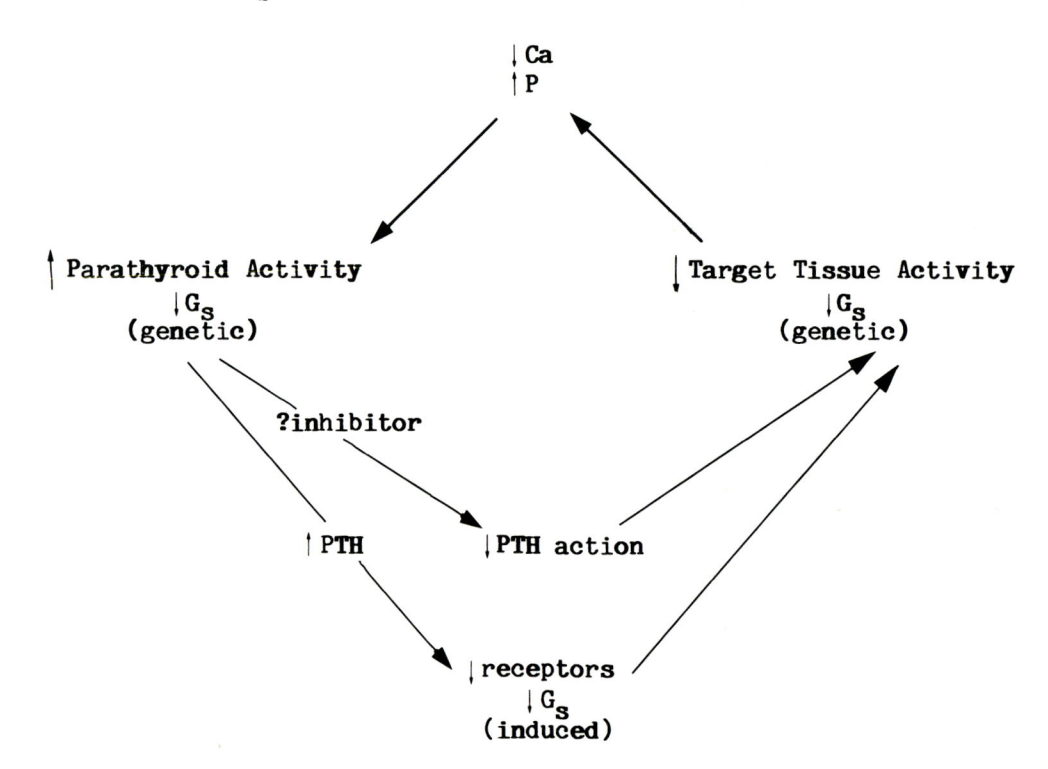

Figure 2. Possible scheme for the initiation and persistance of PTH resistance in pseudohypoparathyroidism type Ia. A widespread genetically-induced reduction in $G_s\alpha$ activity may initiate PTH resistance in this disorder with a resultant increase in parathyroid gland activity and PTH production. The hormone released may be defective, as a result of abnormal parathyroid gland adenylate cyclase activity, and function as a receptor inhibitor, or may be bioactive and induce a receptor reduction and post-receptor defect in $G_s\alpha$ activity in target cells. The latter two mechanisms could then contribute to the maintenance of PTH resistance in the syndrome.

approaches were then used to further delineate this abnormality. In the first approach, renal membranes were labeled with [^{32}P]NAD in the presence of cholera toxin. Cholera toxin is known to catalyze ADP-ribosylation of $G_s\alpha$ [5] and two forms of $G_s\alpha$, a 45 kilodalton form and a 42 kilodalton form, were demonstrated to be [^{32}P]ADP-ribosylated with this technique in rat renal membranes. Cholera toxin-catalyzed [^{32}P]ADP ribosylation of both forms was found to be diminished in renal membranes of D- rats. A second approach was to solubilize renal membranes of vitamin D sufficient rats in order to perform reconstitution studies, but to heat inactivate them prior to use, in order to remove endogenous catalytic unit activity. The absence of catalytic unit activity was confirmed by the inability of forskolin to stimulate adenylate cyclase in these solubilized membranes. When increasing quantities of these solubilized D+ membranes were then added to a fixed concentration of D- membranes, increasing adenylate cyclase stimulation by both Gpp(NH)p and by NaF were observed. These studies demonstrated that stimulated G proteins in the solubilized D+ membranes were capable of restoring adenylate cyclase activity in the D- membranes toward normal. Consequently, the catalytic moiety of the D- renal membranes was capable of being fully activated by a stimulated G binding protein.

Although these studies, therefore, demonstrated that this PTH-resistant state was associated with reduced $G_s\alpha$, it was unclear whether this was due to hypocalcemia, reduced levels of 1,25-dihydroxyvitamin D or to increased PTH concentrations *per se*. To attempt to distinguish among these possibilities, studies were performed in another tissue from the same D- rats, i.e. from testis. This tissue contains 1,25-dihydroxyvitamin D receptors, and was exposed to the same ambient low calcium concentrations as was kidney, but lacks PTH receptors. Membranes prepared from D- testicular tissue were found to have an unimpaired adenylate cyclase response when examined with activators of $G_s\alpha$. Furthermore, cholera toxin-catalyzed [^{32}P]ADP ribosylation of $G_s\alpha$ was not quantitatively or qualitatively different in testicular membranes of D- as compared to D+ animals. Consequently, the post-receptor alteration in association with this PTH-resistant state was present in a target tissue containing PTH receptors but was lacking in a tissue devoid of PTH receptors. Therefore, PTH *per se*, acting through its receptor, appeared to be a major determinant of this phenomenon, with hypocalcemia or 1,25-dihydroxyvitamin D influential, if at all, only as possible modulators of the PTH-receptor interaction.

These studies, therefore, indicate that a reduction in $G_s\alpha$, similar to that seen in pseudohypoparathyroidism, may be induced in the presence of biochemical alterations analogous to that seen in untreated pseudohypoparathyroidism where chronic hypocalcemia, low 1,25-dihydroxyvitamin D levels and elevated PTH levels prevail. Nevertheless, in the acquired disorder the $G_s\alpha$ reduction appears to be restricted to target tissues and would not be expected to persist in cultured target cells (as has been demonstrated in cultured skin fibroblasts from patients with pseudohypoparathyroidism) [19]. However, the influence of chronically elevated circulating PTH would contribute to the genetically-determined $G_s\alpha$ reduction in pseudohypoparathyroidism and perhaps provoke resistance to the hormone by reducing $G_s\alpha$ activity below a critical level required to induce a response.

SUMMARY AND CONCLUSIONS

Pseudohypoparathyroidism is a heterogeneous disorder in which considerable effort has been expended in order to elucidate its pathogenesis. Most success has been achieved with the type I syndrome where a genetically determined reduction in the $G_s\alpha$ component of the adenylate cyclase complex has been defined. This defect appears to correlate best with AHO and is widespread in multiple tissues. A reduction in $G_s\alpha$ within the parathyroid gland could alter adenylate cyclase activity in this gland resulting in abnormal intraglandular processing or metabolism of PTH, such that altered forms of PTH are released. Some may act as peripheral inhibitors to the action of PTH and may be released only intermittently, perhaps in association with specific changes (e.g., normalization) of plasma calcium. Excess parathyroid gland activity, in the presence of hypocalcemia, may be associated with increased circulating levels of bioactive PTH which can in turn further reduce $G_s\alpha$ in target tissues by a "post-receptor" desensitization mechanism. Both mechanisms may, therefore, contribute to the development of hypoparathyroidism, which appears as a predominant manifestation of the endocrinopathy in this multifaceted syndrome.

ACKNOWLEDGEMENTS

This work was supported by grants MT-5775 and MA-9315 to D.G. and G.N.H., respectively, from the Medical Research Council (MRC) of Canada. D.G. is the recipient of a Scientist Award, and G.N.H. is the recipient of a Scholarship from the MRC. We thank Diane Allen for excellent secretarial support.

REFERENCES

1. Albright, F., Burnett, C., Smith, P.H. and Parson, W. (1942): Endocrinology 30, 922.
2. Chase, L.R., Melson, G.L. and Aurbach, G.D. (1969): J. Clin. Invest. 48, 1832.
3. Drezner, M., Neelon, F.A. and Lebovitz, H.E. (1973): N. Engl. J. Med. 289, 1056.
4. Van Dop, C. and Bourne, H.R. (1983): Annu. Rev. Med. 34, 259.
5. Gilman, A.G. (1984): Cell 36, 577.
6. Farfel, Z., Brother, V.M., Brickman, A.S., Conte, F., Neer, R., and Bourne, H.R. (1981): Proc. Natl. Acad. Sci. USA 78, 3098.
7. Levine, M.A., Jap, T.-S., Mauseth, R.S., Downs, R.W., and Spiegel, A.M. (1986): J. Clin. Endocrinol. Metab. 62, 497.
8. Downs, R.W.,Jr., Levine, M.A., Drezner, M.K., Burch, W.M., Jr. and Spiegel, A.M. (1983): J. Clin. Invest. 71, 231.
9. Bourne, H.R., Kaslow, H.R., Brickman, A.S. and Farfel, Z. (1981): J. Clin. Endocrinol. Metab. 53, 636.
10. Carter, A., Bardin, C., Collins, R., Simons, C., Bray, P. and Spiegel, A. (1987): Proc. Natl. Acad. Sci. USA 84, 7266.
11. Levine, M.A., Ahn, T.G., Klupt, S.F., Kaufman, K.D., Smallwood, P.M., Bourne, H.R., Sullivan, K.A. and Van Dop, C. (1988): Proc. Natl. Acad. Sci. USA 85, 617.
12. Fischer, J.A., Bourne, H.R., Dambacher, M.A., Tschopp, F., DeMeyer, F., Devogelaer, J.-P., Werder, E.A., Nagant de Deuxchaisnes, C. (1983): Clin. Endocrinol. 24, 549.
13. Nagant de Deuxchaisnes, C., Fischer, J.A., Dambacher, M.A., Devogelaer, J.-P., Arber, C.E., Zanelli, J.M., Parsons, J.A., Loveridge, N., Bitensky, L. and Chayen, J. (1981): J. Clin. Endocrinol. Metab. 53, 1106.
14. Allgrove, J., Chayen, J., Jawayeera, P. and O'Riordan, J.L.H. (1984): Clin. Endocrinol. 20, 503.
15. Mitchell, J. and Goltzman, D. (1985): J. Clin. Endocrinol. Metab. 61, 328.
16. Goltzman, D., Henderson, B., Loveridge, N. (1980): J. Clin. Invest. 65, 1309.
17. Loveridge, N., Fischer, J.A., Devogelaer, J.-P., Nagant de Deuxchaisnes, C. (1986): Clin. Endocrinol. 24, 549.
18. Loveridge, N., Tschopp, F., Born, W., Devogelaer, J.-P., Nagant de Deuxchaisnes, C. and Fischer, J.A. (1986): Biochim. Biophys. Acta 889, 117.
19. Mitchell, J., Tenenhouse, A., Warner, M. and Goltzman, D. (1988): Endocrinology. In Press.

Discussion:

DR. RIGGS (Rochester, MN): I have a couple of clinical observations. I would be interested in seeing how Dr. Levine might fit this into the general scheme. First, my colleague, Dr. Bob Salasa at the Mayo Clinic, studied a patient with typical pseudo-pseudohypoparathyroidism, normal calcium, normal phosphate. She was about 17 at that time. About three or four years later, she came in with hypocalcemia. At 17, she had an Ellsworth Howard test that was perfectly normal. By the time she was hypocalcemic she had an abnormal Ellsworth Howard test. So, she made a transformation from pseudo-pseudo to pseudo.

The second point is, as you know, some of the patients with pseudohypoparathyroidism actually have hyperparathyroid manifestations in their bones in that they have subperiosteal bone resorption and increased bone turnover on biopsy. So, how does that fit in with the defect that's supposed to be present in all the cells?

DR. LEVINE (Baltimore): I'll respond to the question of pseudo-pseudohypoparathyroidism and hypocalcemia first. I would first ask you, when you say the Ellsworth Howard test, were you measuring urinary excretion of cyclic AMP or just phosphate?

DR. RIGGS: Just phosphate at the time. That was some time ago.

DR. LEVINE: Then you've given me my out. If one uses the urinary cyclic AMP response to PTH to distinguish between pseudo- and pseudo-pseudohypoparathyroidism, we've never seen anyone transform themselves from pseudo-pseudohypoparathyroidism to pseudo or vice versa. Dr. Marc Drezner is standing at the end of this line and I'm going to quote some of his data. So, if I misquote him, he will certainly correct me.

I think that there is an entity called normocalcemic pseudohypoparathyroidism in which, for some reason - perhaps lack of the PTH inhibitor or some other part of the picture- individuals who have deficient alpha GS and an abnormal response to PTH, vis-a-vis deficient urinary cyclic AMP response, are able to maintain a normal serum calcium level. If you look at the evolution of hypocalcemia in individuals with pseudohypoparathyroidism, one finds that at birth and during infancy they have normal serum calcium levels. As they grow older they begin to first show an increase in serum phosphorous; subsequently, when they're seven or eight years old, they develop hypocalcemia.

It therefore appears that there may be an element of an additional, perhaps acquired, defect. In some individuals the defect that causes hypocalcemia may not manifest itself till the teens or later, and they may go back and forth between hypocalcemia and normocalcemia spontaneously.

The second question relates to the bone: there's no doubt that a lot of these patients, typically patients with pseudohypoparathyroidism type 1b, can have osteitis fibrosa cystica, severe metabolic bone disease consistent with a picture of primary hyperparathyroidism. We also see it occasionally in patients with type 1a who have alpha GS deficiency.

I don't think that PTH responsiveness at the level of the bone is inconsistent with the concept of PTH resistance for a number of reasons. Number one, I don't think that we really know what the signal transduction system in the bone is. There's increasing evidence now that PTH receptors are also coupled to phosphoinositol metabolism and activation of phospholipase C and that that may be the signal effector system that produces bone resorption in response to PTH. Accordingly, the alpha GS defect may be present in adenylycyclase of bone cells, but may not manifest itself as a defect in PTH-dependent bone remodeling.

DR. OGATA (Tokyo): I have the third independent way of explanation for the biochemical abnormality in pseudo due to the following reason: both hypoparathyroidism and pseudo are characterized by the decreased production of 1,25. So, if we supplement those patients with physiological doses of active D, patients with pseudo become normocalcemic in sharp contrast to patients with hypoparathyroidism. The normocalcemia that will be obtained in pseudo is quite stable. It is resistant to the calcemic stress by food intake.

It would appear that endogenous PTH is able to act if the physiological amount of active D is supplied. We also could show that the kidneys of a patient with pseudo, at least its calcium reabsorption responses concerned, will be entirely normal, both to endogenous and exogenous PTH. It responds very beautifully with the reabsorptive response of calcium. But, if we supply those patients with adequate amounts of vitamin D, the defect in proximal renal tubules remains.

So, I rather think the functional defect is rather limited to the proximal tubules of kidney in pseudo.

DR. LEVINE: I can respond to that. I'm glad to see that it's been recently published in the Journal of Clinical Endocrinology and Metabolism that patients with pseudohypoparathyroidism appear to resorb calcium normally. Steven Marx, a number of years ago, commented to me that it was a lot easier to treat patients with pseudohypoparathyroidism with vitamin D than it was PTH deficient patients.

DR. OGATA: Not vitamin D, the active vitamin D.

DR. LEVINE: Well, vitamin D or its metabolite because of the absence of hypercalciuria in the pseudo patients.

DR. OGATA: That's right.

DR. LEVINE: I would like to point out that there's now evidence from Keith Hruska's group and other laboratories that PTH is coupled to phospholipase C in the kidney. It may be PTH-dependent resorption of calcium in the distal tubule relies on second messengers other than cyclic AMP. This might explain why GS alpha deficiency would impair certain aspects of PTH action without affecting other actions.

DR. PARFITT (Detroit): This is a question for both speakers. The pathogenetic schemes proposed do not account for the existence of the relatives who have never been hypocalcemic and who have normal cyclic AMP responses, but still have a 50 percent deficiency in the GS alpha. Could either or both speakers explain how they account for that?

DR. LEVINE: I think this may relate to the difficulty of extrapolating from peripheral measurements of GS alpha activity, which are generally done in circulating cells (red cells or platelets) or other non-target cells, to the kidney. There may not be a one-to-one correlation between the absolute levels of deficiency of GS alpha in the target tissue as opposed to other tissues. There may be a general correlation, but the accuracy of the method is not so great as to be able to make fine distinctions. Consequently, I believe it may in part be a problem of making measurements in peripheral tissues and attempting to conclude from these what is occurring in target cells.

DR. MURRAY (Toronto): I have two quick questions, one for each of the speakers. I'd like to ask Dr. Goltzman whether the difference in elution patterns in the PTH on HPLC from hyperparas versus PHP patients can be accounted for by differences in the circulating calcium? It's well recognized that the differences in the serum calcium can change the amount of circulating C terminal fragments.

DR. GOLTZMAN (Montreal): One of the patients, the primary hyperparathyroid patient, was moderately hypercalcemic, and the secondary hyperparathyroid patient, who was vitamin D deficient was moderately hypocalcemic. Although there were slight differences in these two patterns they were relatively minor, with small carboxyl fragments predominating in both. Yet they both differed from the patterns in pseudohypoparathyroidism quite markedly. Consequently, I do not believe differences in calcium would account for what we were seeing in these particular patients. Nevertheless, it is true that there may be alterations in what form of PTH is released from the parathyroid gland, depending on the ambient calcium. Therefore, it may be that indeed different products (perhaps inhibitor fragments or bioactive hormone) are released from pseudohypoparathyroid parathyroid glands depending on ambient calcium levels.

DR. MURRAY: The second question is to Dr. Levine. Is it possible to propagate PHP cells in culture from a PHP patient and still see, in subsequent passages of cells, the defect in GS.

DR. LEVINE: Absolutely. The MRNA that we have examined was extracted from cultured fibroblasts from these patients. Those fibroblasts have gone through many passages, and the defect in alpha GS has been a stable genetic characteristic of those cells.

DR. BELL (Charleston): David, I enjoyed that presentation very much. Do you have any other evidence on whether it's vitamin D deficiency, hypocalcemia, or excess parathyroid hormone that's responsible for the defect? Or could you add 1,25 dihydroxyvitamin D in vitro and correct the defect?

DR. GOLTZMAN: This is obviously a very interesting and critical question. Rather than parathyroidectomizing the animals or adding back vitamin D, we chose to look at this issue differently. Therefore, we selected another tissue, the testes, which was exposed to the same degree of hypocalcemia and vitamin D deficiency, and which reportedly has 1,25 receptors but does not have PTH receptors. In this tissue we did not find any abnormality in adenylate cyclase despite the fact it was in the same milieu of low levels of 1,25 (OH)$_2$D and low levels of calcium that the kidney was exposed to.

Therefore, I would say that it's probably the high PTH acting through its receptor that is responsible for the defect and, if the low calcium and low 1,25 (OH)$_2$D influenced this effect, it's probably at the level of the PTH receptor interaction. That is the only information I have on that at the moment.

DR. BELL: Did you give large doses of parathyroid hormone to animals and produced this?

DR. LEVINE: We did not. I believe Nissenson et al or Martin et al did treat animals with large doses of PTH a number of years ago. They found decreases in receptor numbers, which is what you'd expect. But I don't believe they looked in detail at post-receptor events to see if these were altered as well.

DR. DREZNER (North Carolina): First, a comment with respect to what Larry Riggs said. Most of the patients whom we biopsied, we observed in pseudohypoparathyroidism some elements of increased resorptive activity. I think the end organ resistance at the bone is probably related to the calcemic response, which I won't try to talk about since Dr. Parfitt is next to me and it's his model that would say that they're two different systems in the bone. And one of them may be resistant in patients with pseudohypoparathyroidism.

Secondly, a question for David. What's the functional consequences in your D deficiency state when my own acquaintance with D deficiency is that they maintain hypophosphatemia by virtue of continuous phosphaturia? One, do your rats exhibit hypophosphatemia when they have the deficiency in the G protein? And, if so, is there any functional consequence at the post-cyclic AMP state to the loss of the AG activity?

DR. GOLTZMAN: The animals we studied were not significantly hypophosphatemic. We did not administer parathyroid hormone to see if they did have a defective phosphaturic response. Therefore, we can't tell you for certain whether or not they were resistant from that point of view or not. But they certainly were not hypophosphatemic, so that they did indeed appear to be resistant to the high circulating PTH which did not seem to be causing significant phosphaturia.

DR. BILEZIKIAN (New York): David, I have a question with respect to using another positive control tissue that has parathyroid hormone receptors in this setting, like, for example, lymphocytes or fibroblasts. If you could look at that, are there reductions in GS?

DR. GOLTZMAN: That's a good point. I think those are studies which can readily be done but we have not done them as yet. I believe those tissues are cleaner, actually, to look at than bone, because I would concur that the situation in bone is probably very complex and involves more than a PTH-induced cAMP response. But we haven't done those studies as yet.

DR. MARTIN (Australia): Other questions? Perhaps if I could ask a question of Dr. Goltzman. The circulating inhibitor which inhibits the biological activity of PTH in the cytochemical assay, has that been looked at to see if it influences the cytochemical assay response of other hormones, for example, the TSH cytochemical assay or the LH in the ascorbic acid depletions?

DR. GOLTZMAN: That is an interesting question. We actually have not looked at that because we don't have the cytochemical assay set up for looking at TSH or hormonal responses other than for PTH. Certainly, Nigel Loveridge would be in a position to do this. I don't know if he ever has.

DR. PARFITT: A follow up to my earlier question. What is proposed is that the measurement in the red cells is a good marker of what's going on in the kidney in one class of individuals, namely, those who have hypocalcemia and PTH resistance, but is a poor marker of what is going on in the kidney in the other class of individuals, namely the relatives. The most straightforward interpretation of the data is that deficiency of GS alpha is a good marker for the short metacarpal syndrome but has nothing to do with the hormone resistance.

DR. LEVINE: I would like to respond to that because I wanted to follow up a question asked earlier. Specifically, why should a reduction of alpha GS protein cause hormone resistance in some (i.e., pseudohypoparathyroidism) but not others (i.e., pseudo-pseudohypoparathyroidism). It must be remembered that cyclic AMP metabolism is not just production of cyclic AMP. There's also degradation of cyclic AMP by a specific phosphodiesterase. There might be differences in the activity of phosphodiesterase from patient to patient. You might have sort of a "two-hit" problem going on here. To manifest hormone resistance it might be necessary to inherit an alpha GS defect, but not sufficient unless you also have increased phosphodiesterase activity superimposed on reduced ability to synthesize cyclic AMP. So that we might actually have a convergence of two different defects, metabolic interference, if you will. I would speculate that phosphodiesterase isoenzymes might occur in the population, but unless you also have some deficiency in production of cyclic AMP, the rate of degradation of cyclic AMP will have little or no physiologic (or clinical) manifestation. In general, we can produce much, much more cyclic AMP than is necessary to produce a maximal biologic response.

Another issue is that cyclic AMP dependent protein kinase A is not a well-studied or well-characterized system. The affinity of protein kinase A for cyclic AMP may be variable from patient to patient, or tissue to tissue. This could explain why hormone resistance does not appear in every target tissue in these patients. In summary, deficient GS alpha may be necessary but not sufficient to cause the entire syndrome.

DR. BELL: One comment to you, David, is that more readily available tissue that have cyclic AMP responsive to PTA should be liver cells and also fat cells.

DR. DREZNER: I was just interested in your response, Mike, because I'm not sure you even have to invoke that when you consider that there are some tissues in a given patient with pseudo type 1a, which respond quite normally. Most notably, the adrenal, which, to my knowledge, has never been reported as defective in patients with pseudo 1a but the adrenals have a protein deficiency, G1.

It seems that there have to be other events going on at the end organ which modulate the primary genetic defect and make it expressed as an abnormality or not. It's conceivable that when you have patients that have the decrease, or mothers of affected patients, that they may not have the necessary milieu.

DR. GOLTZMAN: Let me just comment on that. It may be that the down regulation response or resistance induced by different hormones varies in their characteristics. For example, we know that glucagon pre-treatment of target tissues results in a decrease in glucagon receptors and a decrease in GS alpha, i.e., a response very similar to parathyroid hormone. And, indeed, glucagon resistance occurs in type 1a patients when they're injected with glucagon.

We don't know if a marked receptor reduction and postreceptor defect occurs with other hormones which utilize the cyclase system, such as ACTH. It's further complicated by the fact that there may be spare receptors for some of these hormones such as ACTH. Therefore, even if down regulation of receptors occurs this may not be translated into an abnormality. Consequently, not all hormones acting through the adenylate cyclase system may generate a down-regulation response leading to sustained hormone resistance in pseudohypoparathyroidism.

Primary Hyperparathyroidism: The Surgically Cured Patient

SVERKER LJUNGHALL, CHARLOTTE JOBORN, MATS PALMÉR,
JONAS RASTAD, and GÖRAN ÅKERSTRÖM

Departments of Internal Medicine and Surgery
University Hospital
Uppsala, Sweden

Only a few decades ago primary HPT was a rare disease which was generally associated with pronounced symptoms when diagnosed and surgery was usually performed once the diagnosis was established. Since primary hyperparathyroidism (HPT) is nowadays more commonly diagnosed, often in patients with only mild hypercalcemia, and sometimes without obvious symptoms, the optimal management of the disease is no longer unequivocal. It is, however, still generally agreed that patients with high serum calcium values (e.g. above 3 mmol/l) or with symptoms like stone or bone disease should be submitted for surgery. The arguments in favour of parathyroid operations for virtually asymptomatic, elderly patients are less well delineated.

In order to provide a basis for the choice of treatment this paper will attempt to review the short- and long-term consequences for patients operated for primary HPT with regard to operative complications, parathyroid function and serum calcium, clinical symptoms, morbidity and mortality.

I. Effects of surgery on parathyroid function, serum calcium

Experiences underlying this review come from a material of 570 patients with sporadic primary HPT, who underwent primary parathyroid explorations during 1956-1984 at our hospital (1). Among these patients there was a 3:1 female to male ratio, a mean age of 59 years and the patients were postoperatively followed for a mean of 7 years (range of 1-27 years).

In our patient material adenomas were found at operation in 80% and hyperplasia in 17% of the patients. There was, however, an inverse correlation between the values of serum calcium and the proportional incidence of chief cell hyperplasia, i.e. hyperplasia was considerably more common in the patients with the mildest degree of hypercalcemia and adenomas were more frequent in patients with more severe hypercalcemia. Parathyroid carcinoma was diagnosed only in two patients. There was a positive correlation between serum calcium and the glandular weights of both adenomas and hyperplasias (2).

With regard to the short-term (<1 year) operative results normocalcemia was achieved in 93% av the adenomas and 85% of the hyperplasias, with persistent hypercalcemia in 4% and 9%, respectively and hypocalcemia occurring in altogether 3%. These results agree with most other reports from large patient materials and demonstrate that surgery although it is a safe procedure without mortality, may be especially difficult in cases with the mildest hypercalcemia since these patients more often have moderate hyperplasia where the extent of resection maybe difficult to define.

The long-term follow-up showed that among patients with hyperplasia the recurrence rate was altogether 6.5%, gradually increasing with observation time to about 30% after 15 years (3). Recurrences were seen also in 2% of patients operated for adenomas. Such recurrences among adenoma cases were not evident until after 8 years but the frequency increased to 15% after 15 years. All these patients had displayed unequivocal evidence of adenoma at the time of primary surgery, i.e. the glands associated with the adenoma had been visualized and were microscopically in several cases also histopathologically proven to be normal. The findings seem to indicate similar pathophysiologic and perhaps pathogenetic mechanisms in parathyroid adenomatous and hyperplastic disease and may suggest that in some cases adenomas might arise from a general hyperplasia.

The basic pathophysiological disturbance which is responsible for the development of HPT is unknown. A high prevalence of HPT, reaching figures of 1-3% of the population, has been reported from especially the Nordic countries (4) and it has been suggested that a reduced capacity to synthetize active vitamin D, through diminished negative feed-back on the parathyroid glands might ultimately lead to glandular growth and inadequate secretion of PTH. A defect of this kind could be expected first to give rise to diffuse general hyperplasia where one gland subsequently might develop more autonomous function and suppress the other parathyroid glands. Upon removal of the dominant gland uninhibited secretory disorders in the others could, however, be manifest after several years. If so, recurrence of HPT might be prevented by e.g. the long-term postoperative use of active vitamin D.

II. <u>Effects of surgery on subjective symptoms</u>

Thorough investigations have revealed a higher incidence of, often asymptomatic, vertebral compression fractures in primary HPT and also a moderately decreased bone mineral content. A few years following successful parathyroid surgery the bone mineral content is partially restored, but the clinical significance of these findings is not clear since there is no apparently increased fracture rate in HPT and no studies have yet established the effects of surgery on the fracture rate.

The precise cause for renal stone formation in primary HPT is not fully clarified, but it is at least partly linked to the hypercalciuria. In recent patient materials less than 20% have renal stones and only few have frequent recurrent stone episodes. Following parathyroidectomy urinary calcium is markedly lowered and the risk for continued stone formation is virtually eliminated.

The classical symptoms of primary HPT, bone disease and renal stones, are generally considered to constitute indications for surgery. There have, however, been considerable changes in the pattern of clinical presentation of primary HPT over the last few decades and nowadays about half of the patients appear to have no particular symptoms related to the biochemical disturbance (5). An important issue in this context is whether patients who appear asymptomatic really do have no symptoms attributable to HPT, and whether such patients with mild HPT benefit from parathyroid surgery.

Recent studies have revealed that psychiatric disturbances are present in a majority of unselected HPT patients and can also often be found in patients who do not spontaneously report psychiatric symptoms (6, 7). The most common psychiatric symptoms in these patients are fatiguability, lassitude, difficulty in concentration, failing memory, sadness, anxiety, sleep disturbances and irritability (Fig 1). The severity of the symptomatology is not simply related to the degree of hypercalcemia or to the serum PTH concentration and even patients with moderately elevated serum calcium can present with considerable psychiat-

ric disturbances (8). Elderly patients seem to be more sensitive to HPT and can develop severe mental disorders mimicking senile dementia (9).
Parathyroid surgery results in a clear improvement in mental health (Fig 2) in most patients with preoperative symptoms (6-9).

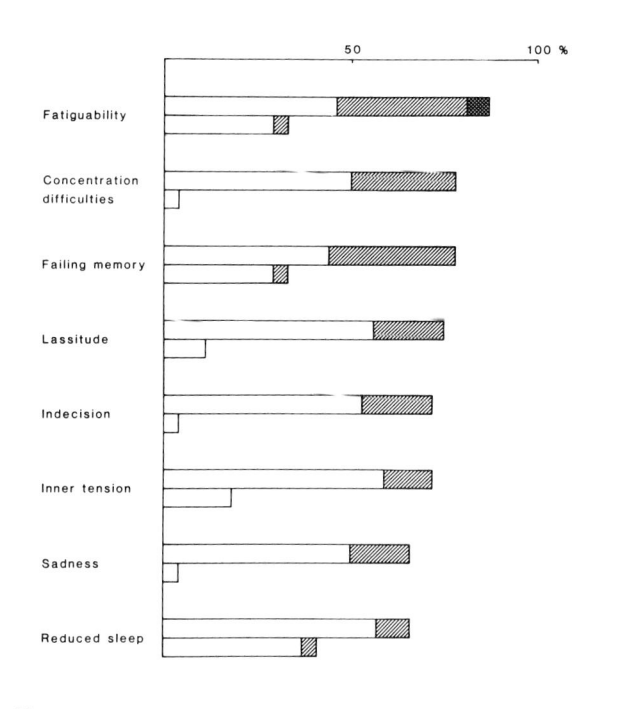

Figure 1.

The most frequent psychiatric symptoms among unselected patients with primary HPT. Proportion of patients (%) who reported each individual symptom prior to (upper bars) and after (lower bars) parathyroid surgery. Scores: 1-1.5 = moderate or periodically occurring symptom (open bars); 2-2.5 = permanent and severe symptom, interfering with normal social functioning (hatched bars); and 3 = extreme degree of symptom (solid bars).

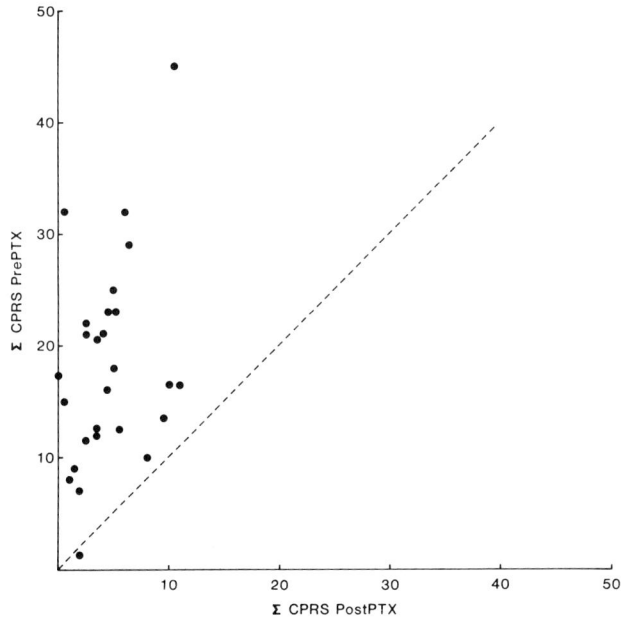

Figure 2.

Total CPRS scores prior to (PrePTX) and after (PostPTX) parathyroid surgery (N = 27). All patients to the left of the dotted line of equality represent improvement (= decrease in CPRS score) from pre- to postoperative investigation. (CPRS = comprehensive psychopathological rating scale).

Patients with primary HPT show increased concentrations of both total and ionized calcium in the cerebrospinal fluid and reduced levels of the monoamine metabolites 5-HIAA and HVA (6, 10). After parathyroid surgery the cerebrospinal fluid levels of monoamine metabolites increase concomitantly with the mental improvement. The findings suggest that calcium per se is the main factor underlying the development of psychiatric symptoms in HPT. Furthermore, there is evidence for a relationship between the central calcium and monoamine metabolism that is of possible importance for the psychiatric symptomatology in primary HPT.

As a group patients with primary HPT also have a muscle contraction defect of possible significance for the feelings of general tiredness (11). After parathyroid surgery there is an improvement in muscle strength (12) but the feelings of tiredness in HPT is probably only partly explained by true muscle weekness but also related to central factors.

III. Cardiovascular risk factors - effects of surgery

Detailed studies have revealed that a majority of, also asymptomatic, HPT patients appear to be at increased risk of acquiring cardiovascular disease. Thus, it is well known that there is an increased prevalence of hypertension and it appears that the entire population of HPT patients has a higher blood pressure than matched controls, i.e. the frequency distribution of blood pressure is shifted to the right with a higher mean value for diastolic blood pressure of around 10 mmHg. The reason for the raised blood pressure is not known and an impairment of renal function is not the only explanation. Influence on sympathetic nerves, on the renin-angiotensin-aldosteron system as well as a direct influence of calcium on the vascular wall have been suggested, but neither of them can be an entirely sufficient explanation.

The direct association between primary HPT and hypertension is questioned by the repeat observation that successful parathyroidectomy will not uniformely normalize blood pressure. Several, also longer term, follow-up studies clearly demonstrate persistent and even aggravated hypertension following parathyroid surgery. Despite the simultaneous occurrence of hypertension and HPT the absence of postoperative improvement suggests that the two disorders may be indirectly associated without a simple cause-and-effect relationship.

Also an impaired glucose tolerance and type II diabetes mellitus are found more often than expected among HPT patients. This appears to be mainly attributed to a reduced peripheral sensitivity to insulin caused by PTH whereas the secretion of insulin in response to glucose is enhanced. Some reports with only a few patients have claimed that there could be a postoperative improvement in already manifest diabetes mellitus of both type I and type II. This is, however, not a uniform experience and larger follow-up studies with regard to glucose tolerance have rather revealed a significant impairment due to a postoperative reduction of the peak insulin response to glucose (13).

Thus, similar to hypertension it seems that the disturbed regulation of glucose metabolism is not a simple consequence of primary HPT and that neither hypertension nor the occurrence of diabetes mellitus or impaired glucose tolerance will strengthen the indication for surgery.

Parathyroid hormone also affects lipolysis and lipoprotein metabolism. Many patients with primary HPT have hyperlipoproteinemia with both hypertriglyceridemia and hypercholesterolemia. In these cases there is generally a normalization after parathyroid surgery (14).

As regards the traditional cardiovascular risk factors all appear to be unfavourably affected in the hyperparathyroid state but without uniform alleviation after parathyroid surgery. Thus, it cannot be simply predicted from the risk factor profile if surgery for primary HPT will affect cardiovascular morbidity and mortality.

IV. Cardiovascular disease in primary HPT

Patients with primary HPT appear to have a higher than expected frequency of diseases of the circulatory organs. In a recent long-term follow-up study of 172 patients with mild hypercalcemia it was found that among those who were below 70 years of age when hypercalcemia was discovered there was a significantly (approximately doubled) increased mortality during a 13-year follow-up (15). Most of the excess mortality could be attributed to cardio- or cerebrovascular disease. In that study the hypercalcemic persons differed from the normocalcemic controls by having significantly higher values for systolic and diastolic blood pressure and there was also a tendency toward higher serum glucose and cholesterol values. However, also after taking these variables into account in a multivariate analysis the estimated effect of hypercalcemia on survival did not disappear. This indicates that the elevated serum calcium concentration had specific influence. Although these, unattended, patients with presumed mild HPT had serum calcium values within a narrow range (mean 2.72 ± 0.14 mmol/l) there was a direct relationship between the level of serum calcium and mortality, i.e. with a higher mortality in those with the highest serum calcium.

It is not clarified whether surgery for HPT will reduce the risk of premature death. In a study where 441 patients were followed after surgery for up to 15 years it appeared that there was an excess death rate throughout the follow-up period (16). This was mainly referrable to a higher than expected death rates during the first postoperative years and the increased risk appeared to be gradually diminished thereafter.

V. HPT and malignant diseases

A number of case reports have described an association between HPT and various malignancies and there are also a few studies which suggest that patients with HPT could be more prone to have a concomitant malignancy. In a recent cohort study (17) over 4,000 patients who had been operated for primary HPT were followed for up to 22 years. The occurrence of malignant disease manifested after the parathyroid operation was investigated through a nationwide Cancer Registry. It was found that the operated HPT patients suffered malignant diseases significantly more often than the background population (relative risk 1.6). The increased risk could not be attributed to any specific site. The findings indicate that HPT either promotes later development of malignant tumours or that HPT and certain malignancies have etiologic factors in common. The increased risk did not diminish with the observation time but it cannot be evaluated if it was affected by the surgery.

Concluding remarks

The cause of primary HPT is unknown. The propensity for long-term recurrence and the lack of a simple cause and effect relationship between prominent symptoms and the biochemical disturbances suggest that so-called primary HPT in fact in some patients could be a secondary compensation for some underlying disturbance. Until the causes of primary HPT can be identified and specific therapy and/or prophylaxis instituted we believe that surgery is the preferred treatment in a majority of the diagnosed cases. Our reasons for a general recommendation for surgery are the common improvement of subjective symptoms and the higher risk of premature death due to circulatory diseases in unattended HPT.

However, it should be remembered that it is often difficult to distinguish with certainty the existence of primary HPT in a patient with only marginally elevated serum calcium levels and that in such cases the surgical procedure is more difficult with a greater risk of both persistent and recurrent hypercalcemia. In view of the great number of patients who have mild primary HPT, the likelihood that they have symptoms related to this disorder and the possibility that surgery can cure them permanently it should be investigated in a prospective, controlled, fashion if the benefit of surgery is worth the costs and the potential risks.

REFERENCES

1   Åkerström G, Bergström R, Grimelius L, Johansson H, Ljunghall S, Lundström B, Palmér M, Rastad J, Rudberg C. Relation between changes in

clinical and histopathological features of primary hyperparathyroidism. World J Surg 1986;10:696-702.
2. Wallfelt C, Gylfe E, Larsson R, Ljunghall S, Rastad J, Åkerström G. Relation between external and cytoplasmic calcium concentrations, parathyroid hormone release and glandular weight in hyperparathyroidism. J Endocrinol 1988;116:457-464.
3. Rudberg C, Åkerström G, Adami H-O, Johansson H, Ljunghall S, Palmér M. Late results of 441 patients operated on for primary hyperparathyroidism. Surgery 1986;99:643-651.
4. Åkerström G, Rudberg C, Grimelius L, Bergström R, Johansson H, Ljunghall S, Rastad J. Histologic parathyroid abnormalities in an autopsy material. Hum Pathol 1986;17:520-527.
5. Palmér M, Ljunghall S, Åkerström G, Adami H-O, Bergström R, Grimelius L, Rudberg C, Johansson H. Patients with primary hyperparathyroidism operated over a 24-year period: temporal trends of clinical and laboratory findings. J Chron Dis 1987;40:121-130.
6. Joborn C, Hetta J, Rastad J, Ågren H, Åkerström G, Ljunghall S. Psychiatric symptoms and cerebrospinal fluid monoamine metabolites in patients with primary hyperparathyroidism. Biol Psychiatry 1988;23:149-158.
7. Joborn C, Hetta J, Lind L, Rastad J, Åkerström G, Ljunghall S. Self-rated psychiatric symptoms in patients with primary hyperparathyroidism. Surgery (in press).
8. Joborn C, Hetta J, Palmér M, Åkerström G, Ljunghall S. Psychiatric symptomatology in patients with primary hyperparathyroidism. Ups J Med Sci 1986;91:77-88.
9. Joborn C, Hetta J, Frisk P, Palmér M, Åkerström G, Ljunghall S. Primary hyperparathyroidism in patients with organic brain syndrome. Acta Med Scand 1985;219:91-98.
10. Joborn C, Hetta J, Niklasson F, Rastad J, Ågren H, Åkerström G, Ljunghall S. Cerebrospinal fluid calcium, parathyroid hormone and the blood-brain barrier in primary hyperparathyroidism. Relation to CSF monoamine and purine metabolism (submitted).
11. Joborn C, Rastad J, Stålberg E, Åkerström G, Ljunghall S. Muscle contractility in patients with primary hyperparathyroidism. Muscle & Nerve (in press).
12. Joborn C, Joborn H, Rastad J, Åkerström G, Ljunghall S. Maximal isokinetic muscle strength in patients with primary hyperparathyroidism before and after parathyroid surgery. Brit J Surg 1988;75:77-80.
13. Ljunghall S, Palmér M, Åkerström G, Wide L. Diabetes mellitus, glucose tolerance and insulin response to glucose in patients with primary hyperparathyroidism before and after parathyroidectomy. Eur J Clin Invest 1983;13:373-377.
14. Ljunghall S, Lithell H, Vessby B, Wide L. Glucose and lipoprotein metabolism in primary hyperparathyroidism. Effects of parathyroidectomy. Acta Endocrinol (Kbh) 1978;89:580-589.
15. Palmér M, Adami H-O, Bergström R, Jakobsson S, Åkerström G, Ljunghall S. Survival and renal function in persons with untreated hypercalcemia: a population-based cohort study with 14 years of follow-up. Lancet 1987;i:59-62.
16. Palmér M, Adami H-O, Bergström R, Åkerström G, Ljunghall S. Mortality after operation for primary hyperparathyroidism: a nation-wide cohort study. Surgery 1987;102:1-7.
17. Palmér M, Adami H-O, Krusemo U-B, Ljunghall S. Increased risk of malignant diseases after operation for primary hyperparathyroidism: a nation-wide cohort study. Amer J Epidemiol (in press).

Primary Hyperparathyroidism in the 1980s

JOHN P. BILEZIKIAN, SHONNI J. SILVERBERG,
and ELIZABETH SHANE

Departments of Medicine and Pharmacology
College of Physicians and Surgeons
New York, NY

The management of primary hyperparathyroidism in the 1980's has become uncertain because of a different clinical profile of the disease that has emerged over the past 15 years (1,2). When primary hyperparathyroidism was accompanied by nephrolithiasis, osteitis fibrosa cystica, neuromuscular disease, or other abnormalities attributable to the disorder, surgical removal of the offending parathyroid adenoma was a reasonable course of action. With routine use of the multichannel autoanalyzer in the late 1960's and early 1970's, primary hyperparathyroidism began to show not only an increasing incidence but also a form of disease characterized only by mild, asymptomatic hypercalcemia. The disease was frequently characterized not by 'bones, stones and groans,' but rather by a lack of specific symptomatology. In the absence of bone and stone disease and other established concomitants of the hyperparathyroid state, asymptomatic primary hyperparathyroidism became and continues to be the most common presentation of this disorder.

Several key questions have resulted from these observations. First, in the patient with primary hyperparathyroidism and mild, asymptomatic hypercalcemia, can other evidence for parathyroid disease be discovered upon more detailed evaluation? Second, does the asymptomatic form of the disorder eventually lead to overt evidence of target organ involvement classically associated with primary hyperparathyroidism (3-4)? If so, can it be established prospectively who is at risk? To answer these questions, a long-term study is needed in which routine clinical assessment of sufficient numbers of patients with primary hyperparathyroidism can be combined with more sensitive methods of analysis. To these ends, we have embarked upon our investigation. Through April, 1988, 67 patients with well-documented primary hyperparathyroidism have joined our study cohort. After the diagnosis of primary hyperparathyroidism is established and routine tests are obtained, a set of more detailed examinations are conducted. These include a detailed neuromuscular examination, dietary calcium analysis, bone densitometry of lumbar, femoral and radial sites, quantitative static and dynamic indices of the percutaneous bone biopsy specimen, as well as circulating markers of parathyroid hormone and vitamin D.

The patient population shows a preponderance of women (58 +/- 2 years) over men (55 +/- 3 years) by 2.5:1. The group of subjects ranges in age from 26 to 77. The average serum calcium is 11.1 +/- 0.1 mg/dl, a value only slightly above the upper limits of normal (10.7 mg/dl). The serum phosphorus is 2.8 +/- 0.1 mg/dl (nl, 2.5-4.5 mg/dl). Utilizing three different immunoassays for parathyroid hormone, increases are found in the vast majority of patients. Determination of parathyroid hormone by 'mid-molecule' radioimmunoassay and by 'intact' immunoradiometric assays show frankly elevated values in 94 and 96% of patients respectively. By comparison, the 'N-terminal' radioimmunoassay shows elevations in a majority but smaller percentage of patients, 79%. 25-Hydroxyvitamin D levels are within normal limits as is the average 1,25-dihydroxyvitamin D concentration. 35% of our patients, however, have frankly elevated levels of the active vitamin D metabolite. 31% of the patients demonstrate urinary calcium excretion greater than 250 mg/g Cr.

The relatively mild biochemical indices of primary hyperparathyroidism in this group are associated with similarly diminished percentages of patients showing overt evidence for involvement of the skeleton and kidneys. In a representative group of patients in whom complete radiographs of the skull, hands, pelvis and spine were obtained, no patient showed specific signs of parathyroid bone disease (osteitis fibrosa cystica, brown tumors, subperiosteal bone resorption). Only 19% of patients had a history of nephrolithiasis and only one patient demonstrated a neuromuscular syndrome consistent with the classical description of the disease.

We are particularly interested to know whether these patients with primary hyperparathyroidism, most of whom conform to the modern day presentation of the disease, will show evidence for bone involvement when a more sensitive set of evaluations is undertaken (5). Bone densitometry was performed at the lumbar spine, distal radius, and hip, sites comprised predominantly of trabecular, cortical, or a mixture of trabecular and cortical bone respectively. As the site monitored corresponded more completely to cortical bone, the evidence for parathyroid involvement became greater. At the distal radius, predominantly cortical bone, 58% of patients showed a reduction in bone mineral density to less than 80% of age and sex-matched control subjects. In contrast, at the lumbar spine, a site of predominantly trabecular bone, only 13% of patients showed a reduction in bone mineral density to less than 80% of expected.

The results suggesting 'asymptomatic' involvement of bones by the hyperparathyroid process are consistent with the preferential physiological actions of parathyroid hormone upon cortical bone but surprising considering the clinical profile presented by these patients. Direct examination of bone biopsy specimens, however, helped to confirm these findings. The vast majority of patients (84%) had mean cortical width determinations below expected whereas an equivalently large number of patients (85%) showed trabecular bone volume greater than average values. The preservation of trabecular bone and loss of cortical bone support the results obtained by bone densitometry.

Insofar as its expectations are concerned, this tudy is still in its infancy. The results, nevertheless, are beginning to call into question the meaning of the term, "asymptomatic primary hyperparathyroidism." If bone involvement by the hyperparathyroid process can be detected by measures not routinely employed in the evaluation of the patient with primary hyperparathyroidism (bone densitometry and bone hystomorphometry), it suggests that one may not be able to know whether or not a patient is free of bone disease until these tests are performed. On the other hand, evidence for a hyperparathyroid process at one point in time does not necessarily predict progression of disease over time. Obviously, the longitudinal aspects of this study will provide needed information along these lines.

An additional insight concerns the postmenopausal woman with primary hyperparathyroidism. It is widely believed that primary hyperparathyroidism places a postmenopausal woman at increased risk for osteoporosis (6). With regard to the vertebral skeleton, the data suggest that this may not be the case for the form of primary hyperparathyroidism seen today. In fact, the data suggest that trabecular bone of the vertebral spine may be preserved in the early phases of primary hyperparathyroidism. On the other hand, preservation of the vertebral spine may occur at the expense of equally vital bone, in the appendicular skeleton. How the effects of parathyroid hormone excess at these different skeletal sites should be evaluated with respect to advice regarding management is going to require much more information than we have at the current time.

Acknowledgements

This project involves a large number of collaborating investigators who are gratefully acknowledged: Luz de la Cruz, R.N., David W. Dempster, Ph.D., Frieda Feldman, M.D., David Seldin M.D., Thomas P. Jacobs, M.D., Ethel S. Siris, M.D., Maureen Cafferty, M.D., May V. Parisien, M.D., Robert Lindsay, M.D., and Thomas L. Clemens, Ph.D. The investigation is supported, in part, by AM32333 from the National Institutes of Health.

References

1. Heath H, Hodgson SF, Kennedy MA. Primary hyperparathyroidism: incidence, morbidity and economic impact in a community. N Engl J Med 1980; 302:189-193.

2. Mundy GR, Cove DH, Fisken R, Sommers S, Heath DA. Primary hyperparathyroidism: changes in the pattern of clinical presentation. Lancet 1980; 1:1317-1320.

3. Bilezikian, JP. Clinical disorders of the parathyroid glands. In: Clinical Endocrinology of Calcium Metabolism (Raisz LG and Martin TJ, eds). Marcel Dekker, New York, 53-97, 1987.

4. Patten BM, Bilezikian JP, Mallette LM, and Aurbach GD. The neuromuscular disease of hyperparathyroidism. Annals Int Med 80:182-194, 1974.

5. Silverberg SS, Shane E, de la Cruz L, Dempster DW, Jacobs TJ, Siris, ES, Parisien MV, Seldin D and Bilezikian JP. Skeletal disease in primary hyperparathyroidism. J Bone Min Res 3:Suppl 1,89A, 1988.

6. Hodgson SF and Heath H, III. Asymptomatic primary hyperparathyroidism: treat or follow? Mayo Clin Proc 56:521-523, 1981.

Discussion:

DR. LANG (New Haven): I'd like to ask both speakers what their experience is in hyperparathyroidism in women who have estrogen versus women who don't have estrogen, either naturally or by replacement. Do they see any difference in bone disease? That's been around in the literature for quite a few years. And, in fact, our studies recently have shown that the only patients who seem to lose bone are women who are low in estrogen.

DR. BILEZIKIAN (New York): Bob, I'm sorry, I didn't get the beginning of your question.

DR. LANG: I'm wondering if the patients who are losing bone are women who are low in estrogen. That's what we have found in our patients. Dr. Melsen spoke earlier in the week and said he doesn't see that. I'm starting to see that in different geographical areas, we're seeing a variety of responses of bone to many different hormones, environmental factors such as renal osteodystrophy, et cetera. I'm wondering what your experience is. You're not very far, geographically. And I'm also interested in what they see in Sweden.

DR. BILEZIKIAN: Right. The overwhelming majority of our patients, interestingly, are, indeed, postmenopausal women within ten years of the menopause, point one. Point two is, with the exception of one patient, none of them is being treated with estrogens.

DR. MARCUS (Palo Alto, CA): My remarks are sort of along the same issue of the possibility of a confound with estrogen. First, I'd like to suggest that maybe it's time that Dr. Bilezikian take some sabbatical leave and go to France where he would learn that duck, actually, is all dark meat and is all type 1 muscle fiber.

I'm a little concerned about your 1,25 measurements. I think that the so-called normal range of 10 to 60 is something which most commercial laboratories will define for you as sort as in the general population. I think that if you look at the normal levels of 1,25 in a postmenopausal non-estrogen-replaced population, they will be substantially lower. We have data in just 20 women where the mean value is 28 picograms per milliliter and two standard deviations goes up only to about 42. So, I would say that your average level for age and estrogen status is probably high.

I'm very alarmed by the data that Dr. Ljunghall presented. I'm not alarmed by the data; I'm alarmed by their implications. And I wanted to ask, in particular, in terms of some of the mortality issues and psychiatric issues what the estrogen status of those women are. Clearly, the data appears to be getting stronger all the time that estrogen replacement is associated with a 40 percent reduction in total mortality. And I wonder how much of the apparent excess mortality compared to what you would have predicted for age might be that you are looking at a uniquely non-estrogen-treated group of subjects.

DR. LJUNGHALL (Sweden): We have the same type of population as Dr. Bilezikian presented: almost all women are postmenopausal. And in Sweden, there is no tradition of a postmenopausal estrogen used for more than, say, six months or one year. So, all of these patients, more less every one of them, are without estrogens.

DR. MARCUS: I just think that it may be that those women who take estrogen may be protected against the emergence of hyperparathyroidism or making the diagnosis of hyperparathyroidism. So, you may have a population selected, just on the basis of their estrogen status, for excess mortality. And that might be a confound. It might not be hyperparathyroidism itself.

DR. LAFFERTY (Cleveland): I'd like to address my remarks to Dr. Ljunghall on his excellent surgical follow up. We've recently completed a five-year follow up on 100 patients operated on in Cleveland and found many of the same things you did, in terms of the response to psychiatric symptoms and lack of response to hypertension.

As you said, 95 percent of these people are cured at one year, but when you get out to five years, the morbidity in terms of recurrence rate, persistence, and the prevalence of hypoparathyroidism approaches 18 percent, the same kind of figures that Sivula found from Helsinke.

What is your prevalence at your 15 and 20-year follow up of hypoparathyroidism? Did you measure the calciums in all these patients?

DR. LJUNGHALL: I think it's in the order of 3 to 5 percent, something like that. We don't have any late cases of hypopara's. They generally occur within the first year or so.

DR. BELL (Charleston): I want to address a comment and a question to both speakers. The first is that the increasing incidence of primary hyperparathyroidism with age looks like the Gompertzian phenomenon that was described for osteoporosis. And, according to Dr. Melsen, this phenomenon has universality. The question is raised therefore whether strategies could be devised to intervene and prevent the development or occurrence of the disease.

A second comment is that there have been some very interesting studies from Vanderbilt on patients with rheumatoid arthritis, concerning morbidity and mortality. An extremely interesting finding is that socioeconomic status has a major effect on morbidity and mortality in rheumatoid arthritis. We normally think of this as being a benign disease but, in fact, there is a surprising degree of mortality associated with it. This phenomenon has been described in other diseases. The question is, have either of you seen any relationship, in your studies, between mortality and morbidity, and socioeconomic status?

DR. BILEZIKIAN: We haven't looked at that, Norman.

DR. LJUNGHALL: As regards your first question, we have thought in these lines as well. And as discussed earlier, I think estrogens and perhaps also vitamin D could be implicated in the pathogenesis of HPT.

And as to your last question, we are conducting such a study now, for the last two years, a case-control study addressing these questions. But I don't have the answers yet.

DR. MALLUCHE (Lexington, KY): Dr. Bilezikian, I enjoyed your presentation. I just would like to ask you one question. You commented on the incidence of renal stones as a complication of hyperparathyroidism. You didn't give us information on nephrocalcinosis. We found that if we induce hypercalciuria in experimental animals for a relatively short period of time, we see rather early a loss in kidney function, most probably related to interstitial nephritis, and nephrocalcinosis. Do you follow your patients for that?

DR. BILEZIKIAN: We are following our patients for that. When I said nephrolithiasis, I meant stone disease, either by history, documented history, or by the presence of a stone. We're not doing CAT scanning on our patients, so I can't say that there isn't nephrocalcinosis. But by routine flat films, we aren't seeing it.

DR. ZIEGLER (Heidelberg): Dr. Ljunghall, I was surprised that you didn't see a correlation between the severity of psychic complaints and the degrees of hypercalcemia, because there are papers documenting such a correlation. Did you try to correct this for age? The reason I ask is that younger persons tolerate hypercalcemia better. So, do you have the same result if choosing, for instance, age groups?

DR. LJUNGHALL: The short answer is yes.

DR. ZIEGLER: And again, no correlation?

DR. LJUNGHALL: There is some impact of age, but the lack of relationship is not due to the various ages. Maybe I will say we have quite a narrow span of both serum calcium and age. I mean, most of our patients are quite mildly hypercalcemic.

DR. BONE (Detroit): I have just a quick comment and short questions. The comment would be that, with the ascertainment being much more incidental, the fact that the patient was discovered to have hypercalcemia may have to do with their being treated for another disease, and this may have something to do with the fact that there is an associated cardiovascular risk. That may be why they were getting a calcium measured in the first place, as a part of their SMAC.

I had a question about methodology for each speaker. First, in the Scandinavian study, what are you doing about different surgical techniques at different centers, whether both sides of the neck are looked at, and that kind of thing?

DR. LJUNGHALL: The first question, our long-term follow up studies, one dealt with patients discovered in the health survey. They had no apparent symptoms at the time of discovery. And yet, they had this increased risk of mortality.

DR. BONE: They had no increased reason to participate in this study? There was no other reason, such as a pre-existing illness, why they might be more likely to - a patient, ill person, might be more likely to participate in that health survey?

DR. LJUNGHALL: That was computer-based, the follow ups. There was 99 percent compliance.

And the question about surgical techniques, there are only a few centers in Sweden that operate for HPT. And I believe they, on the whole, have very similar operative techniques and results. So, I don't think that would influence the data very much.

DR. BONE: I see. And Dr. Bilezikian, how are you following renal function, with respect to Dr. Malluche's question; how are you measuring renal function to look for effects on the interstitium of the kidney?

DR. BILEZIKIAN: Crudely, by creatinine clearance. But that's being measured every three months.

DR. BONE: I see. Thank you.

DR. TALPOS: Comment. The parathyroidectomy that Tiblin does is significantly different in technique from that done by Lindquist of Linkoping or Hamburger or Grandburg in Stockholm. He rarely explores the second side of the neck.

DR. HARRIS (San Francisco): Some years ago, follow up data from the Mayo Clinic suggested that patients who had undergone successful parathyroidectomy in fact had a tendency to show normocalcemia but elevated levels of PTH. I should say a significant minority of patients showed that finding at, I believe it was, five years of follow up. Would either one of the speakers care to comment upon that phenomenon?

DR. LJUNGHALL: I think that's an interesting idea, because the way we have looked at this disease, it is that it's not just a question of one gland becoming diseased and then everything is fixed when it's taken away. So, we're looking at that problem. We have not yet found any patients with elevated PTH during our long-term follow up.

I have a question for Dr. Bilezikian in that area, if I may. My question is if during your follow up any patient normalized parathyroid function.

DR. BILEZIKIAN: 19 of our 62 patients have been operated on, and with all but one have normalized calcium and PTH levels. There is one patient who has normal calciums but elevated PTH's, consistently.

DR. McKENNA (Boston): Regarding the histological finding of increased trabecular bone volume, I just wonder whether that might be a consequence of the thinning of the cortex, which tends to be endosteal bone loss so there's a trabeculization of the cortex, maybe providing thicker trabecular plates, and that might be more consistent with the DPA findings.

DR. BILEZIKIAN: That's an interesting thought. We're right now trying to look at what the basis of that apparent preservation of trabecular bone volume is, whether it's at the level of the trabecular plate, or numbers, or how it's configured. But we really don't have data yet for that.

DR. RAO (Detroit): In your prospective follow up protocol, I heard you say that these were all within ten years of menopause. And if you're measuring, how are you going to make any adjustments, for example, if there is a rapid fall due to early estrogen deficiency during this ten-year period? How do you separate, for example, if the bone density falls with time, whether it is due to the continued accelerated bone loss that has occurred or occurring due to estrogen deficiency or whether it is occurring because of the excess parathyroid hormone secretion?

DR. BILEZIKIAN: That's a long question that has even a longer answer. There are several ways of doing that. Site specific, as well as bone biopsy, we should be able to distinguish these points.

DR. MUCHMORE (LaJolla, CA): For Dr. Ljunghall, a quick question. You found no correlation between the serum calcium and the psychiatric symptoms. Did you try to correlate the parathyroid hormones with the psychiatric symptoms?

DR. LJUNGHALL: No correlation.

VIII
Metabolic Bone Diseases in Children

Overview: Metabolic Bone Disease in Children

MICHAEL P. WHYTE

Division of Bone and Mineral Diseases
Departments of Medicine and Pediatrics
The Jewish Hospital of St. Louis
and Washington University School of Medicine
and Metabolic Research Unit
Shriners Hospital for Crippled Children
St. Louis, MO

The first two presentations of this session concerned inborn errors of metabolism that present during infancy or childhood-carbonic anhydrase II deficiency and hypophosphatasia. Each is a rare but instructive enzymopathy that impairs one "end" of the bone remodeling process.

Dr. William S. Sly, Professor and Chairman, Department of Biochemistry, St. Louis University School of Medicine, St. Louis, Missouri, described how the autosomal recessive syndrome of osteopetrosis/renal tubular acidosis/cerebral calcification, first reported in 1972, was found in 1983 to be a new inborn error of metabolism. Selective absence of the carbonic anhydrase II (CA II) isoenzyme was discovered in patient erythrocytes and half-normal CA II levels were demonstrated in the red cells of obligate carriers. Deficiency of this isoenzyme remains to be shown in bone and kidney tissue. Thirty patients have been reported to date. Clinical expressivity is variable, but generally resembles "intermediate" forms of osteopetrosis. Radiographs show a developmental form of generalized osteosclerosis with features typical of osteopetrosis, that may improve with aging; cerebral calcification is widespread on computed tomography. Most patients have both a proximal and distal renal tubular acidosis. Histopathologic study of bone reveals evidence of unresorbed primary spongiosa - a characteristic feature of all human forms of osteopetrosis. Dr. Sly discussed what this new inborn error of metabolism reveals concerning the physiological role of CA II- including a likely function in osteoclast-mediated bone resorption.

Dr. Michael P. Whyte, Associate Professor of Medicine, Washington University School of Medicine, St. Louis, Missouri, then presented an overview of hypophosphatasia - a heritable form of rickets/osteomalacia that is characterized by deficient activity of the tissue nonspecific (liver/bone/kidney) isoenzyme of alkaline phosphatase (TNSALP); placental and intestinal ALP activity is unaffected. Clinical expressivity is extremely variable and ranges from intrauterine death from profound skeletal undermineralization to onset of recurrent, slowly healing stress fractures in adult life. Premature loss of deciduous teeth is the most sensitive clinical manifestation in children. Rickets occurs although serum levels of calcium and phosphate are not subnormal. There is no effective medical treatment for hypophosphatasia, but early prenatal diagnosis of severe forms is possible. Three phosphocompounds, phosphoethanolamine, inorganic pyrophosphate (PPi), and pyridoxal-5^1-phosphate (PLP) accumulate endogenously. Dr. Whyte reviews how the recent discovery that plasma PLP levels are elevated in all patients with hypophosphatasia indicates that TNSALP functions as an ectoenzyme to regulate extracellular, but not intracellular, levels of a variety of phosphocompounds. Identification in 1988 of a missense mutation in the TNSALP gene in a patient with classic perinatal (lethal) hypophosphatasia provides unequivocal evidence for a role for TNSALP in skeletal mineralization. Absence of ecto-TNSALP activity results in extracellular accumulation of PPi, an inhibitor of hydroxyapatite crystal formation, which could account for the defective skeletal mineralization.

Dr. Russell W. Chesney, Professor and Chairman, Department of Pediatrics, University of Tennessee College of Medicine, Memphis, Tennessee, then described Williams Syndrome. Affected children characteristically have a variety of phenotypic abnormalities including an elfin facies, microcephaly, stellate iris, epicanthal folds, and cardiac defects including supravalvular aortic stenosis. Mental deficiency and characteristic personality traits help to make patients relatively easy to identify. Hypercalcemia occurs in about 15% of subjects and is associated with failure to thrive, calcification of the media of blood vessels, hypercalciuria, and nephrocalcinosis. Williams Syndrome is generally a sporadic disorder, but familial cases have been reported. Dr. Chesney reviewed what is known about the pathophysiology of the hypercalcemia - including evidence for enhanced sensitivity to vitamin D with excessive intestinal absorption of calcium and evidence for a possible defect in calcitropic hormone regulation, since clearance of intravenously administered calcium is decreased in Williams Syndrome.

Dr. Peter H. Byers, Professor of Pathology and Medicine, University of Washington, Seattle, Washington, then presented a discussion of the molecular basis for the clinical heterogeneity of osteogenesis imperfecta (OI). It is now clear that most clinical forms of OI result from mutations that affect the expression or structure of the genes that form type I collagen. Following a description of type I collagen biosynthesis, Dr. Byers summarized the specific biochemical and molecular defects which have thus far been shown to cause the various clinical (Sillence) types of OI. In addition to the rare instances of gene deletion or large rearrangements, more commonly a variety of point mutations are now being identified in the different forms. Previously it was believed that severe type II OI was inherited as an autosomal recessive trait, but now it appears from molecular biological studies that this form results more commonly from sporadic mutation or, when siblings are affected, from gonadal mosaicism. Accordingly, the recurrence risk is considerably less than the 25% for true autosomal recessive disorders. Dr. Byers then reviewed the relationship between the clinical phenotype in OI and the nature of the specific molecular defect. Our rapidly improving comprehension of the molecular basis for this clinically heterogeneous disorder should help to direct potential medical therapies for the various types of OI.

Dr. Laura S. Hillman, Professor of Pediatrics, University of Missouri Medical School, Columbia, Missouri, reviewed the neonatal disorders of mineral metabolism - including early and late neonatal hypocalcemia and mineralization problems in premature and term infants. Controversies regarding the diagnostic criteria for early neonatal hypocalcemia and the need for therapy were discussed. The necessity of using biochemical criteria, based upon serum ionized calcium rather than total calcium determination, was emphasized. The mineral and hormonal changes of early and late neonatal hypocalcemia are reviewed; the role of hypomagnesemia in the latter condition is emphasized. Dr. Hillman discussed how, in term infants, disorders of skeletal mineralization are often related to vitamin D deficiency. However, in premature infants fed breast milk, osteopenia/rickets has resulted from inadequate delivery of mineral to the skeleton. She emphasized the role of both phosphorus and calcium supplementation for correction of this problem and reviewed areas where further research is necessary. Dr. Hillman's presentation was followed by an interesting discussion session which emphasized the regulation of placental function in skeletal mineralization of the fetus.

Dr. Francis H. Glorieux, Professor of Surgery and Human Genetics, McGill University, Montreal, Quebec, discussed the clinical expression, pathogenesis, and medical treatment of vitamin D resistant hypophosphatemic rickets (VDRR). Controversy continues as to whether this most common form of inherited rickets in North America results from the elaboration of a humoral factor that causes selective renal phosphate wasting, or a more generalized cellular defect that involves the gut and bone as well as kidney. The mouse model for VDRR continues to provide useful information. In 1987, the gene for VDRR in humans was mapped to the distal part of the short arm of the X chromosome. Characterization of the aberrant gene and its product now becomes feasible. Dr. Glorieux described how phosphate supplementation together with administration of calcitriol has resulted in improved growth rate, radiographic healing of rickets and, in some subjects, correction of the mineralization defect at trabecular bone surfaces. A lively discussion followed Dr. Glorieux's presentation concerning how hyperparathyroidism provoked by phosphate supplementation can be minimized in VDRR and what effects this medical regimen has on the kidney of these patients.

Osteopetrosis with Renal Tubular Acidosis and Cerebral Calcification: The Carbonic Anhydrase II Deficiency Syndrome

WILLIAM S. SLY

Edward A. Doisy Department of Biochemistry and Molecular Biology
St. Louis University School of Medicine
St. Louis, MO

Introduction

Since osteopetrosis (marble bone disease) was first described in 1904 by Albers-Schonberg, over 300 cases have been reported (1). Two principal types were distinguished. An autosomal dominant form was called the adult, benign form because the benign course is compatible with a normal lifespan. A clinically severe, autosomal recessive, "malignant, lethal" form has its onset in infancy and produces anemia, leukopenia, hepatomegaly, failure to thrive, cranial nerve symptoms, and early death. Although multiple genetic causes produce osteopetrosis, the common mechanism underlying all forms is thought to be failure of bone resorption.

The association of renal tubular acidosis with osteopetrosis was reported in 1972 (2, 3). The initial pedigrees suggested autosomal recessive inheritance. The clinical course, though not entirely benign, was much milder than the course of the recessive lethal form and was compatible with long survival. The hematologic abnormalities associated with the recessive lethal form of osteopetrosis were mild or absent. In 1980, Ohlsson et al. (4) reported the additional finding of cerebral calcification in four children with osteopetrosis and renal tubular acidosis from Saudi Arabia. Calcification of the basal ganglia in the original American kindred was reported independently by Whyte et al. (5) the same year.

In 1983, Sly et al. (6) reported that the three sisters from the original American kindred with this syndrome lacked carbonic anhydrase II (CA II) in their erythrocytes, and that their normal appearing parents had half-normal levels of CA II in erythrocyte lysates. These observations, coupled with the fact that CA II was the only known soluble isozyme of CA in kidney and brain, led them to propose that CA II deficiency is the primary defect in this newly recognized metabolic disorder of bone, kidney, and brain.

In a subsequent report, Sly et al. (7) extended these studies to 18 additional patients in 11 unrelated families of different geographical and ethnic origins. Subsequently, Ohlsson et al. (8) reported four additional Saudi Arabian patients, including the first affected neonate, and summarized the clinical features of 21 reported patients. Recently, Cochat et al. (9) added an additional case and provided an excellent review of the clinical findings on the 30 patients reported to date. Deficiency of CA II was found in erythrocyte lysates of every patient identified with this syndrome.

Clinical Manifestations

There is considerable variability in the age of onset and the severity of clinical manifestations. All have renal tubular acidosis and eventually develop osteopetrosis and cerebral calcification. Additional features include growth failure, mental retardation, and dental malocclusion. Bone fractures and other complications of osteopetrosis have dominated the clinical picture in some patients. Symptoms of metabolic acidosis including failure to thrive, developmental retardation, and growth retardation have been more prominent in others.

Clinical Bone Disease

The osteopetrosis results from a generalized accumulation of bone mass that is secondary to a defect in bone resorption. This defect prevents normal development of marrow cavities, the normal tubulation of long bones, and the enlargement of osseous foramina. Anemia is rarely profound in patients with CA II deficiency, though two patients had sufficient anemia to be referred for bone marrow transplantation. The clinical manifestations of osteopetrosis in the CA II deficiency syndrome tend to be milder than in the recessive, lethal form of osteopetrosis. They appear later, and they also tend to improve over time.

The radiologic findings in patients with the CA II deficiency syndrome are not distinguishable from those in patients with other forms of osteopetrosis. Increased bone density, abnormal modeling, delay or failure of normal tubulation of long bones, transverse banding of metaphyses, fractures, and "bone in bone" appearance are all seen. However, the changes vary with age. In the only neonate studied to date, the radiologic features were too subtle to justify the diagnosis at 23 days of age, even though the hyperchloremic metabolic acidosis and alkaline urine were already prominent findings. This observation suggests that the osteopetrosis is usually a postpartum developmental abnormality. The first patient reported by Gibaud also had no osteopetrosis at age four months, but typical findings evolved and progressed over the first three years of life (9). In at least some patients, the radiologic features of osteopetrosis, which were fully developed in childhood, improved substantially after puberty. The radiographs may normalize as patients move into adulthood (5).

Bone fractures are common in childhood in many patients, with some reporting 15-30 fractures by mid adolescence. After puberty, the frequency of bone fractures decreases. Fractures were the most prominent symptoms in the American patients (5) and the Belgian patient in whom mental retardation was not present (3). Fractures were not seen in Guibaud's patients (2, 9).

Symptoms of cranial nerve compression secondary to osteopetrosis occur in 60% of reported patients, but are milder than in the recessive, lethal form. Although frank optic nerve atrophy is infrequent, optic nerve pallor is common. Strabismus is also common, as is hearing impairment. Facial weakness has been noted in two reports.

Renal Tubular Acidosis (RTA)

The RTA varies in type and severity in different pedigrees. Metabolic acidosis was already present at 23 days of age in the first affected neonate. Although one of the first patients reported had only proximal RTA, evidenced by low bicarbonate threshold, and had normal distal acidification (2), most of the patients have a combination of proximal and distal RTA (9). In most patients, hyperchloremia, a normal anion gap, and inappropriately alkaline urine pH [>6.0] provide evidence of distal RTA. Symptomatic hyperkalemia has been observed in four patients. However, unlike other patients with distal RTA, there is neither hypercalciuria nor nephrocalcinosis. Glomerular filtration rate is not reduced, and serum creatinine and blood urea nitrogen are not elevated.

Most patients also have a proximal RTA with a reduced transport maximum for bicarbonate. Although they have no bicarbonaturia when acidotic, they lose bicarbonate when plasma bicarbonate levels are raised to normal levels by loading. They have no aminoaciduria, glycosuria, or any other manifestations of the Fanconi syndrome.

Mental Retardation The mental retardation was not fully appreciated initially, because affected patients in two of the first four families recognized with this syndrome were not retarded (3, 5). However, over 90% of the patients reported subsequently had significant mental retardation. In affected patients in most families, it has been severe enough to preclude education in regular schools.

Cerebral Calcification Cerebral calcifications were first reported by Ohlsson et al. (4). They were not present at birth, but appeared some time during the first decade (in one case, by 18 months). Calcifications involved the caudate nucleus, putamen, and globus pallidus, and also appeared peripherally in the periventricular and subcortical white matter. The variability in the rate of progression of cerebral calcification in different patients has not been documented. They are much easier to document on CT scan than on X-rays because of the increased bone density.

Growth Retardation Almost all reported patients had short stature and many were underweight. Bone age was retarded, and corresponded to height age. Genu valgum is a common finding in older patients. At least part of the growth retardation is due to the chronic metabolic acidosis. Gibaud reported acceleration of growth following correction of the acidosis (2), but later noted that growth retardation persisted, even after treatment (9).

Dental Malocclusion Dentition was typically delayed and dental malocclusion was a prominent finding in affected patients, complicating dental hygiene. Dental caries may be severe. Enamel hypoplasia has also been noted.

Other Clinical Features Ohlsson has reported a characteristic facies (4). Features include craniofacial disproportion with a prominent forehead and a large cranial vault relative to the size of the face. The mouth is small, and there is micrognathia. The nose is narrow, but prominent. The philtrum is short, the upper lip thin, and the lower lip thick. Squint is common and contributes to the unusual facies.

Ohlsson et al. recently reported findings of restrictive lung disease in two patients (8). Chest films showed no signs of parenchymal lung disease, but the rib cages were very dense.

Optic atrophy has been found in patients in whom the optic foramina were of normal size. The mechanism of optic atrophy in these patients is unclear.

Pathology

Bone biopsies from iliac crest showed histologic features typical of osteopetrosis (5). The cortical bone showed small Haversian systems widely separated by dense bone. Trabeculae were broad and irregular. Osteoid and normal appearing osteoblasts were seen lining trabecular bone in several areas. On routine microscopy, osteoclast morphology was unremarkable. A minute sample of femoral cortex was obtained during open reduction of a femoral fracture. Osteoclasts were normal in appearance on light microscopy. Four osteoclasts were identified on electron microscopy, and showed a normal rim of cytoplasm adjacent to the bone surface. This "clear zone" was free of organelles. The osteoclasts appeared normal, although no "ruffled borders" were seen. In summary, the histologic findings of osteopetrosis were present, but no features appeared to distinguish the osteopetrosis of the CA II deficiency syndrome from other forms of osteopetrosis.

Pathogenesis

In 1983, the three affected sisters reported initially by Sly and described in detail by Whyte et al. (5) were shown to have no detectable CA II activity in their erythrocytes (6). CA I was present in near normal levels. No immunoreactivity was detectable with antibody specific to CA II. The obligate heterozygote parents had half-normal levels of CA II activity. These findings were subsequently extended to 18 similarly affected patients from 11 unrelated families of different geographic and ethnic origins. Every patient with osteopetrosis and renal tubular acidosis since tested had nondetectable levels of CA II activity (8, 9).

CA II deficiency has not yet been demonstrated directly in bone and kidney. However, the deficiency in these tissues can be inferred from the fact that CA II is the only soluble isozyme present in these tissues, and the fact that the observed metabolic abnormalities in the affected patients can readily be explained by the CA II deficiency in these two organs.

Although the complete absence of CA II activity and immunoreactivity has been found in erythrocytes, the residual activity in cells that continue to synthesize protein (such as osteoclasts in bone and cells in the proximal and distal tubules of the kidney) might be significantly higher than in erythrocytes. Some of the clinical heterogeneity in this syndrome may be explained by differences in residual CA II activity in bone and kidney in patients with different mutations in the structural gene for CA II.

Pathophysiology

Osteopetrosis All known forms of osteopetrosis involve the failure to resorb bone. Studies showing inhibition of PTH-induced release of CA^{2+} from bone by CA inhibitors had suggested a role for CA in bone resorption. CA has been demonstrated histochemically in chick and hen osteoclasts and immunohistochemically in rat and human osteoclasts. The osteopetrosis seen in patients with CA II deficiency provided genetic evidence for a role for CA in bone resorption, and specifically implicated the CA II isozyme.

We have proposed that the role of CA II in acidifying the bone resorbing component is an indirect one. It had been suggested that CA aids the resorptive process by mediating the secretion of H^+. It was suggested recently that the acidification of the bone resorbing compartment is mediated by a proton-translocating ATPase, which secretes protons into the lumen (10). This reaction would simultaneously generate an OH^- ion in the cytoplasm for each H^+ translocated to the lumen. Titration of the OH^- ions produced in the cytosol by CA II might be required for the proton translocating ATPase to maintain the pH gradient (7.0-4.5) between the cytosol of the osteoclast and the bone resorbing compartment. This could explain the pharmacologic evidence for a requirement for CA in bone resorption. Since CA II is the only CA isozyme known to be expressed in osteoclasts, it could also explain the osseous manifestations of CA II deficiency.

Renal Tubular Acidosis Three things need explanation. First, most CA II deficient patients have both a proximal and a distal component to the RTA. Second, involvement of the two sites varies in different pedigrees. Some patients have predominantly proximal RTA, while others have predominantly a distal RTA. Third, CA II deficient patients have a nearly normal bicarbonaturia following ingestion or infusion of carbonic anhydrase inhibitors. We explain (11) these findings with a model in which the functions of CA II in the proximal and distal tubules are physiologically and biochemically distinct, and the major role of CA in bicarbonate reclamation is assigned, not to CA II, but to CA IV, the luminal CA in the brush border of the proximal tubule. CA IV is biochemically and immunologically distinct from CA II, and appears to be normal in CA II deficient patients.

First, the explanation for the proximal RTA. Most of the bicarbonate reclamation takes place in the proximal tubule and is blocked by inhibitors of CA. Two distinct CAs participate in bicarbonate reclamation by the proximal tubule, and we suggest that they play separate roles in bicarbonate reclamation.

Bicarbonate reclamation is driven by H^+ secretion, which is mediated by Na^+/H^+ exchange in the proximal tubule. The H^+ secreted into the lumen is titrated by the HCO_3^- in the glomerular filtrate to produce H_2CO_3 which is in contact with the membrane-bound CA IV. The luminal CA IV catalyzes the dehydration of H_2CO_3 to H_2O and CO_2. The bicarbonaturia seen in already acidotic CA II deficient patients in response to infused acetazolamide is attributed to inhibition of this luminal CA IV.

The CO_2 produced by the CA IV catalyzed reaction in the lumen diffuses freely into the cytosol of the proximal tubule. Here in the cytoplasm CO_2 encounters CA II which hydrates the CO_2 to H_2CO_3, which dissociates spontaneously to HCO_3^- and H^+. The HCO_3^- generated from CO_2 in the cytosol is transported from the cytosol to the interstitial fluid or peritubular capillary, completing the reclamation of the filtered bicarbonate. The H^+ regenerated in the cytosol by the CA II-catalyzed reaction can be secreted in exchange for Na^+ to initiate another round of HCO_3^- reclamation.

The fact that CA II deficient patients do not spill HCO_3^- when acidotic, suggests that CA II is not required for HCO_3^- reclamation when patients have low bicarbonate loads, i.e., when acidotic. However, they have a lowered transport maximum for bicarbonate and lose bicarbonate when the filtered load is increased by bicarbonate infusion or ingestion, indicating that CA II is required to regenerate H^+ for bicarbonate reclamation under normal bicarbonate loads. This requirement explains the proximal component of the RTA in CA II deficient patients.

The prominent distal component of the RTA in most CA II deficient patients, evidenced by inappropriately high urine pH values when patients are acidotic, suggests a need for CA II for distal acidification. This is consistent with the immunohistochemical evidence showing a much more intense reaction for CA II in the distal tubule and the intercalated cells of the collecting ducts than in the proximal tubules. The situation is analogous to the distal nephron and collecting system in the amphibian. Here, "CA rich cells" are specialized cells which secrete H+ and are capable of generating a steep pH gradient. However, the acidification of the lumen by these cells is sensitive to inhibition by acetazolamide. This has been explained by the requirement for CA to titrate the OH- produced in the cytosol by the proton-translocating Mg^{2+} ATPase. We have suggested a similar role for CA II in the distal tubule of the human kidney (11). Unless the OH- is titrated by CO_2, the proton-translocating ATPase cannot generate a pH gradient and acidify the lumen. The absence of CA II for this reaction in CA II deficient patients can explain their defect in distal tubular acidification.

The basis for heterogeneity in the renal lesion in CA II deficiency still requires explanation. Why is there variability in prominence of the proximal and distal lesions in different pedigrees? The explanation for this heterogeneity is presently speculative, since the mutational basis for CA II deficiency has not been demonstrated, even in a single patient. However, if one assumes that different structural gene mutations produce CA II deficiency in the different pedigrees of patients with the CA II deficiency syndrome, it is plausible that different mutations could lead to this heterogeneity. First, different mutations could affect the rate of enzyme turnover in proximal and distal tubular cells differentially, resulting in different levels of residual enzyme activity in the two different locations. Second, different structural gene mutations could affect the two different enzymatic activities in the two locations differentially. Hydration of CO_2 to produce H+ and HCO_3^- in the proximal tubule and the condensation of OH- and CO_2 to produce HCO_3^- in the distal tubule might be differentially affected by different mutations in the CA II gene. Delineation of the mutations in different CA II deficient patients should soon be feasible and allow one to test this hypothesis.

Brain Calcification and Cerebral Function

The mechanism of the cerebral calcification is unclear. Carbonic anhydrase II is primarily a glial enzyme that occurs predominantly in oligodendrocytes. It is the only soluble carbonic anhydrase in brain homogenates. As much as 50% of the total carbonic anhydrase II activity occurs in a membrane-bound or myelin-associated form. Its function in the brain is not known. Whether the cerebral calcification in carbonic anhydrase II deficiency is a direct effect of the deficiency of CA II in the brain, or an indirect effect--for example, of carbonic anhydrase deficiency in erythrocytes, or of chronic systemic acidosis--is not clear.

Growth Retardation Growth failure appears to result from the combined effects of the osteopetrosis on bone elongation, and of the chronic metabolic acidosis on general health. Correction of the acidosis has been followed by a growth spurt in one patient, but the dramatic reduction in final height achieved makes it clear that the growth retardation is not due to the acidosis alone.

Inheritance

The CA II deficiency syndrome is inherited as an autosomal recessive trait. Affected patients are offspring of normal appearing heterozygote carrier parents who have half-normal levels of CA II in their erythrocyte lysates. Heterozygotes have no symptoms and no signs of the disorder. Males and females are affected with equal frequency and severity. Consanguinity is very common (87%) in parents of affected offspring.

The geographical distribution of this syndrome is striking, with more than half the known cases observed in families from Kuwait, Saudi Arabia, and north Africa. This probably results from both an increased frequency of the carbonic anhydrase II deficiency allele in these regions, and an increased frequency of consanguineous marriages, particularly in the Bedouin tribes from which many of these patients originated.

Diagnosis

Clinically, CA II deficiency should be suspected in any newborn infant with metabolic acidosis and failure to thrive, especially if the urine pH is alkaline.

Osteopetrosis may not be present initially, but usually develops over the first year of life. If osteopetrosis and renal tubular acidosis coexist, the diagnosis is virtually certain. No patient with this combination has yet been found who does not have CA II deficiency. Cerebral calcification, evident by CT scan, is usually present by the end of the first decade.

Enzymatic confirmation can be made by quantitating the CA II level in erythrocyte lysates. Normally CA I and CA II each contribute about 50% of the total activity, and the CA I activity is virtually completely abolished by inclusion of 8 mM sodium iodide in the assay (12). To quantitate this enzyme, one simply measures the total activity (CA I + CA II), and also the activity seen in the presence of 8 mM sodium iodide (CA II). Patients with CA II deficiency have no iodide-resistant enzyme (i.e., no CA II). Obligate heterozygotes have about half normal levels of iodide resistant activity.

Genetic Counseling

The appropriate counseling for an autosomal recessive trait is indicated. First degree relatives can be tested for heterozygosity (12). Prenatal diagnosis is currently not available. The osteopetrosis does not appear prenatally. Carbonic anhydrase levels in erythrocytes are normally extremely low at birth, and it is not clear that CA II deficiency could be diagnosed by measuring CA II activity in samples of fetal blood. No disease-associated DNA markers are available. Although the cDNA probe for CA II is available, the disease has not yet been linked to the structural gene for CA II, and it is not yet certain that the mutation underlying CA II deficiency involves a structural gene locus.

Treatment

No specific treatment for CA II deficiency is available. Treatment for the metabolic acidosis is recommended, at least until after adolescence. It appears that the renal tubular acidosis may stabilize at a milder level after puberty. Frequent fractures require conventional orthopedic management. Bone healing is usually normal. Most patients require special education because of serious mental retardation. There is no specific treatment for the cranial nerve abnormalities, which may lead to impaired vision, hearing deficits, and facial nerve weakness. Attention to dental hygiene is important because of the susceptibility to caries.

In the American family, treatment with bicarbonate was withheld for fear that the acidosis may be compensating for the osteopetrosis, and that treatment of the acidosis might aggravate the osteopetrosis with further loss of vision and hearing. However, prolonged treatment of several patients by Dr. Gibaud and colleagues appeared to have a beneficial effect on general health without any marked progression of the osteopetrosis and with no aggravation of cranial nerve symptoms. It is not clear whether the development of cerebral calcification is influenced favorably, unfavorably, or not at all by correction of the acidosis.

Bone marrow transplantation is not indicated, since the hematologic manifestations for which this is usually considered appropriate in the infantile, recessive lethal form of osteopetrosis are not present in the CA II deficiency syndrome. Although the bone manifestations might improve following bone marrow transplantation, since CA II-containing osteoclasts would be provided by stem cells from the donor marrow, the renal insufficiency will not improve.

We had the opportunity to replace the CA II deficient red cells with CA II replete blood cells following severe uterine hemorrhage in one of the patients we followed (13). Raising the circulating erythrocyte levels of CA II to the heterozygote range by transfusion with replete erythrocytes had no effect on plasma pH or urine pH. These observations supported the proposal that the metabolic acidosis is due to the renal CA II deficiency, and not a secondary consequence of CA II deficiency in erythrocytes.

Implications for osteopetrosis

CA II is a major enzyme required for the generation of hydrogen ion gradients, and for the normal function of osteoclasts in bone resorption. Although osteopetrosis results from a defect in bone resorption, there are other metabolic disorders in which the reverse is true, and accelerated bone loss is the problem. Can one take advantage of the dependence on CA in the process of bone resorption to inhibit accelerated bone loss? In organ culture, Ca^{2+} release from bones was shown to be hormone responsive (parathormone and dibutyryl cyclic AMP) and sensitive to inhibition by acetazolamide and other inhibitors of CA (14). Animal studies have suggested that bone loss associated with disuse can be partially prevented by CA inhibitors (15). This observation raises hope that CA inhibitors might have a role in treating common causes of bone loss like osteoporosis. One problem, however, is that chronic administration of currently available agents produces a systemic acidosis due to their actions on the kidney, and systemic acidosis itself can lead to calcium mobilization from bone. It has been suggested that development of effective CA inhibitors for metabolic bone disease may require development of agents that act selectively on CA II in bone, or that can be selectively targeted to bone resorbing osteoclasts to avoid inhibition of CA II in kidney and other sites (14).

Summary

1) The carbonic anhydrase II deficiency syndrome is an autosomal recessive disorder which produces osteopetrosis, renal tubular acidosis, and cerebral calcification. Other features include mental retardation, seen in over 90% of reported cases, growth failure, and dental malocclusion.

2) Complications of osteopetrosis include increased susceptibility to fractures which heal normally, and cranial nerve compression symptoms. Anemia and other hematological manifestations of osteopetrosis are absent.

3) The renal tubular acidosis is usually a mixed type. A distal component is evident from inability to acidify the urine, and a proximal component evident from a lowered transport maximum for bicarbonate.

4) Thirty patients have been reported, all of whom have a quantitative deficiency of carbonic anhydrase II activity and immunoreactivity in erythrocytes. Heterozygous carriers can be identified by simple tests, but prenatal diagnosis is not yet feasible.

5) A structural gene mutation at the CA II locus on chromosome 8 is suspected. Although the CA II cDNA has been cloned, the mutational basis for the syndrome has not yet been established.

6) Symptoms of metabolic acidosis improve with treatment, but no specific treatment is available.

References

1. JOHNSTON CC Jr, LAVY N, LORD T, VELLIOS F, MERRITT AD, DEISS WP Jr: Osteopetrosis: A clinical, genetic, metabolic, and morphologic study of the dominantly inherited, benign form. Medicine (Baltimore) 47:149, 1968
2. GUIBAUD P, LARBRE F, FREYCON M-T, GENOUD J: Osteopetrose et acidose renale tubulaire: deux cas de cette association dans une fratrie. Arch Fr Pediatr 29:269, 1972
3. VAINSEL M, FONDU P, CADRANEL S, ROCMANS C, GEPTS W: Osteopetrosis associated with proximal and distal tubular acidosis. Acta Paediatr Scand 61:429, 1972
4. OHLSSON A, STARK G, SAKATI N: Marble brain disease: recessive osteopetrosis, renal tubular acidosis and cerebral calcification in three Saudi Arabian families. Dev Med Child Neurol 22:72, 1980
5. WHYTE MP, MURPHY WA, FALLON MD, SLY WS, TEITELBAUM SL, MAC ALISTER WH, AVIOLI LV: Osteopetrosis, renal tubular acidosis and basal ganglia calcification in three sisters. Am J Med 69:65, 1980
6. SLY WS, HEWETT-EMMETT D, WHYTE MP, YU Y-SL, TASHIAN RE: Carbonic anhydrase II deficiency identified as the primary defect in the autosomal recessive syndrome of osteopetrosis with renal tubular acidosis and cerebral calcification. Proc Natl Acad Sci USA 80:2752, 1983
7. SLY WS, WHYTE P, SUNDARAM V, TASHIAN RE, HEWETT-EMMETT D, GUIBAUD P, VAINSEL M, BALUARTE HJ, GRUSKIN A, AL-MOSAWI M, SAKATI N, OHLSSON A: Carbonic anhydrase II deficiency in 12 families with the autosomal recessive syndrome of osteopetrosis with renal tubular acidosis and cerebral calcification. N Engl J Med 313:139, 1985
8. OHLSSON A, CUMMING WA, PAUL A, SLY WS: Carbonic anhydrase II deficiency

9. syndrome: Recessive osteopetrosis with renal tubular acidosis and cerebral calcification. Pediatrics 77:371, 1986
9. COCHAT P, LORAS-DUCLAUX I, GUIBAUD P: Deficit en anhydrase carbonique II: osteopetrose, acidose renale tubulaire et calcifications intracraniennes. Revue de la literature a partir de trois observations. Pediatrie 42:121, 1987
10. BARON R, NEFF L, LOUVARD D, COURTOY PJ: Cell-mediated extracellular acidification and bone resorption: Evidence for a low pH in resorbing lacunae and localization of a 100-kD lysosomal membrane protein at the osteoclast ruffled border. J Cell Biol 101:2210, 1985
11. SLY WS, WHYTE MP, KRUPIN T, SUNDARAN V: Positive renal response to intravenous acetazolamide in patients with carbonic anhydrase II deficiency. Pediatr Res 19:1033, 1985
12. SUNDARAM V, RUMBOLO P, GRUBB J, STRISCIUGLIO P, SLY WS: Carbonic anhydrase deficiency: Diagnosis and carrier detection using differential enzyme inhibition and inactivation. Am J Hum Genet 38:125, 1986
13. WHYTE MP, HAMM LL, SLY WS: Transfusion of carbonic anhydrase-replete erythrocytes fails to correct the acidification defect in the syndrome of osteopetrosis, renal tubular acidosis, and cerebral calcification (carbonic anhydrase-II deficiency). J Bone Mineral Res 3:385, 1988
14. RAISZ LG, SIMMONS HA, THOMPSON WJ, SHEPARD KL, ANDERSON PS, RODAN GA: Effects of a potent carbonic anhydrase inhibitor on bone resorption in organ culture. Endocrinology 122:1083, 1988
15. KENNY AD: Role of carbonic anhydrase in bone: Partial inhibition of disuse atrophy of bone by parenteral acetazolamide. Calcif Tissue Int 37:126, 1985

Discussion:

DR. KAYE (Montreal): About 30 years ago, we published some experiments in patients with distal RTA, both children and adults. After correcting their acidosis, we gave them a carbonic anhydrase inhibitor, acetazolamide, and they showed an absolutely normal response. Have you challenged any of these people?

DR. SLY (St. Louis): Yes, that is very interesting. The reason that we believe that the membrane-bound form of carbonic anhydrase in these patients is not affected and is normal, is because we gave them an acetazolamide load. We postulated that if the membrane enzyme is normal, they will demonstrate a normal bicarbonate diuresis in response. In fact, this is what was observed. They had an exactly normal bicarbonate diuresis in response to acetazolamide. What we think happens is that the brush border enzyme, which is the product of a different gene, is inhibited.

DR. LANG (New Haven): Very nice work, Bill. You have taken it a long way since we first saw those patients in St. Louis. I would just like to make a comment about one of the things that happened when we first saw this family. After I did a routine workup and found that their urine pH's were not normal I went back and told Lou Avioli. He said, "Oh, they must have carbonic anhydrase deficiency."

DR. SLY: What year was that?

DR. LANG: That was in 1972 when we first saw the patients.

DR. SLY: Right. The thing was, we did not know if this was correct. We considered that idea at that time, but we did not know enough about the gene family to really make a specific hypothesis.

DR. LANG: Yes. Another thing is that I also postulated, when we first saw them, that there was a symbiotic relationship between these two defects, that is, that the RTA protected against the osteopetrosis. That type of relationship was really unprecedented at the time, and remains unproven, but suggestive. Have you looked at carbonic anhydrase in regular osteopetrosis, the recessive lethal type?

DR. SLY: Yes. The classic lethal recessive form, although we have relatively few patients, has been normal. And we have also studied the benign, adult form and the carbonic anhydrase levels are normal.

Let me amplify on one of your points. I alluded to the possibility that maybe the metabolic acidosis protects, to some extent, from the osteopetrosis. If you corrected the acidosis, your osteopetrosis might get worse. One clinical experiment that was done by Dr. Guibaud is of interest in this regard. He treated patients for two years and followed them with serial x-rays, starting at around age nine, and their osteopetrosis did not get worse.

Another important point is that these patients actually tend to get better over time and develop tubulation. If you recall the films on the oldest girl that I showed you, the girl whose leg was broken at age two, she is now age 35 and you would not be able to tell that she ever had osteopetrosis. So, gradually, over time, these patients, radiologically, can improve. Improvement may not take place if you correct their acidosis.

DR. CHESNEY (Memphis, TN): There have been reports from Japan of RTA and deafness with carbonic anhydrase deficiency. Do they have this same syndrome?

DR. SLY: They do not have this syndrome, and they probably do not have carbonic anhydrase deficiency. They reportedly had electrophorectically abnormal carbonic anhydrase. Dr. Richard E. Tashian has examined blood from those patients and has not found a deficiency. They do have deafness and they have a different syndrome.

DR. CHESNEY: With regard to the calcification in the brain, have you done any anatomic studies of this? Is this just simply dystrophic calcification?

DR. SLY: The calcification is in the same distribution as the oligodendrocytes in the normal brain. In fact, most of the carbonic anhydrase II in the normal brain is present in oligodendrocytes. Autopsy studies of CA-II deficiency have not been performed.

DR. CHESNEY: Do these patients have movement disorders?

DR. SLY: None have had movement disorders. Indeed, consulting neurologists who look at their CAT scans are often amazed that they are so normal. However, I must point out that nearly all are mentally retarded and have learning disabilities, about 80 percent.

DR. ARNOLD (Boston): Has a molecular defect been characterized?

DR. SLY: Thank you for that question. We have cloned the CA-II gene. So far we have not found a genetic abnormality by Southern blotting. We are beginning now to isolate the gene from affected patients to characterize the nature of the defect.

DR. ARNOLD: Is the gene for CA-VI distinguishable, and is its chromosomal location known?

DR. SLY: Good question. CA-I, CA-II, and CA-III are all very closely linked on chromosome 8. We are just cloning CA-VI. It has not been characterized yet. That is a very interesting question. CA-VI may be the product of the same gene and produced by alternate splicing. This is a possibility of considerable interest to us.

DR. ARNOLD: Thank you.

DR. WHYTE (St. Louis): The evidence thus far that this is an inborn error of CA-II is based upon demonstration of enzyme deficiency in erythrocytes and saliva. Are there also linkage studies underway which could help to show a defect in CA-II itself?

DR. SLY: It is true CA-II deficiency has not yet been shown in the renal tubule and the osteoclast. But we have not felt justified to biopsy patients to do that. It is very clear from the mutant animal model, however, that the single gene that knocks out the erythrocyte CA-II also reduces CA-II in the kidney tubule, the brain, and in the osteoclast. There is only a single gene product that produces that enzyme.

DR. WHYTE: Thank you, Bill.

Pediatric Forms of Hypophosphatasia

MICHAEL P. WHYTE

Division of Bone and Mineral Diseases
Departments of Medicine and Pediatrics
The Jewish Hospital of St. Louis
and Washington University School of Medicine
and Metabolic Research Unit
Shriners Hospital for Crippled Children
St. Louis, MO

I) INTRODUCTION:

J.C. Rathbun coined the term "hypophosphatasia" in 1948 when he described an infant with severe rickets yet subnormal alkaline phosphatase (ALP) activity in serum and tissue obtained at autopsy (1). Probable cases were reported at least several decades earlier. By 1980, descriptions of 278 patients were available in the medical literature (2). The disorder occurs in all races. The incidence has been estimated to be 1/100,000 live births (3).

Hypophosphatasia is now recognized to be an inborn error of metabolism characterized by deficient activity of the tissue nonspecific (liver/bone/kidney) ALP isoenzyme (TNSALP); activity of the intestinal and placental ALP isoenzymes is normal (2). The molecular defect(s) is unknown. Accordingly, classification of patients remains a clinical one (3). Although distinct separation of the various types is not possible, four forms - perinatal, infantile, childhood, and adult - are reported depending upon the age at which skeletal lesions develop. When only dental manifestations are present, patients are regarded as having "odontohypophosphatasia" (2).

This paper provides an overview of hypophosphatasia, and emphasizes the features of the pediatric forms.

II) CLINICAL FEATURES:

Despite the presence of at least some TNSALP in most normal tissues (4), hypophosphatasia manifests predominantly with skeletal and dental disease. However, the severity of clinical expression is remarkably variable and ranges from death in utero to onset of recurrent fractures late in adult life. Prognosis generally reflects the severity of the skeletal disease which, in turn, correlates inversely with the age at presentation (2,3).

A) Perinatal (lethal) hypophosphatasia is expressed in utero where the pregnancy may be complicated by polyhydramnios. Caput membraneceum and extreme skeletal hypomineralization are present at birth. Limbs are shortened and deformed and rarely unusual spurs may occur at the ends of long bones. Some newborns live a few days but suffer increasing respiratory compromise from rachitic disease of the chest. Failure to gain weight, a high-pitched cry, irritability, periodic apnea with cyanosis and bradycardia, unexplained fever, myelophthisic anemia (perhaps from encroachment on the marrow space by osteoidosis), intracranial hemorrhage, and idiopathic seizures comprise the typical signs and symptoms.

B) <u>Infantile</u> hypophosphatasia presents before age 6 months. Development often seems normal until poor feeding and inadequate weight gain are observed at several months of age; hypotonia and wide fontanels may have been noted earlier. Cranial sutures remain wide and rachitic deformities develop and may progress. Flail chest predisposes to pneumonia. Hypercalcemia and hypercalciuria occur in some subjects and cause recurrent vomiting, nephrocalcinosis, and renal compromise. Functional synostosis of the cranial sutures is the rule and can occur despite widely "open" fontanels and hypomineralized areas of calvarium. Raised intracranial pressure may cause bulging of the anterior fontanel, papilledema, and proptosis, and may be associated with mild hypertelorism and brachycephaly.

C) <u>Childhood</u> hypophosphatasia is highly variable in its clinical expression. Premature loss of deciduous teeth (earlier than age 5) from aplasia or hypoplasia of dental cementum may be the only clinical abnormality. In odontohypophosphatasia, radiographs show no sign of rickets. Incisors are generally lost first, but nearly the entire dentition may be disturbed. Premature tooth loss occurs without inflammatory periodontal disease and with only minimal root resorption. Alveolar bone attrition may occur from lack of mechanical stimulation, since aplasia of the cementum prevents periodontal ligaments from connecting teeth and jaw. Dental radiographs may show enlarged pulp chambers and root canals ("shell teeth"). These patients may account for many cases of "early-onset periodontitis".

When rickets is present, premature loss of teeth, short stature, and delayed walking with a characteristic waddling gait, a dolicocephalic skull with frontal bossing, beading of the costochondral junctions, either bowed legs or knock-knee deformity, and enlargement of the wrists and occasionally knees and ankles are noted.

D) <u>Adult</u> hypophosphatasia usually presents during middle-age with painful recurrent metatarsal stress fractures and/or discomfort in the thighs or hips from femoral pseudofractures. Early loss or extraction of adult teeth is also common. Chondrocalcinosis and calcium pyrophosphate deposition disease, occasionally with attacks of arthritis, occur in some patients. About 50% of affected adults give a history of rickets and premature exfoliation of deciduous teeth during childhood (5).

E) <u>Pseudohypophosphatasia</u> has been documented convincingly in one subject where serum TNSALP activity is consistently normal or increased, yet clinical, radiologic, and biochemical findings are otherwise typical of subjects who survive infantile hypophosphatasia (6). The enzymatic defect appears to involve a mutant TNSALP with substantial enzymatic activity toward artificial substrates at alkaline pH, but defective catalysis for natural substrates at physiologic pH (6). Other reports of pseudohypophosphatasia probably describe individuals with classic hypophosphatasia but transient increases in serum ALP activity or misinterpretation of reference ranges for serum ALP activity and/or urinary phosphoethanolamine (PEA) levels (2).

III) <u>LABORATORY STUDIES</u>:

Hypophosphatasia can usually be diagnosed with confidence from a consistent clinical history and physical findings, radiographic evidence of rickets/osteomalacia, and documentation of hypophosphatasemia (2).

A) <u>Routine Assays</u>: Determination of serum ALP activity on more than one occasion is advisable to establish the diagnosis. Blood specimens must be obtained correctly; chelation of Mg^{++} or Zn^{++} will destroy ALP activity. Furthermore, important age-related changes in serum ALP activity must be kept in mind (4). Infants or children with hypophosphatasia may incorrectly be regarded as having normal serum ALP activity or pseudohypophosphatasia unless the age of the reference population is considered. Hypophosphatasemia occurs in hypothyroidism, starvation, scurvy, severe anemia, celiac disease, Wilson's disease, hypomagnesemia, Zn^{++} deficiency, and from a variety of treatments (glucocorticoids, clofibrate, vitamin D intoxication, milk-alkali syndrome, radioactive heavy metals, massive transfusion of blood) (4). Conditions which increase serum activity of any of the other forms of ALP (e.g., pregnancy) could mask the diagnosis. Occasional reports describe transient increases in serum ALP activity (probably bone enzyme) in hypophosphatasia after fracture or orthopedic surgery. Patients with odontohypophosphatasia generally have the most mild biochemical abnormalities. Quantitation of the individual ALP isoenzymes in serum may be helpful in puzzling cases (7). In perinatal hypophosphatasia, hypophosphatasemia is present in cord blood.

Leukocyte ALP is a form of TNSALP; activity can be subnormal in any clinical form of hypophosphatasia, but is noted regularly only in severe cases (8).

Hypercalciuria and hypercalcemia occur frequently in infantile hypophosphatasia; severely affected children may have hypercalciuria but without hypercalcemia. Circulating levels of $25(OH)D$ and $1,25(OH)_2D$ and iPTH are usually unremarkable. Several patients have been reported to have elevated iPTH, but concomitant hypercalcemia with renal compromise may have explained this finding. Low serum levels of iPTH and the possibility of an abnormality in the Ca^{++}/parathyroid system has been described (2).

Subjects with childhood and adult hypophosphatasia have serum Pi levels that are above the mean value for controls; indeed, about 50% of these individuals are hyperphosphatemic. Enhanced renal reclamation of Pi (increased TMPi/GFR) accounts for this finding (2).

Other routine laboratory tests, including liver function studies and "muscle" enzyme levels in serum are generally unremarkable in all forms of hypophosphatasia.

B) <u>Natural Substrates:</u> The metabolic basis for hypophosphatasia and the physiologic role of TNSALP were clarified by the discoveries of increased endogenous levels of three phosphocompounds (2). In 1955, increased urinary levels were reported of a substance that proved to be phosphoethanolamine (PEA). This discovery provided a useful biochemical marker (9). In 1965 and 1971, high levels of inorganic pyrophosphate (PPi) in urine and blood, respectively, were noted. In 1985, plasma levels of pyridoxal-5'-phosphate (PLP) were found to be markedly elevated (10) - a finding which suggested that TNSALP functions as an ectoenzyme (<u>see Section XI</u>).

Increased urinary PEA level supports the diagnosis of hypophosphatasia, but is not diagnostic. Phosphoethanolaminuria has been noted in a variety of other disorders including several metabolic bone diseases. Furthermore, urinary PEA levels are importantly influenced by age, depend upon diet, follow a circadian rhythm, and have been described as normal in several mild cases of hypophosphatasia (2).

PPi accumulation in hypophosphatasia may play an important role in the pathogenesis of the skeletal disease, but assay of plasma or urine levels is a research technique.

Increased plasma concentration of PLP is a sensitive and specific marker for hypophosphatasia. Even patients with odontohypophosphatasia demonstrate this abnormality. In general, the more severe the disorder, the greater the elevation in plasma PLP level (although overlap among plasma PLP levels for the clinical forms of hypophosphatasia helps to illustrate the clinical spectrum of this condition) (2). Subjects should not be taking vitamin supplements when tested.

IV) RADIOLOGIC FINDINGS:

In perinatal hypophosphatasia, skeletal radiographs are usually diagnostic, since they readily distinguish this form of hypophosphatasia from even the most severe types of osteogenesis imperfecta or congenital dwarfism (11). The skeleton may appear to be almost completely unmineralized, or marked bony undermineralization can occur with severe rachitic changes. Radiolucencies (comprised of growth plate cartilage and unmineralized osteoid) protrude into metaphyses. Diaphyseal defects may also occur. Fractures are common. Cranial bones may be ossified merely at their central portions and give the illusion that sutures are widely separated, although they are functionally closed.

In infantile hypophosphatasia, radiologic changes are characteristic and resemble the perinatal form although they are less extreme (11). Abrupt transition from uncalcified metaphyses to relatively normal diaphyses can occur and suggest a sudden metabolic change. Persistently defective bone mineralization together with progressive skeletal demineralization can occur. Skeletal scintigraphy can reveal premature closure of cranial sutures although they may appear "widened" on conventional radiographs.

In childhood hypophosphatasia, radiographs of joints may reveal well preserved epiphyses but diagnostic "tongues" of radiolucency that project from rachitic growth plates into metaphyses (Figure). True premature bony fusion of cranial sutures can also occur and may cause proptosis, raised intracranial pressure, and brain damage. With this complication, radiographs may show a skull with a "beaten-copper" appearance (11).

Figure: The wrist of this 2-2/3 year old boy with the childhood form of hypophosphatasia shows a characteristic area of radiolucency (arrow) which projects into the distal ulnar metaphysis.

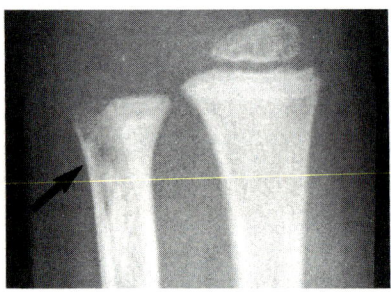

In adult hypophosphatasia, radiographs may reveal osteopenia, chondrocalcinosis, and proximal femoral pseudofractures which are unusual in that they occur most often in the lateral (not medial) cortex (5,12).

V) HISTOPATHOLOGIC FINDINGS:

Histologic abnormalities are primarily skeletal (2,8). In all but the mildest cases, nondecalcified sections of bone reveal defective skeletal mineralization. Unless histochemical studies of ALP activity are performed, however, the changes of hypophosphatasia are like those of other forms of rickets or osteomalacia. The severity of the mineralization defect reflects the clinical severity (8). Osteoblasts, chondrocytes, and matrix vesicles are present; evidence of secondary hyperparathyroidism is generally absent. The number and morphology of osteoblasts and osteoclasts vary from case to case, as does the appearance of unmineralized osteoid. Woven bone may be present. Cranial sutures that are "widened" are not fibrous tissue, but uncalcified osteoid (3).

Electron microscopy of bone from perinatal/infantile hypophosphatasia has revealed normal distribution of proteoglycan granules, collagen fibers, and matrix vesicles in the extracellular chondroid space. However, matrix vesicles are deficient in ALP activity and do not contain hydroxyapatite crystals. Instead, isolated or small groups of crystals, frequently unassociated with matrix vesicles, are noted (13).

Dental findings involve primarily the cementum (2). Premature loss of deciduous teeth occurs in a variety of conditions but, in hypophosphatasia, a characteristic paucity of cementum is observed despite the presence of connective tissue cells which look like cementoblasts. Histopathologic study of exfoliated teeth, demonstrating aplasia or hypoplasia of cementum, is an excellent means for diagnosis. The degree of hypoplasia of the cementum generally reflects the severity of the disease, but does vary from tooth to tooth. Enamel is not affected. Dental tubules may be enlarged, but reduced in number. Big pulp chambers suggest retarded dentinogenesis. There may also be evidence of delayed calcification. The excessive width of predentin, increased amounts of interglobular dentin, and impaired calcification of cementum are analogous to the osteoidosis observed in bone (2).

VI) INHERITANCE:

In 1950, a report of affected sibs provided the first evidence that hypophosphatasia was inherited. Consanguinity has been reported in some families with severely affected cases. Parents of severe cases characteristically demonstrate low or low-normal levels of serum ALP activity and have modest phosphoethanolaminuria. Indeed, perinatal and infantile forms of hypophosphatasia are well documented to be transmitted as autosomal recessive traits (2,4).

Transmission of the milder forms of hypophosphatasia is less clear. Odontohypophosphatasia and adult-onset cases may reflect clinical expression in a heterozygous subject. Mildly affected patients may be heterozygotes for the defect that causes severe disease in homozygotes. Other childhood and adult cases could represent a spectrum of homozygotes and compound heterozygotes with defective TNSALP alleles of lesser severity. In this regard, it is interesting that the clinical expression tends to run true to form in affected sibs in all forms of hypophosphatasia, and vertical transmission of clinically apparent disease seems to be unusual. Further studies of the inheritance pattern of the mild forms of hypophosphatasia are necessary (2). Identification of restriction-fragment-length polymorphisms in the TNSALP gene and close association with the gene locus of TNSALP and the Rh blood group on the short arm of chromosome 1 should facilitate linkage studies (14).

VII) BIOCHEMICAL/GENETIC DEFECT:

The molecular defect(s) which causes hypophosphatasia is unknown. There is no animal model. Hypophosphatasemia is explained by deficiency of both bone and liver ALP activity in serum and does not appear to be due to enhanced loss, degradation, or inhibition of circulating enzyme. Instead it seems to reflect a failure of bone and liver tissue to contribute TNSALP activity into the circulation (2).

Autopsy studies of perinatal and infantile hypophosphatasia have been especially important in clarifying the enzymatic and genetic abnormalities. Profound deficiency of ALP activity has been documented in liver, bone, and kidney, but ALP activity is normal in intestine or placenta (fetal trophoblast). Accordingly, severe forms appear to be due to a defect which diminishes the enzymatic activity of all of the secondary isoenzymes (liver/bone/kidney) of the TNSALP family, but placental and intestinal ALP are unaffected (2).

Autopsy studies of children or adults have not been reported. However, a variety of evidence suggests that clinically mild hypophosphatasia is also due to selective deficiency of activity of TNSALP. In affected children and adults, ALP activity can be deficient in circulating granulocytes and in bone obtained by biopsy (8). ALP in dermal fibroblasts from normal subjects is primarily a TNSALP, and cultivated skin fibroblasts from individuals with all clinical forms of hypophosphatasia have been found to be low in ALP activity (15).

In 1987, linkage of infantile hypophosphatasia with the Rh blood group was described for several Canadian Mennonite kindreds and provided evidence for an abnormality in the TNSALP gene itself (14).

Genetic complementation studies, using cultured skin fibroblasts from 11 individuals from 10 families with perinatal or infantile hypophosphatasia, failed to show correction of TNSALP activity and suggested a defect at the same gene locus (2).

Recent characterization of a cDNA for human TNSALP should help to clarify the molecular basis for hypophosphatasia (16). Chromosomal defects have been reported rarely in hypophosphatasia.

A variety of clinical evidence supports the possibility of a regulatory defect in the biosynthesis of TNSALP in some cases (2). One subject with infantile hypophosphatasia responded to a series of intravenous infusions of pooled normal plasma with a four-month correction of hypophosphatasemia that was associated with remarkable skeletal remineralization (demonstrated both radiologically and histologically) (17). The ALP in his serum during this time appeared to be normal bone TNSALP. Children with hypophosphatasia have somewhat higher levels of serum ALP activity compared to classic adult cases, yet develop clinically overt bone disease earlier. Some patients with adult hypophosphatasia suffer premature loss of deciduous teeth and/or rickets in childhood, but then feel well until middle age; i.e.; clinical remission may occur (5). In infantile hypophosphatasia, some ALP activity is detectable by sensitive methods in liver, bone, and kidney tissue. In most, but not all, of these subjects where the ALP has been partially characterized, it appears to differ from control TNSALP. In one case, enzyme inhibition and isoelectric focusing studies showed that the small amount of ALP activity detected in liver, bone, and kidney was intestinal ALP. This observation was interpreted to reflect compensatory expression of an intestinal ALP gene. Infantile hypophosphatasia fibroblasts in culture, however, seem to produce some TNSALP-like enzyme (15).

VIII) TREATMENT:

There is no established medical therapy (2). Extracellular accumulation of PPi may be a key pathogenetic factor (see Section XI). Promotion of renal PPi excretion with oral Pi supplementation was reported to increase urinary PPi levels and improve radiographic findings in three affected children, however, feeding Pi does not significantly change plasma PPi levels, and increased urinary PPi levels may reflect enhanced renal PPi synthesis. Efficacy of this therapy has not been confirmed.

Intravenous infusions of Paget plasma was of no clinical benefit to four affected infants (17). Administration of fresh normal plasma was reportedly followed by clinical and radiographic improvement in one infant. As described above, pooled plasma infusions were followed by marked temporary improvement in one subject with infantile hypophosphatasia (17). However, a subsequent trial in a different patient did not produce this response (10).

Prolonged challenge with cortisone to a few patients with severe disease has been reported to produce periods of normalization of circulating ALP activity and radiologic improvement, but this is not a consistent finding. Brief treatment with bovine PTH fragment 1-34 to stimulate ALP activity has been unsuccessful (17). Sodium fluoride has not been rigorously tested (2).

Traditional therapies for rickets/osteomalacia are important to avoid since circulating levels of Ca++, Pi, 25(OH)D and 1,25(OH)2D are not reduced. Vitamin D therapy will exacerbate any predisposition to hypercalcemia and hypercalciuria. However, complete restriction of dietary vitamin D or sunshine exposure can cause superimposed vitamin D deficiency rickets (2).

Hypercalcemia in infantile hypophosphatasia responds to glucocorticoid therapy and/or restriction of dietary calcium.

Fractures in children do mend, although delayed healing after femoral osteotomy with casting has been reported. Use of intramedullary rods, rather than load-sparing devices like plates, is probably best for the prophylactic or acute orthopedic management of appropriate fractures and pseudofractures (12). Expert dental care is important.

IX) PROGNOSIS:

Perinatal hypophosphatasia is uniformly fatal. Infantile hypophosphatasia can have a somewhat cyclical clinical course, but about 50% of patients die from their disease; prognosis appears to become more favorable in subjects who survive infancy (2,3). Childhood hypophosphatasia may spontaneously improve, but recurrence of symptoms in adulthood seems likely (5).

X) PRENATAL DIAGNOSIS:

In two cases at risk for childhood hypophosphatasia, where ultrasonography was normal in early pregnancy, hypophosphatasemia was noted in cord blood (personal observation). Only the severe forms of hypophosphatasia have been diagnosed prenatally (18). Ultrasound examination at 16 weeks gestation can reveal an abnormal fetal head, but was judged to be normal at 16-19 weeks gestation in three cases of perinatal hypophosphatasia. Assay of α-fetoprotein in amniotic fluid and ALP activity in cultivated amniotic fluid cells will help to differentiate anencephaly from severe hypophosphatasia. Successful early prenatal diagnosis of a severely affected fetus has been reported with a chorionic villus sample using monoclonal antibodies against TNSALP and placental ALP. Combined techniques - using serial ultrasonography (with attention to the limbs as well as skull), radiologic study of the fetus, and assay of ALP activity in amniotic fluid cells (by an experienced laboratory) - now allow very reliable early prenatal diagnosis of severe cases (18).

XI) PHYSIOLOGIC ROLE OF TNSALP EXPLORED IN HYPOPHOSPHATASIA:

Hypophosphatasia is a valuable model to explore the physiologic role of TNSALP (2,19). Subjects with the severe forms are profoundly deficient in TNSALP activity in all organs; affected children and adults appear to have a more mild deficiency.

The clinical presentation of hypophosphatasia makes clear that, in some way, TNSALP functions importantly in skeletal mineralization and formation of the teeth. However, it also suggests that TNSALP is less important in other tissues, including those that are TNSALP-rich (e.g., liver and kidney). In hypophosphatasia, ALP activity in bone tissue correlates somewhat with the serum ALP activity, but reflects better the degree of skeletal osteoidosis (8). The observation that some hydroxyapatite crystals are found in specimens of bone tissue from severely affected patients, but not within matrix vesicles, indicates that TNSALP conditions the process of "primary" skeletal mineralization (13). Defects in dentin and cementum (histologically similar to bone) show that TNSALP also acts to calcify the dentition.

A variety of evidence indicates that circulating ALP is physiologically inactive (17). Accordingly, deficiency of TNSALP activity in the skeleton itself appears to account for the rickets/osteomalacia of hypophosphatasia. In fact, rachitic rat cartilage has been shown to calcify in serum obtained from an infant with hypophosphatasia, yet slices of the patient's costochondral junction would not mineralize in synthetic calcifying medium or in the pooled serum of healthy children.

Increased PEA levels in plasma and urine provide a useful biochemical marker for hypophosphatasia, and gave the first evidence for a natural substrate for TNSALP. Nevertheless, little insight into the physiologic role of TNSALP resulted from this finding. PEA's metabolic origin is unclear, although it is thought not to be from degradation of phosphatidylethanolamine. The major source of endogenous PEA is reported to be the liver which also degrades PEA to ammonia, acetaldehyde, and Pi. Altered hepatic metabolism may account for the accumulation of PEA in hypophosphatasia (2).

Discovery that PPi levels are increased in the plasma and urine in hypophosphatasia not only indicated that PPi is a natural substrate for TNSALP, but suggested a mechanism for the associated rickets/osteomalacia; PPi was subsequently shown to be an inhibitor of calcium and Pi precipitation. Accumulation of PPi in hypophosphatasia seems to be from defective degradation rather than increased synthesis (2).

Recent discovery that plasma levels of PLP (a cofactor form of vitamin B6) are markedly increased in hypophosphatasia provided evidence for a third natural substrate for TNSALP, and also helped clarify TNSALP's physiologic role (19). Metabolism of vitamin B6 normally involves the conversion of a variety of dietary forms to PLP in the liver. Organ ablation studies show that the liver is the major source of plasma PLP. Apparently, hepatic PLP is then secreted into plasma bound to albumin. Although some PLP circulates freely ($\simeq$ 5%), PLP cannot traverse plasma membranes but must first be dephosphorylated to pyridoxal before entering tissues. Marked increases in the plasma PLP levels in hypophosphatasia indicate that TNSALP acts to dephosphorylate extracellular PLP (20). Increased plasma PLP levels appear to result from deficient activity of plasma membrane-bound TNSALP; accordingly, TNSALP must function as an _ecto_enzyme. Indeed, subjects with hypophosphatasia generally do not have symptoms of vitamin B6 deficiency or toxicity (2). Urinary levels of 4-pyridoxic acid (a PLP degradation product) were normal in four subjects with childhood hypophosphatasia. In three perinatal cases where plasma PLP concentrations were 50-900 fold elevated, tissue levels of PLP, pyridoxal, and total forms of vitamin B6 were essentially unremarkable (10). Finally, children with hypophosphatasia respond normally to an L-tryptophan load (M.P. Whyte and S.P. Coburn; unpublished observation). Subjects with all but the perinatal form of hypophosphatasia have had somewhat elevated plasma pyridoxal levels; i.e., despite deficiency of TNSALP activity, there appears to be sufficient extracellular dephosphorylation of PLP to pyridoxal by some mechanism to account for the normal vitamin B6 status (19).

Recent studies using cultivated perinatal/infantile hypophosphatasia dermal fibroblasts also show that TNSALP is plasma membrane-associated with ectotopography and capable of dephosphorylating physiologic concentrations of PLP and PEA at physiologic pH.

Increased endogenous levels of PEA, PPi, and PLP in hypophosphatasia indicate that TNSALP is an ectoenzyme that is catalytically active toward a variety of phosphocompounds of somewhat variable chemical structure at physiologic pH and physiologic concentration (19,21). In this sense, hypophosphatasia shows that the term "alkaline phosphatase" is a misnomer.

XII) REFERENCES:

1. Rathbun JC: Hypophosphatasia, a new developmental anomaly. Am J Dis Child 71: 822, 1948.
2. Whyte MP: Hypophosphatasia, in _The Metabolic Basis of Inherited Disease_, 6th edition. Ed. by CR Scriver, A Beaudet, WS Sly, D Valle (eds.). McGraw-Hill Book Co., NY (in press, 1989).
3. Fraser D: Hypophosphatasia. Am J Med 22: 730, 1957.
4. McComb RB, Bowers GN Jr., Posen S: _Alkaline Phosphatase_. New York; Plenum Press, 1979.
5. Whyte MP, Teitelbaum SL, Murphy WA, Bergfeld M, Avioli LV: Adult hypophosphatasia: clinical, laboratory, and genetic investigation of a large kindred with review of the literature. Medicine (Baltimore) 58: 329, 1979.

6. Cole DEC, Stinson RA, Coburn SP, Ryan LM, Whyte MP: Increased serum pyridoxal-5'-phosphate in pseudohypophosphatasia (letter). N Engl J Med 314: 992, 1986.
7. Mulivor RA, Boccelli D, Harris H: Quantitative analysis of alkaline phosphatases in serum and amniotic fluid: comparison of biochemical and immunologic assays. J Lab Clin Med 105: 342, 1985.
8. Fallon MD, Teitelbaum SL, Weinstein RS, Goldfischer S, Brown DM, Whyte MP: Hypophosphatasia: clinicopathologic comparison of the infantile, childhood, and adult forms. Medicine (Baltimore) 63: 12, 1984.
9. Rasmussen K: Phosphorylethanolamine and hypophosphatasia. Studies on urinary excretion, renal handling and elimination of endogenous and exogenous phosphorylethanolamine in healthy persons, carriers, and in patients with hypophosphatasia. Dan Med Bull 15: (suppl II): 1-110, 1968.
10. Whyte MP, Mahuren JD, Fedde KN, Cole FS, McCabe ERB, Coburn SP: Perinatal hypophosphatasia: tissue levels of vitamin B6 are unremarkable despite markedly increased circulating concentrations of pyridoxal-5'-phosphate (evidence for an ectoenzyme role for tissue nonspecific alkaline phosphatase). J Clin Invest 81: 1234, 1988.
11. Kozlowski K, Sutcliffe J, Barylak A, Harrington G, Kemperdick H, Nolte K, Rheinwein H, Thomas PS, Uniecka W: Hypophosphatasia: review of 24 cases. Pediatr Radiol 5: 103, 1976.
12. Coe JD, Murphy WA, Whyte MP: Management of femoral fractures and pseudofractures in adult hypophosphatasia. J Bone Joint Surg 68-A: 981, 1986.
13. Ornoy A, Adomian GE, Rimoin OL: Histologic and ultrastructural studies on the mineralization process in hypophosphatasia. Am J Med Genet 22: 743, 1985.
14. Chodirker BN, Evans JA, Lewis M, Coghlan G, Belcher E, Phillips S, Seargeant LE, Sus C, Greenberg CR: Infantile hypophosphatasia - linkage with the RH locus. Genomics 1: 280, 1987.
15. Whyte MP, Rettinger SD, Vrabel LA: Infantile hypophosphatasia: enzymatic defect explored with alkaline phosphatase-deficient skin fibroblasts in culture. Calcif Tissue Int 40: 244, 1987.
16. Weiss MJ, Henthorn PS, Lafferty MA, Slaughter C, Raducha M, Harris H: Isolation and characterization of a cDNA encoding a human liver/bone/kidney-type alkaline phosphatase. Proc Natl Acad Sci USA 83: 7182, 1986.
17. Whyte MP, Magill HL, Fallon MD, Herrod HG: Infantile hypophosphatasia: normalization of circulating bone alkaline phosphatase activity followed by skeletal remineralization (evidence for an intact structural gene for tissue nonspecific alkaline phosphatase). J Pediatr 108: 82, 1986.
18. Kousseff BG, Mulivor RA: Prenatal diagnosis of hypophosphatasia. Obstet Gynecol 57: 6 (supplement): 9-S, 1981.
19. Whyte MP: Alkaline phosphatase: physiologic role explored in hypophosphatasia, in Bone and Mineral Research, Vol. 6, WA Peck (ed). Amsterdam: Elsevier Science Publishers, (in press).
20. Coburn SP, Whyte MP: Role of phosphatases in regulation of vitamin B6 metabolism in hypophosphatasia and other disorders, in Clinical and Physiological Application of Vitamin B6, J.E. Leklem, RD Reynolds (eds). New York, New York: Alan R. Liss, Inc. 1988, pp 65-93.

Discussion:

DR. KAYE (Montreal): Has anybody attempted to do an organ transplant, kidney for example, in severe cases?

DR. WHYTE (St. Louis): Organ transplantation has not been reported in hypophosphatasia, nor has anyone successfully performed a bone marrow transplant.

DR. MARCUS (Palo Alto, CA): That was a beautiful presentation. Could you tell us anything about osteocalcin production, for example, the capacity of the osteoblast to respond to a challenge and make osteocalcin in this disease?

DR. WHYTE: We have preliminary information which indicates that serum BGP levels are normal in this disorder. We have not, however, done any provocative testing.

DR. SANTORA (Detroit): What is the estimate of the gene frequency of the heterozygous state of the severely affected form?

DR. WHYTE: The incidence figure for severe hypophosphatasia of 1 per 100,000 live births that I showed was based on Fraser's experience in Toronto where there is a large inbred Mennonite and Hutterite population affected by this disorder. Accordingly, 1/100,000 is likely to be somewhat of an overestimation of the incidence of the perinatal or infantile form. The incidence of heterozygosity would therefore be somewhat less than 1/316.

DR. SIZEMORE (Maywood, IL): Thank you for a marvelous talk. From time to time, as internists, we see patients with low serum alkaline phosphatase and there are no common causes that we can readily identify. If you saw such a person who is ready to be married would you counsel her in any way? Check her husband-to-be?

DR. WHYTE: That might be worth doing. Certainly, the incidence of this disease, as I mentioned, is very low. Although, in general, serum alkaline phosphatase activity tends to be low-normal and urinary phosphoethanolamine levels tend to be slightly elevated in carriers, there is overlap with normals which makes reliable detection of heterozygotes difficult.

Along the theme of the abnormalities in vitamin B6 metabolism in this disease, we have developed a pyridoxine challenge test to help identify heterozygotes. Patients with all forms of hypophosphatasia have high plasma levels of pyridoxal phosphate, and show really astronomical levels (without symptoms) after a small daily dose of vitamin B6 (pyridoxine) for a six-day period. Heterozygotes also show a clearly abnormal response. This appears to be one way of clearly distinguishing them.

DR. PROESMANS (Belgium): There have been a few reports from France telling us that calcitonin improved the bones of these children. Have you had any experience yourself; have you heard about this therapeutic approch?

DR. WHYTE: Yes. I am aware of a few instances where calcitonin did not appear to be helpful in infantile hypophosphatasia. I can see the rationale for calcitonin treatment in the infantile form where, in addition to the severe mineralization defect, bone resorption continues and the skeleton can dissolve over the course of four or five months. Blocking bone resorption with calcitonin could conceivably be helpful in these select cases, however, it has not been effective to my knowledge.

DR. PROESMANS: I had the opportunity to treat one of two infant siblings. Marked improvement in the skeleton occurred in the child I treated for two years.

DR. WHYTE: Thank you for telling us that. Certainly, there is some cyclicity in the clinical course of infantile hypophosphatasia. Spontaneous improvement has been reported.

Medical intervention is often difficult to evaluate in this disease.

DR. BERGSTROM (Syracuse): Tom Tyree described two perinatal lethal cases several years ago. In his clinical and autopsy material, he called attention to very thick, sticky, viscid bronchial secretions and found them analagous to what is seen in mucoviscidosis. We had a similar experience on our own service, and I wonder if this has been seen by other people and, if so, how it relates to alkaline phosphatase.

DR. WHYTE: That is a very interesting observation. There was some speculation a number of years ago that surfactant, a phospholipid, may in some way be defective in hypophosphatasia because of the absence of alkaline phosphatase activity. This is the only association I could apply to your observation. Of course, mechanical factors appear to account for much of the respiratory disease.

Williams Syndrome

RUSSELL W. CHESNEY

University of Tennessee College of Medicine
Le Bonheur Children's Medical Center
Memphis, TN

WILLIAMS SYNDROME

After the end of the second World War, health authorities in the United Kingdom decided to add vitamin D to milk to correct for what they perceived as a deprivation of this vitamin [1]. British children, they reasoned, had suffered nutritional, emotional, social and economic hardships and deserved to have these wrongs righted. Instead of supplementing each case of evaporated milk with 400 IU (10 µg) as was the practice in the United States, they chose a content of 1800 IU per liter of concentrate. Furthermore, these authorities reasoned that since these cans of milk would be shelved for an extended period prior to use, an additional amount of vitamin D at the level of several hundred units would be prudent. Shortly thereafter an epidemic of hypercalcemia appeared in British infants. An impressive epidemiologic study ultimately uncovered the fallacy of the use of supraphysiologic doses of this fat-soluble vitamin.

Among the infants exhibiting the poor growth, irritability and lethargy of hypercalcemia were a subgroup of children with distinctive clinical features. Prominent among these were a peculiar elfin facial appearance, microcephaly, failure to thrive, feeding problems, hyperactivity once infancy was over, hypercalcemia and supravalvular aortic stenosis. The full blown syndrome was first described in Europe by Buren and in New Zealand by Williams *et al*, hence the name Williams or Williams-Buren syndrome [2]. Additional features include pre-and postnatal growth deficits, mental deficiency, an unusual personality, a medial eyebrow flare contributing to the elfin facies, short palpebral fissures, ocular hypotelorism, a depressed nasal bridge, blue eyes with a stellate or flecked pattern to the iris, prominent lips with an open mouth and epicanthal folds. Patients have a hoarse voice, nail hypoplasia, pectus excavatum, hernias, hypertension, kyphoscoliosis hyperacusis, and numerous cardiac defects, including long segment aortic coarctation, aortic hypoplasia, and cardiac murmurs. Some children are autistic [3].

The disorder is generally sporadic and rarely familial [1]. Some of the psychological characteristics are so prevalent that they deserve mention. Williams syndrome children have hyperactivity, a short attention span, act young for their age, poor motor coordination and clumsiness, talk loudly, have a good memory for people and places, good aural memory, are obsessed with spinning objects such as records and wheels, and also love to close doors and windows. They lack fear of strangers and are very friendly. The term "cocktail-party-patter" has been applied to describe their friendly and loquatious demeanor. A psychological profile has been described, which is somewhat controversial, indicating that these children display wide differences between verbal and motor IQ scores. Children often show an "uneven developmental profile with reading abilities exceeding the expected level and visual-motor skills deficient for overall performance expectations" [3]. When put together this remarkable conglomeration of physical characteristics, personality features, and patterns on cognitive testing make for a child that is difficult for the medical profession to deal with effectively [4].

When first identified, hypercalcemia during infancy was one of the prominent features of this sporadic developmental syndrome. Since its description in the 1950's, the cause and role of hypercalcemia in Williams syndrome has remained an enigma [1]. The etiology of hypercalcemia is uncertain, but it appears to involve an enhanced sensitivity to vitamin D since patients have excessive intestinal absorption of calcium and increased urinary calcium excretion. The fact that massive amounts of vitamin D as high as 10,000 IU per kg body weight when given to pregnant rabbit does lead to calcified supravalvular aortic lesions in their offspring led to further speculation that the syndrome represented the consequence of vitamin D overdose or a hypersensitivity phenomenon [5]. Moreover, as mentioned above, the syndrome was first seen within the setting of the overuse of vitamin D as a national health policy issue [1].

This theory of the importance of vitamin D in causing the features began to fall apart once it was recognized that the offspring of mothers receiving high doses of vitamin D did not have the syndrome and that hypercalcemia was uncommon, perhaps on the order of only 15% of patients with the full blown developmental and phenotypic syndrome [2,3].

Nevertheless, a certain segment of Williams syndrome patients are hypercalcemic and demonstrate clinical features including irritability, poor feeding, lethargy and polyuria suggestive of hypervitaminosis D [1]. Hence the questions remains, what is the cause of hypercalcemia in these children and does the metabolic abnormality leading to hypercalcemia extend to all Williams syndrome patients? Older reports have indicated that the "anti-rachitic" activity of serum of children with Williams syndrome is elevated during periods of hypercalcemia [6]. By contrast, patients with Williams syndrome demonstrate a delayed decline in serum calcium values following an intravenously administered calcium bolus as compared to controls [7]. This finding points to an abnormality in the homeostasis of calcium metabolism and, thus, point to an abnormality in parathyroid hormone (PTH) or calcitonin (CT) secretion. Data relevant to both of these hypotheses, the abnormality in vitamin D or the hormonal imbalance theory, are discussed below.

The first or the vitamin D metabolic abnormality hypothesis is not likely to be due to excessive maternal vitamin D intake, since many infants with Williams syndrome have no history of *in utero* exposure to the secosterol, and infants with such an exposure are not clinically affected [1]. With the development of multiple metabolite assays for vitamin D compounds, several patterns of normal or abnormal metabolite levels have been reported. To date, most patients have normal serum 25(OH)D and 1,25(OH)$_2$D values, except during periods of hypercalcemia when 1,25(OH)$_2$D values are reduced [8]. Taylor *et al* [9] reported that patients with the syndrome who are normocalcemic and have no history of hypercalcemia show a greater rise in serum 25(OH)D values following a dose of 1500 IU per kg daily for 4 days, as compared to normal children given the same dose (Fig 1). These findings suggest an abnormality in vitamin D metabolism. Another pattern was found by French investigators who noted that levels of 1,25(OH)$_2$D were elevated at 160 to 470 pg/ml in hypercalcemic children with the syndrome [10]. These values fell where serum calcium returned to normal and hypercalcemia was controlled with a low calcium diet. These authors suggested that hypercalcemia may be the result of abnormal synthesis or degradation of this active metabolite (Fig 2).

We have examined the circulating values of vitamin D metabolites in 9 children with the phenotypic features of the syndrome and in a pregnant woman who previously gave birth to an affected child. Two of these children had mild hypercalcemia. Two of these children were also given 1500 IU/kg of vitamin D for 4 days to repeat the studies of Taylor *et al* [9]. The results of these determinations are shown in the table, which also indicates the age of each patient and the month during which the blood sample was obtained [12].

Although the number of patients examined is quite small, several features are evident. In patient #1, who remained hypercalcemic during the course of the study, all vitamin D metabolite values were normal. In patient #2, also persistently hypercalcemic, an elevation of vitamin D$_2$ and D$_3$ were found at 7.0 and 129 ng/ml and of vitamin D$_3$ on another occasion of 120 ng/ml. This would be consistent with the idea of high levels of an antirachitic material circulating in the blood

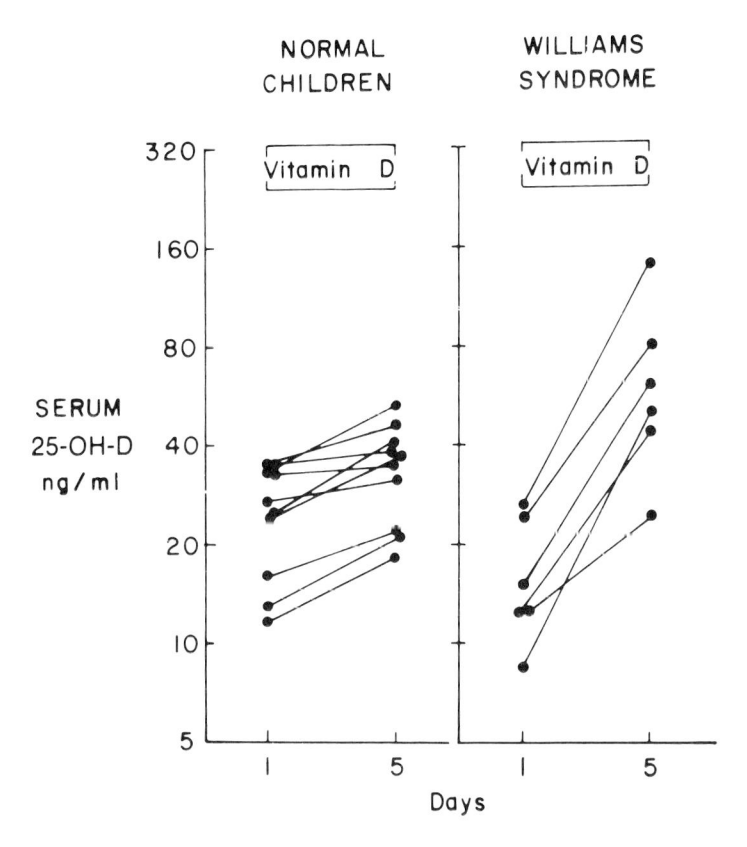

Figure 1. Effects of Vitamin D$_2$ on Serum 25-OH-D in 10 Normal Children and Six Patients with the Williams Syndrome.
Note that the ordinate is drawn on a semi-log plot. The increases in serum 25-OH-D averaged 41 per cent in the normal subjects and 298 per cent in the patients.

Material abstracted from Taylor AB, Stern PH, Bell NH: Abnormal regulation of circulating 25-hydroxyvitamin D in the Williams Syndrome. N Engl J Med 306:972-975, 1982

(6). This patient also had elevated values of 24,25(OH)$_2$D. This patient may have been receiving high levels of vitamin D, although his mother strenuously denied any exposure to vitamin D. As well, the vitamin D$_3$ fraction, presumably of sun exposure origin, was mainly elevated. This child's hypercalcemia was persistent, but was not associated with elevated 25(OH)D or 1,25(OH)$_2$D values.

Patients #3 to 9 had normal values for the age and season of the year. Unfortunately, vitamin D$_2$ and D$_3$ values were not obtained in these 7 children. These findings of normal 25(OH)D$_2$, 25(OH)D$_3$ and 1,25(OH)$_2$D values are consistent with the findings in the literature noted above (8,9).

In a separate study and following the oral dosing with vitamin D$_2$, the serum 25(OH)D$_2$ rose from 4.0 to 37.6 ng/ml and from 7.0 to 56.3 ng/ml in patients 5 and 6 respectively, values similar to those reported by Taylor et al [9]. Total 25(OH)D rose from 47.7 to 63.3 and from 37.8 to 78.9 ng/ml. The rise in 2 control patients was from 6.0 and 9.3 to 28 and 21 ng/ml respectively for the 25(OH)D$_2$ metabolite. Neither patients nor controls had changes in serum calcium, and no alteration in PTH values were noted.

The serum vitamin D profile in a mother of a child with Williams syndrome was normal during pregnancy.

Hence the vitamin D metabolite profile in Williams syndrome patients has a variety of patterns and no single abnormality emerges (Table 2).

Table 1. Circulating Levels of Vitamin D Metabolites in Children with the Williams Syndrome*

Patient No. (Date Obtained)	Age	Serum Calcium mg/dl	25(OH)D$_2$ nanograms/ml	25(OH)D$_3$ pg/ml	24,25(OH)$_2$	1,25(OH)$_2$D
1 (11/80)	10 mo	11.6	21.0	13.2	1.4	6
1 (2/81)	14 mo	10.7	3.0	30.0	2.2	63
2 (3/80)	20 mo	10.9	20.5	28.5	>10	14
2 (3/81)	32 mo	11.2	2.5	28.0	9	48
3 (1/83)	16 yr	9.6	4.9	21.9	1.3	5
3 (4/83)	16 yr	9.5	5.8	29.1	0.9	5
4 (7/83)	5 yr	9.4	2.9	24.3	1.5	32
5 (9/83)	2 yr	10.8	10.0	14.7	1.8	21
6 (7/75)	18 mo	10.2	5.0	31.5	3.3	43
7 (11/82)	8 yr	9.0	4.0	43.7	1.2	30
7 (11/82)	8 yr	9.1	7.6	25.7	1.6	32
8 (6/82)	17 yr	9.4	7.0	30.8	2.2	26
8 (6/82)	17 yr	9.3	7.7	28.9	2.6	22
8 (6/82	17 yr	9.4	7.9	30.9	3.1	21
9 (6/81)	6 yr	9.8	5.6	20.1	lost	44
Controls	(Birth-18)	9.2-10.2	7.3±5.2	23.1±8.7	1.7±0.5	43±12
No. of controls		300	68	68	68	194

*25(OH)D$_2$ denotes 25-hydroxyvitamin D$_2$, 25(OH)D$_3$ denotes 25-hydroxyvitamin D$_3$, 24,25(OH)$_2$D denotes 24,25-dihydroxyvitamin D and 1,25(OH)$_2$D denotes 1,25-dihydroxyvitamin D.

Table 2. Status of Vitamin D in Williams Syndrome

A. Few mothers who have children with Williams syndrome give a history of excessive vitamin D ingestion.

B. Mothers who do take excessive vitamin D during pregnancy do not have offspring demonstrating features of Williams syndrome.

C. Vitamin D metabolite profiles in most children with Williams syndrome shows normal 25(OH)D, 1,25(OH)$_2$D and 24,25(OH)$_2$D circulating values.

D. One child with persistent hypercalcemia showed elevated values for vitamin D$_3$ at 100 times normal.

E. Williams syndrome patients have higher Δ (delta) 25(OH)D values after 4 days of vitamin D at 1500 IU/kg/day as compared to controls.

F. A few hypercalcemic patients have elevated 1,25(OH)$_2$D values which fall into normal range as normocalcemia is achieved.

Compiled from references 8-11.

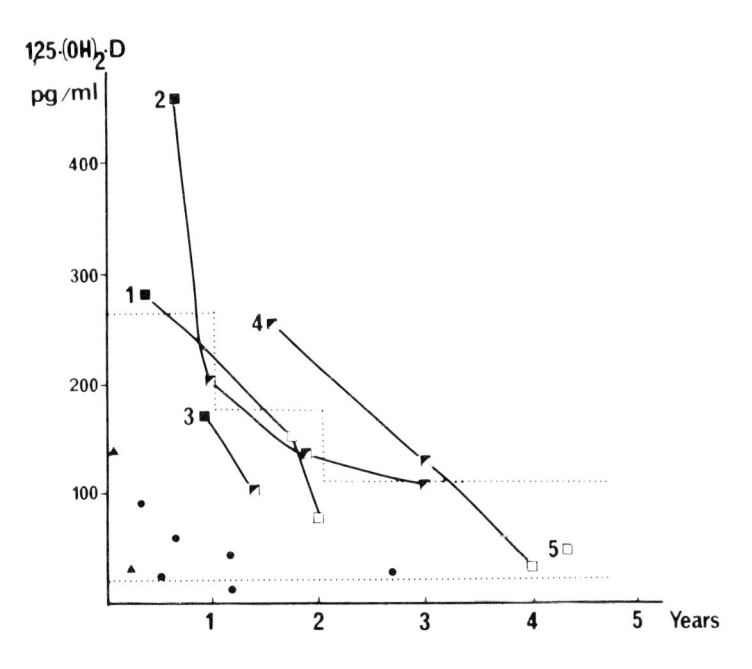

FIGURE 2. Plasma Concentrations of 1,25-Dihydroxyvitamin D (1,25-(OH)$_2$D) in Relation to Age in Children with Hypercalcemia.

Solid dots indicate values in hypercalcemic children with no elfin facies; solid triangles, those in hypercalcemic children after vitamin D intoxication; and squares, those in children with an elfin facies and a history of hypercalcemia. Blood samples were obtained while the children were hypercalcemic (solid squares), normocalcemic under dietary calcium restriction (half-solid squares), and normocalcemic with a normal calcium intake (open squares). Dotted lines show the upper and lower normal limits. Before the age of two years, they show the highest values reported for normal children. [33] After the age of two years, they show the limits found in our laboratory - limits similar to those found by other authors. [32,33]

Garbedian M, JAcqz E, Guillozo H, Grimberg R, Guillot M, Gagnadoux MF, Broyer M, Lenoir G, Balsan S: Elevated plasma 1,25-dihydroxivitamin D concentrations in infants with hypercalcemia and an elfin facies. N Engl J Med 312:948-952, 1985.

The second hypothesis states that a hormonal imbalance results in hypercalcemia and in a delay in the reestablishment of a normal serum calcium concentration following an intravenous bolus in patients with the syndrome [7]. No groups thus far have identified any differences in serum immunoreactive parathyroid values in Williams syndrome patients [8-10,12]. A recent study confirmed the findings of Forbes et al [7] and showed that affected patients had a slower than control value for clearance of calcium after the intravenous delivery of 3 mg/kg of elemental calcium [12] (Fig 3). As noted in Figure 3, the 5 children with Williams syndrome had a blunted calcitonin secretory response after the intravenous calcium bolus. PTH was suppressed equally in both patients and controls, and vitamin D metabolites were normal.

Further information concerning a deficiency in the production or release of calcitonin in Williams syndrome relates to an autopsy report from an adult with the syndrome whose thyroid

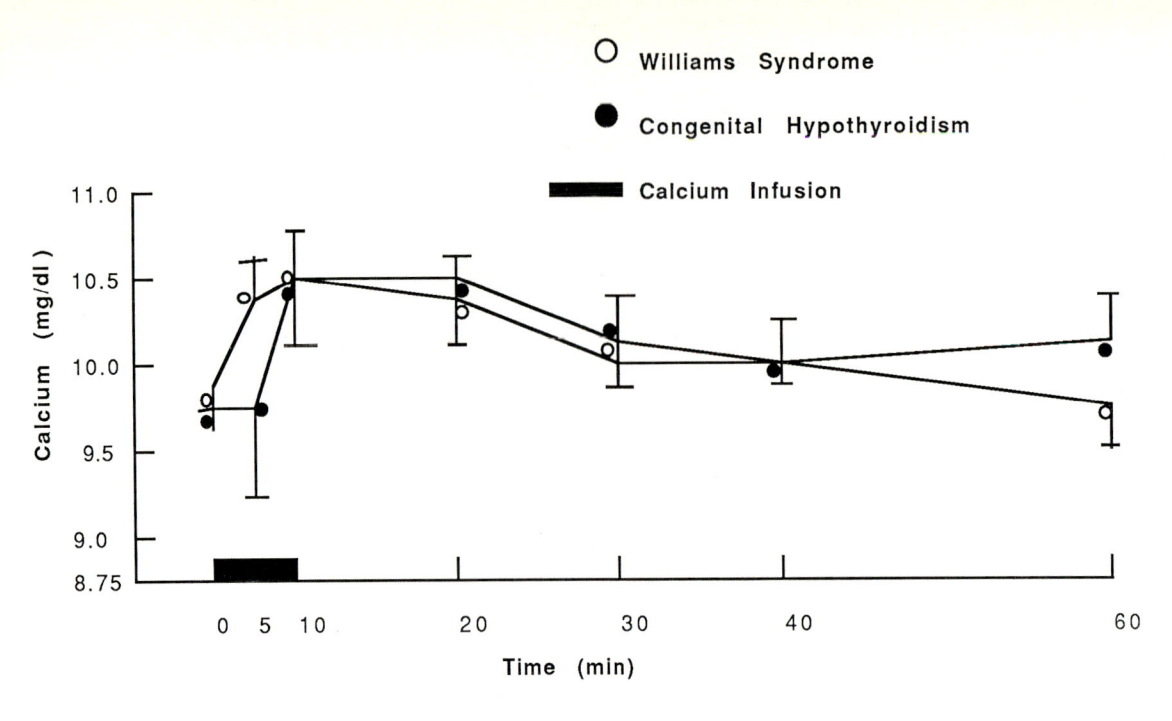

FIGURE 3A Comparison of (mean ± SEM) serum calcium concentrations in five children with Williams Syndrome and eight children with congenital hypothyroidism during calcium infusion study.

Culler FL, Jones KL, and Deftos LJ: Impaired Calcitonin Secretion in Patients with Williams Syndrome. J Pediatr 107:5, 720-723, 1985.

tissues demonstrated C-cell hyperplasia [13]. Whether these glands were hypertrophied because of a delay in CT release is completely speculative.

Culler et al [12] speculate that the calcitonin gene-related peptide, which is encoded on the same gene as calcitonin, may also be disregulated. Since this is a CNS hormone, abnormalities in its production may contribute to central nervous system dysfunction in this syndrome. This hypothesis has no factual supporting data and hence is purely speculative.

To summarize, Williams syndrome is a sporadic dysmorphic condition with phenotypic and developmental features which are readily identifiable. Approximately 15% of patients demonstrate hypercalcemia in infancy. An abnormality in calcium metabolism is also suggested by hypercalcuria, calcification of the media of blood vessels and nephrocalcinosis [1,2]. Two current hypotheses have been put forward to account for the hypercalcemia which relate to either an abnormality in the regulation of vitamin D metabolism or to changes in calcitropic hormone levels. Patients with Williams syndrome may have normal vitamin D metabolite profiles, have elevated vitamin D (prohormone) values, have increased 25(OH)D values following a supraphysiologic dose of the prohormone for 4 days and increased serum 1,25(OH)$_2$D values during periods of hypercalcemia [8-11]. Many of the clinical features fit a defect in vitamin D metabolism in that patients are hypercalcemic, hypercalcuric and show gut hyperabsorption of calcium [7] and thus closely resemble patients who have hypervitaminosis D or a "hypersensitivity" to vitamin D such as that formerly felt for patients with sarcoidosis. Accordingly, it is important to realize that several defects in vitamin D metabolism may underlie the changes in calcium homeostasis in these patients. Until more patients are studied using a comprehensive protocol, the prevalence and importance of the identified defects will remain speculative.

The second hypothesis is supported by the findings of 2 groups that serum calcium values decline slowly after a bolus of intravenous calcium [7,12]. No one has identified parathyroid hypersecretion as a causitive factor, but impaired secretion of calcitonin may be responsible for

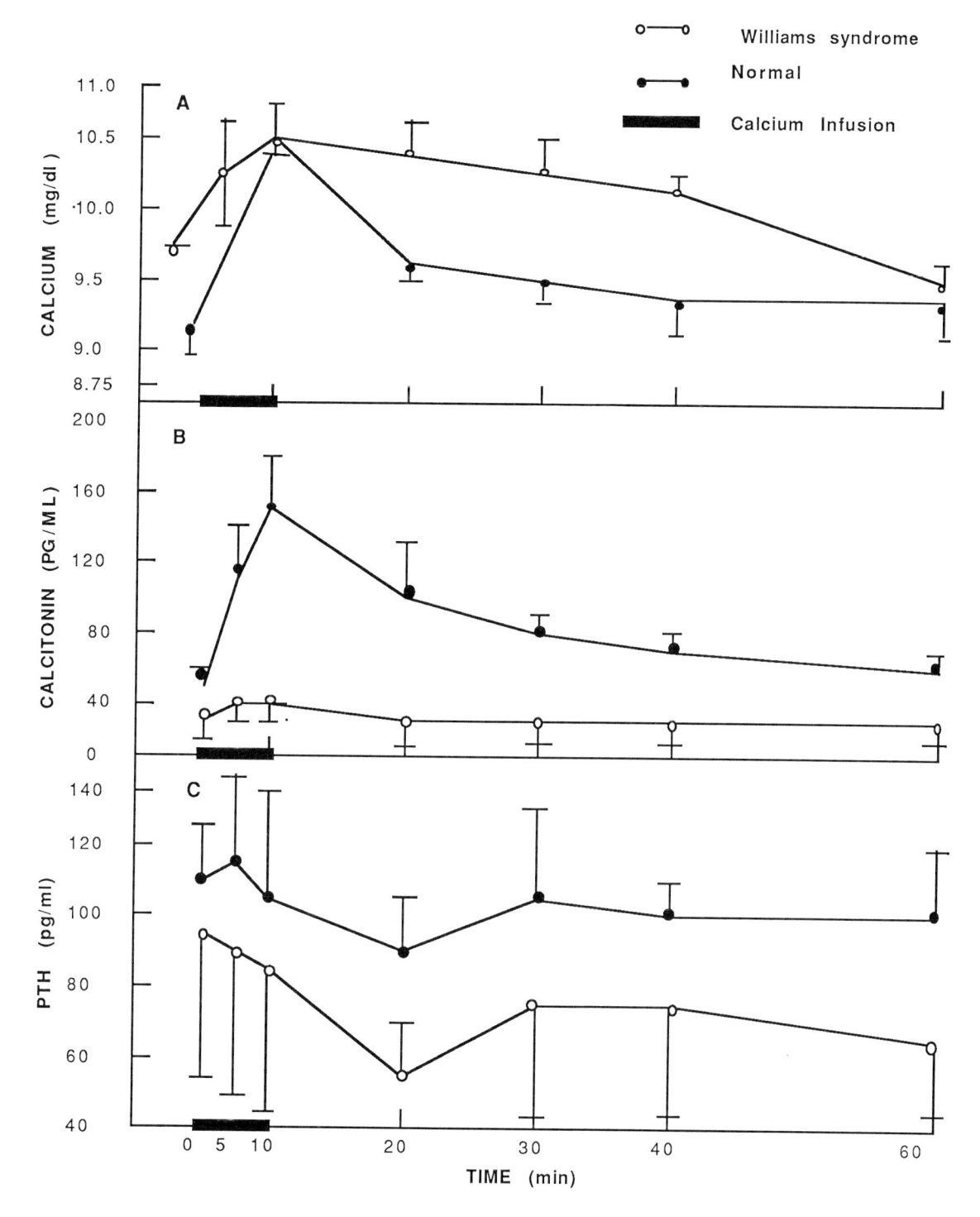

FIGURE 3B Comparison of (mean ± SEM) serum calcium concentration (A) plasma calcitonin concentrations (B) and plasma parathyroid hormone concentrations (C) in 5 children with Williams Syndrome and 7 normal children during calcium infusion study.

*Culler FL, Jones KL and Deftos LJ: Impaired calcitonin secretion in patients with Williams Syndrome. J Pediatr 107:5, 720-723, 1985.

this phenomenon [12]. This hypothesis would not account for the increased intestinal calcium found in Williams syndrome patients nor would calcitonin deficiency result in features resembling hypervitaminosis D. However, the findings of Culler *et al* [12] need to be examined in more patients to understand the magnitude of this calcitonin secretory defect.

Finally, it is important to recognize that hypercalcemia is a small component of the broad clinical and psychosocial features that make up Williams syndrome. Not all children have hypercalcemia, yet virtually all patients have the facial features and personality profile described above, and most have cardiac defects, hyperacusis and delayed growth. Hence it is very unlikely that hypercalcemia plays any role in the pathogenesis of the syndrome other than in the development of nephrocalcinosis and calcification of the media of arteries. The frustration described by parents persists and Williams syndrome remains an enigma for the clinician, psychologist and student of calcium metabolism.

REFERENCES:

1. Greer FR and Chesney RW: Disorders of calcium in the neonate. In Moore ES, Kurtzman NA (eds). Seminar in Nephrology: Role of the kidney in mineral homeostasis in early life. 1983. Grune and Stratten, New York. pp 110-115.
2. Jones KL and Smith DW: The Williams elfin facies syndrome. J Pediatr 86:718-723-1975.
3. Pagon RA, Bennett FC, LaVeck B, Stewart KS and Johnson J: Williams syndrome: Features in late childhood and adolescence. Pediatr 80:85-91, 1987.
4. Anonymous: Case history of a child with Williams syndrome. Pediatr 75:962-968, 1985
5. Friedman WF and Roberts WC: Vitamin D and the supravalvular aortic stenosis syndrome. The transplacental effect of vitamin D on the aorta of the rabbit. Circulation 34:77-86, 1966.
6. Fellers FX and Schwartz R: Etiology of the severe form of idiopathic hypercalcemia of infancy. N Engl J Med 259:1050-1058, 1958.
7. Forbes GB, Bryson MF, Manning J, Amirhakimi GH and Reina JC: Impaired calcium homeostasis in the infantile hypercalcemia syndrome. Acta Pediatr Scand 61:305-309, 1972.
8. Aarskog D, Aksnes L and Maskestad T: Vitamin D metabolism in idiopathic infantile hypercalcemia. Am J Dis Child 135:1021-1024, 1981.
9. Taylor AB, Stern PH, Bell NH: Abnormal regulation of circulating 25-hydroxyvitamin D in the Williams syndrome. N Engl J Med 306:972-975, 1982.
10. Garbedian M, Jacqz E, Guillozo H, Grimberg R, Guillot M, Gagnadoux MF, Broyer M, Lenoir G, Balsan S: Elevated plasma 1,25-dihydroxyvitamin D concentrations in infants with hypercalcemia and an elfin facies. N Engl J Med 312:948-952, 1985.
11. Chesney RW, DeLuca HF, Gertner JM and Genel M: Circulating levels of vitamin D metabolites in children with the Williams syndrome. N Engl J Med 313:888-890, 1985.
12. Culler FL, Jones KL and Deftos LJ: Impaired calcitonin secretion in patients with Williams syndrome. J Pediatr 107:720-723, 1985.
13. Hutchins GM, Mirvis SE, Mendelsohn G, Bulkley GH: Supravalvular aortic stenosis with parafollicular cell (C-cell) hyperplasia. Am J Med 64:967-973, 1978.

Discussion:

DR. BOUILLON (Belgium): At what age can you recognize the diagnosis and, if you can recognize it soon after birth, has anyone looked at vitamin D levels in the mothers, because vitamin D intoxication usually remains detectable for a long time.

DR. CHESNEY (Memphis, TN): That is a very good point. It is very hard to recognize these children immediately after birth because babies look so similar. Michelle Garabedian's numbers and data were from very young children. It may well be that we would have missed this in looking at this ourselves. However, we did have the opportunity to measure D metabolite levels in a pregnant woman who subsequently delivered a child with Williams' Syndrome, and her vitamin D profiles were completely normal.

DR. BOUILLON: If you will allow me a second question? Some of these children have reached adult age; is something known about their offspring? Is Williams' Syndrome transmittable?

DR. CHESNEY: Women with Williams' Syndrome have successfully delivered and their offspring are normal. There have not been many, however.

DR. PEACOCK (Lexington, KY): The cause of the hypercalcemia is either the gut, the bone, or the kidney, or a combination. I am not sure, from your presentation, what is the cause of the hypercalcemia at that level. I presume it is absorption, but you have not shown any absorption data.

DR. CHESNEY: There is some very old absorption data which would indicate that it is from the gut. But the findings that infusion of calcium remains in the serum or plasma for a long period of time is very interesting. I believe there are at least two reports of increased intestinal absorption. But the methods used were certainly not state-of-the-art.

DR. PEACOCK: But is this not a fundamental part of the examination of the hypercalcemia before you explore what the pathogenesis of the hypercalcemia might be?

DR. CHESNEY: I would agree.

DR. GAGEL (Houston): I have two brief questions. First, did you look at calcium metabolism including vitamin D and parathyroid hormone and calcitonin in the children in whom you transplanted kidneys, before and after transplantation?

DR. CHESNEY: Yes, and we did not detect any gross abnormalities.

DR. GAGEL: So, whatever defects they had before were persistent after renal transplantation?

DR. CHESNEY: They had low 1,25's consistent with renal failure, and then, once they were transplanted, their 1,25's rose. But they had no other defects that we could see crudely. Admittedly, we did not do a calcium absorption test.

DR. GAGEL: Second question, do you know whether the children who had been reported to have a low serum calcitonin value after a calcium infusion were hypercalcemic at the time they were studied? I ask that question because there is an evolving literature in the calcitonin field which suggests, although it is still not completely proven, chronic hypercalcemia may actually suppress calcitonin gene expression, resulting in lowered calcitonin production. It would be important to know whether these children were hypercalcemic.

DR. CHESNEY: The children that were described by Dr. Culler had a mean serum calcium of 9.5 at the beginning of the loading test. The level rose to 10.5 after ten minutes of calcium infusion, and then fell into the normal range after about an hour. The normal subjects rose to the same degree, but fell back within about ten minutes.

DR. COLE (Halifax): You have commented on the frustrations, obviously, with our understanding of the etiology and pathogenesis of the disorder, but you did not discuss treatment. This is certainly another problem for clinicians. When the hypercalcemia is recognized, do you have any guidelines about its treatment?

DR. CHESNEY: The basis of treatment of hypercalcemia in Williams' Syndrome is purely anecdotal. It consists of putting the child on no vitamin D and a low calcium diet, using a meat-based formula or similar diet. This type of experience has been empirical. There really are no controlled studies that have looked at this problem.

DR. COLE: The British experience suggests that many of these patients develop rickets on that kind of treatment. Do you think there is any role for calciotropic hormone treatment such as PTH antagonists?

DR. CHESNEY: Potentially. But careful studies will be necessary.

DR. McKENNA (Boston): Regarding fortification of foodstuffs with vitamin D and the risk of developing the Williams' Syndrome, you alluded to the history of a temporal relationship between fortification of foodstuffs and identification of the syndrome. This association, among other reasons, has still inhibited the fortification of foodstuffs in Great Britain. Now that one understands better the relative contributions of sunlight and diet to vitamin D status, is there a safe level of vitamin D intake?

DR. CHESNEY: There is no answer to this. But the point is that the RDA of 400 international units is a safe level in more than 99.9 percent of children. There are no studies that really have shown any impairment of growth or hypercalcemia at that level, except in a child who might have something like sarcoidosis, et cetera.

It is probable that a child could get by, at least in the United States, with about 100 international units a day. And, indeed, some recommendations for pre-term infants are suggesting 100 international units a day. There are studies from as long ago as the 1930s that suggest that if a child receives 1800 international units a day in foodstuffs, it will impair linear growth. But, again, the measurement techniques and statistical analyses are not as we would have used today. And nobody is going to repeat those studies.

DR. BONE (Detroit): I have two parts to my question and they both relate to earlier questions. Firstly, have any children been treated with calcitonin chronically while hypercalcemic?

DR. CHESNEY: I am not aware that they have.

DR. BONE: Secondly, are the children who are hypercalcemic, hypercalcemic when they have been fasted from calcium?

DR. CHESNEY: Again, there is some older literature on that. And we did that, but did not see any great differences. They were hypercalcemic but when put on a low calcium diet for about four days, we did not observe any major differences.

DR. BONE: That would suggest at least some of the calcium is not coming from the gut, I would think?

DR. CHESNEY: Right.

DR. SANTORA (Detroit): You mentioned that precocious puberty was occasionally a feature of the disease. How often is this observed, and is it a true precocious puberty or a pseudopuberty?

DR. CHESNEY: The precocious puberty is a true precocious puberty. It is seen in about ten percent of the patients.

DR. GREEN: There were some reports that vitamin A levels were also high in these children, a finding that suggests an additional mechanism.

DR. CHESNEY: Exactly. I am glad that you brought that up. There was an isolated report of elevated levels of vitamin A which, of course, could increase bone resorption. That observation needs to be explored as well.

The Molecular Basis of Clinical Heterogeneity in Osteogenesis Imperfecta

PETER H. BYERS, DANIEL H. COHN, BARBRA J. STARMAN, GILLIAN A. WALLIS, and MARCIA C. WILLING

*Departments of Pathology and Medicine
and Center for Inherited Disease
University of Washington
Seattle, WA*

It is now clear that most forms of osteogenesis imperfecta (OI), ranging from very mild phenotypes to those which are lethal in the perinatal period, result from mutations that affect the expression or the structure of the genes that encode the chains of type I collagen. In those disorders, the phenotypic heterogeneity results from the nature and location of mutations in the genes of type I collagen.

Biosynthesis of type I procollagen: a complex process (Table I)

Type I procollagen, the biosynthetic precursor of type I collagen which is the major protein of bone, is composed of two proα1(I) chains and one proα2(I) chain that are the products of the distinct genes COL1A1 and COL1A2, respectively. COL1A1 is located on chromosome 17 and COL1A2 is on 7. Each gene has a complex structure that consists of more than 50 exons. The expression of the two genes is coordinated, splicing occurs in the nucleus and the mature mRNAs are transported to the cytoplasm where translation occurs on membrane-bound polysomes. The precursor chain has a signal sequence that directs insertion into the lumen of the rough endoplasmic reticulum during synthesis, an amino-terminal propeptide extension, a long triple-helical domain that contains the repeating $(Gly-X-Y)_{338}$ structure, and a carboxyl-terminal propeptide domain. Each of the domains has a specific structure and, presumably, a discrete function or functions. During chain elongation virtually all prolyl residues in the Y-position (about 100 in each chain) are enzymatically hydroxylated to form 4-hydroxyproline, several Y-position lysine residues are hydroxylated and some of the hydroxylysyl residues are glycosylated, and an asparagine-linked oligosaccharide group is added in each carboxyl-terminal propeptide domain. Only chains in random coil conformation are substrates for the modifying enzymes; once chains are assembled into molecules posttranslational modification ceases. Each completed proα chain of type I procollagen contains about 1450 residues. The chains assemble through domains located in the carboxyl-terminal ends and formation of triple-helix propagates from the carboxyl-terminal end of the molecule toward the amino-terminal end. The formation of a stable triple-helix depends on the presence of glycine in every third position and is stabilized by the presence of hydroxyproline in many Y-position sites. The stabilizing character of hydroxyproline is illustrated by the relative thermal stabilities, 27°C and 42°C, of the unhydroxylated and hydroxylated procollagen molecules, respectively. The assembly and modification of the molecule occurs in the lumen of the rough endoplasmic reticulum (RER).

Once assembled, the procollagen molecule is transferred to the Golgi where the oligosaccharide is modified to a high-mannose structure and the molecule is

TABLE I. Events during collagen biosynthesis.

Event	Enzyme	Location
Transcription	Many	Nucleus
Splicing	"Splicesome-complex"	Nucleus
Transport	Unknown	Nucleus-cytoplasm
Translation	Many	Cytoplasm/RER
Signal cleavage	Signal peptidase	RER Membrane
Prolyl hydroxylation	Proline 4-hydroxylase	RER lumen
Proline 3-hydroxylase		RER lumen
Lysyl hydroxylation	Lysyl hydroxylase	RER lumen
Hydroxylysyl glycosylation	Collagen glucosyl transferase	RER lumen
	Collagen galactosyl transferase	RER lumen
Heterosaccharide addition and modification	Many	RER lumen
Intrachain disulfide bond formation	Disulfide isomerase	RER lumen
Chain assembly	Not known	RER lumen
Interchain disulfide bond formation	Disulfide isomerase	RER lumen
Triple-helix propagation	Prolyl cis-trans isomerase	RER lumen
Transport to golgi	Many (unknown)	RER/golgi
Modification of heterosaccharide	Many	Golgi
Sulfation	Sulfotransferase	Golgi
Exocytosis	Many	Cell surface
Amino-terminal processing	Procollagen amino-protease	ECM
Carboxyl-terminal processing	Procollagen carboxyl-protease	ECM
Fibril formation	Non-enzymatic	ECM
Cross-link formation	Lysyl oxidase	ECM

then secreted. Outside the cell the amino-terminal and carboxyl-terminal propeptide extensions are cleaved by specific proteases, and the collagen molecule assembles into a fibrillar array which is stabilized by covalent, lysine-derived, crosslinks. Mineralization of collagen in bone occurs subsequent to fibril formation.

The many steps required for transcription, processing, and post-translational modification provide many sites for mutations to act; many mutations that affect the structure of the collagen genes result in the phenotypes of osteogenesis imperfecta (see Table II).

Clinical heterogeneity of osteogenesis imperfecta (OI)

Until the past 10 years it was not clear whether the clinical heterogeneity apparent in the OI phenotypes was the result of the different expression of a single mutation or due to different mutations in one or multiple genes. The clinical studies of OI completed by Sillence and his colleagues demonstrated

Table II. Osteogenesis imperfecta, clinical heterogeneity and biochemical defects

OI type	Clinical features	Inheritance*	Biochemical defects
I	Normal stature, little or no deformity, blue sclerae, hearing loss in about 50% of individuals, dentinogenesis imperfecta (DI) is rare and may distinguish a subset	AD	Decreased production of type I procollagen Substitution for glycine residue in the carboxyl-terminal telopeptide of α1(I)
II	Lethal in the perinatal period, minimal calvarial mineralization, beaded ribs, compressed femurs, marked long bone deformity, platyspondyly	AD (new)	Rearrangements in the COL1A1 and COL1A2 genes Substitutions for glycyl residue in the triple-helical domain of the α1(I) chain
		AR (rare)	Small deletion in α2(I) on the background of a null allele Non-collagen mutations
III	Progressively deforming bones, usually with moderate deformity at birth. Sclerae variable in hue, often lighten with age. DI is common, hearing loss common. Stature very short.	AR	Frame-shift mutation that prevents incorporation of proα2(I) into molecules Non-collagen mutations
		AD	Point mutations in the α1(I) or α2(I) chain
IV	Normal sclerae, mild to moderate bone deformity and variable short stature, DI is common and hearing loss occurs in some	AD	Point mutations in the α2(I) chain Rarely, point mutations in the α1(I) chain Small deletions in the α2(I) chain

*AD, autosomal dominant; AR, autosomal recessive.

clearly that the different phenotypes of OI, identified by clinical and radiographic features were distinct entities, a formulation that has been amply demonstrated by the subsequent biochemical and genetic investigations. Although it is clear that the Sillence classification of OI has some limitations, it is used here to illustrate the manner in which classes of mutations give rise to a limited array of phenotypic consequences.

OI type I, a mild dominantly inherited phenotype with blue sclerae, usually results from mutations that decrease the synthesis of proα1(I)

OI type I is the mildest of the OI phenotypes; most affected individuals are of normal or near normal stature and deformity is rare. Unfortunately, a minor clinical feature, blue sclerae, is often used to identify individuals with OI type I when the more relevant clinical features of height and bone deformity may suggest a different diagnosis. Genetic linkage studies, using polymorphic restriction endonuclease cleavage sites within or adjacent to the genes that encode both chains of type I collagen, suggest that the phenotype is genetically heterogeneous, that is, may result from mutations in either gene. This apparent heterogeneity may be due, in part, to inclusion of individuals with blue sclerae when the majority of clinical features would be most compatible with another form of OI.

Cultured fibroblasts from the majority of individuals with OI type I synthesize about half the normal amount of structurally normal type I procollagen as a result of synthesis of about half the normal amount of normal proα1(I) chains. Several types of mutations have been identified so far which appear to account for the decreased synthesis of normal type I procollagen; these include deletion of one COL1A1 allele, synthesis of proα1(I) chains which cannot be incorporated into mature type I procollagen molecules, and defects in the splicing and maturation of the precursor proα1(I) mRNA which prohibit transport to the cytoplasm. Because type I procollagen molecules cannot be assembled with more than a single proα2(I) chain, the amount of proα1(I) chains available effectively titrates the amount of intact type I procollagen than can be synthesized and secreted.

Structural alterations in the chains of type I procollagen are less common causes of the OI type I phenotype but small deletions near the amino-terminal end of the triple-helical domain of proα2(I) and substitutions of cysteine (probably for glycine) in the amino-terminal 400 residues of the triple-helix of the proα1(I) chain have been observed among such individuals.

Perinatal lethal osteogenesis imperfecta, OI type II: a heterogeneous disorder that results from new dominant mutations which affect the structure of proα1(I) or proα2(I)

OI type II is generally lethal in the perinatal period. Increasing numbers of affected fetuses are being recognized early in pregnancy by routine ultrasound examinations. Affected infants are dwarfed, have a paucity of calvarial mineralization and small thoracic cavities. Radiologically the long bones are markedly osteopenic, ribs are beaded, and long bones are short and deformed; the femurs are generally markedly telescoped. Although originally considered to be a recessively inherited disorder it is now clear that OI type II usually results from new dominant mutations and that recurrence in a family is usually the result of mosaicism for the mutation in the germ line (but not in somatic cells) of one of the parents.

Cells from most infants with OI type II synthesize some normal type I procollagen and type I procollagen molecules which are secreted inefficiently, are overmodified along a part or all of the triple-helical domain, and are less stable to thermal denaturation than their normal counterparts. In all such cell strains in which the basic defect has been identified there has been substitution for a single glycyl residue in the triple-helical domain of some proα1(I) chains. All molecules that incorporate the abnormal chain (either one or two copies) are abnormal so that fully three-quarters of the molecules synthesized by such cell strains do not have a normal structure. The substitution for a glycine appears to affect the propagation of triple-helix during assembly and leaves the portion of the molecule amino-terminal to the site of mutation available for extensive further posttranslational modification. Because the efficiency of secretion is less than normal, and because the abnormal molecules adversely affect fibrillogenesis, the amount of collagen secreted is low and the structure of the matrix is abnormal. To date, substitutions for glycyl residues in the triple-helical domain between 391 and the carboxyl-terminal end of the α1(I) chain are known to produce the OI type II phenotype. It is likely that not all amino acids substituted for glycine in that domain produce the OI type II phenotype and it is possible that point mutations in the COL1A2 gene that result in substitutions for glycyl residues can also result in OI type II.

Rarely, large rearrangements have been identified that result in the OI type II phenotype. Two intron-to-intron deletions, one in the triple-helical domain of proα1(I) that deletes 84 amino acids, and the other in the triple-helical domain of proα2(I), which deletes 180 residues, and an insertion in one COL1A1 allele which results in duplication of about 60 amino acid residues were all lethal in the newborn period. Of more than 150 infants with the OI type II phenotype that have been evaluated at the biochemical level fewer than five percent appear to have rearrangements in the genes of type I collagen.

One infant has been identified in which a single exon deletion, apparently on the background of non-expression of the other COL1A2 allele results in the lethal phenotype.

Finally, family and linkage studies suggest that rarely the OI type II phenotype may result from a recessively inherited disorder of genes other than those which encode the chains of type I procollagen.

Progressive deforming OI, OI type III, is a genetically and biochemically heterogeneous disorder that results from point mutations and frameshift mutations

OI type III is characterized by dwarfism, striking and progressive bone deformity with considerable kypho-scoliosis that may interfere with normal cardio-pulmonary function, and marked bone fragility. Sclerae are often blue early in childhood but lighten following puberty; dentinogenesis imperfecta is common.

The progressive deforming phenotype of OI has been the most difficult to understand from the biochemical point of view. Several of the initial clinical studies suggested that OI type III was inherited in an autosomal recessive fashion because the condition was known to recur among sibs, and because consanguinity was recognized in some families. A small number of families were identified in which the condition was inherited in an autosomal dominant fashion.

In the first individual studied with a recessively inherited disorder, the condition was found to result from a frame-shift mutation near the 3' end of both COL1A2 alleles. The mutation changed the last several amino acids of the carboxyl-terminal propeptide, a change that was sufficient to interfere with incorporation of the chain into molecules. As a result, cells from the affected individual secreted type I procollagen molecules that contained only proα1(I) chains. To date, this is a unique family.

Biochemical findings in the majority of individuals with OI type III are similar to those in infants with OI type II. That is, cells synthesize normal and abnormal collagen molecules. The abnormal molecules are overmodified along part or all their length, are secreted less efficiently than the normal molecules synthesized by the same cells, and have a slightly decreased thermal stability. It appears that these alterations in molecular conformation and stability are often the result of point mutations in either the COL1A1 or the COL1A2 gene. Substitution of cysteine for glycine at position 526 in the triple-helical domain of the α1(I) chain and the de novo appearance of cysteine between residues 3 and 327 in the α2(I) chain of type I collagen lead to similar OI type III phenotypes. These substitutions are readily detectable because cysteine does not normally appear within the triple-helical domain of either chain. It is likely that substitution by other residues for glycine residues in selected domains of both chains and, possibly, small deletions or insertions toward the amino-terminal end of either chain could also result in the OI type III phenotype.

Mild to moderately severe OI, OI type IV, usually results from point mutations in the COL1A2 gene

Originally thought to be rare, OI type IV may be one of the more common varieties of OI although controversy still surrounds the precise clinical phenotype. We have chosen to use the term in a slightly broader sense than Sillence originally intended. Rather than limiting the phenotype to those with "white" sclerae we use the OI type IV designation to include the mild-to-moderate phenotype with normal or grey sclerae and mild to moderate short stature, all inherited in an autosomal dominant fashion or due to new dominant mutations. Dentinogenesis imperfecta is far more common in this group than OI type I.

The first studies using polymorphic restriction sites within the genes of type I collagen demonstrated linkage of the OI type IV phenotype to the COL1A2 gene. Subsequent studies have demonstrated that point mutations which result in substitution for glycine in the triple-helical domain of the α2(I) chain and small deletions in the α2(I) chain can result in the OI type IV phenotype. Further, in one family the appearance of cysteine in the triple-helical domain of α1(I) (between residues 123 and 401) results in the same clinical picture.

Molecular-phenotype correlation

Despite the apparent diversity of mutations encountered among individuals with different forms of OI, there is a relationship between the clinical phenotype and the nature of the underlying molecular defect. Mutations which affect the "expression" of the COL1A1 gene are milder in their clinical effect than those which affect the structure of chains synthesized by either COL1A1 or COL1A2. Point mutations in the COL1A1 gene that result in substitutions for glycine residues in the triple-helix are, in general, more severe than those which affect the COL1A2 gene. This is a consequence both of the stoichiometry of the chains in the molecule and the roles of the chains. There is a gradient of phenotypic effect in the COL1A1 gene such that mutations toward the carboxyl terminal end of the triple-helix are more severe than those near the amino-terminal end. The gradient probably has a distinct "slope" for each residue capable of substituting for the glycyl residues and, with the exception of cysteine, substitution at any given position with a bulky residue probably produces a more severe phenotype than substitution by a smaller residue. The relationship between location in the gene and phenotypic outcome may be different for the COL1A2 gene and, further, because so few mutations have been characterized to date, it is likely that some of the lethal point mutations will be found in the COL1A2 genes (bulky substitutions near the carboxyl-terminus of the triple helix). Large rearrangements, expressed in protein, are generally lethal. Some mutations can interfere with several functional domains, disturb several important functions (eg. secretion, cleavage of the amino-terminal propeptide, and cross-link formation), and thus result in complex mixed clinical phenotypes (Ehlers-Danlos type VII and OI, for example). The vast majority of individuals with OI result from mutations in only a single collagen allele; rarely non-collagen mutations result in an OI phenotype.

Biochemical heterogeneity: implications for rational medical therapies

Most medical therapies have failed to increase bone mass, decrease fracture frequency or normalize height among individuals with different forms of OI. It is clear that no one treatment could reasonably be expected to alter the course of OI given the molecular heterogeneity. More rational therapies might be designed to increase the synthesis of chains not made (eg, in OI type I), to alter the extent of posttranslational overmodification in the more severe deforming varieties of OI, or to decrease the synthesis of the abnormal chains while maintaining synthesis of the normal chains. Both pharmacologic manipulation of modifying enzymes and genetic manipulation of the biosynthetic machinery might be expected to alter the clinical outcome of different types of mutations. Such intervention might increase the range of therapies available so that the surgical treatment currently available can be reserved for peoptle with severe and deforming bone disease recalcitrant to other medical approaches.

Annotated References

Byers, P. H. Disorders of collagen structure and biosynthesis. In <u>Metabolic Basis of Inherited Disease</u>, 6th edition, Scriver C. R., Beaudet A. L., Sly, W. S., and Valle, D., eds. McGraw-Hill, New York, 1988, in press.

> The most recent complete review of collagen biosynthesis and the characterization of mutations that affect collagen synthesis and structure.

Prockop, D. J. and Kivirikko, K. I. Heritable disease of collagen. New Engl. J. Med. 311:376-386, 1984.
> An excellent review of collagen biosynthesis.

Byers, P. H. and Bonadio, J. F. The molecular basis of clinical heterogeneity in osteogenesis imperfecta: mutation in type I collagen genes have different effects on collagen processing. In _Genetic and Metabolic Disease in Pediatrics_, Lloyd, J. K. and Scriver, C. R. eds. Butterworths, London, 1985.
> A detailed description of the mechanisms by which OI can be produced.

Sillence, D. O., Senn, A., and Danks, D. M. Genetic heterogeneity in osteogenesis imperfecta. J. Med. Genet. 16:101-116, 1979.
> The most recent and best description of the clinical heterogeneity of OI.

Discussion:

DR. WHYTE (St. Louis): Perhaps I could ask the first question? Because of the high incidence of new mutations, but also the presence of gonadal mosaicism, what would the recurrence risks be for families with severely affected cases?

DR. BYERS (Seattle): For the OI type II phenotype, which is due almost entirely to new mutations, there is an empiric recurrence risk of about six percent in looking across the board at families. We routinely recommend, however, that all subsequent pregnancies be studied by ultrasound. Prenatal diagnosis by ultrasound is extremely effective. There are rare instances where it has been missed, but these reports are almost always in the older literature and when people have not been looking appropriately. If limb length measurements are made at 14 to 16 gestational weeks the diagnosis can be made.

It is possible to make a diagnosis prenatally by analysis of collagens in chorionic villi directly, or by growing the mesenchymal cells from chorionic villi and looking at their collagens. But, with the exception of the direct chorionic villus analysis, there is only a few days advantage with cultured cells in terms of prenatal diagnosis.

DR. GLORIEUX (Montreal): Peter, you whet our appetite by alluding briefly, at the end, to mutations in noncollagenous proteins. Is that still speculation or have you actually identified one?

DR. BYERS: No, mutations have not been identified. The way in which the analysis has been done is basically by linkage analysis with recessive phenotypes, looking to determine whether or not both infants have the same array of collagen genes. Now, there are two explanations for that. And, also, by looking at the collagens that are made by those cells. The collagens made by them are often normal. And in those cases, it has not been possible to show that both infants have the same set of collagen genes, which would be necessary for recessive inheritance of a collagen defect. So, linkage studies are highly suggestive of their being non-collagen defects, particularly in the South African OI type III group and in very rare individuals with the perinatal lethal form of OI.

Petros Tsipouras has said that, in a few families with dominantly inherited OI, there may be non-collagen mutations. But the data have not been fully presented yet.

Neonatal Disorders of Mineral Metabolism

LAURA S. HILLMAN

Department of Child Health
University of Missouri Medical School
Columbia, MO

MINERAL PROBLEMS IN THE NEONATE

A) <u>Early Neonatal Hypocalcemia</u>

Early neonatal hypocalcemia is defined as hypocalcemia occurring during the first 72 hours of life. There is no consensus as to what level of serum calcium defines early neonatal hypocalcemia, (7.0, 7.5, or even 8.0 mg/dl) however, even at the lowest serum calcium level, early neonatal hypocalcemia is a very common problem in the neonatal intensive care unit. The reason for the rather arbitrary definition based on serum calcium is that there is not a recognizable symptom complex associated with the entity. Infant are almost always asymptomatic, rarely showing lethargy or jitteriness, and almost never demonstrating seizures (asphyxiated infants may have both hypocalcemia and seizures secondary to the asphyxia, however, these seizures are not caused by nor responsive to intravenous calcium). The reason for this appears in part to be a relative sparing of the ionized calcium such that ionized calcium falls below 3.0 mg/dl in <10% of cases and less than 2.5 mg/dl in only a handful of cases. (1) Immaturity of the premature brain may also contribute to the lack of symptom. Indeed, the high frequency of this entity and the lack of symptoms have caused different neonatologists to react in very different ways. Many neonatologists opt to add significant amounts of calcium to the intravenous fluids of all infants at risk of early neonatal hypocalcemia and thus to avoid the problem, stating that the risks of I.V. calcium are low enough to be less than any potential risks of undiagnosed significant hypocalcemia. Other neonatologists, especially those who have had access to measurements of ionized calcium and who have become tired of rarely finding a low ionized calcium, choose to ignore the frequent low total serum calcium and allow the entity to resolve itself without treatment. We have advocated an intermediate approach of screening with a total serum calcium and obtaining an ionized calcium on infants with a total calcium <6.0 mg/dl, with treatment of infants with a serum ionized calcium <3.0 mg/dl, for sure less than 2.5 mg/dl, or infants who do not begin to correct their calcium within 24-48 hours. (1)

The pathophysiology of early neonatal hypocalcemia is of physiologic interest if not clinically relevant. Early neonatal hypocalcemia is an exaggeration of the normal fall in serum calcium that occurs in all infants as they go from in utero to extra utero life. The three groups of risk are: 1) premature infants, 2) infants of diabetic mothers, and 3) "asphyxiated infants" (this commonly used and misused term is applied to infants who have suffered some sort of a stress during labor and delivery which results in depression and acidosis) and the relative importance of various factors varies within these groups. In the normal infant calcium is actively transported across the placenta and cord blood total and ionized calcium is high (>10 mg/dl or >5 mg/dl) with an appropriately physiologically suppressed or normal level of PTH. When the placental supply of calcium is taken away, serum calcium falls and PTH increases to normal or high levels over the first 48 hours with the expected parallel increase in serum 1,25-dihydroxyvitamin D. (2) This picture is complicated by an elevated serum calcitonin at birth (and probably in utero) which surges further after 2 hours of life, peaking at 12 hours, and slowly falling to normal over several days probably blunting the effects of PTH and 1,25(OH)$_2$D on mobilization of calcium from bone, necessitating gastrointestinal absorption of calcium. In premature infants in general this calcitonin surge is exaggerated both in the height and duration of the peak. (2) Although the stimulus for this surge remains unclear, the catecholamine surge related to birth is a likely stimulus and "asphyxiated" infants have markedly elevated calcitonin surges. In these "asphyxiated" infants a clear exaggeration of the increase in PTH is seen. Most but not all PTH assays also show an exaggerated increase in PTH in premature infants, however, Tsang et al clearly showed that PTH responsiveness to the calcium fall during an exchange transfusion increases both with increasing postnatal age and with increasing gestational age so that "inadequate" PTH compensation relative to calcitonin may play a role in some premature infants. In infants of diabetic mothers, the calcitonin surge is much less impressive and the data to support a blunting of PTH response is stronger although not supported in all studies. The lower magnesium seen in diabetics especially during pregnancy and transiently in many infants of diabetic mothers has been postulated to play a role in the slower PTH response. Finally, an obvious factor in many of the sicker infants is decreased or absent oral intake of both calcium and magnesium.

B) <u>Late Neonatal Hypocalcemia</u>

Late neonatal hypocalcemia is defined as hypocalcemia occurring after 72 hours of life, usually at 5-10 days of life. Although less common than early neonatal hypocalcemia, it's presentation is far more dramatic and the need for urgent treatment is almost always the case. Late neonatal hypocalcemia usually presents as frank seizures which are responsive to intravenous calcium although it may occasionally present as extreme jitteriness or apnea. Since serum calcium is not routinely measured in well infants of this age, there may well be a larger asymptomatic population. Follow-up of infants presenting with late neonatal hypocalcemia seizures is very good with uniformly normal neurological examinations, however, frequent abnormalities are seen in enamel formation of the molars which are calcifying at this point in development. This entity has best been studied in the Asian population residing in the British Isles which is a well described vitamin D deficient population. Late neonatal hypocalcemia seizures have been reported in over 2% of therm infants in this population. Vitamin D supplementation of the mothers during pregnancy markedly reduces the incidence of this entity and thus vitamin D deficiency certainly plays a role. (3) However, the pathophysiology is certainly more complicated than just vitamin D deficiency in the infant and in the United States most cases of late neonatal hypocalcemia do not have a component of vitamin D deficiency. (4) In most cases the hypocalcemia is accompanied by hyperphospatemia (the entity is more common in infants with high phosphorus intakes such as infants eating cows milk or cows milk derived formulae) and hypomagnesemia. This triad would suggest a failure of PTH function and indeed several series have shown PTH values which are low relative to the degree of the hypocalcemia. (4) Late neonatal hypocalcemia was an unrecognized common cause of death in infant's of mothers with primary hyperparathyroidism during pregnancy and has more recently been recognized in mothers with secondary hyperparathyroidism secondary to renal disease who are now becoming pregnant post renal transplant. Here an exaggerated suppression of the fetal parathyroid secondary to very high maternal and thus fetal serum calcium in utero results in a delayed increase in PTH postnatally. The hypomagnesemia, whether secondary to a delayed rise in PTH or primary for reasons which remain unclear, certainly plays a role in causing or propagating, the PTH suppression by decreasing the release of PTH. Hypomagnesemia also blocks the effectiveness of PTH in bone resorption and thus may also play a role in blunting end-organ responsiveness even in cases where serum PTH appears appropriate. It is mandatory that the hypomagnesemia be corrected in order to achieve a sustained increase in serum calcium after giving intravenous and/or oral calcium. PTH levels have been seen to rapidly return to normal after correction of the hypomagnesemia. Infants of diabetic mothers, who are usually term, also have an increased chance of developing late neonatal hypocalcemia probably related to the magnesium problems already illuded to. Infants who are term but who are small secondary to in utero growth retardation have been described to increase their serum magnesium more slowly after birth than do appropriately grown infants who usually normalize serum magnesium by 48 hours of life and these infants are also at increased risk of late neonatal hypocalcemia. (2) We have recently described another high risk group, infants who have surgery in the immediate neonatal period. In these infants one can observe the development of hypomagnesemia and secondarily PTH suppression and hypocalcemia. Although decreased magnesium intake postoperatively clearly plays a role the effect of the surgical stress on magnesium homeostasis is intriguing. (4)

As discussed, treatment of these infants involves immediate control of symptoms with intravenous calcium and support of serum calcium by oral calcium and correction of any hypomagnesemia with I.M. Magnesium sulfate. In many infants the hyperphosphatemia (>9 mg/dl) may require treatment by switching to a low phosphorus containing infant formula or ideally breast milk. After a few weeks supplemental calcium can usually be stopped and the infant rechallenged with reasonable phosphorus intakes. Infants should certainly be receiving the recommended 400 IU of vitamin D per day, which is provided by a quart of all U.S. made infant formulae or in standard vitamin supplements, since this will rapidly correct low 25-OHD serum concentrations in most term infants. If significant maternal vitamin D deficiency is suspected on epidemiologic or clinical ground the use of 1,000 - 2,000 IU vitamin D per day for several days may be indicated, however, high dose vitamin D or 1,25 $(OH)_2D$ treatment is usually not indicated (Infants with persistent hypocalcemia certainly need to be worked up for the rare inborn errors of vitamin D metabolism and $1,25(OH)_2D$ receptor function).

C) <u>Mineralization Problems in Term and Premature Infants</u>

In the term infant mineralization problems almost always relate to vitamin D deficiency or are secondary to another obvious disease process such as renal disease or an inborn error of metabolism. Vitamin D deficiency remains common in many parts of the world where dietary supplementation is not routine and where sun exposure is hindered by environmental conditions and clothing habits (it is very common in Saudi Arabia where sun is abundant but religious custom require complete covering of the woman's body). Severely vitamin D deficient mothers will give birth to infants with very low circulating and probably negligibly stored 25-hydroxy-vitamin. This can readily be corrected by providing the infant with an oral intake of vitamin D (over and above that contained in relatively deficient breast milk) or adequate sun exposure, however, the same conditions which led to the maternal vitamin D deficiency may perpetuate deficiency in the infant. Vitamin D deficiency is on the upswing in the U.S. with the emergence of groups who believe in 1) prolonged unsupplemented breast feeding, 2) vegetarian diets and 3) occlusive dress usually for religious reasons (5). The high incidence of vitamin D deficiency in the Asian population of the British Isles has already been commented upon. In these populations major educational campaigns to encourage adequate vitamin D intake and/or sun exposure for both the mother and the infant are needed and have been successful. Unfortunately, infants are usually diagnosed late when they have manifested obvious bony abnormalities and/or have clear rickets on x-ray. Treatment with vitamin D (not 1,25(OH)$_2$D or 25-OHD) usually produces changes in the biochemical abnormalities (↓ Ca ↓ P ↑ alk. phos. ↑ PTH) within days and resolution of x-ray changes within weeks.

In premature infants vitamin D deficiency can certainly exaggerate problems and vitamin D requirements are markedly increased if considered on a per kg basis, however, problems of mineralization are rarely as simple as providing vitamin D. (6,7,8,9) The major problem is providing an adequate supply of minerals; comparable to the large amounts of minerals that are transported across the placenta during the third trimester. Even with adequate vitamin D and maximal calcium and/or phosphorus absorption the amounts of calcium and/or phosphorus available in standard formulae designed for term infants or human breast milk cannot allow for absorption of amount of minerals even approaching the amounts required to match in utero accretion. Because of the marked differences in the regulation of calcium and phosphorus and the different proportions of these two minerals in human versus cows milk (and thus unmodified formulas) it is important to address calcium and phosphorus separately in the premature infant. We will begin with phosphorus.

1. <u>Phosphorus deficiency</u> (Human milk and soy formulae)

Phosphorus absorption from the intestines in the premature infants as in the adult is excellent (>90%) and is minimally effected by vitamin D. As in the adult, the premature infants regulates this phosphorus need through renal reabsorption of phosphorus. Infants fed cows milk based formula where phosphorus is abundant relative to calcium (1.2:1 Ca:P) infants excrete large amounts of phosphorus and do not have problems of excessive phosphorus retention. Converse premature infants fed phosphorus limited milk such as human milk are able to reabsorb essential all of the phosphorus such that urinary phosphorus is undetectable. (6) Thus since both absorption and reabsorption are maximal, the phosphorus content of the milk is the limiting factor. Human milk containing about 150 mg/dl only provide about 1/4 to 1/3 of the in utero phosphorus accretion and because phosphorus is necessary for soft tissue as well as bone accretion, a severe deficiency of phosphorus available for bone mineralization can be predicted. Indeed almost all premature infants < 1,000 gms fed unsupplemented human milk will develop classical phosphorus deficiency which often leads to classical phosphorus deficiency rickets. (6) These infants will have a low serum phosphorus, usually less than 4 mg/dl (normal is 6.5 - 7.5 mg/dl) and an undetectable urine phosphorus. 1,25(OH)$_2$D will be stimulated by the hypophosphatemia and be quite high and PTH is suppress, possibly by the 1,25(OH)$_2$D directly or the increased calcium. If calcium is not also limited, hypercalcemia may be seen. Since there is a lack of phosphorus for bone mineralization (as evidence by an elevated alkaline phosphatase) absorbed calcium cannot be adequately used for mineralization and presents as hypercalciuria.

Treatment with additional phosphorus rapidly corrects the

hypophosphatemia and the hypercalciuria and alkaline phosphatase decreases with more time. (6) Currently, attempts at prevention focus on "fortification" of human milk by mixing with or alternating with premature formula or liquid fortifier or by adding powdered minerals and protein to the human milk. Although all of these methods appear to prevent severe phosphorus deficiency rickets, none of these methods match radiographic or bone mineral content measurements of in utero curves or even infants fed a premature formula. It is clear that additional attempts to increase the effective quantity of fortification are needed. The question of the necessary duration of supplementation poses even greater problems since the goal is to have an infant nursing at the breast yet there is no way to increase the phosphorus content of human milk as excreted.

Early formulations of soy formulae contained large amounts of phosphorus which was not bioavailable and a similar phosphorus deficiency rickets was well described in premature infants. (9) Aggravation of the situation by vitamin D deficiency is occasionally the case with human milk and may have been very frequent with the soy formulae (6,9). Although use of newer formulations of soy formula and attention to vitamin D sufficiency may decrease problems, the cautious and time limited use of soy formulae in premature infants may still be warranted.

2. Calcium Deficiency (Standard formulae, vitamin D deficiency)

In the adult or term infant, both calcium gastrointestinal absorption and renal reabsorption are regulated, primarily through $1,25(OH)_2D$ and thus availability of vitamin D and its metabolic conversion is crucial to maximizing calcium absorption and reabsorption. How crucial this classical vitamin D regulation is in the premature infant remains unclear. Animal data would suggest that early in the neonatal period calcium absorption is primarily passive and that the development of an actively regulated system depends on the development of adequate numbers of $1,25(OH)_2D$ receptors at a later time. Comparable data cannot be obtained in the human infant but several factors suggest that this may also be the case. Balance data would suggest that within solubility limits increasing calcium content results in increased calcium absorption. Although many factors differ between "standard" and "premature" formulae, our studies using stable isotopes of calcium show comparable precent true calcium absorptions with double the calcium content (10). Calcium homeostasis and mineralization does not appear to be improved by giving premature infants either 25-OHD or $1,25(OH)_2D$ and production of $1,25(OH)_2D$ appears adequate from very small amounts of 25-OHD in the premature infant. At high mineral intakes no benefit is seen in increasing vitamin D intake. However, at low calcium intakes, a positive effect of giving the parent compound, vitamin D, has been seen both on calcium absorption by balance and mineral homeostasis and mineralization (8). It is possible that this effect, seen with vitamin D but not 25-OHD, does not operate through a receptor mechanism. From the practical point of view, while it is important to assure adequate vitamin D intake (400 - 800 IUD/day which in the 1,000 gm infant is 400 - 800 IUD/kg), it is probably easier to increase total calcium intake than to try to alter percent calcium absorption. To this end, a number of "premature" formulae have been created with 2 to 3 times the calcium content of standard formulae. Many factors of formula composition (fat content and composition, sugar composition, protein content, and phosphorus) may modify calcium absorption, however, these remain unstudied using methods which measure true calcium absorption. Unclear but probably similar factors result in a much higher percent calcium absorption from human milk which partially compensates for the lower calcium content (about 300 mg/dl). However, as phosphorus and protein are added to human milk, calcium may now become limiting and most of the "fortification" regimens also strive to increase calcium content to levels comparable to premature formulae. The effect of this on calcium absorption and other unique properties of human milk is largely unstudied. Premature infants fed either fortified human milk or premature formulae have increased urinary calcium excretion suggesting some limitation of renal reabsorption. Both fortification of human milk and use of premature formulae increase bone mineral content (BMC) in premature infants, however, following of the in utero BMC curve is not yet seen. Whether this represents a developmental delay in some facet of bone mineralization or a continued failure to provide adequate mineral intake remains unclear.

Modern day neonatology in reality presents even far greater problems complicated by 1) total parenteral nutrition, 2) chronic calcium loosing diuretics, 3) abnormal acid-base status, 4) potential trace mineral deficiencies, and 5) many other unknown factors. Clearly much more work remains to be done in this important area.

REFERENCES

1. Scott SM, Ladenson JH, Aguanna JJ, Walgate J, Hillman LS: Effect of calcium therapy in the sick premature infant with early neonatal hypocalcemia. J Pediatr. 104:747-751, 1984.
2. Hillman LS, Rojanasathit S, Slatopolsky E, Haddad JG: Serial measurements of serum calcium, magnesium, parathyroid hormone, calcitonin, and 25-hydroxy-vitamin D in premature and term infants during the first week of life. Pediatr Res. 11:739-744, 1977.
3. Brooke OG, Brown IRF, Cone CDM, Carter ND, Cleeve HJN, Maxwell J, Robinson VP, Windes SM: Vitamin D supplements in pregnant Asian women: effects on calcium status and fetal growth. BMJ 280:751-754, 1980.
4. Fakhraee S, Bell M, Hillman L: Hypomagnesemia and parathyroid hormone (PTH) deficiency in classical late neonatal hypocalcemia (CLNH) and surgically related late neonatal hypocalcemia (SLNH). Pediatr Res. 114:571, 1980.
5. Bachrach S, Fisher J, Parks JS: An outbreak of vitamin D deficiency rickets in a susceptible population. Pediatr. 64:871-877, 1979.
6. Hillman LS, Salmons SH, Slatopolsky E, McAlister WH: Phosphorus deficiency in very premature infants fed preterm human milk: Relationship to 25-hydroxyvitamin D, birthweight, and postconceptional maturity. J Pediatr. Gastroenterol Nutr. 4:762-770, 1985.
7. Hillman LS, Hoff N, Salmons S, Martin L, McAlister W, Haddad J: Mineral homeostasis in very premature infants: Serial evaluation of serum 25-hydroxyvitamin D, serum minerals, and bone mineralization. J Pediatr. 106:970-980, 1985.
8. Hillman LS, Hollis B, Salmons S, Martin L, Slatopolsky E, McAlister W, Haddad J: Absorption, dosage, and effect on mineral homeostasis of 25-hydroxycholecalciferol in premature infants: Comparison with 400 IU and 800 IU vitamin D supplementation. J Pediatr. 106:981-989, 1985.
9. Hoff N, Haddad J, Teitelbaum S, McAlister W, Hillman L: Serum concentration of 25-hydroxyvitamin D in rickets of extremely premature infants. J Pediatr. 94:460-466, 1979.
10. Hillman L, Tack E, Viera N, Yergy A: Use of intravenous ^{46}Ca and oral ^{44}Ca to measure true calcium absorption in premature infants. Ped. Res. in press.

Discussion:

DR. PETTIFOR (Transvaal, South Africa): Laura, that was a very nice presentation. I have two questions. First, what do you think is the role of the 1,25 production in the placenta; do you think it has a role in vivo?

DR. HILLMAN (Columbia, MO): I am not sure if it has a major role. I think the transport of calcium across the placenta probably is under the control of 1,25. Evidence that it is under the control of the 1,25 produced by the infant, more so than the placenta, is available there, but far from complete.

DR. PETTIFOR: My second question relates to calcium/phosphorus ratios in the diet. Do you believe there is much to be said for a two-to-one ratio of calcium/phosphorus in the diets of premature infants?

DR. HILLMAN: That is a good question. One of the reasons I investigated a number of different calcium and phosphorus ratios is that I had initially studied one of the first premature formulas, Ross' Special Care, which had a very high level of calcium and phosphorus. What we observed appeared like classic phosphorus deficiency. Furthermore, the other studies that have been done, even with the newest formulation, show much lower phosphorus absorption than one is used to seeing. So, I think that, very clearly, when you get to high levels of calcium, you interfere with phosphorus absorption as you have this type of competition.

I then had Mead-Johnson make a number of different ratios, but the highest I took the calcium content of the formula up to, was about 1,000 milligrams. At the lower levels of calcium, the calcium/phosphorus ratio does not seem to make much difference, and the serum phosphoruses are nice and normal. So, I think that at reasonable ranges these two constituents are fairly independently absorbed and it does not make a difference. But when you go up to very high levels of calcium, there are problems of phosphorus absorption.

Whether or not the very low phosphorus content of breast milk, that started this whole line of investigation, is a component of why calcium is so well absorbed from human milk, again, I do not know. I think there are multiple other factors besides phosphorus.

DR. GLORIEUX (Montreal): Just a comment about Dr. Pettifor's question and the role of fetal 1,25 production. We have observed a series of newborns with the Potter Syndrome, that is, born with renal agenesis. We found that bone mineralization was perfectly normal. So, I do not believe that the 1,25 produced in the fetal kidney is of critical importance for bone mineralization.

Another comment concerns the high calcitonin levels that are observed in utero. It is striking to see the close correlation with the very minimal amount of bone resorption that takes place in fetal bone. We are currently looking, with Bernard Salle, at about 50 bone specimens spanning a period from 20 weeks of gestation until three months of life. It is obvious that in the postnatal period, bone resorption takes off very rapidly.

DR. HILLMAN: Yes, I think calcitonin clearly is "the" hormone in utero, in terms of promoting bone mineralization. I was interested that, very early on, when we looked at the falloff in calcitonin in premature infants we found that it remains elevated. It slowly decreases but does not reach normal adult levels until post-conceptual term.

Also of interest, it was the infants that had the worst bone disease that had the higher calcitonins. It was almost as if there was some factor that was feeding back to increase calcitonin levels to preserve bone in this setting of abnormally low mineral intakes.

DR. SIZEMORE (Maywood, IL): Dr. Hillman, in the early neonatal hypocalcemia, presumed to be due to hypercalcitoninemia, are you able to correlate the decrements in serum calcium, from normal down, with the calcitonin concentration, and is the phosphate low in those infants, as you would expect?

DR. HILLMAN: I cannot do this from the sketchy data that you have seen. However, the late Dr. Constantine Anast did some very nice work which showed this kind of an inverse relationship; the higher the calcitonin, the lower the serum calcium level.

I do not think that phosphorus load really plays much role at all in early neonatal hypocalcemia.

DR. SIZEMORE: I am sorry, I was not implying that. It is just that calcitonin, in very high concentrations, would be a phosphaturic hormone, and that is why I was asking the question.

DR. MARTIN (Australia): Could I comment on the question of placental transport of calcium, which is necessary for maintaining the fetal calcium and for providing calcium to the fetal skeleton? You pointed to the suppressed PTH levels in utero, but, in fact, the cytochemical assay for PTH, as you probably know from Tony Care's work and Nigel Loveridge, points to elevated bioactive PTH levels in the fetus, and that has now been shown in man and presented at the ASBMR last year.

We will present, at the ASBMR meeting, evidence to suggest that the PTH-related protein that has been isolated from cancers is able to restore the placental calcium transport mechanism in the fetal lamb, in the operated fetal lamb that has been parathyroidectomized, and that this is a function that cannot be carried out by PTH or any vitamin D metabolites or calcitonin. We suggest, on the basis of evidence, that it is a function for this PTH-like hormone. The hypothesis would be that the mechanism of calcium metabolism changes dramatically at around the time of birth, and that can contribute to some of the abnormalities that we see. It is easy, of course, for us to have the hypothesis until we have sensitive enough assays to be able to test it.

DR. HILLMAN: That is interesting. I very carefully said, "immunoreactive PTH," when I talked about that early data because I know this data and I share your opinion that, maybe, we are talking about a fetal parathyroid function. I am glad to hear that you are able to restore it with the same tumor factor because it had been one of my hypotheses that tumors, being a kind of uncontrolled fetal cell, might reflect re-expression of a fetal property and a fetal PTH.

Since bone formation does not quite get where it ought to be until post-conceptual term, some say perhaps it is a problem intrinsic to bone. I emphasize that bones normally mineralize beautifully in utero, and I think have nearly matched the in utero conditions in terms of at least adult-type PTH and everything else. There may be something that is still missing, perhaps a fetal PTH, and that is why we cannot quite mimic the in utero situation.

DR. HARMEYER (Germany): I would like to make a brief comment on the role of 1,25 for the transplacental transport of calcium and phosphorus. We have done some work with pigs who have pseudo-vitamin D deficiency type 1.

When we look at the mothers, who are clearly subnormal in 1,25, the newborn piglets also have unphysiologically low 1,25 levels, yet their plasma calcium and phosphorus are normal. And, in fact, the concentration differences for calcium and phosphorus between the mother and the piglets are much higher in the homozygous piglets which have normal calcium due to the low plasma calcium and phosphorus concentration in the mother. So, I do not think that 1,25 plays a major role, at least in the pigs, for the transport of calcium and phosphorus across the placenta.

DR. HILLMAN: Thank you. Of course I was quoting other people's suggestions. I have not studied this question directly. Both your data and the previous questioner's data would seem fairly convincing, and, of course, Dr. Glorieux has told about the data in the Potter Syndrome babies.

QUESTIONER: When is it safe to introduce whole milk, cow's milk, to infants, considering the economics?

DR. HILLMAN: I think that, as long as you have a functioning PTH system, it is probably acceptable from very early on. These infants can excrete the phosphorus and therefore handle it fairly well. But given all the other benefits, of course, of human milk, I think that waiting until at least six months of age is probably wise. But it is not the phosphorus, particularly, that is worrisome.

Vitamin D Resistant Hypophosphatemic Rickets (VDRR): Pathogenesis and Medical Treatment

FRANCIS H. GLORIEUX

Departments of Surgery and Human Genetics
McGill University
and Genetics Unit
Shriners Hospital
Montreal, Quebec, Canada

The most frequent of the hypophosphatemic syndromes was described more than 50 years ago (1) and still awaits clarification of its pathophysiologic mechanisms. It is inherited as an X-linked dominant trait (2) with the mutant gene being located in the distal part of the short arm of the X chromosome (3). In 1976, an homologous mutation was discovered in the mouse (Hyp) (4). Despite chromosomal rearrangement during evolution, the high degree of conservation of the mammalian X chromosome and comparative mapping of the man and mouse gonosomes (5) support the contention of a close analogy between the VDRR and Hyp mutations. Active studies are in progress in parallel to better understand the phenotypic expression of the abnormal genes.

Clinical expression

The classic triad, fully expressed in hemizygous male patients, is made of: a) hypophosphatemia, b) lower limb deformities, and c) stunted growthrate. Although low serum phosphate (P) is evident early after birth, it is only at the time of weight bearing that leg deformities and progressive departure from normal growthrate become sufficiently striking to become call signs for medical opinion. Isolated hypophosphatemia can be found in some heterozygous females, thus this trait is considered as the marker for the mutation. There has not yet been a thorough study of the biochemical and histologic characteristics of these apparently healthy trait carriers. They provide, however, evidence that hypophosphatemia and renal P wasting cannot solely explain the abnormal phenotype.

Basic defect

The original Albright theory linking the renal P leak to secondary hyperparathyroidism was discarded in favor of the hypothesis of a primary inborn error of phosphate transport probably located in the proximal nephron (6). It is noteworthy that the defect is less severe in heterozygotes than it is in hemizygotes. This gene-dose effect indicates that the abnormality is close to the abnormal gene product. The abnormality in the Hyp mouse has been localized in the brush border of the proximal tubular cells (7). Suggestions that the abnormality would be secondary to the presence of an humoral "hypophosphatemic factor" have not received conclusive experimental support, so far (8).

Because of the close link between phosphate repletion status and 1,25-dihydroxyvitamin D (1,25 D) synthesis, the metabolism of this hormone has been extensively

---

Work supported by the Shriners of North America.

studied. It should be pointed out that there is no evidence of simple 1,25 D deficiency, as seen in vitamin D dependency type I. The reported inappropriate response of 1,25 D synthesis to dietary phosphate restriction (9) [there is no abnormality in the response to a low calcium challenge (10)], points towards the vitamin D metabolism abnormality being secondary to the primary P transport defect and its consequences on intracellular P economy.

Response to treatment

Based on the established renal P wasting, therapy has centered on often aggressive P replacement (1-3 g elemental P/d in 4-5 doses). To offset the hypocalcemic effect of P supplementation, that has caused sometimes severe secondary hyperparathyroidism, large (20-75,000 IU/d) amounts of vitamin D were added to the regimen. With adequate compliance to such a combined treatment, growthrate was markely improved and there was radiologic evidence of healed rickets (11). However, histologic studies of iliac crest bone biopsies showed that the osteomalacic component of the bone disease was hardly improved (12). It was only by substituting 1,25 D for vitamin D at the dose of 30-70 ng/kg/d that improvement and sometimes healing of the mineralization defect was observed at the trabecular surfaces (13-16). Interestingly, the hypomineralized periosteocytic lesions (HPL) which are a hallmark of XLH, never completely disappear even after active mineralization has been restored at the endosteal surfaces. After more than 2 years of efficient therapy, HPL are still present around 20% of the osteocytes in the newly formed osteons (17). As HPL are never present in other chronic hypophosphatemic states, this observation gives substance to the early proposal that there may be an osteoblastic primary metabolic defect in XLH (18). The lesions are also present in the Hyp mouse (19), and we have recently demonstrated that there was an intrinsic defect in Hyp osteoblasts leading to defective bone formation (20).

Long-term effects of treatment

P loading, except for occasional osmotic diarrhea, has not caused any harmful effects. We prefer to use coated tablets containing a mixture of sodium and potassium salts in order to avoid excessive sodium load.

For many years, large amounts of vitamin D were administered with P to offset its hypocalcemic effect and consequent hyperparathyroidism. Major difficulties were encountered leading in several cases to "tertiary" hyperparathyroidism that could only be controlled surgically (11). The substitution of 1,25 D for vitamin D, initiated 10 years ago, has greatly improved this situation. It is clear that 1,25 D may through its direct effect on PTH release maintain a state of euparathyroidism compatible with adequate bone modeling and remodeling (16).

One major problem with long term administration of 1,25 concerns its possible deleterious effects on renal function following repeated episodes of hypercalciuria. One recent report indicates that echodense renal pyramids were found in 11/23 patients who received vitamin D or 1,25 D, and P for more than 3 years (21). The findings were not related, however, to evidence of decreased renal function. High doses of 1,25 D will cause frequent episodes of hypercalcemia and/or hypercalciuria (16), after initial bone healing has occured. It is our experience that smaller ($\leq 1\mu g/d$) doses of 1,25 D, even if control of the mineralization defect is slower and not always complete, should be preferred as episodes of hypercalciuria are rare (less than 1 day/year over 139 patient/year) with such a regimen, and with frequent monitoring of urinary calcium excretion. Long term continuous administration of 1,25 D and P can be maintained without measurable negative effects on renal function.

Treatment of adult patients

When compliance has been adequate throughout the growth period, in a patient in whom treatment was initiated early (before age 4), clinical results are usually satisfactory in terms of height achieved and extent of lower limb deformities. Since most of these effects are the consequence of the aggressive P supplementation, the question arises whether one should maintain such a demanding regimen after fusion of the epiphyses or not. If compliance is unlikely to be maintained, it is doubtful if the irregular and variable use of phosphate supplements will have any significant effect on the osteomalacia of the affected adult. Because bone growth has ceased and bone turnover is reduced in the adult, the high demand for phosphate is probably reduced. Thus one could envisage that continuation of 1,25 D alone, through its effects on bone turnover and intestinal P absorption would maintain the good results obtained by the combined therapy. Our preliminary observations in 6 adult VDRR patients indicate that 1,25 D alone (at 1-2 µg/d) has a significant beneficial effect on the parameters of bone mineralization over a period of 11-17 months. The study is still in progress and should allow us to answer the question of long-term treatment of adult VDRR.

Conclusion

Although the pathogenesis of VDRR is still elusive, the medical treatment of its clinical expression has made significant progress in the past ten years. The combination of P supplements and supraphysiologic doses of 1,25 D is able to allow normal growth and adequate bone mineralization. If carefully monitored, such a regimen should not have adverse effects on renal function.

References

1. Albright F, Butler AM and Bloomberg E. Rickets resistant to vitamin D therapy. Am J Dis Child 54, 529, 1937.

2. Winters RW, Graham JB, Williams TF, McFalls VW and Burnett CH. A genetic study of familial hypophosphatemia and vitamin-D resistant rickets with a review of the literature. Medicine 37, 97, 1958.

3. Thakker RV, Read AP, Davies KE, Whyte WP, Weksberg R, Glorieux FH, Davies M, Mountford RC, King A, Kim GS, Harris R and O'Riordan, JLH. Bridging markers defining the map position of X-linked hypophosphatemic rickets. J Med Genet 24, 756, 1987.

4. Eicher EM, Southard JL, Scriver CR and Glorieux FH. Hypophosphatemia: mouse model for human familial hypophosphatemic (vitamin D-resistant) rickets. Proc Natl Acad Sci (USA) 73, 4667, 1976.

5. Davisson MT. X-linked genetic homologies between Mouse and Man. Genomics 1, 213, 1987.

6. Glorieux F and Scriver CR. Loss of a PTH sensitive component of phosphate transport in X-linked hypophosphatemia. Science 175, 997, 1972.

7. Tenenhouse HS, Scriver CR, McInnes RR and Glorieux FH. Renal handling of phosphate in vivo and in vitro by the X-linked hypophosphatemic male mouse (Hyp/Y). Evidence for a defect in the brush border membrane. Kidney Intern 14, 236, 1978.

8. Bonjour J-P, Caverzasio J, Muhlbauer R, Trechsel U and Troehler. Are 1,25(OH)$_2$D$_3$ production and tubular phosphate transport regulated by one common mechanism which would be defective in X-linked hypophosphatemic rickets? In: Vitamin D, Chemical, Biochemical and Clinical Endocrinology of Calcium Metabolism. AW Norman, K Schaefer, D v.Herrath, Grigoleit H-G, eds. Walter de Gruyter, Berlin, New York, 427-433, 1982.

9. Lobaugh B and Drezner MK. Abnormal regulation of renal 25-dihydroxyvitamin D-1α-hydroxylase activity in the X-linked hypophosphatemic mouse. J Clin Invest 71, 400, 1983.

10. Meyer RA Jr, Gray RW, Roos BA and Kiebzak GM. Increased plasma 1,25-

dihydroxyvitamin D after low calcium challenge in X-linked hypophosphatemic mice. Endocrinology 111, 174, 1982.

11. Glorieux F, Scriver CR, Reade TM, Goldman H and Roseborough A. The use of phosphate and vitamin D to prevent dwarfism and rickets in X-linked hypophosphatemia. New Engl J Med 281, 481, 1972.

12. Glorieux FH, Bordier PJ, Marie P, Delvin EE and Travers R. Inadequate bone response to phosphate and vitamin D in familial hypophosphatemic rickets. In: Homeostasis of phosphate and other minerals. S Massry, E Ritz and A Rapado, Eds. Plenum, 227-232, 1978.

13. Glorieux FH, Marie PJ, Pettifor JM and Delvin EE. Bone response to phosphate salts, ergocalciferol and calcitriol in hypophosphatemic vitamin-D resistant rickets. N Engl J Med 303, 1023, 1980.

14. Costa T, Marie PJ, Scriver CR, Cole DEC, Reade TM, Nogrady B, Glorieux FH and Delvin EE. X-linked hypophosphatemia. Effect of calcitriol on renal handling of phosphate, serum phosphate, and bone mineralization. J Clin Endocr Metab 52, 463, 1981.

15. Drezner MK, Lyles, KW, Haussler MR and Harrelson JM. Evaluation of a role for 1,25-dihydroxyvitamin D in the pathogenesis and treatment of X-linked hypophosphatemic rickets and osteomalacia. J Clin Invest 66, 1020, 1980.

16. Harrell RM, Lyles KW, Harrelson JM, Friedman NE and Drezner MK. Healing of bone disease in X-linked hypophosphatemic rickets/osteomalacia. Induction and maintenance with phosphorus and calcitriol. J Clin Invest 75, 1858, 1985.

17. Marie PJ and Glorieux FH. Relation between hypomineralized periosteocytic lesions and bone mineralization in vitamin D resistant rickets. Calcif Tissue Int 35, 443, 1983.

18. Frost HM. Some observations on bone mineral in a case of vitamin D resistant rickets. Henry Ford Hosp Med Bull 6, 300, 1958.

19. Glorieux FH and Ecarot-Charrier B. X-linked vitamin-D resistant rickets: Is osteoblast activity defective? In: Calcium Regulation and Bone Metabolism. Volume 9. DV Cohn, TJ Martin, PJ Meunier, eds. Excerpta Medica, Amsterdam, New York, Oxford, 227-231, 1987.

20. Ecarot-Charrier E, Glorieux FH, Travers R, Desbarats M, Bouchard F and Hinek A. Defective bone formation by transplanted Hyp mouse bone cells into normal mice. Endocrinology. In press.

21. Goodyer PR, Kronick JB, Jequier S, Reade TM and Scriver CR. Nephrocalcinosis and its relationship to treatment of hereditary rickets. J. Pediatr. 111, 700, 1987.

Discussion:

DR. OGATA (Tokyo): You said the addition of 1,25-dihydroxyvitamin D3 gave better results than vitamin D2. Do you think this is due to the direct effect of calcitriol on bone cells, or is it just a reflection of improved blood calcium levels or suppression of PTH?

DR. GLORIEUX (Montreal): This is a question that is often debated among those interested in hypophosphatemic rickets. I would say that it is probably a combination of both. I showed you that we can obtain better serum phosphate values with 1,25-dihydroxyvitamin D3. What I did not have time to show you is that if you give large doses of calcitriol to an adult, and we have done this in six subjects who received two micrograms/day for periods from 5 to 17 months without phosphate supplementation, there is significant improvement in the osteomalacia at the trabecular surface that occurs without significant changes in the serum phosphate concentration. They were still clearly hypophosphatemic and hyperphosphaturic, yet their bone was improved with 1,25-dihydroxyvitamin D3 therapy alone. Nevertheless, I believe that we do not fully understand if 1,25 has a direct effect at the bone level.

DR. OGATA: My second question concerns the occurrence of hyperparathyroidism during the medical control of these patients. I have the impression that the incidence of hyperparathyroidism has increased since we have used activated vitamin D as compared to the use of plain vitamin D. What is your view?

DR. GLORIEUX: Our experience has been the opposite. Before we used 1,25, we had considerable problems with secondary hyperparathyroidism induced by phosphate therapy. We have had two episodes of so-called tertiary hyperparathyroidism and have had to surgically control the situation. In the past ten years, we have been using 1,25 and phosphate supplementation and although we have patients who have higher serum levels of immunoreactive PTH, we have not reached a point where we had to remove hyperplastic glands. We can control PTH secretion by adjusting treatment.

DR. HAUSSLER (Tucson, AZ): Francis, has any progress been made in the isolation and cloning of the phosphate transport protein that is presumably defective in this disorder?

DR. GLORIEUX: Not yet. But I hope it will come soon.

DR. MEUNIER (France): When they are adults, these patients have usually a dramatic osteosclerosis. We have recently measured the bone mineral density by DPA in five subjects. They scored at plus three, or between plus three and plus five. How do you explain this major osteosclerosis?

DR. GLORIEUX: First, I wish to say that you are not the only ones who have observed this osteosclerosis. The finding has been in the literature for a while, now. I alluded to it when I said that this form of osteomalacia is not accompanied by a decrease in bone volume. Actually, bone volume, if anything, even in the young age, is higher than in age-matched controls. Perhaps this is explained by bone with a mineralization defect yet not coupled to increased resorption activity. There is hardly any resorption going on. Maybe this is because there are not many surfaces to resorb.

DR. MEUNIER: Is it the progressive accumulation of matrix that leads to the osteosclerosis?

DR. GLORIEUX: It is possible.

DR. DREZNER (Raleigh-Durham, NC): I would like to make several comments about some data that we have accumulated relative to what you have presented. We have observed hyperechogenicity of the renal pyramids in a goodly number of our patients who have been treated. Most of them, in fact, before we have had any incidence of hypercalcemia or hypercalciuria. Interestingly, most of those patients are children, and we very rarely see renal hyperechogenicity in adults. However, we have observed no deterioration of renal function over quite long periods of time, in spite of the hyperechogenicity. So, we are not exactly sure what importance to put on this finding.

DR. GLORIEUX: I completely share your view. We have not been following our patients by ultrasound. But we certainly have followed, very closely, renal function over the years. We have not observed any decrease in renal function parameters over the time of our observations.

DR. DREZNER: A second point where we tend to disagree a little is that we are observing a tremendous incidence of immunoreactive hyperparathyroidism, if you will, in virtually 100 percent of our treated patients at this time. We have seen one subject go on to intractable hypercalcemia, requiring removal of the parathyroids, but, by and large, we see creeping increases in PTH in every one of the patients treated with phosphate and 1,25-dihydroxyvitamin D3.

Lastly, with respect to the dose of 1,25, what we have observed as we lowered the dose in the latter periods of therapy is that, if we go low enough (in an adult, say one microgram, which is not one microgram in a child, obviously) that they actually unheal. And there is an obvious threshold dose for the 1,25, which we believe is approximately 30 nanograms per kilogram body weight, for a maintenance dose.

DR. GLORIEUX: I have always had difficulty in evaluating calcitriol doses in nanograms per kilogram, because we have access to only 250 nanograms capsules. In a growing child it is a little ludicrous to try to do it. I welcome your remarks about adults. As you know, I am a pediatrician, so adults drift away from our facility. It is interesting to learn that you can maintain patients on a lower dose.

Now, concerning the PTH levels, we have looked at this carefully and repeatedly, and do not see significant increases in serum PTH levels. Could our observation be linked to the doses of 1,25. We work with lower doses than yourself. I also know that in Japan they use higher doses of 1-alpha or 1,25 than we use. Perhaps there could be a relation.

DR. DREZNER: Is it not paradoxical to your premise that 1,25 is effective in suppressing parathyroid hormone levels? How then, could greater doses of 1,25 not be "more effective"?

DR. GLORIEUX: I cannot explain your data just mentioned to me. The only thing I can say is that, with the type of dosages and the protocol we use, over the time period of observation, we have not seen problems of severe secondary hyperparathyroidism. Furthermore, we did see this often before changing to 1,25 therapy.

DR. KANIS (England): Francis, to return to the question of dose, it has been my impression, in adults anyway, that these patients can tolerate enormous doses of 1,25 compared to healthy adults. And my impression from looking at the literature is that it is also the case in children. I wonder whether you could confirm this? And secondly, what do you think this means in terms of abnormal target tissue response to 1,25 in this disorder?

DR. GLORIEUX: Thank you for raising this point, John. This is something that we have observed. We, in fact, have about as many patients with vitamin D dependency type 1 as children with hypophosphatemic rickets. We follow 24 patients with VDDR, type I.

It is clear that to correct completely the phenotype of VDDR type 1 we use lower doses of 1,25 than those that are tolerated by the hypophosphatemic children. So my impression is similar to yours. I am convinced that XLH patients tolerate much more 1,25 than you would expect if there was a simple 1,25 deficiency. We have thus to consider some form of resistance at the target cell level.

DR. HARMEYER (Germany): My question follows this theme and concerns the etiology of XLH. Is the primary cause the defective transport mechanism in the kidney, or is the deficiency in some regulatory mechanism? There is one report in the literature concerning a kidney transplant into one of these patients. The defective transport of phosphate developed in this transplanted kidney.

DR. GLORIEUX: I know that paper. My major reservation about it is that the donor kidney was taken from a sister of the patient, and that she may very well have been an heterozygote for the disease. Therefore, I do not think that the observation is convincing for a regulatory defect.

DR. LAFFERTY (Cleveland): Would you elaborate on the six adults that you treated? You said their serum phosphorus did not change. You gave them two micrograms per day. Were they given phosphorus as well?

DR. GLORIEUX: No, they were not. They received only 1,25.

DR. LAFFERTY: So, you do not feel that it is necessary to give phosphorus?

DR. GLORIEUX: This was just a pilot study. First, I should mention that the same findings were reported from Durham a few years ago. It is our feeling that if you cannot reasonably count on compliance with the fairly demanding schedule of phosphate administration, it is probably better not to give it, because we will end up with spikes of phosphate concentration in the serum that will not last long enough to change the steady-state level of phosphate concentration. They may also have some major adverse effects on hormonal secretion.

DR. LANG (New Haven): Very nice work, and particularly the treatment. It has really come a long way in the last 15 years.

I have a question about the pathogenesis. Why do you feel that this is a defect in the reabsorption of phosphate? How about the possibility that there is a problem getting phosphate out of the cell? This does not look like phosphate depletion, or is it akin to the rare syndromes of phosphate wasting seen with some tumors?

DR. GLORIEUX: This is a very good point. If you remember the model I showed, there was a white arrow coming from the cell to the tubular lumen indicating one of the hypotheses we consider, namely, that the control of the phosphate out of the cell into the extracellular space is disturbed.

DR. LANG: I meant getting it out of the cell in the other direction. If the patients were phosphate-depleted, you would expect the 1,25 to be much higher than what you measure, correct? Perhaps intracellular phosphate is not very low, but is actually high.

DR. GLORIEUX: That is a possibility.

DR. SUH (Hawaii): Francis, I enjoyed your presentation very much. I have two questions. One concerns your earlier report on a possible defect in the PTH response in terms of a phosphaturic effect. What do you think about it now?

DR. GLORIEUX: I think it still holds. We have not repeated those studies, and if somebody else has, I would like to hear about it. Our patients certainly do not respond like normal people in terms of phosphate excretion when you infuse them with PTH.

DR. SUH: The second question concerns the urinary

calcium/creatinine ratio. You test the morning urine. Is that a fasting urine sample?

DR. GLORIEUX: We use the second specimen of the day. That means that we have the patients empty their bladder when they wake up, and we then use the specimen produced in the clinic, which is, therefore, from the time they wake up until they come fasting to the hospital.

DR. SUH: Is not this urinary calcium/creatinine ratio of 0.3 too high? Earlier, I had a discussion with Dr. Charles Pak. He mentioned that in adults, calcium/creatinine ratio in the fasting urine is 0.11.

DR. GLORIEUX: The 0.3 limit is based on specimens collected with the same conditions in 45 normal children. The highest value we observed was 0.3.

DR. PROESMANS (Belgium): Francis, I am not aware of any studies in which the intracellular phosphate was measured in the renal tubular cells. How is it in the mouse model?

DR. GLORIEUX: It has been measured, and found to be normal. The technology, I think, may still improve, and we should expect to have new findings along those lines. The first attempts did not indicate any apparent differences between the normal and the abnormal cells.

DR. PROESMANS: Do the mice also have normal 1,25 levels?

DR. GLORIEUX: Yes. I'm sure that you will hear about that this afternoon from the speakers who will discuss phosphate and vitamin D metabolism.

IX
Vitamin D in Health and Disease

Overview:
Vitamin D Metabolism in Health and Disease

NORMAN H. BELL

*Medical University of South Carolina
and Veterans Administration Medical Center
Charleston, SC*

In this portion of the program, the most recent information concerning factors that regulate the production and biologic action of 1,25-dihydroxyvitamin D, the most active metabolite of vitamin D, in normal and disease states, was presented.

Mark Haussler described the structure and functional domains of the receptor for 1,25-dihydroxyvitamin D. The human receptor is a polypeptide containing 427 amino acids with an N-terminal DNA binding domain (150 amino acids) and a C-terminal hormone binding domain (226 amino acids) that are separated by a "hinge" (51 amino acids) ( ). Importantly, the DNA binding region contains two "zinc fingers" that are thought to be important in binding of the 1,25-dihydroxyvitamin D-receptor complex to DNA (see below). The vitamin D receptor bears a striking resemblance to other nonpolypeptide hormone receptors including the glucocorticoid receptor, estrogen receptor, retinoic acid receptor and thyroid receptor (1). Not surprising is the finding that there is a high degree of homology among the receptors at the DNA binding site. Haussler indicates that 1,25-dihydroxyvitamin D_3 upregulates its receptor, that phosphorylation may occur in this process and that upregulation may be physiologically important by amplifying gene regulation and biologic action. Although the mechanisms by which 1,25-dihydroxyvitamin D regulates gene expression are not known, he proposes a model in which phosphorylation of the vitamin D receptor is catalyzed by casein kinase, and the hormone-receptor-DNA complex initiates transcription (1).

Uri Liberman indicated that five defects in hereditary vitamin D-dependent rickets type II have been described based on studies of cellular uptake and nuclear binding of ^{3}H-1,25-dihydroxyvitamin D_3(2). These are outlined as follows:

Type I	no binding of hormone to soluble cell extract or nuclei
Type II	reduced binding capacity with normal binding affinity to soluble cell extract and nuclei (reduced number of receptors)
Type III	reduced binding affinity with normal binding capacity (normal number of receptors)

Type IV   normal binding affinity and capacity to soluble cell extract and no nuclear uptake

Type V   near normal binding affinity and capacity to soluble cell extract and abnormal elution of hormone-receptor complex from heterologous DNA-cellulose

Type VI was not described but would include patients with post-transcription defects who should show normal binding and nuclear uptake of 1,25-dihydroxyvitamin D_3 and normal elution of hormone-receptor complex from heterologous DNA-cellulose. Patients with type III and IV disease respond to large doses of 1,25-dihydroxyvitamin D_3, whereas patients with types I, II and V disease respond poorly or not at all.

Based on these findings and assuming that receptor defects are qualitative (and result from point mutations) and are not quantitative (and do not result from lack of expression), it can be predicted that the structure of the 1,25-dihydroxyvitamin D-binding domain of the receptor is abnormal in patients with type I disease and that structure of the DNA binding domain is abnormal in patients with type V disease. It is now known that two separate mutations exist in type V disease. Point mutations have been identified in each of the two "zinc fingers" which account for the lack of response to 1,25-dihydroxyvitamin D_3 in vivo and abnormal nuclear uptake of the 1,25-dihydroxyvitamin D_3-receptor complex in vitro in two different families with vitamin D-dependent rickets type II (Pike, J.W., personal communication). These results emphasize the importance of the structure of the cysteine-containing loops or "zinc fingers" in binding of the 1,25-dihydroxyvitamin D_3-receptor complex for biologic function of the vitamin. Studies are in progress in Dr. Pike's laboratory to determine whether abnormal structure of the 1,25-dihydroxyvitamin D-binding domain of the receptor or abnormalities in post-transcription events are responsible for expression of the disease in other patients. He proposes to transfect cells that have an abnormal receptor with the gene for the normal vitamin D receptor to determine whether a defective receptor fully accounts for the disease in a given patient.

Previous studies in rats showed the importance of dietary phosphate in regulating the production of 1,25-dihydroxyvitamin D (3). Thus, phosphate intake varied directly with renal production of the metabolite. Also, previous studies demonstrated the importance of restriction of phosphate intake in preventing secondary hyperparathyroidism in chronic renal failure (4). Curtis Morris showed that changes in phosphate intake regulate the renal production of 1,25-dihydroxyvitamin D and serum 1,25-dihydroxyvitamin D in normal subjects (5). Also, he showed that phosphate restriction prevents inhibition of the renal synthesis of 1,25-dihydroxyvitamin D and secondary hyperparathyroidism even in patients with modest reductions in glomerular filtration rate. His studies indicate, therefore, that dietary intake of phosphorus should be limited early in the course of renal disease to prevent the development of secondary hyperparathyroidism and its sequelae.

Marc Drezner and his colleagues presented evidence that the renal tubular reabsorption of phosphate and renal synthesis of 1,25-dihydroxyvitamin D are closely linked (6). Thus, TmP/GFR or tubular phosphate reabsorption and plasma 1,25-dihydroxyvitamin D varied directly with each other in patients with X-linked hypophosphatemic rickets, tumor-induced osteomalacia and tumoral calcinosis. However, there was poor correlation between TmP/GFR and plasma 1,25-dihydroxyvitamin D in patients with hereditary hypophosphatemic rickets and hypercalciuria. In this disorder, circulating 1,25-dihydroxyvitamin D was increased and was responsible for the hypercalciuria. They suggest that the proximal renal tubular site at which phosphate is reabsorbed may be important in the regulation of renal synthesis of 1,25-dihydroxyvitamin D and that the interrelation of these two processes, which appear to be linked, is complex.

Hypercalcemia caused by increased circulating 1,25-dihydroxyvitamin D is a potentially preventable cause of renal failure and death in patients with sarcoidosis. Yair Liel and his colleagues developed a means to identify patients who may be at risk to develop hypercalcemia. His method is based on the fact that feedback regulation of circulating 1,25-dihydroxyvitamin D normally occurs in response to increases in dietary calcium (7). He found in a small number of patients with sarcoidosis and active disease that, in contrast to normal subjects in whom serum 1,25-dihydroxyvitamin D declined in response to increases in dietary calcium, serum 1,25-dihydroxyvitamin D did not change. These results were interpreted to mean that since the production of 1,25-dihydroxyvitamin D is not normally regulated, it must be synthesized at extrarenal sites in patients with active disease. Thus, patients with active disease may be at risk for developing hypercalcemia. In fact, one of the patients developed hypercalcemia in the course of a summer.

Sol Epstein indicated that blacks and obese subjects have a greater bone mass than Caucasians and nonobese individuals and are at less risk for developing osteoporosis and fractures of the hip (8). Blacks and obese white subjects also show decreases in serum 25-hydroxyvitamin D and urinary calcium and increases in serum 1,25-dihydroxyvitamin D and urinary cyclic adenosine 3',5'-monophosphate as compared to nonobese white men and women. As he indicates, it remains to be seen whether the altered vitamin D endocrine system in these subjects is related to the increased bone mass.

References

1. Haussler, M.R. 1,25-Dihydroxyvitamin D_3 receptor structure and function. In Clinical Disorders of Bone and Mineral Metabolism. (Kleerekoper, M., and Krane, S.M., eds). Mary Ann Liebert, Inc., New York. In press.

2. Liberman, U.A., Marx, S.J. Hereditary resistance to 1,25-dihydroxyvitamin D: pathophysiology, diagnosis and treatment. In Clinical Disorders of Bone and Mineral Metabolism. (Kleerekoper, M., and Krane, S.M., eds). Mary Ann Liebert, Inc., New York. In press.

3. Tanaka, Y., and DeLuca, H.F. (1973) The control of 25-hydroxyvitamin D metabolism by inorganic phosphorus. Arch. Biochem. Biophys. 154:566-574

4. Slatopolsky, E., Caglar S, Pennell, J.P., Taggart, D.D., Canterbury, J.M., Reiss, E., and Bricker, N.S. (1971) On the pathogenesis of hyperparathyroidism in chronic experimental renal insufficiency in the dog. J. Clin. Invest. 50:492-499

5. Morris, R.C., Jr. Regulation of vitamin D metabolism by phosphorus in health and disease. In Clinical Disorders of Bone and Mineral Metabolism. (Kleerekoper, M., and Krane, S.M., eds). Mary Ann Liebert, Inc., New York. In press.

6. Nesbitt, T., Davidai, G.A., Brazy, P.C., Drezner, M.K. Clinical disorders of phosphorus and vitamin D metabolism. In Clinical Disorders of Bone and Mineral Metabolism. (Kleerekoper, M., and Krane, S.M., eds). Mary Ann Liebert, Inc., New York. In press.

7. Liel, Y., Basile, J., Bell, N.H. Abnormal vitamin D and calcium metabolism in sarcoidosis and related diseases. In Clinical Disorders of Bone and Mineral Metabolism. (Kleerekoper, M., and Krane, S.M., eds). Mary Ann Liebert, Inc., New York. In press.

8. Epstein, S., Bell, N.H. The effects of race and body habitus on the vitamin D endocrine system. In Clinical Disorders of Bone and Mineral Metabolism. (Kleerekoper, M., and Krane, S.M., eds). Mary Ann Liebert, Inc., New York. In press.

1,25-Dihydroxyvitamin D_3 Receptor Structure and Function

MARK R. HAUSSLER

Department of Biochemistry
University of Arizona College of Medicine
Tucson, AZ

Introduction

The functional metabolism and target cell actions of vitamin D via its 1,25-dihydroxyvitamin D_3 (1,25$(OH)_2D_3$) hormonal form are depicted in Fig. 1. 1,25$(OH)_2D_3$ is classified as a hormone both because its production by the kidneys is regulated and because it operates biochemically at the level of the target cell nucleus in a fashion analogous to that of the steroid hormones (1). As summarized in Fig. 1, the effects of the 1,25$(OH)_2D_3$ hormone are mediated by a nuclear receptor molecule which controls the transcription of genes coding for proteins that modify the functions of vitamin D target cells.

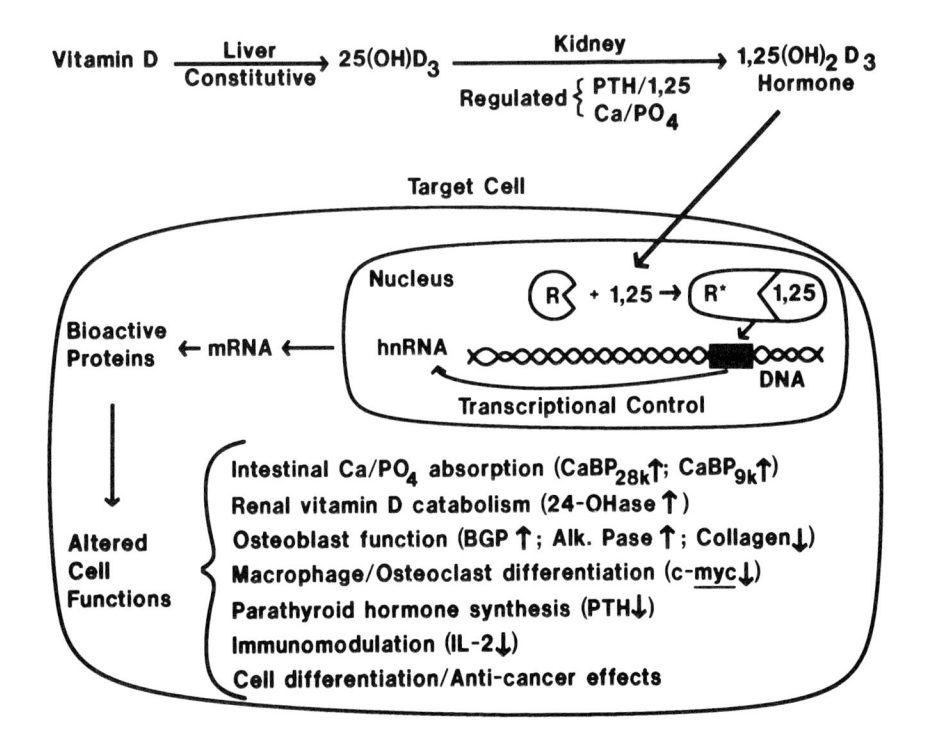

Fig. 1. The vitamin D endocrine system. R = receptor for 1,25$(OH)_2D_3$; activated receptor is denoted as R*.

The number of proteins that are known to be induced or repressed by 1,25(OH)$_2$D$_3$ is now approaching 50, but only several key examples of proteins regulated at the point of transcription and their associated biological actions are shown in Fig. 1. The biochemical mode of action of 1,25(OH)$_2$D$_3$ resembles not only that of structurally related steroid hormones like estradiol, cortisol, etc., but also that of chemically distinct compounds such as thyroid hormones and the vitamin A metabolite, retinoic acid (2).

Structure of the 1,25(OH)$_2$D$_3$ Receptor

The 1,25(OH)$_2$D$_3$ receptor is localized in the target cell nucleus and it binds 1,25(OH)$_2$D$_3$ with high affinity ($K_d = 10^{-10}$M) and selectivity over other vitamin D metabolites. Our laboratory (3,4) has identified avian and mammalian 1,25(OH)$_2$D$_3$ receptors as proteins of MW 58/60 kDa and 52-55 kDa, respectively, through immunoblotting and in vitro translation of mRNA. Based upon a number of biochemical experiments (5) we have constructed a map of the avian 1,25(OH)$_2$D$_3$ receptor protein as illustrated in Fig. 2. The 58 kDa avian receptor form differs from the 60 kDa species by apparently lacking an N-terminal fragment estimated to be 2 kDa by denaturing gel electrophoresis. These data are consistent with the in vitro translation results yielding both forms (4) and the existence of internal (alternate) translation start sites in the avian 1,25(OH)$_2$D$_3$ receptor amino acid sequence (see Fig. 3 below). The 1,25(OH)$_2$D$_3$ hormone binds in a hydrophobic pocket encompassing the C-terminal half of the protein, although removal of only a few amino acids by carboxypeptidase causes dissociation of 1,25(OH)$_2$D$_3$ (6). The center of the molecule contains a domain that is immunogenic and extremely sensitive to limited proteolysis; this region probably constitutes an exposed "hinge" between the hormone binding domain and the N-terminal DNA binding domain (Fig. 2). The DNA binding region (~ 8 kDa) is characterized by two fingers anchored via Zn atoms coordinated by sulfhydryl groups of cysteine residues.

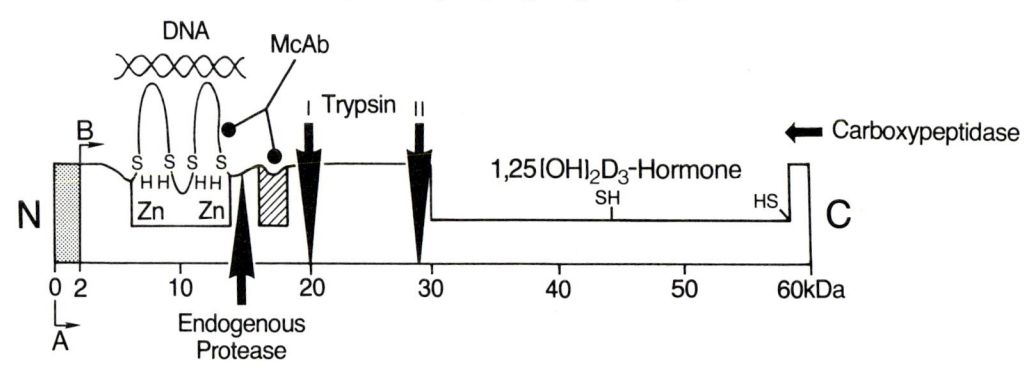

Fig. 2. Biochemical anatomy of the avian 1,25(OH)$_2$D$_3$ receptor. SH=sulf hydryl of cysteine; McAb=monoclonal antibody; A=60 kDa form; B=58 kDa form.

Accordingly, we have shown that sulfhydryl reagents dissociate the 1,25(OH)$_2$D$_3$ receptor from DNA and chelators such as EDTA destroy the DNA binding function of the receptor; the latter phenomenon is prevented by the presence of free zinc ions (7). Molecular cloning of this region of both the chicken (8) and human (9) 1,25(OH)$_2$D$_3$ receptor reveals that the deduced amino acid sequences are virtually homologous (see Fig. 3) and similar to that of the oncogene v-erbA and steroid hormone receptors like the glucocorticoid receptor and the estrogen receptor (10). Most striking is the high content of basic amino acids and the nine cysteines positionally conserved in all sequences. The conservation of this region in steroid receptors indicates that it performs a critical general function. Because it is similar to the multiple zinc finger DNA binding domain of transcription factor IIIA and a host of other transcriptionally active DNA binding proteins like GAL4, SP1 and the testes determining factor (11), the molecular genetics of the vitamin D receptor are

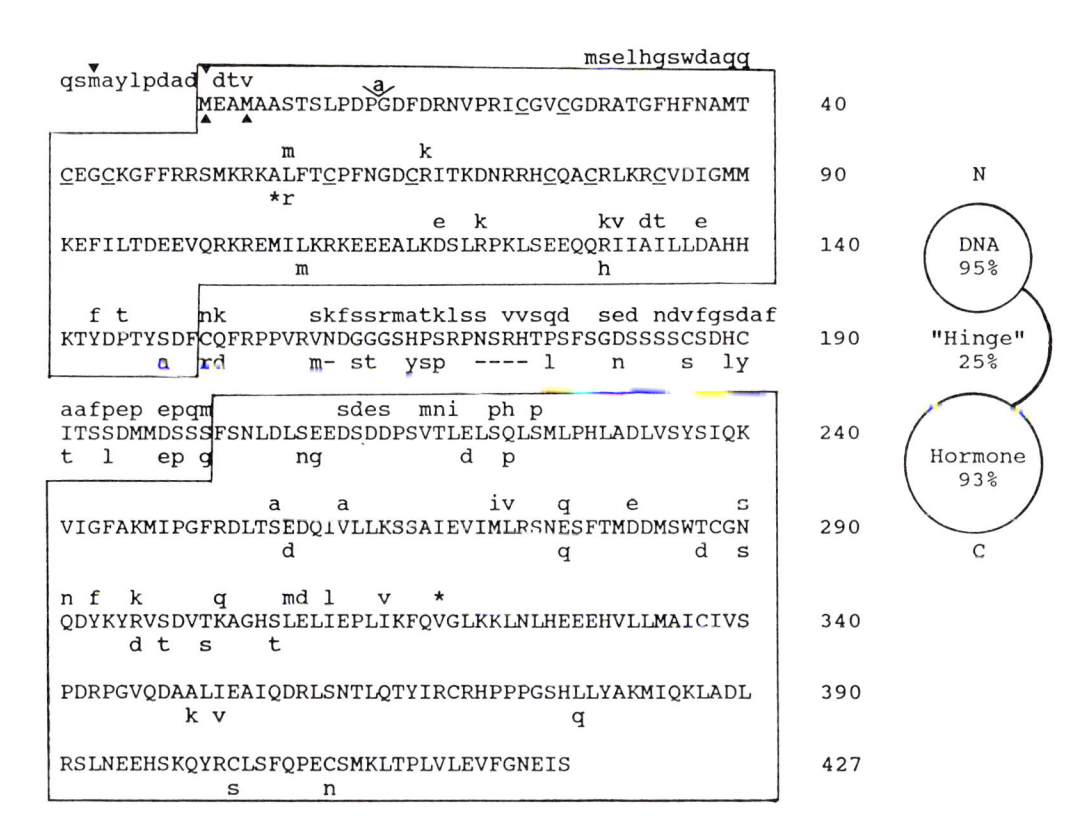

```
                                mselhgswdaqq
   qsmaylpdad dtv         a
            ▼MEAMAASTSLPDPGDFDRNVPRICGVCGDRATGFHFNAMT          40
            ▲▲
            m           k
   CEGCKGFFRRSMKRKALFTCPFNGDCRITKDNRRHCQACRLKRCVDIGMM           90
         *r
                 e   k          kv dt  e
   KEFILTDEEVQRKREMILKRKEEEALKDSLRPKLSEEQQRIIAILLDAHH          140
                 m               h

    f t     nk      skfssrmatklss vvsqd  sed ndvfgsdaf
   KTYDPTYSDFCQFRPPVRVNDGGGSHPSRPNSRHTPSFSGDSSSSCSDHC          190
         a   rd        m- st  ysp ---- l   n   s ly

   aafpep epqm      sdes  mni  ph p
   ITSSDMMDSSSFSNLDLSEEDSDDPSVTLELSQLSMLPHLADLVSYSIQK          240
    t l  ep g       ng         d p

               a    a       iv  q  e    s
   VIGFAKMIPGFRDLTSEDQIVLLKSSAIEVIMLRSNESFTMDDMSWTCGN          290
               d            q       d s

    n f  k   q      md l  v    *
   QDYKYRVSDVTKAGHSLELIEPLIKFQVGLKKLNLHEEEHVLLMAICIVS          340
        d  t    t

   PDRPGVQDAALIEAIQDRLSNTLQTYIRCRHPPPGSHLLYAKMIQKLADL          390
         k v                               q

   RSLNEEHSKQYRCLSFQPECSMKLTPLVLEVFGNEIS                       427
          s     n
```

N

DNA 95%

"Hinge" 25%

Hormone 93%

C

Fig. 3. Comparison of chick, human and rat 1,25(OH)$_2$D$_3$ receptor. Amino acids are given by the single letter code and the 9 conserved cysteines are underlined. The complete human sequence is depicted in capital letters and refers to the numbers at the right. The partial chicken sequence (ending with glutamine 317) is listed in lower case letters above the human sequence. The partial rat sequence (beginning with arginine 57) is denoted in lower case letters below the human sequence. Vertical arrows indicate methionine coded for by the nucleotide consensus for the start of translation. Homology percentages listed in the hinge model at the far right allow for conservative replacements and are the average of differences between the chick/human or rat/human sequences.

consistent with the biochemical conclusions that this domain recognizes control regions of vitamin D modulated genes.

The complete amino acid sequence of the human 1,25(OH)$_2$D$_3$ receptor (9) is depicted in Fig. 3 and it is compared to partial sequences of the chicken (8) and rat (12) receptor. Two areas of extremely high homology are revealed, the N-terminal region containing the DNA binding domain (95% identity) and the C-terminal domain possessing the 1,25(OH)$_2$D$_3$ hormone binding site (93% identity). The two conserved domains are separated by a 50 amino acid region of low homology that apparently consists of a generic "hinge" motif without strict sequence constraints. This hinge could permit the transduction of information between the hormone and DNA binding domains and transmit conformational changes analogous to those occurring in antibodies and in many prokaryotic DNA binding proteins (i.e., LexA). It is also noteworthy that the avian 1,25(OH)$_2$D$_3$ receptor deduced so far has 24 more amino acids than the human receptor; 22 of those constitute an N-terminal extension in the chicken receptor. This is in concert with the larger MW of the chicken 1,25(OH)$_2$D$_3$ receptor. Also, methionine residues with the Kozak nucleotide consensus (13) for the start of translation are present at positions 15 and 23 in the avian receptor as a potential alternative start sites for translation and could account for the occurrence of the 58 kDa isoform (see Fig. 2).

Finally, it is of interest to contrast the structure of the $1,25(OH)_2D_3$ receptor with other members of this superfamily of gene regulatory proteins. Fig. 4 illustrates several key receptors and compares their structures. The vitamin D receptor is the smallest of the receptors cloned to date. It is most similar in size and sequence to the thyroid hormone receptor (hcerbA), indicating that the vitamin D hormone is actually more closely linked evolutionarily to the thyroid hormone than to its chemical relatives, the steroid hormones.

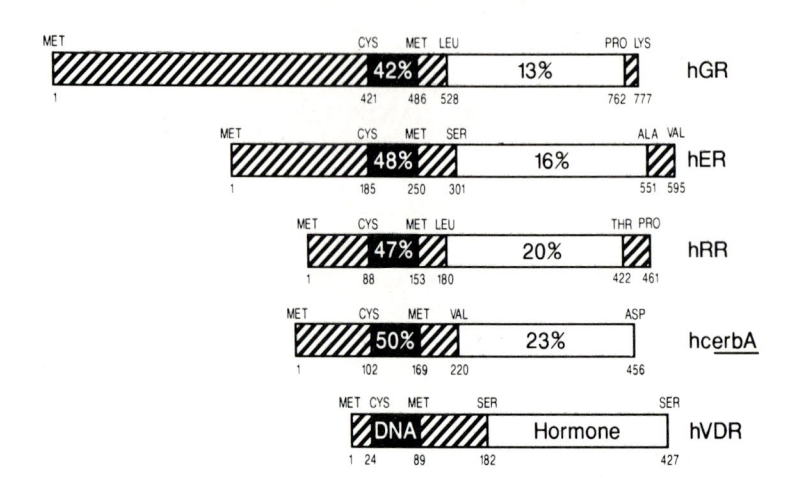

Fig. 4. Comparison of human vitamin D receptor (hVDR), thyroid hormone receptor (hcerbA), retinoic acid receptor (hRR; ref. 29), estrogen receptor (hER) and glucocorticoid receptor (hGR). Homology listed as percentages versus hVDR and cross-hatched areas are of unknown function.

Regulation of the Vitamin D Receptor

Our laboratory (4,7,8) and others (14) have observed upregulation in the amount of $1,25(OH)_2D_3$ receptor when cultured cells and animals are treated with $1,25(OH)_2D_3$. Phosphorylation of the receptor has also been detected in 3T6 mouse fibroblasts exposed to physiologic levels of $1,25(OH)_2D_3$ (15) and this phosphorylation occurs primarily on serine residues (16). We suggest an important role for receptor regulation in the action of $1,25(OH)_2D_3$. For example, by upregulating the amount of receptor protein, the $1,25(OH)_2D_3$ hormone could amplify the response of gene regulation in target cells. Phosphorylation may play a significant part in the transcriptional activation property of the receptor or, alternatively, it might mark the receptor for turnover or degradation. As discussed in the next section, we propose that $1,25(OH)_2D_3$ elicited receptor phosphorylation on serine(s) is a crucial biochemical modification that confers the receptor with the ability to trans-activate genes via the interaction with proteins of the transcription machinery.

Molecular Mode of Action of the $1,25(OH)_2D_3$ Receptor

Although it is certain that the $1,25(OH)_2D_3$ receptor binds hormone and DNA, the molecular mechanism whereby it induces or represses genes is not known. Based upon data with other steroid receptors such as estrogen, it is likely that simple binding to vitamin D regulatory elements in controlled genes is not sufficient to modulate transcription (17). Instead, it now appears that transcriptional regulation in higher eukaryotes biochemically resembles that in yeast (18), which involves acidic domains in enhancer binding proteins that interact with other proteins to create an active transcription complex (19,20). Of particular interest is the control of the GAL1 gene for galactose catabolism, in which galactose binds to the GAL80 protein to remove it from enhancer bound GAL4, thereby exposing acidic regions of GAL4 that in turn activate transcription of GAL1 via protein-protein interactions (21). The acidic, trans-activating sequences of GAL4 bear strong domain homology with five regions of the human vitamin D receptor, namely amino acids 1-17, 85-101, 112-128, 202-218 and 253-269 (see Fig. 3). These sequences are analogous to those in GAL4 in that they are rich in acidic and hydrophobic amino acids. The first three sequences straddle the DNA binding domain. The last two sequences are located in the 1,25(OH)$_2$D$_3$ hormone binding domain and may be similar to the amphipathic helix in that region of the estrogen receptor that is proposed to positively control transcription (17). A fascinating feature of these acidic-hydrophobic domains is that they are impregnated with serines and threonines which are candidate phosphorylation sites for casein kinases. Casein kinases I and II are known to phosphorylate ser/thr when they are flanked by acidic amino acids on the N-terminal and C-terminal sides, respectively (22). Casein kinases phosphorylate RNA polymerase II, transcription factors, topoisomerase and are required for the transforming activity of the SV-40 large T antigen (22,23). Thus, it is possible that casein kinase catalyzed phosphorylation of the vitamin D receptor generates hyperacidic hydrophobic regions for the purpose of transcriptional activation.

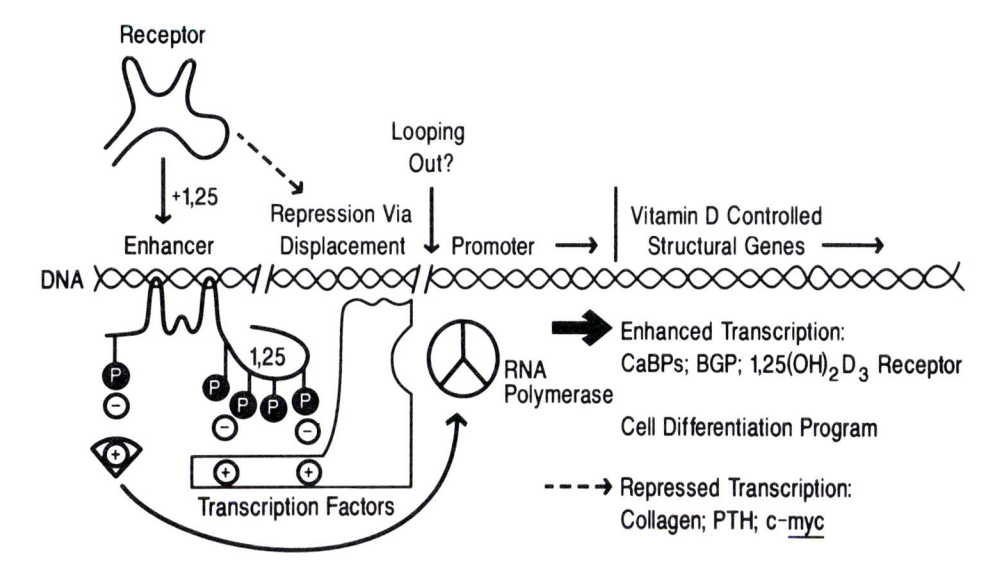

Fig. 5. Proposed model for the control of gene transcription by the 1,25(OH)$_2$D$_3$ receptor.

Figure 5 presents a model for the participation of hormone occupied vitamin D receptor in gene control. The unoccupied receptor is envisioned as a molecule with the trans-activation domain(s) silent and the DNA binding fingers repressed or contorted such that optimal binding to vitamin D responsive enhancer elements is not achieved. The binding of the 1,25(OH)$_2$D$_3$ ligand is proposed to render the DNA binding fingers competent for tight and specific DNA binding and concomitantly to alter the conformation of the putative acidic/hydrophobic motifs saturated with serines. Hormone elicited phosphorylation could create highly acidic patches on the receptor that attract or complex with positive domains in rate limiting transcription factors. If the enhancer elements are far upstream, looping out of DNA (shown as a break in the DNA) would allow the formation of a transcriptosome, or a large complex of proteins analogous to the replication complex in DNA synthesis. The results of such a process would be a stimulation of the expression of genes such as CaBP and BGP that have been shown via nuclear run-off technology to be controlled at transcription (24). Negative gene control by 1,25(OH)$_2$D$_3$, which is documented by nuclear run-off data for collagen, PTH, and c-myc (24), probably occurs when the cis-regulatory element is positioned such that occupied receptor binding interferes with the transcription machinery by displacing a crucial transcription factor. The next step in testing the model pictured will be the elucidation of the vitamin D regulatory element and pinpointing its location in the genes orchestrated by the $1,25(OH)_2D_3$ receptor complex.

The $1,25(OH)_2D_3$ Receptor in Diseases of Bone and Mineral Metabolism

Type II vitamin D-dependent rickets is the clinical syndrome caused by a genetic defect in the $1,25(OH)_2D_3$ receptor and is characterized by either a mutation in the hormone binding domain or the DNA binding domain of the receptor in the kindreds evaluated to date (2). Because such patients have excessive circulating levels of $1,25(OH)_2D_3$ coexisting with rickets, this disease verifies the obligatory role of the receptor in vitamin D action. Type II inherited rickets is analogous to androgen resistance in complete testicular feminization. The new basic information presented above predicts that other varients of Type II rickets will include genetic defects in the transcription control/phosphorylation domain(s) of the receptor as well as mutated structural genes or D-responsive elements in $1,25(OH)_2D_3$ modulated genes. These latter genetic abnormalities will appear as postreceptor defects, with $1,25(OH)_2D_3$ hormone and DNA binding being normal by the receptors. A second primary disorder involving the $1,25(OH)_2D_3$ receptor is the possibility that certain neoplasms possess overexpression of an oncogenic homologue of the receptor, as is the case in hepatic cancer and the expression of an altered version of the retinoic acid receptor (25).

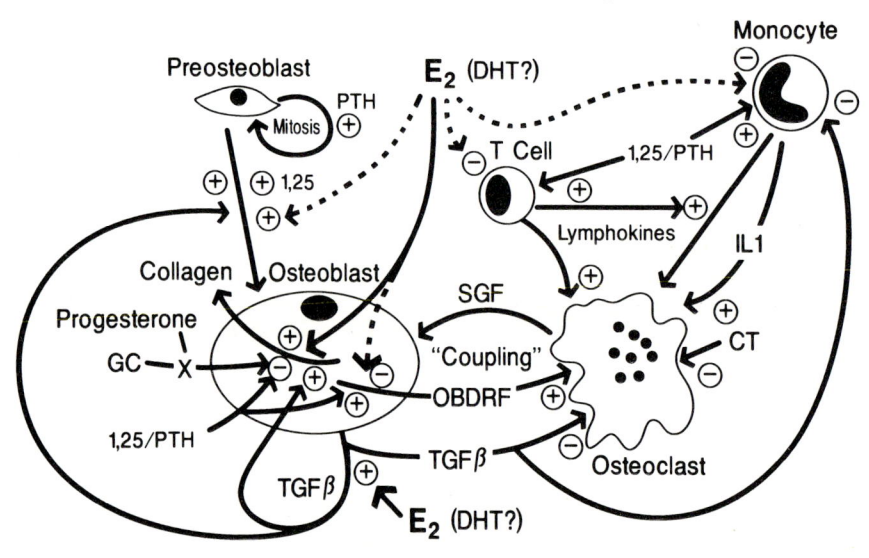

Fig. 6. Control of bone remodeling by steroid and peptide hormones.

Other clinical disorders associated with secondary defects in $1,25(OH)_2D_3$ receptors or regulation thereof have not been examined in detail. An obvious candidate for $1,25(OH)_2D_3$ receptor overexpression is renal stones caused by intestinal hyperabsorption of calcium in the face of normal $1,25(OH)_2D_3$ levels. Conversely there is some evidence for vitamin D resistance and osteopenia in Type I diabetes, suggesting that insulin could control $1,25(OH)_2D_3$ receptor levels. Moreover, osteoporosis is a relevant disease elicited by deranged bone remodeling (Fig. 6). $1,25(OH)_2D_3$ is a key player in controlling bone remodeling via direct actions on osteoblasts and indirect actions to cause the differentiation and recruitment of osteoclasts. Altered $1,25(OH)_2D_3$ receptor levels could contribute to osteoporosis in terms of hyporesponsiveness of intestine and bone to $1,25(OH)_2D_3$, although the dominant cause of osteoporosis is a sex hormone deficit. Our group (26) and another (27) have recently observed estrogen (E_2) receptors and biological effects in osteoblast-like cells. Thus, while estrogens could prevent osteoporosis by affecting monocytic precursors or T-cells to dampen osteoclastogenesis, we propose (Fig. 6) that they modulate osteoblast activity by increasing collagen and TGF-beta. Further we postulate that estrogen may oppose the effect of $1,25(OH)_2D_3$ and PTH to release osteoblast derived resorptive factors (OBDRF) and this could serve to attenuate bone resorption and keep it coupled to the formation rate. When estrogens diminish at menopause, the delicate balance is probably lost and $1,25(OH)_2D_3$ and PTH take over to reduce collagen and augment resorption via the secretion of resorptive factors from osteoblasts. Finally, the enhancement of TGF-beta by estrogen might simply mediate its effect to increase collagen, or could inhibit existing osteoclasts to limit resorption while blunting the differentiation of new osteoclasts (28). The net result of this hypothetical scenario is that estrogen builds bone by increasing collagen matrix, and by shifting the balance toward formation via a reduction in total osteoclast number and by suppressing the activity of existing osteoclasts. It is evident that understanding the interplay between the sex steroids and hormones such as $1,25(OH)_2D_3$ in bone cell physiology and pathology may be the key to preventing and treating postmenopausal osteoporosis. It will be of interest to evaluate the level of both $1,25(OH)_2D_3$ and estrogen receptors as an index of the interaction of these two hormones in the pathogenesis of osteoporosis.

References

1. Haussler, M.R., and McCain, T.A. (1977) N. Engl. J. Med. 297, 974-983 and 1041-1050
2. Haussler, M.R. (1986) Ann. Rev. Nutr. 6, 527-562
3. Pike, J.W., Sleator, N.M., and Haussler, M.R. (1987) J. Biol. Chem. 262, 1305-1311
4. Mangelsdorf, D.J., Pike, J.W., and Haussler, M.R. (1987) Proc. Natl. Acad. Sci. USA 84, 354-358
5. Allegretto, E.A., Pike, J.W., and Haussler, M.R. (1987) J. Biol. Chem. 262, 1312-1319
6. Allegretto, E.A., Pike, J.W., and Haussler, M.R. (1987) Biochem. Biophys. Res. Commun. 147, 479-485
7. Haussler, M.R., Mangelsdorf, D.J., Yamaoka, K., Allegretto, E.A., Komm, B.S., Terpening, C.M., McDonnell, D.P., Pike, J.W., and O'Malley, B.W. (1988) J. Cellular Biochem. in press
8. McDonnell, D.P., Mangelsdorf, D.J., Pike, J.W., Haussler, M.R., and O'Malley, B.W. (1987) Science 235, 1214-1217
9. Baker, A.R., McDonnell, D.P., Hughes, M., Crisp, T.M., Mangelsdorf, D.J., Haussler, M.R., Pike, J.W., Shine, J., and O'Malley, B.W. (1988) Proc. Natl. Acad. Sci. in press
10. Weinberger, C., Thompson, C.C., Ong, E.S., Lebo, R., Gruol, D.J., and Evans, R.M. (1986) Nature 324, 641-646
11. Evans, R.M., and Hollenberg, S.M. (1988) Cell 52, 1-3
12. Burmester, J.K., Maeda, N., and DeLuca, H.F. (1988) Proc. Natl. Acad. Sci. 85, 1005-1009
13. Kozak, M. (1980) Cell 22, 7-8
14. Costa, E.M., Hirst, M.A., and Feldman, D. (1985) Endocrinology 117, 2203-2210
15. Pike, J.W., and Sleator, N.M. (1985) Biochem. Biophys. Res. Commun. 131, 378-385
16. Haussler, M.R., Mangelsdorf, D.J., Komm, B.S., Terpening, C.M., Yamaoka, K., Allegretto, E.A., Baker, A.R., Shine, J., McDonnell, D.P., Hughes, M., Weigel, N.L., O'Malley, B.W., and Pike, J.W. (1988) Recent Prog. Horm. Res. 44, in press
17. Kumar, V., Green, S., Stack, G., Berry, M., Jin, J.R., and Chambon, P. (1987) Cell 51, 941-951
18. Webster, N., Jin, J.R., Green, S., Hollis, M., and Chambon, P. (1988) Cell 52, 169-178

19. Ma, J., and Ptashne, M. (1987) *Cell* 51, 113-119
20. Struhl, K. (1987) *Cell* 49, 295-297
21. Ma, J. and Ptashne, M. (1987) *Cell* 50, 137-142
22. Edelman, A.M., Blumenthal, D.K., and Krebs, E.G. (1987) *Ann. Rev. Biochem.* 56, 567-613
23. Paucha, E., Kalderon, D., Harvey, R.W., and Smith, A.E. (1986) *J. Virol.* 57, 50-64
24. Pike, J.W. (1987) *Steroids* 49, 3-27
25. deThe, H., Marchio, A., Tiollais, P., and Dejean, A. (1987) *Nature* 330, 667-670
26. Komm, B.S., Terpening, D.M., Benz, D.J., Graeme, K.A., Gallegos, A., Korc, M., Greene, G.L., O'Malley, B.W., and Haussler, M.R. (1988) *Science* in press
27. Eriksen, E.F., Colvard, D.S., Berg, N.J., Graham, M.L., Mann, K.G., Spelsberg, T.C., and Riggs, B.L. (1988) *Science* in press
28. Pfeilschiffer, J., Seyedin, S.M. and Mundy, G.R. (1988) *Calcif. Tissue Int.* 42(Suppl) A34 (Abstr 133)
29. Giguere, V., Ong, E.S., Segui, P., and Evans, R.M. (1987) *Nature* 330, 624-629

Hereditary Resistance to 1,25-Dihydroxyvitamin D: Pathophysiology, Diagnosis, and Treatment

URI A. LIBERMAN[1,2] and STEPHEN J. MARX[2]

[1]Metabolic Diseases
Beilinson Medical Center
Petah Tiqva, Israel
and Division of Physiology and Pharmacology
Sackler School of Medicine
Tel Aviv University, Tel Aviv, Israel
[2]Mineral Metabolism Section
Metabolic Diseases Branch
National Institute of Diabetes and Digestive and Kidney Diseases
National Institutes of Health
Bethesda, MD

We define resistance to a factor as a state in which normal concentrations of the factor are associated with subnormal biological response. In the case of 1,25-dihydroxyvitamin D (1,25-$(OH)_2D$) resistance the relevant biological responses are serum calcium concentrations, reflecting mainly the effect on net intestinal transcellular calcium transport. This is often measured as changes in plasma calcium, pertubations in parathyroid gland function, or bone matrix mineralization.

CLINICAL AND BIOCHEMICAL FEATURES: Hereditary resistance to 1,25$(OH)_2D$ is a rare inborn error in vitamin D metabolism (1). There are up to now about 33 kindreds with this disorder, including some that have not yet been published. The characteristic clinical features are the following: early onset rickets (in the majority of patients) and osteomalacia cause bone deformities and growth retardation; there is no history or biochemical evidence for vitamin D deficiency and patients do not respond to replacement doses of 1,25$(OH)_2D_3$; in about two thirds of the kindreds alopecia is a prominent feature (Fig. 1); parental consanguinity and multiple siblings with the same defect occur in about half of the kindreds, suggesting an autosomal recessive mode of inheritance in these and perhaps in all kindreds. There is a striking clustering of patients close to the Mediterranean, most of the patients reported from Europe and America are descendants in families originating from around the Mediterranean as well. Notable exceptions are several kindreds reported for Japan. The typical biochemical features are depicted in Figure 2 and consist essentially of hypocalcemia, secondary hyperparathyroidism, and elevated serum concentrations of 1,25$(OH)_2D$ (particularly during therapy). The combination of hypocalcemic rickets, secondary hyperparathyroidism, and elevated 1,25$(OH)_2D$ serum levels fits the definition of resistance to 1,25$(OH)_2D$. We suggest therefore the term hereditary resistance to 1,25$(OH)_2D$ as a term more appropriate than vitamin D dependency type II to describe this entity. Moreover, the fact that more than half of the patients did not respond to therapy with calciferol makes the term vitamin D dependency inappropriate.

A peculiar feature of the syndrome that appears in about two

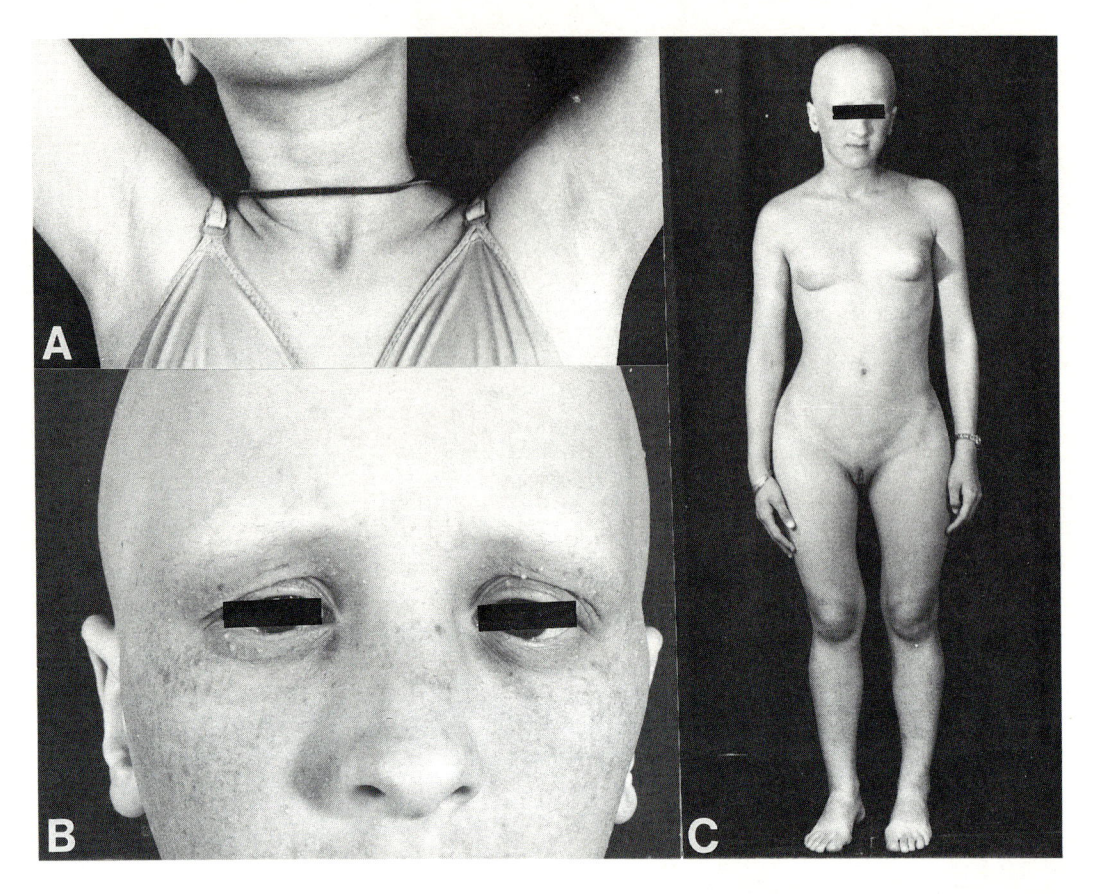

Figure 1: A patient with hereditary resistance to 1,25(OH)$_2$D and total alopecia. Note the lack of scalp hair, absence of eyelashes and multiple milia and epidermal cysts in (B), lack of axillary hair (A) and pubic hair (C).

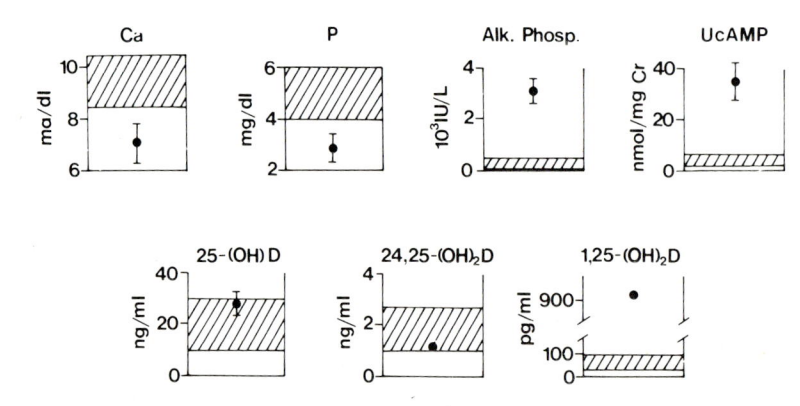

Figure 2.: Biochemical data of a patient with hereditary resistance to 1,25(OH)$_2$D.

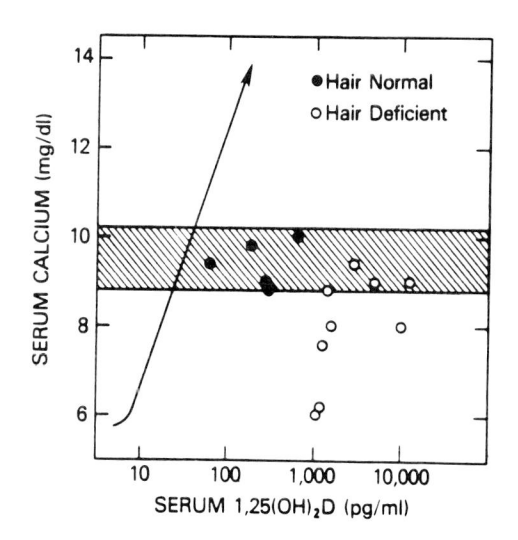

Figure 3.: Relation between serum concentrations of calcium and 1,25(OH)$_2$D in patients with hereditary resistance to 1,25(OH)$_2$D during calciferol therapy. Stippled area is normal range for calcium. Solid curve is theoretical normal relation between calcium and 1,25(OH)$_2$D. (●) Hair normal (o) alopecia (From Marx et l. (1986) Clin. Endocrinol. 25: 373-381).

thirds of the kindreds is alopecia (1,2) that varies from sparse hair to total alopecia without eye lashes (Fig. 1). In some patients multiple milia with multiple epidermal cysts appear (Fig.1). The alopecia may be obvious at birth or develop during the first months of life. Alopecia seems to be a marker of a more severe form of the disease as judged by the earlier age of presentation of the disease and extraordinarily high serum 1,25-(OH)$_2$D levels during therapy with high doses of calciferol (Fig. 3).

INTRACELLULAR DEFECTS: Studies on the nature of the intracellular defect in the 1,25(OH)$_2$D receptor-effector system became possible with the demonstration that cells originating from tissues easily accessible for biopsy contain receptors for 1,25(OH)$_2$D; and thus may serve as a model system to study gene defects in target tissues. The cells used are mainly dermal fibroblasts, but keratinocytes, bone cells, and recently peripheral blood mononuclear (PBM) cells have been used as well (3-6). The following methods have been used to characterized the interaction among hormone, receptor and nuclei (3-11): 1) [^{3}H]1,25(OH)$_2$D$_3$ uptake by intact cells at 37°C and then (a) receptors are extracted by hypertonic lysis or (b) the plasma membrane is dissolved with detergent and nuclear associated hormone is measured. 2) Measurements of binding affinity and/or capacity with soluble (high KCl) cell extract at 0-4°C by [^{3}H]1,25(OH)$_2$D$_3$ binding 3) Properties of [^{3}H]1,25(OH)$_2$D$_3$ bound specifically to nuclei and/or soluble cell extract (i.e. receptor bound [^{3}H]1,25(OH)$_2$D$_3$) has been analyzed by continuous sucrose gradient centrifugation and by adsorption to and elution from heterologus DNA-cellulose). 4) The following markers have been used to measure the in vitro bio-effect of 1,25(OH)$_2$D$_3$ on the various cells: (a) induction of the enzyme 25-hydroxyvitamin D$_3$ 24-hydroxylase (24-hydroxylase) in dermal fibroblasts or bone cells; (b) induction of osteocalcin (bone gla protein or BGP) production in bone cells; (c) inhibition of cell proliferation, mainly in mitogen stimulated PBM cells and in one case in dermal fibroblasts.

Using the above mentioned methods, at least five separate defects in the 1,25(OH)$_2$D$_3$ receptor-effector system have been demonstrated (2-11): Type I - no binding of hormone to soluble cell extract or nuclei. Type II - reduced binding capacity with normal affinity to soluble cell extract and nuclei. Type III - decreased binding affinity to 1,25(OH)$_2$D$_3$ with normal capacity. Type IV - normal affinity and capacity of [^{3}H]1,25(OH)$_2$D$_3$ binding to soluble cell extract, unmeasurable nuclear localization under the assay condition, and normal elution profiles from DNA-cellulose columns of the hormone-receptor complex from soluble cell extract. Type V nearly normal binding affinity and capacity of [^{3}H]1,25(OH)$_2$D$_3$ to soluble cell extract and homologus nuclei but abnormal elution of the hormone-receptor complex from heterologus DNA-cellulose.

SIMILAR INTRACELLULAR DEFECTS IN VARIOUS TISSUES: Measurements of the intracellular 1,25(OH)$_2$D$_3$ receptor-effector system in dermal fibroblasts and cells derived from bone of two patients (with type I and IV defects) revealed a similar if not identical defect in both cell types (5). Moreover, the similarity of the bioresponse in the various cells to 1,25-(OH)$_2$D$_3$ in vitro and of the patients' calcemic response to calciferols in vivo, supports the notion that a similar defect exists in the intestinal epithelium as well. In another study performed on PBM cells and dermal fibroblasts from patients with type I and V defects, similar disturbance in the 1,25(OH)$_2$D$_3$ receptor and the bioresponse to the hormone has been demonstrated (Fig. 4) (6). Thus it could be concluded that: (a) probably the same gene is responsible for the expression of the 1,25(OH)$_2$D$_3$ receptor-effector system in various tissues, (b) the effect of 1,25(OH)$_2$D$_3$ in these various tissues is receptor mediated, and (c) PBM cells can be used as a model for 1,25(OH)$_2$D$_3$ target organs. This system can offer an easy, inexpensive and rapid (4-5 days) method of diagnosis of patients with hereditary defects in the 1,25(OH)$_2$D$_3$ receptor-effector system.

IN VIVO AND IN VITRO RESPONSES TO HIGH 1,25(OH)$_2$D$_3$ CONCENTRATIONS: Though the number of patients with hereditary resistance to 1,25(OH)$_2$D is small in each subgroup (categorized by type of receptor defect), it seems to be that: patients with type III (deficient affinity) and type IV (deficient hormone-binding nuclear localization) defects will respond to high doses of calciferols with complete clinical and biochemical remission; patients with type II defect (low capacity) and most patients with types I (receptor negative) and V (receptor positive) defects could not be cured with high doses of calciferol. However, it should be emphasized that not all of these patients received the treatment for a long enough period and with sufficiently high doses of calciferols (see below). Measurements of an in vitro bioresponse of cells to 1,25(OH)$_2$D$_3$ were carried only in about one third of the kindreds with hereditary resistance to 1,25(OH)$_2$D. Induction of 24-hydroxylase by 1,25(OH)$_2$D$_3$ in cultured dermal fibroblasts showed an invariable correlation to the therapeutic response to calciferols in vivo (7-9) (Fig. 5). The inhibitory effect of 1,25(OH)$_2$D$_3$ on mitogen induced lymphocyte proliferation was tested in a smaller number of patients (Fig. 4) (6) but may also have predictive value for responsiveness to treatment with calciferols.

THERAPY OF HEREDITARY RESISTANCE TO 1,25(OH)$_2$D: If the predictive therpeutic value of the in vitro bioresponse to 1,25(OH)$_2$D$_3$ could be substantiated, it may eliminate the need for expensive and time-consuming therapy trials with calciferols. In the meantime, it is mandatory to treat every patient with hereditary resistance to 1,25(OH)$_2$D, regardless of the intracellular type of defect in the receptor-effector mechanism. The treatment consists of vitamin D$_2$ alone for the mildest cases; in more severe typical cases therapy should be initiated with high

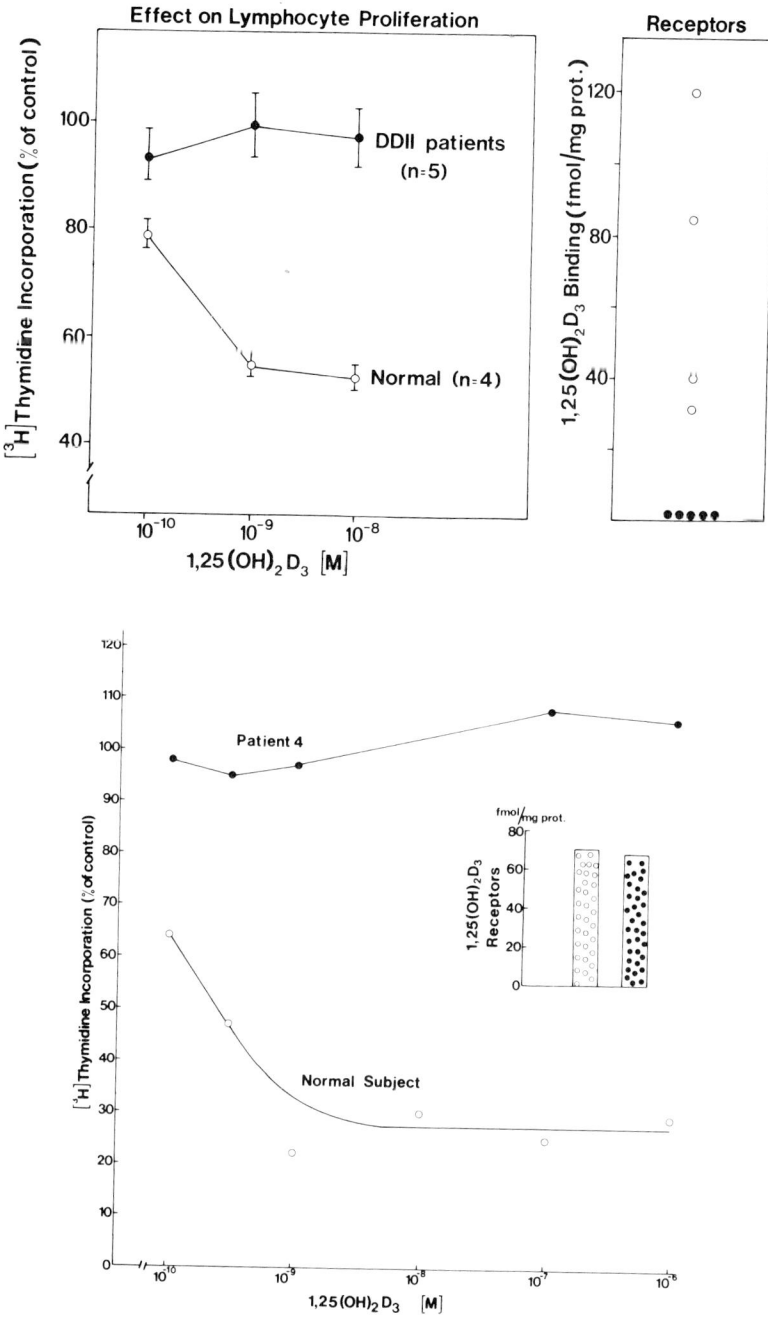

Figure 4.: Effect of 1,25(OH)$_2$D$_3$ on mitogen induced stimulation of PBM cell from normal subjects (open circles) and patients with hereditary resistance to 1,25(OH)$_2$D (closed circles). In right upper panel and inset of lower panel, number of high affinity binding sites for [^{3}H]1,25(OH)$_2$D$_3$ in soluble cell extract. Patients presented in upper panel have type I receptor defect, patient in lower panel suffers from type V receptor defect (Based on data from Koren et al (1985) J. Clin. Invest. 76: 2012-2015, and Liberman et al. (1987) in Calcium Regulation and Bone Metabolism, vol. 9, pp. 501, with permission).

doses of 1,25(OH)$_2$D$_3$ or 1-alpha hydroxy D$_3$ up to 6 µg per kg body weight per day, or a total of 50 µg/day, with calcium supplementation (up to 2 g of elementary calcium per day), and for a period of at least 4-5 months. A close followup is essential and consists of clinical signs and symptoms, serum levels of calcium,

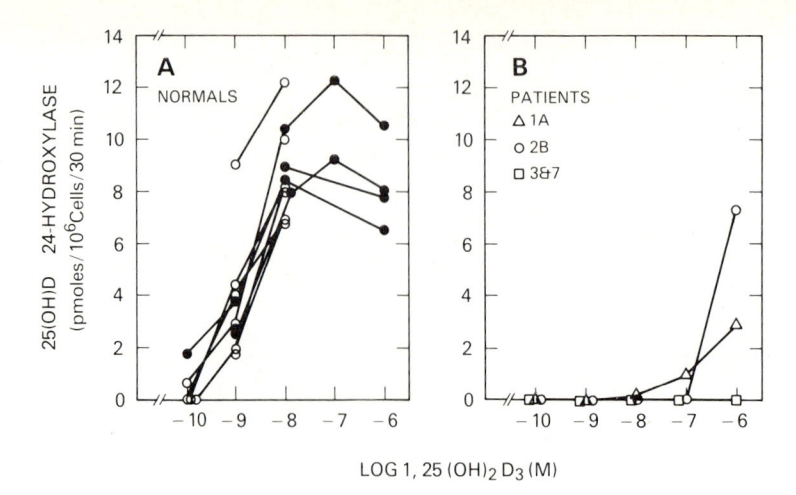

Figure 5.: 25OHD$_3$24-hydroxylase response to 1,25(OH)$_2$D$_3$ in cultured normal dermal fibroblasts (panal A and shaded area in panel B), and patients with hereditary resistance to 1,25(OH)$_2$D (curves in panel B). Patients 1A and 2B had type IV receptor defect with a calcemic response to high doses of 1,25(OH)$_2$D$_3$ in vivo. Patients 3 and 7 had type V receptor defect and neither showed a calcemic response to high doses of calciferol (based on data from Gamblin et al. (1985) J. Clin. Invest. 75:954-960).

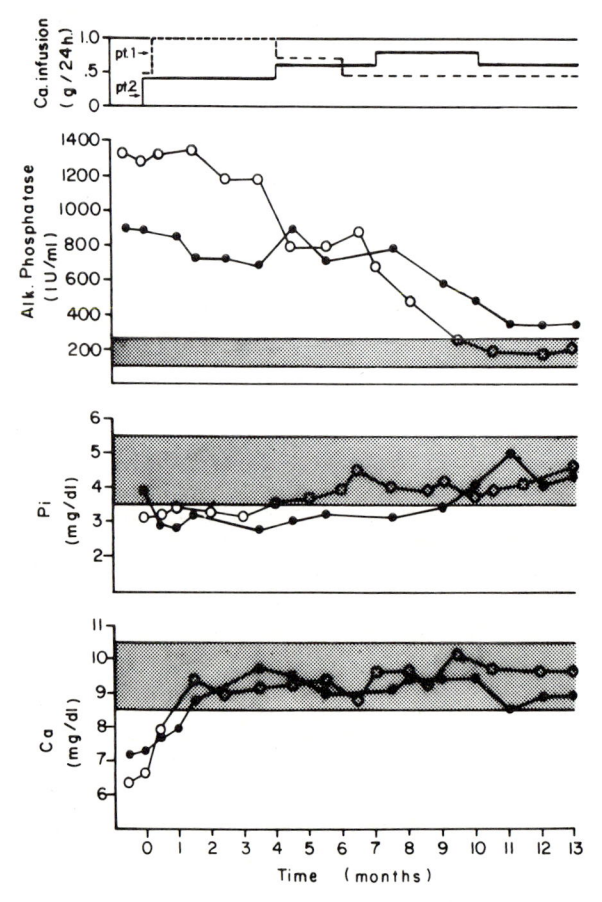

Figure 6.: Serum levels of calcium, phosphorus and alkaline phosphatase in two patients with hereditary resistance to 1,25(OH)$_2$D, before and during a year of intracaval calcium infusions (doses indicated in the upper panel). Shaded areas represent the normal range (From Weisman et al. (1987) Am. J. Med. 83: 984-990, with permission).

phosphorus, alkaline phosphatase and creatinine, urinary excretion of calcium, phosphorus and creatinine, parameters of parathyroid gland function, and serum 1,25(OH)$_2$D levels. Failure of therapy may be considered if no change in any of these parameters occurs during 4-5 months of therapy while 1,25(OH)$_2$D serum levels are maintained above 100 times the mean normal range.

It was reported recently that remarkable clinical and biochemical remission including catch-up growth and histological healing of defective osteoid mineralization, was achieved by long term intracaval infusion of calcium in several unusual patients with hereditary resistance to 1,25(OH)$_2$D that did not respond at all to calciferol therapy (Fig. 6) (12). Even long term therapy with high dose oral calcium is possible (13). These important studies imply that (a) clinical remission could be achieved by calcium administration even in the most resistant patients and (b) it is conceivable that 1,25(OH)$_2$D has no direct effect on bone matrix mineralization.

References

1. Marx, S.J., Liberman, U.A., Eil, C., Gamblin, G.T., DeGrange, D., Balsan, S. (1984) Rec. Prog. Horm. Res. 40:589-615.
2. Marx, S.J., Bliziotes, M.M., Nanes, M. (1986) Clin. Endocrinol. Metab. 25:373-381.
3. Eil, C., Liberman, U.A., Rosen, J.F., Marx, S.J. (1981) N. Eng. J. Med. 304: 1588-1591.
4. Liberman, U.A., Eil, C., Marx, S.J. (1983) J. Clin. Invest. 71: 192-200.
5. Balsan, S., Garabedian, M., Larchet, M., Gorski, A.M., Cournot, G., Tau, C., Bourdeau, A., Silve, C., Ricour, C. (1986) J. Clin. Invest. 77: 1661-1667.
6. Koren, R., Ravid, A., Liberman, U.A., Hochberg, Z., Weisman, Y., Novogrodsky, A. (1985) J. Clin. Invest. 76: 2012-2015.
7. Griffin, J.E., Zerwekh, J.E. (1983) J. Clin. Invest. 72: 1190-1199.
8. Chen, T.L., Hirst, M.A., Cone, C.M., Hochberg, Z., Tietze, H.U., Feldman, D. (1984) J. Clin. Endocrinol. Metab. 59: 383-388.
9. Gamblin, G.T., Liberman, U.A., Eil, C., DeGrange, D.A., Marx, S.J. (1985) J. Clin. Invest. 75: 954-960.
10. Hirst, M., Hochman, H., Feldman, D. (1985) J. Clin. Endocrinol. Metab. 60: 490-495.
11. Liberman, U.A., Eil, C., Marx, S.J. (1986) J. Clin. Endocrinol. Metab. 62: 122-126.
12. Weisman, Y., Bab, I., Gazit, D., Spirer, Z., Jafe, M., Hochberg, Z. (1987) Am. J. Med. 83: 984-990.
13. Sakati, N., Woodhourse, N.J.Y., Niles, N., Harfi, H., deGrange, D.A., Marx, S. (1986) Horm. Res. 24:280-287.

The Role of Phosphorus in Modulating Vitamin D Metabolism in Health and Disease

R. CURTIS MORRIS, JR., BERNARD P. HALLORAN, and ANTHONY A. PORTALE

Departments of Medicine and Pediatrics
General Clinical Research Center
University of California
San Francisco, CA

That phosphorus can modulate the metabolism of vitamin D was first demonstrated by DeLuca and his co-workers (1, 2). In studies of thyroparathyroidectamized (TPXed) vitamin D-deficient rats, this group demonstrated that the apparent production of 1,25-dihydroxyvitamin D (1,25-(OH)$_2$D) in vivo, correlated inversely with serum concentrations of phosphorus induced to vary over a broad range by dietary manipulations (1). In the vitamin D-deficient chick, this group demonstrated that severe depletion of phosphorus stimulated the activity of 25-hydroxyvitamin-D-1-alpha-hydroxylase (1-hydroxylase) (in vitro) despite inducing hypercalcemia (2), which of itself (3), and by suppressing release of parathyroid hormone (PTH) (4), can dampen the activity of this enzyme in other metabolic circumstances. Employing their then newly developed technique to measure serum concentrations of 1,25-(OH)$_2$D, Haussler and his colleagues (5) demonstrated that its level was increased in intact and TPXed rats rendered chronically hypophosphatemic by dietary restriction of phosphorus. Lemann and his colleagues (6) subsequently demonstrated in normal women that dietary restriction of phosphorus over days induced an increase in the serum concentration of 1,25-(OH)$_2$D which occurred in the absence of changes in either the serum concentration of iPTH or urinary excretion of cyclic AMP (6). They attributed the increase in 1,25-(OH)$_2$D to an increase in its production rate caused by the attendant decrease in serum concentration of phosphorus, as measured in the morning fasting state (6). That the serum concentration of phosphorus could regulate the activity of 1-hydroxylase rapidly and independently of parathyroid hormone, was suggested by observations made by Booth and her colleagues (7). In the parathyroidectomized vitamin D-deficient chick in which continuous intravenous administration of calcium prevented worsening of hypocalcemia throughout the 24-hr period after PTX, this group demonstrated that the activity of 1-hydroxylase correlated inversely with serum concentrations of phosphorus (r = -0.91, P<0.001) induced to vary over a broad range by intravenously administered glucose.

A few years later Van den Berg and his colleagues (8) demonstrated in patients with idiopathic hypercalciuria that supplementation of dietary phosphorus induced a decrease in the circulating concentrations of 1,25-(OH)$_2$ to normal values, despite inducing a further increase in the serum concentration of iPTH. These investigators interpreted these findings as suggesting that "a primary change in PO$_4$ metabolism can override PTH as a regulator of renal 1,25-(OH)$_2$D production." Although they observed no increase in the morning fasting serum concentration of phosphorus during PO$_4$ therapy, these investigators suggested that "the integrated (12-hr) serum phosphorus level probably increased during this therapy." In patients with primary hyperparathyroidism Broadus and his colleagues (9) also observed that supplementation of dietary phosphorus induced a decrease in the serum levels of 1,25-(OH)$_2$D to normal values, while inducing a substantial further increase in serum iPTH. They suggested that such phosphorus supplementation was capable of "short-circuiting the PTH-1,25-(OH)$_2$D axis."

Portale and his colleagues (10) subsequently reported a positive test of the hypothesis that in patients with moderate renal insufficiency in whom the dietary intake and serum concentration of phosphorus are not increased, a phosphorus-mediated suppression of the activity of 1-hydroxylase still dampens the renal synthesis and hence the plasma concentration of 1,25-(OH)$_2$D, and thereby contributes to the pathogenesis of the hyperparathyroidism of these patients. They found that in children with moderate renal insufficiency, short term (5 d) restriction and supplementation of dietary phosphorus induced an increase and a further decrease, respectively, in the plasma concentration of 1,25-(OH)$_2$D, and induced a decrease and further increase, respectively, in the serum concentration of iPTH. With restriction of dietary phosphorus, the circulating concentrations of both 1,25-(OH)$_2$D and iPTH became normal.

Thus, with both restriction and supplementation of dietary phosphorus, the circulating concentrations of iPTH varied inversely with those of 1,25-(OH)$_2$D. When the hormonal changes induced in each of the 13 studies were analyzed as a single set, the changes induced in the circulating concentrations of iPTH correlated strongly, but inversely, with those induced in 1,25-(OH)$_2$D (r = -0.88, P<0.001) (10). Had the changes in circulating iPTH induced by manipulating dietary phosphorus been primary and mediating of those induced in the level of 1,25-(OH)$_2$D, one would have expected the relationship between these changes to be direct, not inverse. The phosphorus-induced changes in the circulating concentration of 1,25-(OH)$_2$D were then primary, and the oppositely directed changes induced in iPTH their consequence. Recent evidence indicates that in men, manipulation of dietary phosphorus induces changes in the serum concentrations of 1,25-(OH)$_2$D by inducing changes in its production rate (11). Accordingly, the studies of Van den Berg (8), Broadus (9), and Portale (10), each in a different clinical setting, all demonstrate that dietary phosphorus can exert a dampening effect on the renal production of 1,25-(OH)$_2$D that overrides the potentially stimulatory effect of even greatly increased circulating concentrations of parathyroid hormone.

In the children with moderate renal insufficiency studied by Portale et al., the increase in serum concentration of 1,25-(OH)$_2$D induced by dietary phosphorus restriction was attended by no decrease in the serum concentration of phosphorus, as measured in the morning fasting state (10). Similarly, in a group of normal men studied by Lemann and his colleagues (12), moderate dietary phosphorus restriction combined with aluminum hydroxide (Al(OH)$_3$) (to bind intestinal phosphorus) induced a 30% increase in circulating 1,25-(OH)$_2$D but no persisting change in the serum concentration of phosphorus, as measured in the morning fasting state. Lemann et al. suggested that a decrease in the serum concentration of phosphorus might have been demonstrated with "multiple measurements throughout the day".

In fact, the usually measured morning fasting value of serum phosphorus can substantially underestimate the severity of hypophosphatemia that obtains throughout most of the day, as when dietary restriction of phosphorus is combined with ingestion of Al(OH)$_3$ (vide infra). In normal subjects under normal metabolic conditions the serum concentration of phosphorus undergoes a circadian variation: a decrease in the morning to a nadir shortly before noon, followed by a rapid increase to an extended plateau in the afternoon, and a modest further increase to a peak shortly after midnight (13). Employing spectral analysis, Portale and his associates recently reported that the normal circadian rhythm in serum concentration of phosphorus can be described as the sum of sinusoidal functions with periodicities of 24 and 12 hours (14). Dietary restriction of phosphorus, combined with orally administered Al(OH)$_3$, induced within 10 days a striking change in the character of the circadian rhythm of serum phosphorus. Although inducing only a modest decrease in the morning fasting value of serum phosphorus, such extreme restriction of dietary phosphorus, to less than 100 mg/day, abolished the 12-hr periodic component of the time series that normally includes the afternoon rise in serum phosphorus, and thus induced a 40% reduction in the 24-hr mean serum level of phosphorus. Indeed, the magnitude of reduction in the serum level of phosphorus induced throughout the afternoon was twice that induced at 0800, the values decreasing to 2.0 and 2.6 mg/dl, respectively. Even with phosphorus restriction, the nocturnal peak in phosphorus concentration persisted in each subject, if at a lower level, i.e., the 24-hr periodicity was maintained. Extreme phosphorus supplementation, 3 gm/day for 10 days, which induced no persisting change in the morning fasting serum of phosphorus level, induced a 14% increase in the 24-hr mean serum level of phosphorus by exaggerating the afternoon rise in serum phosphorus.

Within 10 days, such extreme restriction and supplementation of dietary phosphorus induced striking changes in the plasma concentration of 1,25-(OH)$_2$D, an 80% increase and 30% decrease, respectively, changes entirely accounted for by changes in the production rate of 1,25-(OH)$_2$D (11). The changes induced in the 24-hr mean serum level of phosphorus varied inversely and significantly with those induced in the production rate (and plasma concentration) of 1,25-(OH)$_2$D (r = -0.88, P<0.001) (14). Thus with phosphorus restriction, modest, diet-induced reductions in the morning fasting serum level of phosphorus are predictably attended by later, larger reductions in its level in the afternoon and evening that appear to be critical in mediating the observed large increases in the production rate and plasma concentration of 1,25-(OH)$_2$D.

1,25-(OH)$_2$D is the most active metabolite of vitamin D known with respect to stimulating not only intestinal absorption of phosphate and calcium but also, as demonstrated by Raisz and his colleagues, bone resorption (15). At least in part by stimulating bone resorption, administered 1,25-(OH)$_2$D increases the plasma concentration of phosphorus in phosphorus-depleted, hypophosphatemic vitamin D deficient rats, a state in which intestinal absorption of phosphorus is negligible and renal reabsorption of phosphorus near complete (16). Even moderate hypophosphatemia enhances bone resorption in the rat, and vitamin D deficiency mitigates this enhancement (15). In premature infants in whom insufficient intake of phosphorus causes hypophosphatemia, rickets occurs in association with strikingly increased serum concentrations of 1,25-(OH)$_2$D; supplementation of phosphorus that corrects the hypophosphatemia and normalizes the serum levels of 1,25-(OH)$_2$D heals the rickets (18, 19). In the premature infant with hypophosphatemic rickets studied by Raisz and his colleagues (18), "the serum contained the highest bone-resorbing activity yet seen with this assay." Accordingly, and given that 1,25-(OH)$_2$D stimulates bone resorption (15), these investigators proposed that the increased circulating concentration of 1,25-(OH)$_2$D was an important pathogenetic determinant of hypophosphatemic rickets of prematurity (18).

These facts and this proposal bear directly on the syndrome of hypophosphatemic metabolic bone disease induced in humans over time by phosphorus-binding antacids, e.g., aluminum hydroxide (Al(OH)$_3$). As usually described, and induced experimentally in human subjects by Bartter and his colleagues (20), this syndrome is characterized biochemically by severe hypophosphatemia, near disappearance of urinary phosphorus, striking hypercalciuria that is caused in part by bone resorption, and greatly increased values of serum alkaline phosphatase. It has generally been held that the syndrome of antacid-induced metabolic bone disease does not occur without severe hypophosphatemia. But as judged from a number of published observations, phosphorus-responsive metabolic bone disease can result from antacid-induced hypophosphatemia that is not severe, at least as traditionally measured in the morning fasting state (21-24). In all reported cases of the syndrome, with one notable exception (21), the reported values of serum phosphorus concentration are either morning fasting values or their timing is not specified. In that exception, the index case, a woman self-medicated with aluminum hydroxide, Bloom and Finchum were at pains to point out that whereas the morning fasting value of serum phosphorus was hardly reduced at 2.9 mg/dl, the afternoon value was distinctly if not severely reduced at 2.0 mg/dl, and persistently so for as long as aluminum hydroxide was continued. With discontinuance of Al(OH)$_3$, her bone pain stopped and her osteomalacia healed.

Of particular interest are two recently described men with antacid-induced, histomorphometrically documented osteomalacia, who complained only of incapacitating bone pain (22, 23), both denying muscle weakness, malaise or anorexia, symptoms described by Bartter as being characteristic of severe hypophosphatemia (20). Neither patient had severe hypophosphatemia, as judged by morning fasting values of serum phosphorus, 3.2 and 2.0 mg/dl, respectively. In both, the values of the serum concentration of 1,25-(OH)$_2$D were extremely high, more than twice the upper limit of the normal range, and urinary phosphorus was negligible, findings that strongly suggest that throughout much of the day the concentration of serum phosphorus was much lower than the morning fasting value measured in both men. Predictably, the plasma alkaline phosphatase and urinary excretion of calcium were greatly increased, and in both men, discontinuance of antacid combined with dietary supplementation of phosphorus, rapidly normalized the serum concentration of 1,25-$(OH)_2D$, stopped the bone pain, and healed the osteomalacia.

Those observations would seem to bear on the use of phosphorus binders, either Al(OH)$_3$ or calcium carbonate (CaCO$_3$), in patients with chronic renal insufficiency to attenuate or prevent the otherwise invariably associated secondary hyperparathyroidism and its baleful skeletal consequences. In a recently reported study of children with chronic renal insufficiency in whom the daily ingestion of either Al(OH)$_3$ or CaCO$_3$ had completely corrected secondary hyperparathyroidism for a year, presumably by inducing the consistently "supranormal" serum values of 1,25-$(OH)_2D$ that were measured (25), Turner and his colleagues (26) reported several seriously untoward skeletal changes: "In contrast to the improvement in histological indices related to hyperparathyroidism, the mild mineralization defect present before treatment deteriorated during the year of study. There was a significant decrease in mineral appositional rate and increase in mineralization lag time. Before treatment two patients had some quantitative histological osteomalacia, while after treatment four patients had evidence of this disease." They went on to state: "It is not possible to completely exclude phosphate depletion as the cause of impaired mineralization in our patients; however, their plasma phosphate levels, while low, remained within the normal range. Since plasma calciums were towards the upper limit of normal, no patient's calcium x phosphate product fell below 2.5 at any time during the study. Impaired mineralization due to hypophosphatemia therefore seems unlikely."

All of the children studied by Turner and his colleagues had been treated for some time beforehand with Al(OH)$_3$. Serum aluminum levels were within the range in which aluminum-related osteodystrophy has been reported. Having found weakly positive histological staining for skeletal aluminum in 9 of the 11 children studied, and having discounted the possibility that hypophosphatemia had impaired mineralization, the investigators attributed the deterioration of the mineralization defect to aluminum toxicity and recommended CaCO$_3$ as a phosphorus-binder to suppress secondary hyperparathyroidism. But in the children studied by Turner et al., the morning fasting values of serum phosphorus decreased some 20% throughout administration of apparently either of the phosphorus-binders. It seems likely that this decrease in morning fasting serum phosphorus level was followed by the occurrence of hypophosphatemia throughout much of the day. This phenomenon is described in adult patients with chronic renal insufficiency receiving Al(OH)$_3$ (27). It would seem likely that chronic post-matutinal hypophosphatemia contributed to the further deterioration of the mineralization defect, particularly in light of the chronically "supranormal" circulating concentrations of 1,25-$(OH)_2D$ that were induced. In an adult patient with moderate renal insufficiency, we have recently observed that short term administration of Al(OH)$_3$ which normalized the circulating concentrations of 1,25-$(OH)_2D$ and iPTH, while inducing only a modest decrease in the morning fasting value of the serum concentration of phosphorus, induced clear-cut if moderately severe hypophosphatemia throughout most of the day. It would seem prudent to document that therapeutic administration of phosphorus-binders to suppress secondary hyperparathyroidism does not induce chronic post-matutinal hypophosphatemia of a severity and duration sufficient to exacerbate bone mineralization defects. Hypophosphatemia sufficient to induce chronically "supranormal" serum concentration of 1,25-(OH)$_2$D may well be sufficient to exacerbate bone mineralization defects. It is apparent that aluminum-related osteodystrophy and hypophosphatemic metabolic bone disease are not mutually exclusive.

Metabolic bone disease caused by chronic hypophosphatemia of moderate severity does not also require chronic ingestion of aluminum hydroxide. The phosphate-responsive hypophosphatemic rickets of premature infants might be considered a special case, given the unique metabolic circumstances of prematurity. But in a particularly pristine instance of chronic moderate hypophosphatemia that occurs in both adults and growing children, the hereditary hypophosphatemia rickets with hypercalciuria (HHRH) recently described by Tieder and his colleagues (28, 29), an apparently isolated impairment in the renal reabsorption of phosphate seemingly gives rise to all metabolic abnormalities through the single agency of chronic hypophosphatemia of moderate severity. In addition to metabolic bone disease, these abnormalities include increased plasma concentrations of 1,25-(OH)$_2$D, muscle weakness and hypercalciuria (28, 29). In patients with HHRH, continued phosphorus therapy alone readily normalizes serum concentrations of phosphate and 1,25-(OH)$_2$D, and within months, stops the bone pain, reverses the radiographic signs of rickets and accelerates linear growth in those children whose growth plate has remained open. Phosphorus therapy alone also rapidly improves muscle strength and normalizes the urinary excretion of calcium and serum level of alkaline phosphatase.

Tieder et al. proposed that phosphorus may be a "fine modulator" of 1,25-(OH)$_2$D production in humans, based on their finding of a significant inverse relationship between morning fasting serum levels of phosphorus and 1,25-(OH)$_2$D in a group comprised of the patients with HHRH, their less hypophosphatemic relatives with only hypercalciuria, and normal subjects (27). However, in this study, as in the earlier study of Gray et al. (4), the observed inverse relationship depends on the inclusion of values from subjects with hypercalciuria in whom the concentrations of serum phosphorus and 1,25-(OH)$_2$D were abnormally decreased and increased, respectively. When only those values from normal subjects are considered, no relationship is apparent in either study. Thus, the question remains: In normal humans under normal metabolic and physiological conditions, is either the dietary intake or serum concentration of phosphorus a determinant of the metabolism of 1,25-(OH)$_2$D?

We have recently demonstrated that restriction of dietary phosphorus within a normal range can increase the serum concentration of 1,25-(OH)$_2$D and decrease the serum concentration of phosphorus, both within their normal ranges, the decrease in serum levels of phosphorus occurring only after the morning fasting state. When the values obtained on both the high- and the low-normal intakes of phosphorus were analyzed as a single set, the serum concentrations of 1,25-(OH)$_2$D varied inversely and significantly with the 24-hr mean serum concentrations of phosphorus (r = -0.80, P<0.001). When these data are combined with those from our prior study (14) of healthy men in whom dietary phosphorus was manipulated over an extreme range from approximately zero to more than 3 gm per day, serum levels of 1,25-(OH)$_2$D extending over a 4-fold range, varied inversely with 24-hr mean serum levels of phosphorus (r = -0.90, P<0.001). These findings provide compelling evidence that normal dietary intakes of phosphorus physiologically regulate the renal production and serum concentration of 1,25-(OH)$_2$D, and suggest that the regulation is mediated through dietary modulation of the serum concentration of phosphorus.

Where does phosphorus fit in the hierarchy of regulation of 1,25-(OH)$_2$D production? For the rat, bird, and human, the stimulating effect of dietary restriction of phosphorus on the production of 1,25-(OH)$_2$D can override any dampening effect of the absence of PTH, and in the rat and vitamin D-deficient bird at least, any dampening effect of hypercalcemia per se. In humans with renal insufficiency, dietary restriction of phosphorus increases the production rate of 1,25-(OH)$_2$D even when greatly increased circulating concentrations of PTH do not. Conversely, in patients with idiopathic hypercalciuria and in those with primary hyperparathyroidism, dietary supplementation of phosphorus dampens the production rate of 1,25-(OH)$_2$D, despite further increasing the circulating concentrations of PTH. Thus, phosphorus can be a more potent determinant of the production rate of 1,25-(OH)$_2$D than PTH, or Ca^{++}. In the normal chick, under normal metabolic circumstances, the normal circulating concentration of 1,25-(OH)$_2$D physiologically dampens 1-hydroxylase (30). With dietary restriction of phosphorus in normal humans, the fact of an increased circulating concentration of 1,25-(OH)$_2$D indicates that restriction of phosphorus stimulates the production rate of 1,25-(OH)$_2$D more than the increased circulating concentration of 1,25-(OH)$_2$D can dampen it. When dietary phosphorus is manipulated in normal men over a broad range so that the values of mean 24-hr serum concentration of phosphorus extend throughout the normal range and beyond, these values vary inversely with those of the serum concentration of 1,25-(OH)$_2$D. Clearly, dietary phosphorus can regulate the metabolism of 1,25-(OH)$_2$D in health and disease. The evidence seems persuasive that dietary phosphorus regulates the production and hence the serum concentration of 1,25-(OH)$_2$D by modulating the serum concentration of phosphorus throughout a large part of the day.

REFERENCES:
1. Tanaka, Y., and H.F. DeLuca. 1973. The control of 25-hydroxyvitamin D metabolism by inorganic phosphorus. Arch. Biochem. Biophys. 154:566-574.
2. Baxter, L.A., and H.F. DeLuca. 1976. Stimulation of 25-hydroxyvitamin D$_3$-1-alpha-hydroxylase by phosphate depletion. J. Biol. Chem. 251:3158-3161.
3. Trechsel, U., J.-P. Bonjour, and H. Fleisch. 1979. Regulation of the metabolism of 25-hydroxyvitamin D$_3$ in primary cultures of chick kidney cells. J. Clin. Invest. 64:206-217.
4. Henry, H.L., R.J. Midgett, and A.W. Norman. 1974. Regulation of 25-hydroxyvitamin D$_3$-1-hydroxylase in vivo. J. Biol. Chem. 249:7584-7592.
5. Haussler, M.R., D.J. Baylink, M.R. Hughes, P.F. Brumbaugh, J.E. Wergedal, F.H. Shen, R.L. Nielsen, S.J. Counts, K.M. Bursac, and T.A. McCain. 1976. The

assay of 1-alpha, 25-dihydroxyvitamin D_3: Physiologic and pathologic modulation of circulating hormone levels. <u>Clin. Endocrinol.</u> 5(Suppl.): 151s-161s.

6. Gray, R.W., D.R. Wilz, A.E. Caldas, and J. Lemann, Jr. 1977. The importance of phosphate in regulating plasma 1,25-$(OH)_2$-vitamin D levels in humans: Studies in healthy subjects, in calcium-stone formers and in patients with primary hyperparathyroidism. <u>J. Clin. Endocrinol. Metab.</u> 45:299-306.

7. Booth, B.E., H.C. Tsai, and R.C. Morris, Jr. 1977. Parathyroidectomy reduces 25-hydroxyvitamin D_3-1-alpha-hydroxylase activity in the hypocalcemic vitamin D-deficient check. <u>J. Clin. Invest.</u> 60:1314-1320.

8. Van den Berg, C.J., R. Kumar, D.M. Wilson, H. Heath III, and L.H. Smith. 1980. Orthophosphate therapy decreases urinary calcium excretion and serum 1,25-dihydroxyvitamin D concentrations in idopathic hypercalciuria. <u>J. Clin. Endocrinol. Metab.</u> 51:998-1001.

9. Broadus, A.E., J.S. Magee, L.E. Mallette, R.L. Horst, R. Lang, P.S. Jensen, J.M. Gertner, and R. Baron. 1983. A detailed evaluation of oral phosphate therapy in selected patients with primary hyperparathyroidism. <u>J. Clin. Endocrinol. Metab.</u> 56:953-961.

10. Portale, A.A., B.E. Booth, B.P. Halloran, and R.C. Morris, Jr. 1984. Effect of dietary phosphorus on circulating concentrations of 1,25-dihydroxyvitamin D and immunoreactive parathyroid hormone in children with moderate renal insufficiency. <u>J. Clin. Invest.</u> 73:1580-1589.

11. Portale, A.A., B.P. Halloran, M.M. Murphy, and R.C. Morris, Jr. 1986. Oral intake of phosphorus can determine the serum concentration of 1,25-dihydroxyvitamin D by determining its production rate in humans. <u>J. Clin. Invest.</u> 77:7-12.

12. Maierhofer, W.J., R.W. Gray, and J. Lemann, Jr. 1984. Phosphate deprivation increases serum 1,25-$(OH)_2$-vitamin D concentrations in healthy men. <u>Kidney Int.</u> 25:571-575.

13. Stanbury, S.W. 1958. Some aspects of disordered renal tubular function. <u>Adv. Inter. Med.</u> 9:231-282.

14. Portale, A.A., B.P. Halloran, and R.C. Morris, Jr. 1987. Dietary intake of phosphorus modulates the circadian rhythm in serum concentration of phosphorus. <u>J. Clin. Invest.</u> 80:1147-1154.

15. Raisz, L.G., C.L. Trummel, M.F. Holick, et al. 1972. 1,25-dihydroxycholecalciferol: A potent stimulator of bone resorption in tissue culture. <u>Science</u> 175:768-769.

16. Castillo, L., Y. Tanaka, and H.F. DeLuca. 1975. The mobilization of bone mineral by 1,25-dihydroxyvitamin D_3 in hypophosphatemic rats. <u>Endocrinology</u> 97:995-999.

17. Baylink, D.J., J.E. Wergedal, and M. Stauffer. 1971. Formation, mineralization, and resorption of bone in hypophosphatemic rats. <u>J. Clin. Invest.</u> 50:2519-2530.

18. Rowe, J.C., D.H. Wood, D.W. Rowe, and L.G. Raisz. 1979. Nutritional hypophosphatemic rickets in a

premature infant fed breast milk. <u>N. Engl. J. Med.</u> 300:293-296.

19. Greer, F.R., J.J. Steichen, and R.C. Tsang. 1982. Calcium and phosphate supplements in breast milk-related rickets. <u>Am. J. Dis.Child.</u> 136:581-583.

20. Lotz, M., E. Zisman, and F.C. Bartter. 1968. Evidence for a phosphorus-depletion syndrome in man. <u>N. Engl. J. Med.</u> 278:409-415.

21. Bloom, W.L. and D. Flinchum. 1960. Osteomalacia with pseudofractures caused by the ingestion of aluminum hydroxide. <u>J.A.M.A.</u> 174:1327-1330.

22. Carmichael, K.A., M.D. Fallon, M. Dalinka, et al. 1984. Osteomalacia and osteitis fibrosa in a man ingesting aluminum hydroxide antacid. <u>Am. J. Med.</u> 76:1137-1143.

23. Godsall, J.W., R. Baron, and K.L. Insogna. 1984. Vitamin D metabolism and bone histomorphometry in a patient with antacid-induced osteomalacia. <u>Am. J. Med.</u> 77:747-750.

24. Saadeh, G., T. Bauer, A. Licata, et al. 1987. Antacid-induced osteomalacia. <u>Cleve. Clin. J. Med.</u> 54:214-216.

25. Slatopolski, E., C. Weerts, G. Thielan, K. Martin, and H. Harter. 1983. Marked suppression of secondary hyperparathyroidism (SH) by intravenous 1,25-(OH)$_2$D$_3$ in uremic patients. In <u>Clinical Disorders of Bone and Mineral Metabolism</u>, edited by Frame, B. and J.T. Potts. Amsterdam, Excerpta Medica, pp. 267-270.

26. Turner, C., J. Compston, R.H.K. Mak, S. Vedi, R.W.E. Mellish, G.B. Haycock, and C. Chantler. 1988. Bone turnover and 1,25-dihydroxycholecalciferol during treatment with phosphate binders. <u>Kidney Int.</u> 33:989-995.

27. Cam, J.M., V.A. Luck, J.B. Eastwood, and H.E. DeWardener. 1976. The effect of aluminum hydroxide orally on calcium, phosphorus and aluminium metabolism in normal subjects. <u>Clin. Sci. Molec. Med.</u> 51:407-414.

28. Tieder, M., D. Modai, R. Samuel, et al. 1985. Hereditary hypophosphatemic rickets with hypercalciuria. <u>N. Engl. J. Med.</u> 312:611-617.

29. Tieder, M., D. Modai, U. Shaked, et al. 1987. 'Idiopathic' hypercalciuria and hereditary hypophosphatemic rickets. <u>N. Engl. J. Med.</u> 316:125-129.

30. Booth, B.E., H.C. Tsai, and R.C. Morris, Jr. 1985. Vitamin D status regulates 25-hydroxyvitamin D$_3$-1-alpha-hydroxylase and its responsiveness to parathyroid hormone in the chick. <u>J. Clin. Invest.</u> 75:155-161.

Discussion:

DR. DREZNER (Raleigh-Durham, NC): My question is for Mark Haussler. I wish to know if work has been done in vitro relative to the zinc fingers and the 1,25-dihydroxyvitamin D receptor showing dependence on available zinc, and whether zinc deficiency in vivo might induce a relative resistance to 1,25-dihydroxyvitamin D. You did not mention this as a possible means of modifying the receptor. Zinc deficiency, I have learned, is a common consequence of total parenteral nutrition so that we could extrapolate from the in vitro to the in vivo situation.

DR. HAUSSLER (Tucson, AZ): That is a good extrapolation. Zinc deficiency does compromise developmental aspects. And, as you noted, all of the zinc finger proteins are involved, somehow, in either development or the regulation of development. That is as far as it has gone. If one wishes to wildly speculate, there are syndromes, such as the fetal alcohol syndrome, which are developmental problems that are associated with low levels of zinc. So, there are a few clinical hints. Careful studies to test the effects of zinc deficiency on the actions of vitamin D have not been done. I think the point you raised is an interesting one.

It may also be necessary to include, a consideration of zinc economy within the cell. There is an intracellular protein metalothionine, function unknown, that is thought to detoxify cadmium and zinc. It, in fact, may be a protein that buffers zinc and allows the amount of zinc to always be adequate for these developmentally important proteins. This is another consideration that needs to be examined.

DR. DREZNER: If you cultured cells in the total absence of zinc for a long period of time, would it be possible to examine the structure of the receptor for 1,25-dihydroxyvitamin D to determine if the zinc fingers were still present?

DR. HAUSSLER: We have considered culturing cells with zinc-deficient serum and media. However, it has proven to be a formidable technical problem that we have not been able to solve. Zinc-deficient serum and media are not available. It would be a good experiment.

DR. PHELPS (Brooklyn, NY): I have a question for Dr. Morris. Has it been determined that a reduction in the mean serum phosphorus over 24 hours is necessary to increase serum 1,25-dihydroxyvitamin D and to reduce serum immunoreactive parathyroid hormone values in patients with renal insufficiency? I thought that Dr. Portali, your colleague, had shown, in fact, that phosphate restriction achieved these changes in renal insufficiency without changing the mean serum phosphorus over 24 hours.

DR. MORRIS (San Francisco): In the article that we wrote several years ago, we found that phosphorus restriction, in fact, normalized circulating 1,25-dihydroxyvitamin D and immunoreactive parathyroid hormone without changing the morning fasting phosphate concentration.

DR. PHELPS: Are there any studies that reproduce the alterations in serum phosphate you showed in normal subjects in which measurements of the serum phosphorus were performed throughout a period of 24 hours in patients with renal insufficiency? I seem to recall an abstract that was presented last year at the annual meeting of the ASBMR by Dr. Portali showing a similar effect of phosphate restriction on serum 1,25-dihydroxyvitamin D in patients with renal failure who had no change in mean serum phosphorus.

DR. MORRIS: No, the mean serum phosphorus always changes, both in patients with moderate renal insufficiency, normal young people and normal old people. This latter finding was something of a surprise. Of course, the point I was trying to make is that the changes in phosphorus will not be evident if only a single morning fasting sample is obtained. The change is apparent if serum phosphorus is determined, later in the day, at 1:00 or 2:00 p.m. in the afternoon.

DR. BERGMANN (Belgium): I have a question for Dr. Liberman. I understood that patients with complete absence of binding of 1,25-dihydroxyvitamin D responded to the treatment with calcitriol although those with low binding did not respond. What is your explanation for that?

DR. LIBERMAN (Israel): I said that, of the group of patients that had no binding of 1,25-dihydroxyvitamin D to the receptor there was one that did respond. This may represent a case of an extreme affinity defect. It is possible that with a very high dose of calcitriol, a response is evident.

The patient with the low capacity is a very interesting one because it means that if ten percent of so-called normal receptors are occupied the response is not optimal. There is some precedent in animal studies showing a linear relationship between receptor occupancy and biological response. So one may conclude that ten percent occupancy of "normal" receptors is not enough to elicit a full normal response. For the study of the biochemistry of the receptors, it might be interesting to determine what regulates receptor occupancy assuring that the receptor is normal.

DR. KAYE (Montreal): My question is to Dr. Morris. Your beautiful data on the variation in serum phosphorus is very persuasive for the normal subjects, and the effect of amphogel in inducing a mineralizing defect in patients. My question is, have you or anybody else clearly demonstrated a mineralizing defect in patients with renal failure as a result of attempting to lower the serum phosphorus with aluminum hydroxide?

DR. MORRIS: I tried to touch on that at the latter part of my talk. In the current issue of Kidney International, a group led by Chandler described their experience in attempting to prevent the development of secondary hyperparathyroidism by administration of, first, aluminum hydroxide and then calcium carbonate. They found a mineralization defect that became worse with the successful control of the secondary hyperparathyroidism and specifically commented on the problem. Neither they nor anyone else have solved the problem that administration of a phosphorus-binding agent sufficient to control secondary hyperparathyroidism produces a mineralization defect. However, I do not say that it cannot be done. On the other hand, I do not know of anyone who has been able to solve this dilemma.

DR. MALLUCHE (Lexington, KY): I want to ask Dr. Morris whether the effects of lowering serum phosphorus can be dissociated from the effects of aluminum that you administered?

DR. MORRIS: For the acute studies, I am not sure that I need to sort out an effect of aluminum, unless you suggest that aluminum has an effect on the synthesis of 1,25-dihydroxyvitamin D.

DR. MALLUCHE: This point is not entirely established. However, some in vitro studies suggest that aluminum does, indeed, affect renal 25-hydroxyvitamin D-1-hydroxylase.

DR. MORRIS: Well, my data do not address this possibility directly. Our studies, perhaps, will need to be repeated with the administration of calcium carbonate as a way of reducing the serum phosphorus concentration. This is readily doable, of course. I cannot say, for certain, that the aluminum hydroxide that was given in our studies did not have an effect on renal 25-hydroxyvitamin D-1-hydroxylase, as you suggest.

DR. WOODHOUSE (Saudi Arabia): Dr. Liberman, you demonstrated beautifully how intravenous calcium can correct all the abnormalities in some of the patients with vitamin D-dependent rickets type II that you described. As you know, this is also possible when very high doses of calcium are given by mouth. What will happen to the child when infusions of calcium are stopped? What type of management do you propose to use? Have you considered the possibility of carrying out a parathyroidectomy which might prevent skeletal deformities so that the patient subsequently could be more easily treated with oral calcium?

DR. LIBERMAN: The method of treatment is quite new. The followup is only about a year after stopping the treatment with intravenously administered calcium. What will happen, I assume, is there will be a relapse of the disease. I think probably the important thing is to treat these children during the accelerated growth period. Some of the deformities would be avoided and those that were not could then be surgically corrected after the growth spurt. The question of parathyroidectomy is an interesting suggestion. I do not know. Intuitively, I feel uneasy about it, but the idea could be entertained.

DR. GLORIEUX (Montreal): My question is for Dr. Morris. In my recollection of the Gray and Leeman study in normal subjects deprived of phosphate, the first alteration that was observed was not a change in serum phosphate, but in urinary phosphate, which rapidly declined to zero. The serum 1,25-dihydroxyvitamin D increased before any change in serum phosphate. Do any observations of that sort in your studies indicate that the changes in urinary phosphate were a triggering mechanism for altering the activity of renal 25-hydroxyvitamin D-1-hydroxylase?

DR. MORRIS: Our study was not designed to sort that out, and I did not mean to imply that the changes we found in serum phosphorus were not mediated through a change in renal handling of phosphorus. This point will be addressed later this afternoon in Dr. Drezner's presentation.

DR. MARCUS (Palo Alto, CA): I am interested in the implications of Dr. Morris' findings, not in terms of phosphate restriction in patients with renal insufficiency, but, perhaps, the influence of modest increases in phosphorus intake in normal people. I thought that the concept of the importance of the dietary calcium-to-phosphorus ratio for osteoporosis was one whose time had come and gone. It seems to me that, since an increased intake of phosphorus of the amount that you described in your studies caused reductions in serum 1,25-dihydroxyvitamin D that you found, a high intake of phosphorus could lower the serum 1,25-dihydroxyvitamin D and reduce calcium absorption in elderly subjects.

On the other hand, there is a large body of literature from Herter-Spencer, Robert Heaney and others, in which calcium balance was determined over a wide range of phosphorus intake. In these studies, alterations in dietary phosphate had little effect on calcium balance. Could you reconcile those two findings and have you given some thought to this issue?

DR. MORRIS: I do not know that I can reconcile them. I am attracted to the notion that you have just described, that over a period of time, large intakes of dietary phosphorus could act to suppress 1,25-dihydroxyvitamin D and possibly could contribute to the development of metabolic bone disease. Of course, other factors are important. As people age, there is loss of renal mass and, therefore, glomerular filtration rate tends to fall. A modest reduction in renal mass together with an increased phosphate load could combine to cause a reduction of the rate of synthesis of 1,25-dihydroxyvitamin D and plasma 1,25-dihydroxyvitamin D that could play a role in the pathogenesis of osteoporosis. But I cannot resolve the discrepancies in the results of the two kinds of studies that you describe.

DR. PEACOCK (Indianapolis): My comments are directed to Mark Haussler and to Uri Liberman. Is the value for serum 24,25-dihydroxyvitamin D in plasma useful in the conditions you describe, and can the values be used as an indication of a biological response? How is vitamin D metabolized if the 25-hydroxyvitamin D-24-hydroxylase is not working?

DR. LIBERMAN: This is an interesting point. I did not discuss this during my talk as I did not have enough time. The serum 24,25-dihydroxyvitamin D is usually low or even normal in patients with vitamin D-dependent rickets. These values may be considered to be inappropriately low because the values of serum 1,25-dihydroxyvitamin D are very high, as 1,25-dihydroxyvitamin D is supposed to stimulate the 25-hydroxyvitamin D-24-hydroxylase. Thus the concentration of 24,25-dihydroxyvitamin D in serum is not a reliable indicator of biologic response. On the other hand the relative low serum levels may be an indicator that the effect of 1,25-dihydroxyvitamin D on 25-hydroxyvitamin D-24-hydroxylase is receptor mediated. Therefore if the receptor is defective, serum values for 24,25-dihydroxyvitamin D would not correlate with serum values for 1,25-dihydroxyvitamin D and would reflect low activity of the enzyme.

DR. BELL: I want to thank the first three speakers for their excellent presentations.

Clinical Disorders of Phosphorus and Vitamin D Metabolism

TERESA NESBITT, GIORA A. DAVIDAI, PETER C. BRAZY, and
MARC K. DREZNER

Duke University Medical Center
Durham, NC

A variety of diseases, including the genetic and acquired forms of hypophosphatemic (vitamin D resistant) rickets and tumoral calcinosis, have as their characteristic feature an abnormality of phosphate homeostasis occurring alone or in combination with a derangement of vitamin D metabolism. In these disorders, the disturbance of the inorganic phosphate (Pi) status results from a pathophysiological alteration of the renal tubular Pi reabsorptive capacity, a primary control mechanism maintaining phosphorus homeostasis. When present, the associated defect of vitamin D metabolism (an inability to normally regulate calcitriol production) represents a failure to effect an appopriate adaptive response to the resultant hypophosphatemia. This concomitant abnormality contributes to the disturbed phosphate economy.

In spite of this association between disordered renal phosphate transport and vitamin D metabolism, the mechanism(s) linking these defects remains unknown. Although phosphate availability is a primary factor regulating renal 25 hydroxyvitamin D-1-hydroxylase activity, it is unclear if this is a function of the plasma phosphate concentration or the rate of phosphate transport through the tubules. Changes in the serum phosphate concentration per se may initiate compensatory modifications in renal calcitriol production. Alternatively, the regulation of renal calcitriol production may be linked to the rate of phosphate transport through the cells containing the 25 hydroxyvitamin D-1-hydroxylase enzyme. Previous studies have established that dietary phosphate deprivation or loading leads to substantial and parallel modifications of both renal phosphate transport capacity and calcitriol production that are independent of parathyroid hormone (1-5). However, these studies do not define the role of plasma phosphate or phosphate transport in modulating the effects of Pi deficiency/excess on $1,25(OH)_2D$ production. Nevertheless, evidence has begun to emerge which suggests that an alteration of phosphate flux across renal proximal convoluted tubular cells may influence renal 1-hydroxylase activity. In this regard, our studies of the hypophosphatemic rachitic diseases and tumoral calcinosis have provided data which define a potential relationship between renal Pi transport and vitamin D metabolism. The remainder of this chapter presents an overview of our investigations. This information provides the basis for proposing an integrated model for regulation of renal phosphate transport and calcitriol production, while highlighting questions which must be addressed.

<u>Renal Phosphate Transport and Vitamin D Metabolism</u>
    <u>Human Diseases</u>
    Initially we studied X-linked hypophosphatemic rickets (XLH), the prototypic form of the vitamin D resistant disorders. Characteristic

abnormalities of this disease include impaired renal tubular reabsorption of phosphate, hypophosphatemia, defective calcification of cartilage and bone, and refractoriness to vitamin D therapy. The primary inborn error of this disorder results in an expressed abnormality in the renal proximal tubule which impairs phosphate reabsorption. An associated abnormality of vitamin D metabolism has also been discovered in affected patients. Data supporting this conclusion include the presence of: 1) a circulating level of the active vitamin D metabolite, $1,25(OH)_2D$, which is apparently low for the prevailing hypophosphatemia (6); 2) a significantly lesser increment of the serum calcitriol level in response to parathyroid hormone stimulation in affected patients compared to that in age-matched controls (7); and 3) a subnormal increase of the serum $1,25(OH)_2D$ concentration after dietary phosphorus deprivation (8). While these data are in accord with the presence of an apparent defect in calcitriol production, they do not establish that the abnormality represents an acquired derangement secondary to decreased renal phosphate transport.

However, complementary observations in related clinical disorders favor the possibility that altered renal Pi reabsorption does influence calcitriol production. In this regard, we have investigated the biochemical abnormalities manifest in patients with tumor-induced osteomalacia (TIO) (9,10) and Fanconi's syndrome (FS) (unpublished observations). These diverse diseases of both acquired and genetic origin share with XLH multiple biochemical abnormalities (Table 1). Most notably, the expressed hypophosphatemia in affected patients with these disorders is not associated with an increased serum $1,25(OH)_2D$ level. Rather, abnormally regulated renal 25 hydroxyvitamin D-1-hydroxylase activity is manifest concomitantly with a primary defect in renal phosphate transport. Such a shared linkage of these defects in this collectively diverse group of diseases suggests that the aberrant calcitriol production is a consequence of the abnormal phosphate transport which is the primary disturbance common to all of these disorders.

Further support for a potential relationship between $1,25(OH)_2D$ production and renal phosphate transport derives from studies in patients with tumoral calcinosis. This disorder is a rare genetic disease characterized by the presence of periarticular tumorous calcifications. Affected patients traditionally manifest the biochemical markers of hyperphosphatemia and an elevated serum $1,25(OH)_2D$ concentration (11) which are paradoxical when compared to a state of dietary phosphate loading. However, the pathophysiological basis for this disease is a primary abnormality of the renal tubule which results in enhanced phosphate reabsorption (12), a characteristic of dietary phosphate depletion. Thus, patients with tumoral calcinosis manifest increased renal tubular phosphate transport and enhanced $1,25(OH)_2D$ production, concordant alterations which are similar to the non-reciprocal changes in these variables observed in patients with the various hypophosphatemic disorders. Collectively, these data indicate an apparent dependence of renal 25(OH)D-1-hydroxylase activity on renal phosphate transport. Indeed, we have observed that the renal TmP/GFR (an index of phosphate transport capacity) bears a strikingly linear correlation with the plasma calcitriol levels in normal subjects as well as those with XLH, TIO and tumoral calcinosis (13,14) (Figure 1).

While these data indicate that a causal linkage exists between renal Pi transport and $1,25(OH)_2D$ production, the relationship of these observations to the previously reported data regarding phosphate availability and renal 25(OH)D-1-hydroxylase activity is not immediately apparent. The difficulty in demonstrating this relationship may involve the presence of heterogeneity in rates of phosphate transport and metabolic processes among the different segments of proximal renal tubules (S1, S2 and S3). We believe that a more complete characterization of the contribution of phosphate transport rates to phosphate availability for cellular metabolism in each of these tubule segments will provide the basis for understanding phosphate homeostasis and vitamin D metabolism during selected physiologic or pathophysiologic conditions.

In any case, although these observations strongly support the possibility that $1,25(OH)_2D$ production is dependent upon changes in renal Pi transport, several recent reports indicate that the relationship may be far more complex than initially appreciated. In this regard, Lieberman and his colleagues (15) have described a newly recognized genetic form of hypophosphatemic rickets [hereditary hypophosphatemic rickets and hypercalciuria (HHRH)] which exhibits significant biochemical differences from XLH (Table 1). Affected subjects with this disorder manifest diminished renal phosphate transport and hypophosphatemia in association with an elevated serum $1,25(OH)_2D$ level. Such a coexistence of decreased phosphate flux and apparent enhanced calcitriol production is antithetical to the predicted relationship between these processes which we have suggested. However, recently completed studies in animal models of the hypophosphatemic rachitic disorders have allowed resolution of this apparent paradox and provide data which confirm and extend our understanding of the role which renal Pi transport plays in the regulation of renal 25(OH)D-1-hydroxylase activity.

Animal Models of XLH

Over the past several years we have investigated two murine homologues of the human disease XLH, the Hyp- and Gy-mouse. These species are the result of two distinctly different mutations in the family of genes on the X-chromosome which regulate renal phosphate transport (16). Biochemical abnormalities shared by these murine models include defective renal Pi transport and consequent hypophosphatemia. In our investigations we have examined the control mechanisms influencing $1,25(OH)_2D$ production.

Initially we observed that the Hyp-mouse manifests abnormal Pi/PTH (cAMP) regulated renal 25(OH)D-1-hydroxylase activity. In this regard, this mutant displayed enzyme function which was: 1) fourfold less in the basal state than that of phosphate-depleted mice (17); and 2) one-third of that achieved in normal and phosphate-depleted mice after PTH (or cAMP) stimulation (18). While these data suggest that Hyp-mice have a generalized derangement of renal $1,25(OH)_2D$ production, we could not be certain if this defect is a consequence of the abnormal renal Pi transport. However, recent studies by Kurakowa and his associates (19,20) permitted us to establish this linkage. In their investigations they demonstrated the presence of two distinct and uniquely regulated 1-hydroxylase systems in the mammalian kidney located in the proximal convoluted (PCT) and proximal straight tubules (PST). Recognition of such axial heterogeneity along the nephron revealed that we had tested regulation of enzyme function only in the PTH (cAMP) and Pi sensitive PCT, the locus of abnormal Pi transport. Thus, in further studies of Hyp-mice, we examined the effects of calcitonin on the 25(OH)D-1-hydroxylase of the PST to determine if, in the absence of impaired Pi transport at this site, abnormal enzyme regulation is similarly evident. Surprisingly, in response to this stimulus enzyme activity in the mutants increased to levels that were no different from those of normal mice (21). These data established that defective regulation of renal 25(OH)D-1-hydroxylase activity in the Hyp-mice is confined to the PCT. More importantly, selective localization of this defect to that segment of the renal tubule which exhibits abnormal Pi transport represents strong evidence that the aberrant enzyme responsiveness is a consequence of this primary defect.

While these data clearly link abnormal phosphate transport to defective regulation of $1,25(OH)_2D$ production, they do not explain the paradoxical occurrence of elevated serum calcitriol levels in patients with HHRH. However, our studies in Gy-mice, the second murine homologue of XLH, provide insight into this dilemma. In these investigations we discovered that the Gy-mutants unexpectedly maintain normal regulation of vitamin D metabolism in spite of abnormal renal Pi transport. Indeed, consistent with an expressed hypophosphatemia these mutants maintain enhanced renal 25(OH)D-1-hydroxylase activity (9.3 ± 0.6 fmoles/mg kidney/min) in the basal state, similar to that of phosphate-depleted mice (9.3 ± 1.3), but significantly greater than that of controls (2.8 ± 0.3). Moreover, PTH stimulation of the Gy-mice increased the enzyme activity to a level (59.3 ± 7.7) equivalent to that obtained by both normals (65.8 ± 7.7) and phosphate-depleted animals (58.4 ± 7.4). Similarly, calcitonin administration enhanced enzyme function comparably in Gy- and normal mice. These observations establish that increased $1,25(OH)_2D$ production can occur in association with abnormal renal phosphate transport.

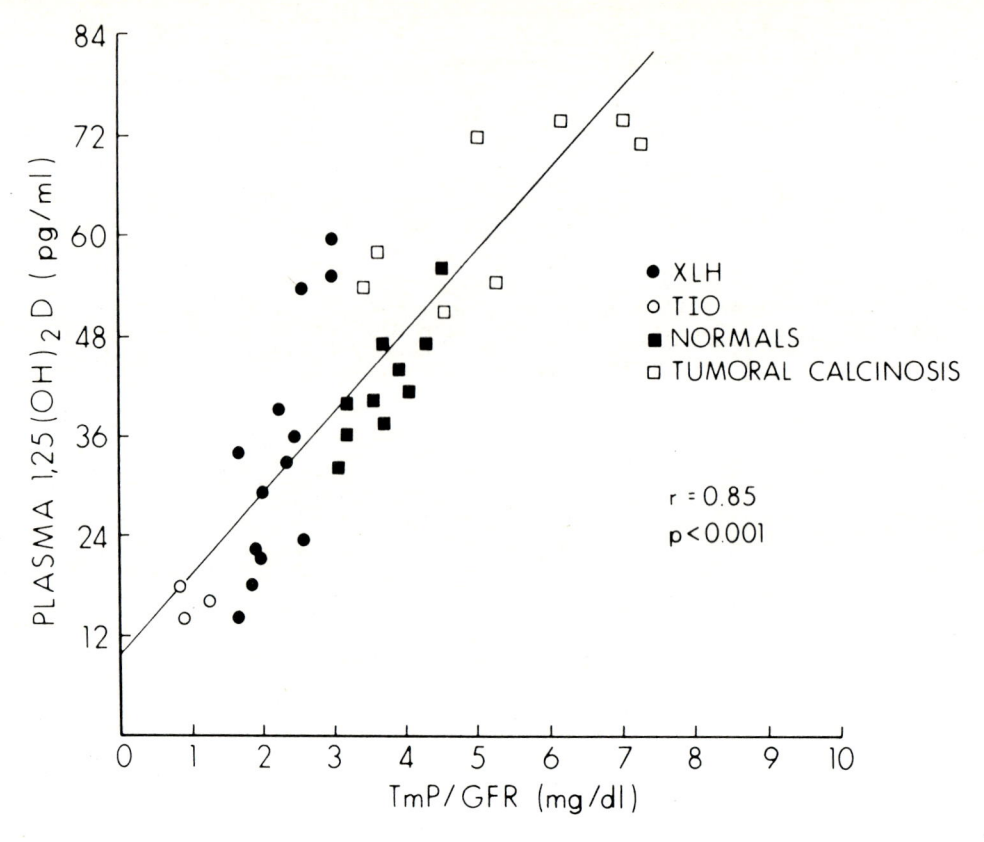

Figure 1. Correlation between renal TmP/GFR and plasma 1,25(OH)$_2$D levels in normals and patients with XLH, TIO and tumoral calcinosis. Significant linear correlation is evident, suggesting a potential relationship between renal phosphate transport and the prevailing plasma levels of active vitamin D. [From Drezner MK (13) and Lyles et al (14) with permission.]

TABLE 1

Biochemical Abnormalities In Diseases Characterized By Abnormal Renal Phosphate Transport

		XLH	T1O	FS	HHRH	P-Depleted
TMP/GFR		↓	↓	↓	↓	↑
S	P	↓	↓	↓	↓	↓
S	1,25(OH)$_2$D	↓	↓	↓	↑	↑
S	Ca	N	N	N	N	↑
GI Absorption						
	P	↓	↓	↓	↑	↑
	Ca	↓	↓	↓	↑	↑
U	Ca/24h	↓	↓	↓	↑	↑
U	P/24h	↑	↑	↑	↑	↓

The pathophysiological basis for such biochemical diversity in the Hyp- and Gy-mice and for the similar non-comparable defects in human diseases, however, is not immediately apparent. Nevertheless, if we consider that renal phosphate transport does, in fact, influence renal 25(OH)D-1-hydroxylase activity, a potential explanation becomes evident. Indeed, previous studies have established that an array of mitochondrial functions in the renal proximal tubule are dependent upon phosphate availability (22). Therefore, abnormal phosphate flux secondary to decreased transport may impair the 1-hydroxylase activity in these cells by effecting a structural or functional alteration in the enzyme or varying NADPH availability. Regardless, such a potential influence on $1,25(OH)_2D$ production provides the basis for understanding the observed differences in renal 25(OH)D-1-hydroxylase activity in Hyp- and Gy-mice as well as the human diseases. In this regard, we propose that $1,25(OH)_2D$ production, like other biochemical processes within the tubular cells, may not be a universal function in all segments of the proximal convoluted tubule. Thus, a difference in the site of abnormal phosphate transport within the proximal convoluted tubule may variably influence enzyme activity. In Hyp-mice, for example, localization of abnormal phosphate transport in the S1 segment, in which 25 hydroxyvitamin D-1-hydroxylase activity has been definitively demonstrated, may negatively influence calcitriol production. Such a site specific defect, diminished S1 segment brush border membrane alkaline phosphatase activity, has been previously identified in Hyp-mice by Brunnette et al (23). In contrast, in the Gy-mice, similarly impaired phosphate transport, confined to the S2 segment, may not affect vitamin D metabolism if cells in this segment of the nephron do not normally manifest enzyme activity. Confirmation of this hypothesis of course awaits further study. In any case, a similar hypothetical construct may explain the apparent paradoxical relationship between phosphate transport and $1,25(OH)_2D$ production in human diseases such as HHRH. Thus, we believe that a model does exist which effectively provides for integrated regulation of renal phosphate and $1,25(OH)_2D$ production. Accordingly, alterations of renal phosphate transport at different sites along the proximal convoluted tubule may variably express renal 25(OH)D-1-hydroxylase activity. Regardless, it seems evident that variation in phosphate flux is an important determinant of $1,25(OH)_2D$ production.

References:
1. Pastoriza-Munoz E, Mishler DR, Lechene C. Effect of phosphate deprivation on phosphate reabsorption in rat nephron: Role of PTH. Am J Physiol 244:F140-F149, 1983.
2. Beck N, Webster SK, Reineck H. Effect of fasting on tubular phosphorus reabsorption. Am J Physiol 237:F241-F246, 1979.
3. Tanaka Y, DeLuca HF. The control of 25-hydroxyvitamin D metabolism by inorganic phosphorus. Arch Biochem Biophys 154:566-574, 1973.
4. Gray RW, Napoli J. Dietary phosphate deprivation increases 1,25-dihydroxyvitamin D_3 synthesis in rat kidney in vitro. J Biol Chem 258:1152-1155, 1983.
5. Gray RW, Wilz DR, Caldas AE, Lemann, Jr J. The importance of phosphate in regulating plasma $1,25-(OH)_2$-vitamin D levels in humans: Studies in healthy subjects, in calcium-stone formers and in patients with primary hyperparathyroidism. J Clin Endocrinol Metab 45:299-306, 1977.
6. Lyles KW, Clark AG, Drezner MK. Serum 1,25-dihydroxyvitamin D levels in subjects with X-linked hypophosphatemic rickets and osteomalacia. Calcif Tissue Int 34:125-130, 1982.
7. Lyles KW, Drezner, MK. Parathyroid hormone effects on serum 1,25 dihydroxyvitamin D levels in patients with X-linked hypophosphatemic rickets: Evidence for abnormal 25-hydroxyvitamin D-1-hydroxylase activity. J Clin Endocrinol Metab 54:638-644, 1982.
8. Insogna KL, Broadus AE, Gertner JM. Impaired phosphorus conservation and 1,25 dihydroxyvitamin D generation during phosphorus deprivation in familial hypophosphatemic rickets. J Clin Invest 71:1562-1567, 1983.

9. Drezner MK, Feinglos MN. Osteomalacia due to 1,25 dihydroxycholecalciferol deficiency: Association with a giant cell tumor of bone. J Clin Invest 60:1046-1053, 1977.
10. Lyles KW, Harrelson JM, Drezner MK. Hypophosphatemic osteomalacia: Association with prostatic carcinoma. Ann Int Med 93:275-278, 1980.
11. Lyles KW, Burkes EJ, Ellis GJ, Lucas KJ, Dolan EA, Drezner MK. Genetic transmission of tumoral calcinosis. Autosomal dominant with variable clinical expressivity. J Clin Endocrinol Metab 60:1093-1096, 1985.
12. Zerwekh JE, Sanders LA, Townsend J, Pak CYC. Tumoral calcinosis: Evidence for concurrent defects in renal tubular phosphorus transport and 1,25 dihydroxycholecalciferol synthesis. Calcif Tissue Int 32:1-6, 1980.
13. Drezner MK. Understanding the pathogenesis of X-linked hypophosphatemic rickets: A requisite for successful therapy. A CPC Series: Cases in Metabolic Bone Disease Vol 2, No 1, March, 1987.
14. Lyles KW, Halsey DL, Friedman NE, Lobaugh B. Correlations of serum concentrations of 1,25 dihydroxyvitamin D, phosphorus and parathyroid hormone in tumoral calcinosis. J Clin Endocrinol Metab Vol 67, 1988, In Press.
15. Tieder M, Modai D, Shaked U, Samuel R, Arie R, Halabe A, Weissgarten J, Averbukh Z, Cohen N, Edelstein S, Liberman U. "Idiopathic" hypercalciuria and hereditary hypophosphatemic rickets: Two phenotypical expressions of a common genetic defect. N Engl J Med 316:125-129, 1987.
16. Lyon MF, Scriver CR, Baker LRI, Tenenhouse HS, Kronick J, Mandia S. The Gy mutation: Another cause of X-linked hypophosphatemia in the mouse. Proc Natl Acad Sci USA 83:4899-4903, 1986.
17. Lobaugh B, Drezner MK. Abnormal regulation of renal 25-hydroxyvitamin D-1α-hydroxylase activity in the X-linked hypophosphatemic mouse. J Clin Invest 71:400-403, 1983.
18. Nesbitt T, Drezner MK, Lobaugh B. Abnormal parathyroid hormone stimulation of 25-hydroxyvitamin D-1-hydroxylase activity in the Hyp-mouse: Evidence for a generalized defect of vitamin D metabolism. J Clin Invest 77:181-187, 1986.
19. Kawashima H, Torikai S, Kurokawa K. Localization of 25-hydroxyvitamin D_3-1α-hydroxylase and 24-hydroxylase along the rat nephron. Proc Natl Acad Sci USA. 78:1199-1203, 1981.
20. Kawashima H, Torikai S, Kurokawa K. Calcitonin selectively stimulates 25-hydroxyvitamin D-1α-hydroxylase in the rat kidney. J Clin Invest 70:135-140, 1982.
21. Nesbitt T, Lobaugh B, Drezner MK. Calcitonin stimulation of renal 25-hydroxyvitamin D-1α-hydroxylase activity in Hyp-mice: Evidence that the regulation of calcitriol production is not universally abnormal in X-linked hypophosphatemia. J Clin Invest 75:15-19, 1987.
22. Brazy PC, Mandel LJ, Gullans SR, Soltoff SP. Interactions between phosphate and oxidative metabolism in proximal renal tubules. Am J Physiol 247:F575-F581, 1984.
23. Brunette MG, Chan M, Lebrun M. Phosphatase activity along the nephron of mice with hypophosphatemic vitamin D resistant rickets. Kid Int 20:181-187, 1981.

Acknowledgements:
Work reported in this manuscript from the authors' laboratory was supported in part by grants from the National Institutes of Health (AR27032 and DK38015) and the National Kidney Foundation.

Abnormal Vitamin D and Calcium Metabolism in Sarcoidosis and Related Diseases

YAIR LIEL, JAN BASILE, and NORMAN H. BELL

*VA Medical Center
and Departments of Medicine and Pharmacology
Medical University of South Carolina
Charleston, SC*

Hypercalcemia and hypercalciuria resulting from increased circulating 1,25-dihydroxyvitamin D are known to occur in sarcoidosis and a number of other diseases. It is proposed a) to review the disorders in which abnormal vitamin D and calcium metabolism occur, b) to review the mechanisms for abnormal vitamin D metabolism in nonrenal tissue that are responsible for the ensuing hypercalcemia and hypercalciuria that is apparent clinically in patients with sarcoidosis and c) to present evidence that abnormal vitamin D metabolism may be present in normocalcemic patients with sarcoidoisis and that these patients are at risk for developing hypercalcemia and its sequelae, the most important of which is impairment of renal function.

Diseases with abnormal vitamin D and calcium metabolism

The diseases in which hypercalcemia was reported to be associated with elevated serum 1,25-dihydroxyvitamin D are summarized in Table 1 (1). In each of them, suppression of serum immunoreactive parathyroid hormone and urinary cyclic adenosine 3',5'-monophosphate characteristically occur.

Table 1. Diseases Associated with Elevated Serum 1,25-Dihydroxyvitamin D and Hypercalcemia

A. Granulomatous diseases
   1. Sarcoidosis
   2. Tuberculosis
   3. Leprosy
   4. Silicone-induced
B. Lymphoma and Solid Tumors
   1. Hodgkins disease
   2. Non-Hodgkins lymphoma
      a. Histiocytic
      b. Mixed histiocytic-lymphocytic
      c. T-cell
      d. B-cell
   3. Plasma cell granuloma
   4. Leiomyoblastoma
   5. Seminoma
C. Miscellaneous causes
   1. Idiopathic
   2. Hypercalcemia of infancy

The group of granulomatous diseases include sarcoidosis, tuberculosis, disseminated candidiasis, leprosy, silicone-induced granulomas and rheumatoid arthritis. Hypercalcemia was also reported to occur in patients with disseminated coccidioidomycosis, tuberculosis and leprosy in whom serum 1,25-dihydroxyvitamin D was suppressed. It is evident, therefore, that abnormal calcium metabolism is not always caused by abnormal vitamin D metabolism in these disorders.

The group of lymphoma, leukemia and solid tumors include Hodgkin's disease, T-cell leukemia-lymphoma, B-cell lymphoma, histiocytic lymphoma, plasma cell granuloma, and the solid tumors leiomyoblastoma and seminoma. Other patients with hypercalcemia and T-cell leukemia were found to have suppressed serum 1,25-dihydroxyvitamin D so that abnormal vitamin D metabolism in them was not responsible for the abnormal calcium metabolism.

Three patients were reported with hypercalcemia caused by increased serum 1,25-dihydroxyvitamin D in whom there was no apparent associated disease. All of them were males. The site of production and mechanism for abnormal vitamin D metabolism in these individuals is not known.

Four infants with elfin facies were described in whom hypercalcemia was associated with increased circulating 1,25-dihydroxyvitamin D (2). However, another child was described in whom hypercalcemia was associated with a low serum 1,25-dihydroxyvitamin D. Thus, the mechanism for hypercalcemia in this disorder may be multifactorial. The hypercalcemia is often associated with the Williams syndrome which is characterized by an elfin facies, supravalvular aortic stenosis and mental retardation.

In all of the diseases except tuberculosis, hypercalcemia is life threatening and aggressive treatment is required. Each of the diseases characteristically responds to treatment with glucocorticoids which lower both the serum 1,25-dihydroxyvitamin D as well as the serum calcium. In infants with hypercalcemia, the abnormal calcium metabolism may be particularly severe and rapidly lead to renal insufficiency. However, the hypercalcemia is self limited and usually occurs within the first two years of life. In contrast to the clinical course in the other diseases which may be protracted, hypercalcemia in tuberculosis is transient, not life threatening and may be treated by forcing fluids.

Abnormal vitamin D metabolism in sarcoidosis

a. In vitro metabolism

Sarcoidosis is a disease of activated T lymphocytes which begins as an alveolitis and an accumulation of lymphocytes within the alveolar intestinum and along the alveolar surfaces. There is an enhanced rate of proliferation of T lymphocytes because of the enhanced production of interleukin 2, a lymphocyte growth factor, and antigen-driven macrophage stimulation (3,4). Other factors are produced that also are important in the development and maintenance of the inflammatory response including macrophage chemotactic factor, leukocyte inhibitory factor, γ-interferon but not interleukin 1 (5). The macrophages in granulomas are derived from peripheral monocytes. Monocyte chemotactic factor from activated T lymphocytes attracts the monocytes and leukocyte inhibitory factor prevents neutrophil accumulation at the site of inflammation.

1,25-Dihydroxyvitamin D was produced by cultured alveolar macrophages from patients with sarcoidosis and hypercalcemia. The structure of the metabolite was confirmed by mass spectral analysis (6). Production of the metabolite was enhanced in a dose-response fashion by γ-interferon and interleukin 2 (7,8). Conversely, 1,25-dihydroxyvitamin D_3 was shown to inhibit proliferation and to suppress γ-interferon synthesis and interleukin 2 activity by phytohemaglutinin-stimulated human peripheral monocytes (9,10). If receptors are present for

1,25-dihydroxyvitamin D in activated pulmonary T lymphocytes and if 1,25-dihydroxyvitamin D acts in a similar manner on activated T lymphocytes in granulomas to inhibit proliferation and the production of interleukin 2 and γ-interferon, production of 1,25-dihydroxyvitamin D by alveolar macrophages could provide a means to inhibit inflammation (11). It is evident that the compensatory production of 1,25-dihydroxyvitamin D by the granulomatous tissue is responsible for the abnormal calcium metabolism in sarcoidosis.

Kinetic analysis of the synthesis of 1,25-dihydroxyvitamin D_3 by pulmonary alveolar macrophages from patients with sarcoidosis demonstrated a Km that ranged from 52 to 210 nM, a range similar to values from homogenenates of mouse kidney, cultured mouse renal cells, rat renal cortical cells and partially purified 25-hydroxyvitamin D-1α-hydroxylase from rat kidney (7). In addition, the production of 1,25-dihydroxyvitamin D by alveolar macrophages varied with the extent of disease determined clinically. Thus, little conversion of ^{3}H-25-hydroxyvitamin D_3 to ^{3}H-1,25-dihydroxyvitamin D_3 occurred in patients with stage I disease (hilar adenopathy alone) whereas considerably more conversion occurred in patients with more extensive disease, stage II or III (pulmonary infiltrates) as determined from radiographs (11).

The production of 1,25-dihydroxyvitamin D_3 by pulmonary alveolar macrophages from patients with sarcoidosis was inhibited in a stepwise fashion only modestly and at high concentrations by 1,25-dihydroxyvitamin D_3, and production was not influenced by parathyroid hormone in alveolar macrophages from normal subjects (8). On the other hand, production was inhibited by dexamethasone and by chloroquine, both of which are known to be effective clinically in correcting the abnormal vitamin D and calcium metabolism in sarcoidosis. These findings taken together indicate that the control of synthesis of 1,25-dihydroxyvitamin D in sarcoid granuloma is regulated in a fashion that is different from that in the kidney.

b. In vivo metabolism

Recent studies show that whereas the production rate of 1,25-dihydroxyvitamin D is abnormally increased, the metabolic clearance rate is normal in patients with sarcoidosis (12). As shown in Table 2, of five patients studied, three had hypercalcemia and two had a normal serum calcium. Other studies show that increases in serum 1,25-dihydroxyvitamin D occur in normocalcemic patients with sarcoidosis. In one study, three groups of individuals were evaluated, those with hypercalcemia alone, those with hypercalcemia and hypercalciuria and those with hypercalciuria alone. The range of values for serum 1,25-dihydroxyvitamin D were similar in the three groups and the mean value was abnormally elevated (13). These and other studies indicate that abnormal vitamin D metabolism occurs in normocalcemic patients.

Table 2. Metabolic Clearance and Production Rates of 1,25(OH)$_2$D in Sarcoidosis

Patient	Serum Ca mg/dl	Serum 1,25(OH)$_2$D pg/ml	Metabolic clearance rate ml/min	Production rate pg/day
A	11.3	114	53	8,700
B	11.8	99	42	6,000
C	11.4	50	44	3,200
D	9.4	77	31	3,460
E	9.3	99	31	4,460
Patients (5)		88 + 12	40 + 5	5,166 + 1,104
Normals (13)		42 + 2	37 + 2	2,250 + 144
P value		<0.001	NS	<0.001

Modified from Insogna KL et al (12).

We found abnormal regulation of serum 1,25-dihydroxyvitamin D in patients with sarcoidosis who had no history of hypercalcemia. Thus, in response to vitamin D, 100,000 units a day for four days, mean serum 1,25-dihydroxyvitamin D increased by threefold in a group of six patients with sarcoidosis and a normal serum calcium and did not change in a group of normal subjects (14). These findings indicate the potential for nonrenal production of 1,25-dihydroxyvitamin D in the patients.

Table 3. Effects of vitamin D, 100,000 units/day for 4 days, in normal subjects and patients with sarcoidosis

Treatment	Serum Ca mg/dl	Serum P mg/dl	Serum Creatinine mg/dl	Serum 25-OHD ng/ml	Serum 1,25(OH)$_2$D pg/ml
Normals (17)					
Control	9.5 ± 0.1	4.1 ± 0.1	0.9 ± 0.1	30 ± 4	32 ± 3
Vitamin D	9.6 ± 0.1	4.1 ± 0.1	1.0 ± 0.1	99 ± 15	29 ± 3
P value	NS	NS	NS	<0.001	NS
Patients (6)					
Control	9.4 ± 0.2	3.9 ± 0.3	1.0 ± 0.1	19 ± 3	40 ± 7
Vitamin D	9.8 ± 0.2	4.2 ± 0.3	1.0 ± 0.1	65 ± 19	120 ± 24[+]
P value	<0.01	<0.01	NS	<0.05	NS

Serum 25-OHD was determined in 12 normals before vitamin D and 9 normals after vitamin D.
[+]P <0.001 vs. normals.
Adapted from Stern PH et al (14).

More recently, we conducted studies to determine whether nonrenal production of 1,25-dihydroxyvitamin D occurs in patients with sarcoidosis who are normocalcemic and did not have a history of abnormal calcium metabolism (15). Under normal circumstances, circulating 1,25-dihydroxyvitamin D regulates the intestinal absorption of calcium and varies inversely with calcium intake. To evaluate the relationship between serum 1,25-dihydroxyvitamin D and dietary calcium, we compared the response of serum 1,25-dihydroxyvitamin D to increases in calcium intake from 400 to 1,000 mg per day in a group of six normocalcemic patients with biopsy-confirmed, active sarcoidosis and in 14 age-matched normals (15). We found that whereas an increase in calcium intake significantly lowered mean serum 1,25-dihydroxyvitamin D from 34 ± 1 to 20 ± 1 pg/ml (P <0.001) in the 14 normal subjects, it did not change mean serum 1,25-dihydroxyvitamin D in the six patients (41 ± 5 vs. 39 ± 5 pg/ml, N.S.). Further, one of the patients developed hypercalcemia as a result of increased serum 1,25-dihydroxyvitamin D in the course of a summer. These results provide evidence that extrarenal synthesis of 1,25-dihydroxyvitamin D frequently occurs in normocalcemic patients with active sarcoidosis and that these patients are at risk for developing hypercalcemia and its consequences.

In summary, abnormal calcium metabolism results from increased circulating 1,25-dihydroxyvitamin D in a number of diseases. In sarcoidosis, a number of laboratories have shown that this occurs because of synthesis of the metabolite in granulomatous tissue which appears to be a compensatory mechanism to reverse inflammation. The abnormal calcium metabolism apparently occurs because nonrenal synthesis of 1,25-dihydroxyvitamin D is not regulated by normal physiologic mechanisms.

References

1. Bell, N.H. Sarcoidosis and related diseases in Metabolic Bone Disease. 2nd edition. (Avioli, L.V., and Krane, S.M., eds.) W. B. Saunders Company, Philadelphia. In press.

2. Garabedian, M., Jacqz, E., Guillozo, H., Grimberg, R., Guillot, M., Gagnadoux, M.F., Broyer, M., Lenoir, G., Balsan, S. (1985) Elevated plasma 1,25-dihydroxyvitamin D concentrations in infants with hypercalcemia and an elfin facies. N. Engl. J. Med. 312:948-952

3. Pinkston, P., Bitterman, P.B., Crystal, R.G. (1983) Spontaneous release of interleukin 2 by lung T-lymphocytes in active pulmonary sarcoidosis. N. Engl. J. Med. 308:793-800

4. Venet, A., Hance, A.J., Saltini, C., Robinson, B.W.S., Crystal, R.G. (1985) Enhanced alveolar macrophage-mediated antigen-induced T lymphocyte proliferation in sarcoidosis. J. Clin. Invest. 75:293-301, 1985

5. Robinson, B.W.S., McLemore, T.L., Crystal, R.G. (1985) Gamma interferon is spontaneously released by alveolar macrophages and lung T lymphocytes in patients with pulmonary sarcoidosis. J. Clin. Invest. 72:1488-1495

6. Adams, J.S., Singer, F.R., Gacad, M.A. (1985) Isolation and structural identification of 1,25-dihydroxyvitamin D_3 produced by cultured alveolar macrophages in sarcoidosis. J. Clin. Endocrinol. Metab. 60:960-966

7. Adams, J.S., Gacad, M.A. (1985) Characterization of 1α-hydroxylation of vitamin D_3 sterols by cultured alveolar macrophages from patients with sarcoidosis. J. Exp. Med. 161:755-765

8. Reichel, H., Koeffler, H.P., Barbers, R., Norman, A.W. (1987) Regulation of 1,25-dihydroxyvitamin D_3 production by cultured alveolar macrophages from normal human donors and from patients with pulmonary sarcoidosis. J. Clin. Endocrinol. Metab. 65:1201-1209

9. Tsoukas, C.D., Provvedini, D.M., Monalagas, S.C. (1984) 1,25-Dihydroxyvitamin D_3: a novel immunoregulatory hormone. Science 224:1438-1440

10. Reichel, H., Koeffler, H.P., Tobler, A., Norman, A.W. (1987) 1α,25-Dihydroxyvitamin D_3 inhibits γ-interferon synthesis by normal human peripheral blood lymphocytes. Proc. Natl. Acad. Sci. USA 84:3385-3389

11. Adams, J.S., Gacad, M.A., Singer, F.R., Sharma, O.P. (1986) Production of 1,25-dihydroxyvitamin D_3 by pulmonary alveolar macrophages from patients with sarcoidosis. Ann. N. Y. Acad. Sci. 465:585-594

12. Insogna, K.L., Dreyer, B.E., Mitnick, M., Ellison, A.F., Broadus, A.E. (1988) Enhanced production rate of 1,25-dihydroxyvitamin D in sarcoidosis. J. Clin. Endocrinol. Metab. 66:72-75

13. Meyrier, A., Valeyre, D., Bouillon, R., Paillard, F., Battesti, J-P., Georges, R. (1985) Resorptive versus absorptive hypercalciuria in sarcoidosis: correlations with 25-hydroxyvitamin D_3 and 1,25-dihydroxyvitamin D_3 and parameters of disease activity. Quart. J. Med. 215:269-281

14. Stern, P.H., De Olazabal, J.D., Bell, N.H. (1980) Evidence for abnormal regulation of circulating 1α,25-dihydroxyvitamin D in patients with sarcoidosis and normal calcium metabolism. J. Clin. Invest. 66:852-855

15. Basile, J.N., Liel, Y., Miller, S., Shary, J., Bell, N.H. (1988) Evidence for extrarenal production of 1,25-dihydroxyvitamin D in patients with active sarcoidosis and normal calcium metabolism. J. Bone Min. Res. In press (abstract)

The Effects of Race and Body Habitus on the Vitamin D Endocrine System

S. EPSTEIN and N.H. BELL

Albert Einstein Medical Center
Temple University School of Medicine
Philadelphia, PA
and VA Medical Center and Medical University of South Carolina
Charleston, SC

It is now established that black subjects have advanced skeletal development in childhood, increased bone mass in adulthood and a decreased incidence of osteoporosis and fractures of the hip with increasing age compared to white subjects [1]. To establish whether these skeletal changes could be attributed to alterations in vitamin D metabolism, we studied 12 black subjects, 7 men and 5 women, and 14 white subjects, 8 men and 6 women, aged 20-35 years [2]. On a daily diet of 400 mg calcium, 900 mg phosphorus, and 110 meq sodium we found that serum immunoreactive parathyroid hormone (iPTH) (350±34 vs 225±26 pg/ml, p<0.01) and 1,25 dihydroxyvitamin D (1,25(OH)$_2$D) (41±3 vs 29±2 pg/ml p<0.01) were significantly higher and serum 25 dihydroxyvitamin D (25(OH)$_2$D) was significantly lower in blacks than in whites (Table I).

Table 1: <u>Serum Values in Normal Black and White Subjects</u>

Subjects	Serum calcium	Serum Ca^{2+}	Serum phosphate	Serum magnesium	Serum iPTH*	Serum 25-OHD	Serum 1,25(OH)$_2$D
	mg/dl	mg/dl	mg/dl	meq/liter	pg/ml	ng/ml	pg/ml
Black (12)	9.0±0.1	4.9±0.1	3.9±0.1	1.80±0.03	350±34	6±1	41±3
White (14)	9.0±0.1	4.8±0.1	3.9±0.2	1.85±0.04	225±26	20±2	29±2
P value	NS	NS	NS	NS	<0.01	<0.001	<0.01

Results are given as mean±SE. Figures in parentheses are the number of subjects. * Serum immunoreactive PTH (iPTH) was measured in 9 blacks and 11 whites.

Urinary calcium (101±14 vs 166±13 mg/d, p<0.01), urinary phosphate (688±44 vs 938±37 mg/day, p<0.001), urinary potassium and magnesium were lower and urinary cAMP was higher (3.11±0.47 vs 1.84±0.25 nM/dl glomerular filtrate, p<0.01) in the blacks than in the whites (Table 2).

Table 2: <u>Urinary Values in Normal Black and White Subjects</u>

Subjects	Urinary calcium	Urinary phosphate	Urinary sodium	Urinary potassium	Urinary magnesium	Urinary cAMP	Creatinine clearance
	mg/d	mg/d	meq/d	meq/d	meq/d	nM/dl GF	liter/d
Black (12)	101±14	688±44	124±8	40±2	7.2±0.6	3.11±0.47	170±9
White (14)	166±13	938±37	124±8	62±4	9.2±0.4	1.84±0.25	173±6
P value	<0.01	<0.001	NS	<0.001	<0.02	<0.01	NS

Results are given as mean±SE of the average urinary values of the first 2 d of the study. Figures in parentheses are the number of subjects.

An IV calcium load (15 mg/kg body weight) when given to black subjects was excreted as efficiently as the whites, serum bone gla protein (BGP) was lower in the blacks than the whites. (14±2 vs 24±3 ng/ml p<0.02) and increased significantly in both groups after 1,25(OH)$_2$D$_3$ administration, 4 ug per day for 4 days. However, blacks excreted less calcium after 1,25(OH)$_2$D and serum calcium did not change. Generally in both groups no difference was observed in serum total and ionized calcium and phosphate (Table 3).

Table 3: **Effects of 1,25(OH)$_2$D$_3$ on Serum Calcium, Serum Phosphate, and Serum Bone Gla Protein in Normal Black and White Subjects**

Subjects	Serum calcium Control	1,25(OH)$_2$D$_3$	Serum phosphate Control	1,25(OH)$_2$D$_3$	Serum Gla protein Control	1,25(OH)$_2$D$_3$
	mg/dl	mg/dl	mg/dl	mg/dl	ng/ml	ng/ml
Black (12)	9.1±0.1	9.4±0.1*	3.8±0.2	4.2±0.1‡	14±2	22±3§
White (14)	9.0±0.1	9.0±0.1	3.7±0.2	4.3±0.2§	24±3	32±3‡
P value	NS	NS	NS	NS	<0.02	<0.05

Results are given as mean±SE of values obtained before and after 1,25(OH)$_2$D$_3$, 4 μg/d. Figures in parentheses are the number of subjects.
* NS vs. mean control value. ‡ P < 0.02 vs. mean control value. § P < 0.001 vs. mean control value.

This study provides evidence that in normal young black adult subjects a state of secondary hyperparathyroidism exists as shown by increases in serum iPTH, urinary CAMP and serum 1,25(OH)$_2$D. Serum BGP was lower but rose appropriately after exogenous 1,25(OH)$_2$D$_3$, showing that the osteoblast respond normally.

We feel that the lower serum 25(OH)D is probably a result of diminished dermal synthesis of vitamin D known to occur in black subjects. Unanswered questions still remain to be elucidated as regards the reduction in urinary phosphate, potassium and magnesium in black as compared to white subjects. Explanations for the increased bone density with the altered response of the skeleton to PTH, i.e., decreased serum bone gla protein and the presumed enhanced intestinal absorption of calcium and tubular calcium reabsorption because of the increased 1,25(OH)$_2$D production may all be associated with increased muscle mass and strain on the skeleton in some manner producing these changes.

Because of these findings of increased serum iPTH in blacks as compared to whites and similar elevations of serum iPTH in obese subjects, the vitamin D-endocrine system was studied in 12 obese subjects to see if a state of secondary hyperparathyroidsm exists [3]. The 12 obese subjects had a mean weight of 106±6 kg vs 68±2 kg in nonobese subjects on a daily diet of 400 mg calcium and 900 mg of phosphorus. It was observed that mean serum iPTH (518±48 vs 243±33 pg/ml, p<.001), 1,25(OH)$_2$D (37±2 vs 24±2 ng/ml, p<0.01) and serum BGP (33±2 vs 24±3 ng/ml, p<0.02) were significantly higher but serum 25(OH)$_2$D (8±1 vs 20±2 ng/ml, p<0.001) was significantly lower in the obese than in the nonobese men and women (Table 4).

Table 4: **Serum Values in Obese and Nonobese White Subjects**

Subjects	Serum calcium	Serum Ca^{2+}	Serum phosphorus	Serum magnesium	Serum Gla protein*	Serum iPTH‡	Serum 25-OHD	Serum 1,25(OH)$_2$D
	mg/dl	mg/dl	mg/dl	meq/liter	ng/ml	pg/ml	ng/ml	pg/ml
Obese (12)	9.0±0.1	4.8±0.1	4.0±0.1	1.88±0.02	33±2	518±48	8±1	37±2
Nonobese (14)	9.0±0.1	4.8±0.1	3.9±0.2	1.85±0.04	24±3	243±33	20±2	29±2
P value	NS	NS	NS	NS	<0.02	<0.001	<0.001	<0.01

Results are given as mean±SE. Figures in parentheses are the number of subjects. * Serum Gla protein was measured in 11 obese and 14 nonobese subjects. ‡ Serum immunoreactive PTH (iPTH) was measured in 12 obese and 13 nonobese subjects.

Urinary cyclic AMP and creatinine clearance were significantly higher in the obese than in nonobese individuals. Urinary calcium was significantly lower in the obese than in nonobese subjects (115±10 vs 166±13 mg/d, p<0.01) (Table 5).

Table 5: Urinary Values in Obese and Nonobese White Subjects

Subjects	Urinary calcium	Urinary phosphorus	Urinary sodium	Urinary potassium	Urinary magnesium	Urinary cyclic AMP	Creatinine clearance
	mg/d	mg/d	meq/d	meq/d	meq/d	nM/dl GF	liter/d
Obese (12)	115±10	1,043±50	104±8	62±3	9.3±0.9	3.18±0.43	216±17
Nonobese (14)	166±13	938±37	124±8	62±4	9.2±0.4	1.84±0.25	173±6
P value	<0.01	NS	NS	NS	NS	<0.01	<0.01

Results are given as mean±SE of the average of two consecutive 24-h urine values in each subject. Figures in parentheses are the number of subjects.

These biochemical abnormalities resemble the changes observed in nonobese black subjects, i.e., secondary hyperparathyroidism. As in black subjects, the increase in serum iPTH and 1,25(OH)$_2$D and enhanced tubular reabsorption of calcium in obesity be related to body mass and strain on the skeleton. However, we feel, that a vitamin D deficiency is a more likely etiology in obese white subjects since the observed changes are reversed by 25(OH)D$_3$ administration. These changes are peculiar to obesity since after weight reduction serum iPTH values decrease [4] and serum 25(OH)$_2$D values increase to the normal range. In our study, serum BGP was increased in the obese subjects which was different from the lowered serum BGP values in black subjects and may reflect the effect of increased circulating 1,25(OH)$_2$D values in the obese subjects. The important influence of excess weight stimulating bone formation similar to the condition of increased muscle mass in body builders where both serum BGP and bone density are increased [5] may override the vitamin D deficiency. The next question posed by these observations is whether obesity in black subjects produces alterations in the vitamin D-endocrine system that are over and above the changes present in nonobese black subjects. We studied 10 obese black subjects (3 men and 7 women) and compared them to 12 nonobese black subjects (7 men and 5 women) and the same dietary protocol as described previously was followed [6]. The results showed that except for a higher mean serum bone gla level in obese black subjects there was no significant alteration in any of the biochemical measurements of the vitamin D-endocrine system produced by obesity per se in black subjects (Tables 6 and 7).

Table 6: Serum Values in Obese and Nonobese Black Subjects

Subjects	Serum calcium (mg/dl)	Serum Ca²⁺ (mg/dl)	Serum phosphorus (mg/dl)	Serum magnesium (meq/l)	Serum Gla protein (ng/ml)	Serum iPTH[a] (pg/ml)	Serum iPTH[b] (pg/ml)	Serum 25 OHD (ng/ml)	Serum 1,25-(OH)$_2$D (pg/ml)
Obese (10)	8.8 ± 0.1	4.8 ± 0.1	4.1 ± 0.2	1.82 ± 0.04	23 ± 4	379 ± 23	357 ± 26	5 ± 1	43 ± 3
Nonobese (12)	9.0 ± 0.1	4.9 ± 0.1	3.9 ± 0.1	1.80 ± 0.03	14 ± 2	312 ± 26	392 ± 27	6 ± 1	41 ± 3
p value	NS	NS	NS	NS	<.05	NS	NS	NS	NS

Results are given as mean ± SE. Figures in parentheses are the number of individuals. NS, not significant.
[a]Serum immunoreactive PTH (iPTH, "midmolecule" assay) was measured in 9 obese and 11 nonobese subjects.
[b]Serum immunoreactive PTH (iPTH, "carboxy-terminal" assay) was measured in 10 obese and 11 nonobese subjects.

It thus appears that in black subjects in contrast to white subjects obesity does not influence the vitamin D-endocrine system but that obesity itself

Table 7: **Urinary Values in Obese and Nonobese Black Subjects**

Subjects	Urinary calcium (mg/d)	Urinary phosphorus (mg/d)	Urinary sodium (meq/d)	Urinary potassium (meq/d)	Urinary magnesium (meq/d)	Urinary cAMP[a] (nmols/dl GF)	Urinary clearance (l/d)
Obese (10)	105 ± 13	755 ± 63	115 ± 14	39 ± 3	7.5 ± 0.8	3.12 ± 0.24	194 ± 16
Nonobese (12)	101 ± 14	688 ± 44	124 ± 8	40 ± 2	7.2 ± 0.6	3.11 ± 0.47	170 ± 9
p value	NS	NS	NS	NS	NS	NS	NS

Results are given as mean ± SE of the average of two consecutive 24-h urine values in each subject. Figures in parentheses are the number of individuals. NS, not significant.
[a]Urinary cyclic AMP was measured in 8 obese and in 12 nonobese subjects.

increases the serum values of BGP. The cause of low serum 25(OH)D values in obesity may have important clinical implications as bone biopsies of obese patients have revealed evidence of secondary hyperparathyroidism and mild osteomalacia. The low serum 25(OH)D values are not due to impaired dermal production of precursors but may be related to impaired metabolic clearance and enhanced uptake of vitamin D by adipose tissue as has been demonstrated in rats and in vivo human studies.

Because racial differences exist in adults as regards regulation of the vitamin D-endocrine system the issue was raised whether similar differences exist in children. Accordingly, 27 white children, 23 white adults, 14 black children and 25 black adults were studied on a metabolic ward on a daily diet consisting of 400 mg calcium, 900 mg phosphate, 18 meq of magnesium, 110 meq sodium and 65 meq potassium [7]. Our findings revealed that black children differed from white children in that serum 25(OH)D was significantly lower in black vs white children (15±1 vs 10±1 pg/ml p<0.02) and urinary phosphate (558±34 vs 679±21 mg/d, p<0.001) potassium (34±2 vs 49±2 meq/d, p<0.001) and urinary cAMP (1.69±0.16 vs 2.22±0.16 nM/dl/GF, p<0.05) were significantly lower in the black than in the white children.

Compared to adults, children of both races had significantly higher serum total and ionized calcium, phosphate, bone gla protein, somatomedin C and iPTH, and significantly lower urinary calcium and phosphate. Serum 1,25(OH)$_2$D was higher in the white children than in white adults (41±2 vs 29±2 ng/ml, p<0.001) but values for black children did not differ from those for black adults.

When calcium was increased to 1600 mg/day, failure to suppress serum 1,25(OH)$_2$D occurred in some but not all the children. Balance studies on 2 of the children showed that children on a higher calcium intake of 1000 mg/day failed to suppress serum 1,25(OH)$_2$D and had enhanced intestinal absorption and retention of calcium [8]. This finding in black children of a higher set point for 1,25(OH)$_2$D suppression may have the beneficial effect of allowing enhanced intestinal absorption and retention of calcium and possibly lead to increased bone mass during adulthood.

Geography and nutrition also appear to play a part in the vitamin D status of different racial groups. In the United Kingdom the British Asian population have the lowest values for serum 25(OH)D concentrations when compared to white and West Indian children [9]. The West Indian children have lower serum 25(OH)$_2$D values than the white children. Diets rich in unleavened bread and ultraviolet deprivation have been cited as etiological factors but this is not conclusively established as Asian children on a western diet and with the same sunlight exposure still have lower values for serum 25(OH)D than their white counterparts. However, Asian adults in Pakistan have significantly higher values for serum 25(OH)D than Asian adults in the U.K. (74 vs 18 nmol/l, p<0.001) despite similar dietary and cultural habits. In the Kashmir region of India severe osteomalacia has been described despite high sun exposure as well as in Iran and in the rural Bantu areas in South Africa. So although skin pigmentation appears to be correlated with diminished dermal production of 25(OH)D from a given dose of irradiation, it does not appear to be the sole explanation for the low serum 25(OH)D values in Asians. West Indian immigrants with darker skin do not suffer clinical vitamin D deficiency despite the same environment as the Asians in the U.K. [10]

In conclusion, the regulation of the vitamin D endocrine system appears to be different in different racial groups as well as being influenced by obesity. These differences may be protective in counteracting osteoporosis in black subjects and in obese individuals. Evidence for this protective effect is seen in the increased bone mineral density studies of the radius, hip and spine in premenopausal black and obese women as well as the decreased incidence of symptomatic osteoporosis in such individuals [11].

REFERENCES

1. Cohn SH, Abesamis C, Yasamura S, Aloia JF, Zanzi I, and Ellis, KJ 1977 Comparative skeletal mass and radial bone mineral content in black and white women. Metab. Clin. Exp. 26:171-178.

2. Bell NH, Greene A, Epstein S, Oexmann MJ, Shaw S, and Shary J 1985 Evidence for alteration of the vitamin D endocrine system in Blacks. J. Clin. Invest. 76:470-473.

3. Bell NH, Epstein S, Greene A, Shary J, Oexmann MJ, and Shaw S 1985 Evidence for alteration of the vitamin D endocrine system in obese subjects. J Clin Invest 76:370-373.

4. Atkinson RL, Dahms WT, Bray GA, and Schwartz AA 1978 Parathyroid hormone levels in obesity. Effects of intestinal bypass surgery. Miner. Electrolyte Metab. 1:315-320.

5. Bell NH, Godsen RN, Henry DP, and Epstein S. The effects of body building on vitamin D and mineral metabolism. Bone and Mineral Res. In Press.

6. Epstein S, Bell NH, Shary J, Shaw S, Greene A, Oexmann MJ 1986 Evidence that obesity does not influence the vitamin D endocrine system in Blacks. J. Bone Mineral Res. 1:181-184.

7. Epstein S, Liel Y, Bell NH, Oexmann MJ, Shary J, Greene V. Effects of race on the vitamin D endocrine system in children and adults. Submitted for publication.

8. Liel Y, Greene A, Shary J, Shaw S, Bell NH 1987 Demonstration that calcium intake does not regulate circulating 1-25 dihydroxyvitamin D in black children. J. Bone and Mineral Res. 2 Suppl 1, Abstract #396.

9. Ford JA, McIntosh WB, Butterfield R, Preece MA, Pietrek J, Arrowsmith WA, Arthurton MW, Turner W, O'Riordan JLH, and Dunnigan MG 1976 Clinical and subclinical vitamin D deficiency in Bradford children. Arch. Dis. Child 51:939-953.

10. Clemens TL, Adams A, Henderson SL, and Holick MF 1982 Increased skin pigment reduces the capacity of the skin to synthesize vitamin D. Lancet 1:74-76.

11. Liel Y, Edwards J, Shary J, Spicer KM, Gordon L, Bell NH. The effects of race and body habitus on bone mineral density of the radius, hip and spine in premenopausal women. J. Clin. Endo. Metab. In press.

Discussion:

DR. LANG (New Haven): Sol, I really enjoyed your presentation. I would like to know who is abnormal and who is normal. White women get osteoporosis and black women do not. So, maybe the abnormality is in the white people and not in the blacks. It may be in the genes, but it may not be. Therefore, I wonder about other things that might increase bone resorption and whether white women have bone loss from smoking, caffeine or other factors, that might alter circulating parathyroid hormone or 1,25-dihydroxyvitamin D. What are your thoughts about that?

DR. EPSTEIN (Philadelphia): We cannot determine who is normal and who is abnormal. For example, the decadence of white society and the luxury of their living may be abnormal. We can argue that.

This question obviously has cropped up as whether the black population that we studied in Charleston is unique? They appear to be a population of stable, well settled black subjects, as were the white subjects.

I take your point that perhaps adaptively the blacks may have fared much better than the whites so that they may be normal and we may be abnormal.

DR. LANG: Could I ask one more question, please? Marc, your presentation leaves a lot of room for speculation. I want to ask whether the problem in some of these conditions is not related to the tubular reabsorption of phosphorus, but to the transport of phosphorus out of the renal tubular cell so that the intracellular concentration of phosphate may actually be high. This may not be the case in hypophosphatemic rickets with hypercalciuria. In that disease a low intracellular concentration of phosphate seems likely.

DR. DREZNER (Raleigh-Durham, NC): We have measured the intracellular concentration of phosphate, as have others, in the hyp-mouse, and now more recently in the gy-mouse, and the values are not elevated. We have also measured the intracellular ATP concentrations. On the mean they are low. If you believe that phosphate is necessary for the synthesis of high energy phosphate bands, our findings suggest that, on the mean, there is a low prevailing cellular phosphate concentration.

DR. LANG: Well, the intracellular concentration of phosphate is not elevated, but the values are not low either. It may be that the intracellular phosphate concentration can only increase to a certain level.

DR. DREZNER: The other aspect is that, in the in vitro studies of the renal tubule, marked increases in phosphate concentration on the serosal side do not influence mitochondrial function. The influence of phosphate on mitochondrial function is totally a function of changing the phosphate concentration in the bathing medium that faces the brush border. Therefore, I would be surprised if increasing the phosphate concentration on the serosal side would make a difference, regardless of the rate of egress.

DR. LIBERMAN (Israel): I have two questions for Dr. Epstein and a comment for Dr. Drezner, if I may. The questions are, in both black and obese white subjects, you have elevated serum levels of 1,25-dihydroxyvitamin D. What is the intestinal calcium absorption in those subjects? And second, what happens in the black subjects when you infuse calcium, as far as parathyroid hormone is concerned?

DR. EPSTEIN: As regards your first question, we assume that there may be enhanced intestinal calcium absorption, but this has not been determined. Studies will be done to answer this question. The effects of calcium infusion on serum immunoreactive parathyroid hormone have not been determined in blacks.

DR. LIBERMAN: A comment. You may know, Marc, that we are going to present, in New Orleans, studies in a family that has the Fanconi Syndrome and hereditary hypophosphatemic rickets. Serum phosphate is low, serum 1,25-dihydroxyvitamin D is elevated, and hypercalciuria is present. These findings fit very nicely with those in your gy-mice. In the hereditary hypophosphatemic rickets, we do not know where the defect is. In the family to be presented it must reside in the proximal tubule, because of the features of the Fanconi Syndrome.

DR. GLORIEUX (Montreal): Marc, I very much enjoyed your presentation and am fascinated by your use of the gy-mouse model. You did not give us the serum values for 1,25-dihydroxyvitamin D in those mice for comparison with hereditary hypophosphatemic rickets. Are the values elevated, compared to normal, or compared to those of the hyp-mouse?

DR. DREZNER: We do not know yet. We have not had the opportunity to collect enough blood from the existing mice to perform the measurements.

DR. GLORIEUX: My second question concerning the gy-mice is with regard to their inheritance. The gy gene, if I remember correctly, is very close to the hyp gene on the murine X chromosome. The mode of inheritance of hereditary hypophosphatemic rickets on the other hand, is probably a little broader, with the disorder in some families reported as being autosomal dominant. Do you see any conflict in these observations?

DR. DREZNER: I do not think that the gy-mouse is a model for the human disease in the sense that it fits all the criteria. It simply has the same biochemical abnormalities. It seems to me, however, that as little as we know about the control of phosphate transport, it is quite conceivable that there are multiple enzyme systems that interplay at the brush border, regulating phosphate transport. And one of those enzyme systems or proteins might be controlled by an X-linked dominant gene, whereas another contributing factor could be contributed by an autosomal factor.

DR. OGATA (Tokyo): I would like to ask a question to Dr. Drezner. You indicated that the abnormal 25-hydroxyvitamin D-1-alpha hydroxylase function in the mitochondria might be due to phosphate depletion. How do you explain this with specificity? I think that the abnormality, rather, results from defective 25-hydroxyvitamin D-1-alpha hydroxylase. There are many reactions that require NADPH in mitochondria. For example, 25-hydroxyvitamin D-24-hydroxylase. What is the evidence for a specific abnormality in 25-hydroxyvitamin D-1-alpha hydroxylase reaction in the hyp-mouse?

DR. DREZNER: I do not think that we have examined mitochondrial function as well as we might. The kind of abnormalities I anticipate might be evident in the mitochondria of the hyp-mouse would be abnormalities in calcium or phosphate transport or the transport of malate, succinate, and the like, which are defects that have been reported in response to phosphate deficiency in in vitro systems.

I am not exactly certain how those defects would manifest themselves in the in vivo circumstance. I believe, however, that the changes in phosphate and calcium transport that are known to occur in response to the phosphate deficiency could well have an influence on 25-hydroxyvitamin D-1-hydroxylase. So, it is a matter of extrapolation from the in vitro circumstance.

DR. OGATA: Have you measured the 25-hydroxyvitamin D-24-hydroxylation reactions?
DR. DREZNER: In the hyp-mouse, we have, yes, and it, too, shows a defect.
DR. OGATA: A defect?
DR. DREZNER: A defect in regulation.
DR. PETTIFOR (South Africa): Sol, you presented some intriguing results. I have a couple of comments and a question. In South Africa, in children, certainly, skeletal development is not increased in blacks and is about one and a half years behind that of white children. This is confirmed by studies of bone density as measured by metacarpal indices and of bone mineral density as measured by single-photon absorptiometry. So, I think diet does have a major role. This may relate to your findings in your black adults. Two days on a constant low calcium diet may be insufficient to correct for different calcium intakes prior to that time. Is it possible that the results in your subjects is a reflection of long-term changes in calcium intake?
DR. EPSTEIN: As I mentioned at the outset, this was obviously a concern whether these people were chronically deprived of adequate intake of calories, nutrients or vitamin D. From their dietary histories and life styles, this did not appear to be the case. Our black children and adolescents in America tend to have higher body mass and thicker skeletons compared to their white counterparts. So, we do not think that chronic nutritional vitamin D deficiency accounts for the findings in our black subjects. In the obese white subjects, vitamin D depletion may be important.
DR. PETTIFOR: I am not concerned about vitamin D deficiency. A lower calcium intake is all that is needed to increase the serum 1,25-dihydroxyvitamin D.
DR. EPSTEIN: As far as we could gather, there appeared to be no difference in the intakes of calcium between the two groups. However, this was not systematically evaluated.
DR. BELL: We performed a small number of studies in black adult subjects. If you maintain them for two weeks on a low calcium diet, 400 mg per day, serum 1,25-dihydroxyvitamin D values remain elevated. If you administer a higher calcium intake, 1,000 mg per day, serum 1,25-dihydroxyvitamin D declines. Therefore, I am not convinced that our black subjects have calcium deficiency. The changes in their vitamin D-endocrine system we felt may be caused by deficiency of 25-hydroxyvitamin D, which I think has a metabolic role in modestly regulating calcium absorption.
DR. BOUILLON (Belgium): Well, first of all, I would like to congratulate you for drawing the attention of everyone on the aspects of calcium and vitamin D metabolism that have not been looked at before: obesity, race and muscle strength. However, the data you have in your blacks differ totally from the data we obtained in blacks in Africa. I think that is mainly due to the difference in 25-hydroxyvitamin D levels.
The main conclusion of your observations in blacks is that you have a major problem of vitamin D deficiency. I see levels of 5 and 6 nanograms per milliliters of 25-hydroxyvitamin D. Those values are extremely low. They are even lower than the mean levels in our country. That is the first comment.
In Africa, we see that the population has 25-hydroxyvitamin D levels between 30 and 40 nanograms per milliliter, a low calcium intake, and a low calcium excretion. But instead of increasing the production of 1,25-dihydroxyvitamin D, they maintain 1,25-dihydroxyvitamin D levels as in Caucasians on a higher calcium intake. They "prefer", instead, a lower serum calcium, even when

corrected for serum protein concentrations.

This is a situation that resembles observations in the hypertensive rat model, and, as you know, hypertension is very frequent in blacks. So, it might have something to do with the transport of calcium across the cell membrane, and represent a link between hypertension and disturbances in vitamin D metabolism.

DR. EPSTEIN: It may also appear that, for example, the autoregulation of serum 25-hydroxyvitamin D, 1,25-dihydroxyvitamin D and calcium absorption may be set differently depending upon the nutritional status and the environment. What really surprised us is, with the low serum 25-hydroxyvitamin D in the group of blacks that we studied, that they may be truly deficient in 25-hydroxyvitamin D because administration of 25-hydroxyvitamin D3 lowered the serum 1,25-dihydroxyvitamin D and increased the urinary calcium.

The differences in your findings and my findings points to the difference that environment, geography, and diet may play. It's also interesting that the West Indians in Britain, when compared to Asian counterparts, tend to have higher serum 25-hydroxyvitamin D despite the fact that they were exposed to the same degree of sunlight. The Asians, even when they were exposed to the same standardized diet, still had lower serum 25-hydroxyvitamin D values. The West Indians, despite their increased skin pigmentation, do not suffer from clinical vitamin D deficiency.

DR. ZIEGLER (Heidelberg): Dr. Epstein, could you exclude an inference of different caloric intake in your results comparing normal weight and overweight people? As you gave the same amount of calcium and phosphorus, did you also give the same amount of calories? The amount of 400 milligrams of calcium will be, presumably sufficient for a normal weight person to stay in balance. But for overweight people, this intake may not be sufficient and could cause a negative calcium balance.

DR. EPSTEIN: Yes. The duration of the study was too short for this possibility. As was evident in the presentation, there were positive correlations between urinary cyclic AMP and serum immunoreactive parathyroid hormone and body weight. So, in obese subjects the changes appear to be related to body weight.

As I mentioned in my presentation, weight loss does correct the elevated serum immunoreactive parathyroid hormone in obese subjects. I don't think that an intake of 400 milligrams per day of calcium in an obese subject over such a short period of time would produce a negative calcium balance. I do not think it would be a factor.

DR. ZIEGLER: With respect to your last table: were the black normal and overweight people also on a standardized diet like the white ones?

DR. EPSTEIN: Yes, they were. These studies were conducted on a metabolic ward so that the intakes of calcium, phosphorus, sodium, potassium and magnesium were rigorously controlled.

DR. WOODHOUSE (Saudi Arabia): Dr. Epstein, this is a follow-on to Dr. Bouillon's question to you. I, too, was very impressed by how low the serum 25-hydroxyvitamin D values were in your group. They are about the same as they are in subjects in Saudi Arabia, extremely low. What I wanted to know is did you give the obese subjects physiologic doses of 25-hydroxyvitamin D3 and what did that do to any of the parameters you measured?

DR. EPSTEIN: I did not perform that study. Dr. Bell, perhaps, could answer, because he was the one who gave the 25-hydroxyvitamin D3 and observed the return of values to normality after administration. I will defer that question to the Chairman, who administered the 25-hydroxyvitamin D3 to the obese subjects.

DR. BELL (Charleston): The dose varied from 40 to 100 micrograms per day of 25-hydroxyvitamin D3. It was administered for a week before subjects were admitted for a second study. Subjects were tested individually. The end point was the dose required to increase both the serum 25-hydroxyvitamin D and the urinary calcium. In these studies, the serum 25-hydroxyvitamin D values remained within the normal range in each subject. The doses used were clearly pharmacologic, therefore it is possible that there may be increased metabolic clearance of 25-hydroxyvitamin D in obese subjects. This possibility has not been examined.

DR. KRANE (Boston): I would just like to make a couple of comments. One is that we are all looking for reasonable markers of bone formation. I think that to take it for granted that measurements of bone gla protein in serum is the gold standard for measuring osteoblastic function is not critically looking at the issue.

After all, bone gla protein was found in EGTA extracts of the mineral phase of bone. So, it is obviously in the mineral phase and is destroyed by proteases. It is produced by osteoblasts and incorporated into matrix. And it is cleared in organs in a manner we do not fully understand.

Since we know nothing about any of these rate constants, to assume that a given manipulation, or differences in two populations, between the circulating levels of bone gla protein at any one time are indices of bone formation, in view of the other reservations we have to have is, I would say, at the least, overstating the issue.

DR. EPSTEIN: I would tend to disagree on some of the aspects, because most of the studies that we've done with bone gla, we have compared to dynamic indices of bone histomorphometry and found (as others have) a very good correlation with bone formation.

DR. KRANE: Do you have measurements of any of those rate constants?

DR. EPSTEIN: No, we don't, but as stated, in the rat model, we compared bone formation determined histomorphometrically with serum gla protein and found a very good correlation. Given the state of the art today, and the limitations of alkaline phosphatase and other markers of bone metabolism, measurement of serum gla protein appears in our hands to be the best one available at the present time. As mentioned previously, we found that there is a very good correlation between serum gla protein and osteoblast number, bone formation, and bone accretion on bone histomorphometry.

DR. KRANE: There are data suggesting correlations. But since all these other rate constants are totally unknown, any manipulation you make that will alter these other factors will alter your steady-state levels. We know that there are ways in which serum gla protein does not correlate and that there are other markers that correlate differently. So, I am just saying that it could be that a fat person metabolizes more or less BGP than a skinny person. And you do not have any data for that.

DR. EPSTEIN: No. We accept your point that we do not have any correlation between serum gla protein and bone histomorphometry in obese subjects. But, at the present state of the art, serum gla protein is the best marker that we have of bone formation.

DR. KRANE: It is only one marker, and you should not be using it too literally. That is my only point.

The other question, for Dr. Liel, was that in the study from Dr. Reikel in which interleukin 2 was used to increase the 25-hydroxylation 1-hydroxylation, was recombinant interleukin 2 used or some commercial soup that was called interleukin 2, since there are other factors such as GMCSF, interleukin 4, and interleukin 5 that would also be present in those preparations?

DR. LIEL (Israel): It was the human recombinant interleuken 2.

DR. BELL: Steve, to answer the question about the gla protein, the only instance where we can be certain that gla protein is a marker of bone formation is in the nonobese black subjects who have a low serum gla protein. Dr. Weinstein found, by histomorphometric analysis, that normal adult blacks have a low bone turnover. One might argue that bone resorption is reduced as well.

DR. KRANE: There is no point in arguing about this, but there are exceptions. And the most striking one to me, in my experience, is what we have seen in Paget's disease. When we look at other markers such as the carboxy terminal peptide of type 1 procollagen, which is hard to measure because the assays are not readily available and we have trouble getting antigen, the correlations are excellent with the level of circulating 1,25-dihydroxyvitamin D. We do not have metabolic clearance data for this peptide, I grant you. In response to treatment, the values initially are elevated and then decline. And this is not what is seen with serum gla protein. Therefore, I want everybody to be aware that maybe what you are measuring is not what you think you are measuring.

DR. EPSTEIN: This is going to become a to-and-fro see-saw. And I do not think it's really worthwhile pursuing to the nth degree. There are instances where measurement of serum bone gla protein is useful, and where it is not useful. Paget's disease is a clear example of where measurement of serum gla protein is not a useful index of bone formation.

In the experimental rat after oophorectomy we found that with measurement of bone formation, bone resorption, and bone turnover by histomorphometric methods, there is very good correlation with serum bone gla protein. But I will accept the fact that looking at any parameter of bone remodeling, one measurement does not appear to make the case.

X
Clinical Disorders of Bone and Mineral Metabolism

Overview:
Miscellaneous Disorders of Calcium and Bone Metabolism

GREGORY R. MUNDY

Division of Endocrinology and Metabolism
University of Texas Health Science Center
San Antonio, TX

During this section of the meeting, a miscellaneous group of disorders affecting calcium homeostasis and bone metabolism were reviewed by investigators with special experience with these particular disorders. The session began with a discussion of the pathophysiology of hypercalcemia by Dr. John Kanis. Dr. Kanis discussed the distribution of calcium in normal plasma, the importance of binding to plasma proteins and the effects that this has on interpretation of measurements of total plasma calcium. He then discussed the transport of calcium between the extracellular fluid and the gut, bone and the kidney. He stressed the importance of the kidney and in particular renal tubular calcium reabsorption in calcium homeostasis. He then reviewed how careful determination of urine calcium excretion may give insights into calcium fluxes from the skeleton and calcium absorption from the gut.

One of the commonest causes of hypercalcemia is malignant disease. Dr. Kanis indicated that hypercalcemia occurs in malignant disease in a number of different settings. Professor T.J. Martin then described a newly described factor associated with one of these settings, namely the humoral hypercalcemia of malignancy. In this syndrome, a solid tumor produces a humoral factor which alone or in concert with other factors stimulates osteoclastic bone resorption, enhances renal tubular calcium reabsorption and increases urinary cyclic AMP. Dr. Martin described a biological activity from one of these tumors which stimulated adenylate cyclase activity in bone cells and in renal membranes, whose effects were blocked by synthetic antagonists to PTH and which was not affected by antisera to PTH. He described the purification and molecular cloning of this factor and then the biological effects of synthetic fragments. This factor, which was referred to as the PTH-related protein, has considerable homology to authentic parathyroid hormone in the N-terminal region since 8 of the first 13 amino acids are identical. It binds to the PTH receptor and activates it. It stimulates bone resorption and renal tubular calcium reabsorption and increases plasma calcium in vivo. Immunoreactive PTH-rP was found in a variety of tumors, some of which are associated with hypercalcemia and some of which are not.

Dr. Mundy then described factors which are implicated in the hypercalcemia associated with hematologic malignancies. In myeloma, hypercalcemia occurs as a consequence of increased bone resorption usually associated with decreased glomerular filtration. In this malignancy, the tumor cells produce a cytokine (lymphotoxin) which stimulates osteoclastic bone resorption in vitro and in vivo and increases plasma calcium in vivo. In some lymphomas associated with hypercalcemia, there is increased production of 1,25 dihydroxyvitamin D. This has been found in association with adult T-cell lymphomas, with B-cell lymphomas and in occasional cases with Hodgkin's disease. It seems likely in these circumstances that the neoplastic lymphoid cells have developed the capacity to synthesize 1,25 dihydroxyvitamin D.

Dr. Olav Bijvoet then gave an update of Paget's disease of bone. This bone disorder is characterized by a primary abnormality in the osteoclast which is accompanied by morphologic abnormalities which include increased multinucleation, increased functional capacity and the presence of intranuclear inclusion bodies. These intranuclear inclusion bodies seem likely to be due to a slow virus which is probably the primary cause of this disorder. Paget's disease which is associated with pain or deformity can be treated with calcitonin or with one of the drugs of the bisphosphonate family. Dr. Bijvoet stressed the utility of the newer bisphosphonates, particularly the amino bisphosphonates, which are more potent than the first generation agents, produce fewer side effects and may lead to better and more prolonged therapeutic responses.

Dr. Charles Pak discussed the current status of pathophysiology, diagnosis and medical management of renal calculi. He reviewed the history of the pathophysiologic approach to diagnosis and treatment of recurrent renal calculi. He then discussed the three major mechanisms thought responsible for hypercalciuria, namely absorptive hypercalciuria, resorptive hypercalciuria and renal leak hypercalciuria. He then discussed other less common mechanisms for hypercalciuria including the primary renal phosphate leak group, the group associated with primary enhancement of 1,25 D production and the group with combined renal tubular disturbances which lead to hypercalciuria. He then reviewed the role of hypocitrituria which is present in 70-80% of patients with recurrent renal calculi and hypercalciuria. Hypocitraturia has multiple causes, is easily diagnosed and readily corrected by potassium citrate, an effective drug which reduces stone formation in these patients. Finally, he discussed the utility of medical prevention of recurrent renal calculi with the use of thiazides and potassium citrate. He suggested that despite the recent striking advances in the surgical approach to recurrent renal stones, medical therapy had a useful place in prevention of further development of stones, reduction of the need for further surgery and as a cost-effective form of therapy. However, he stressed that medical therapy did not cure the underlying defect responsible for this disorder and still required diagnostic evaluation for careful choice of therapy.

Recent concepts of the pathophysiology of renal bone disease were discussed by Dr. Brendan Boyce. Renal bone disease is comprised of three main pathologic entities, osteitis fibrosa (secondary hyperparathyroidism), osteomalacia responsive to vitamin D metabolites and aluminum bone disease. Dr. Boyce concentrated on aluminum bone disease. He showed that aluminum is an important pathophysiologic agent in bone disease associated with chronic renal disease, and is responsible for a syndrome characterized by resistance to therapy with 1,25 dihydroxyvitamin D, a relative decrease in serum immunoreactive PTH, a relative decrease in alkaline phosphatase and the bone biopsy picture of osteomalacia. There are several variants to the bone biopsy picture. These include pure osteomalacia with low mineralization rates, thick osteoid seams and no evidence of osteitis fibrosa, a mixed picture of osteomalacia and osteitis fibrosa and an aplastic or adynamic biopsy appearance associated with low bone turnover. He pointed out that patients who are particularly at risk for aluminum intoxication were those who were hyperabsorbers of aluminum, those who used dialysis water in which aluminum was not removed by treatment of water with reverse osmosis or deionization, and those who ingest large amounts of aluminum binders. He then reviewed the difficulties in diagnosis of aluminum bone disease without a bone biopsy.

This can be made with the desferrioxamine test followed by measurement of the serum aluminum response, although this test is not uniformly reliable. He then indicated the potential problems of patients with aluminum bone disease who were subjected to parathyroidectomy. He concluded by indicating that hypercalcemia in a patient with chronic renal disease should not be treated by parathyroidectomy unless aluminum bone disease has been carefully excluded, that aluminum toxicity is still an important cause of renal bone disease and that the role of parathyroidectomy in exacerbating aluminum bone disease in a patient with underlying increased aluminum content in bone remains unclear.

The session concluded with a review of the multiple endocrine neoplasia Type 2a syndrome by Dr. Robert Gagel. This syndrome comprises medullary thyroid carcinoma, pheochromocytoma and parathyroid hyperplasia. It was first described by Sipple in 1961. Dr. Gagel showed how this syndrome has gone through three phases beginning with the clinical description in the the 1960s, followed by the use of calcitonin measurement in the diagnosis and screening of asymptomatic patients in the 1970s, and then by recent advances in understanding the abnormalities in gene function which lead to the molecular derangements in patients with this syndrome. He pointed out that the thyroid disease almost always occurs first and that the adrenal disease is a particularly difficult problem because it is frequently diffuse and bilateral. However, the adrenal tumors are rarely malignant, are almost always intra-adrenal and usually secrete epinephrine. His preference is that a patient with evidence for disease in only one adrenal should undergo unilateral adrenalectomy initially. Thyroidectomy should be performed on individuals with abnormalities in calcitonin secretion at the earliest feasible time. Recently, the gene responsible for this disorder has been mapped to chromosome 10 at a point near the centromere. It appears most likely that oncogenesis in this disorder is due to a deletion of a regulatory gene similar to that which has been described in patients with retinoblastoma. In MEN 2a, this deletional mutation is present near the centromere of chromosome 10. It is hoped that these studies will lead soon to the ability to diagnose this disease at birth which may lead to changes in the therapeutic approach (particularly with respect to timing of thyroidectomy) and an improvement in the overall prognosis. At the present time, in patients who are screened and diagnosed as having underlying thyroid disease before the onset of symptoms, about 90% are disease-free at 5 years if they are subjected to total thyroidectomy.

Pathophysiology of Hypercalcaemia

JOHN A. KANIS, EUGENE McCLOSKEY, NEVEEN HAMDY,
DECLAN O'DOHERTY, and DEREK BICKERSTAFF

Department of Human Metabolism and Clinical Biochemistry
University of Sheffield Medical School
Sheffield, UK

Serum calcium homeostasis is effected by the exchange of calcium to and from the extracellular fluid (ECF) and the factors which modulate this. Since disorders of calcium homeostasis alter these normal processes it is appropriate to consider hypercalcaemia in terms of the way in which these are disturbed.

Serum calcium

Calcium is widely distributed throughout living tissue, but the intracellular concentration is comparatively low and in the adult comprises 1% or less of total body calcium. Extracellular calcium accounts for a further 1% of total body calcium and the remaining 98% is found in bone. The concentration of plasma calcium in health is maintained within a narrow range despite large movements of calcium across gut, bone, kidney and cells. Several hormones, including parathyroid hormone (PTH) and calcitriol regulate the ionised fraction of plasma calcium (approximately 50% of total plasma calcium) by modulating calcium fluxes to and from the extracellular fluid. In turn the secretion rate of these hormones is regulated by the calcium concentration in the ECF.

Changes in the concentration of serum calcium are usually accompanied by changes in the total amount of calcium in the ECF since there is a passive distribution of ionised calcium throughout this compartment. Within the plasma compartment, however, 40% of calcium is bound to proteins, mainly albumin, and the binding is pH dependent. Major changes in plasma protein concentration, the presence of abnormal proteins and large shifts in extracellular pH may, therefore, affect the proportion of total plasma calcium that is bound. A further 5-10% of total plasma calcium is bound to small anions such as citrate, phosphate and bicarbonate, and the extent of binding may vary as the concentration of these anions change. For these reasons the estimation of total plasma calcium may not accurately reflect the ionised calcium concentration which is the fraction of biological relevance.

Changes in the binding of calcium in plasma have some important clinical consequences. Thus, the paresthesiae found in patients with hyperventilation syndrome are due to a decrease in ionised calcium concentration because of alkalosis; but the total plasma calcium is normal. In the absence of severe acidosis or alkalosis, the major factor influencing the amount of calcium bound is the quantity of albumin present, since the proportion of calcium which is bound varies little. Failure to account for protein binding may result in the erroneous diagnosis of hypercalcaemia in conditions where there is an increased concentration of albumin (eg dehydration). Conversely, in hypoproteinaemic states such as disseminated carcinoma a normal total plasma calcium may mask hypercalcaemia of the ionised calcium. Rarely, hypercalcaemia may be due to the presence of an abnormal protein which binds serum calcium so that whereas total serum calcium is high the ionised fraction is normal. Such pseudohypercalcaemia has been reported in myeloma.

Since estimations of total serum calcium are at best an index of the ionised fraction, ionised plasma concentrations should ideally be measured. Several formulae have been proposed for predicting the ionised calcium from the total plasma calcium or 'correcting' the total plasma calcium to a normal protein value (1), but none are entirely satisfactory and are more appropriate for the study of populations rather than individuals (1,2).

A small proportion of total plasma calcium is complexed with anions such as phosphate, citrate and bicarbonate. The calcium which is normally filtered by the kidney includes this complexed calcium as well as ionised calcium and can be measured by passing plasma through membrane filters which retain the protein bound calcium. The measurement of ultrafiltrable or dialysable calcium may be of value in assessing hypercalcaemia.

Sites of calcium exchange

The major movements (fluxes) of calcium to and from the extracellular fluid occur across bone, gut and kidney (Fig 1).

Calcium enters the body by intestinal absorption. The true absorption of calcium is greater than the net absorption because some calcium is returned to the gut lumen in biliary, pancreatic and intestinal secretions. Thus, from an average daily dietary intake of 25mM (1g), approximately 10mM are absorbed. This is offset by intestinal secretions amounting to 5mM daily leaving a net transport into the ECF of 5mM. Intestinal absorption of calcium is regulated by a variety of factors including the extracellular concentration of calcitriol, and hypercalcaemia may arise because of increased production of calcitriol, for example in sarcoidosis and adult onset T-cell lymphoma.

The kidney is a major site for calcium excretion from the body. A large

Major sites of action of PTH, calcitonin & vitamin D

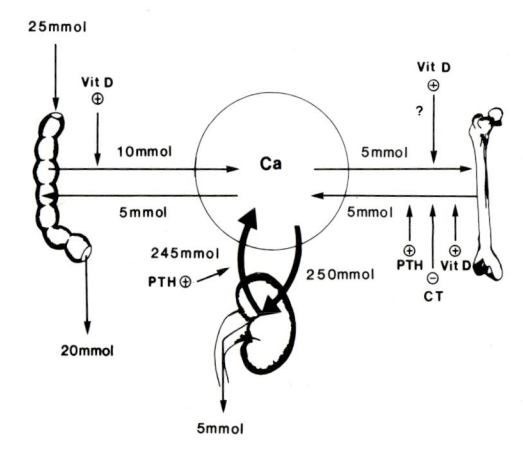

Figure 1.
Major fluxes of calcium (mmol/day) in healthy adults. Exchange of calcium to and from the extracellular fluid occurs across bone, gut and kidney. The net balance for calcium equals the net absorption minus the losses of calcium in faeces and urine which in the healthy adult is zero. The fluxes of calcium are regulated by the major calcium regulating hormones. PTH increases renal tubular reabsorption of calcium and bone resorption. Calcitonin inhibits bone resorption and vitamin D augments intestinal absorption of calcium. In addition, vitamin D stimulates bone resorption and the mineralisation of bone.

amount of calcium is filtered (Fig 1) but most of this is re-absorbed so that only 1-3% is excreted into urine. These large fluxes to and from the ECF mean that small changes in renal tubular reabsorption may have profound effects on the ECF concentration of calcium. Since reabsorption is under hormonal control, principally by PTH, this has led to the view that the kidney is a major organ in the regulation of serum calcium.

In the mature adult who is neither gaining nor losing calcium, bone and soft tissues contribute neither a net gain nor loss of calcium from the extracellular fluid. Thus, the amount of bone resorbed (approximately 5mM daily) matches the amount formed. This turnover of calcium needs to be distinguished from the more rapid and much larger exchange of calcium which occurs within bone and soft tissues. Studies with radioisotopes have shown that in normal human adults the exchangeable pool of calcium is approximately 1-2% of total body calcium, in the region of 2mM/Kg during the first few days after injection. This represents approximately 125mM, which is a substantial amount considering that the ECF contains somewhat less than 20mM as ionised calcium. This exchangeable pool of calcium is, therefore, very important in plasma calcium homeostasis, and movements of calcium between body fluid cells and surfaces of bone occur continuously. These exchanges of calcium between ECF and bone are independent of bone resorption or formation and there is some evidence that they are under endocrine control and therefore contribute to serum calcium homeostasis (3).

Calcium balance is a function of these integrated fluxes across bone, gut and kidney. The concentration of calcium in the ECF is set by the relative size of the various fluxes, in turn under the influence of controlling agents including several hormones. These hormones can be divided into the major calcium regulating hormones and the influencing hormones. The major calcium regulating hormones include PTH, calcitonin and calcitriol, the production of each of which is altered in response to changes in the plasma ionised calcium concentration. The influencing hormones are those other hormones such as thyroid hormones, growth hormone and adrenal and gonadal steroids which have effects on calcium transport, but the production of which is determined primarily by factors other than changes in plasma calcium.

Set point and error correction
It is useful to draw a distinction between the way in which plasma calcium is set at a particular concentration, and the way in which movements of calcium in and out of the ECF are controlled. The plasma calcium level is set close to a particular value in different individuals in normal and diseased states. Deviations from this value are corrected by hormone induced changes in the relative fluxes of calcium in and out of the extracellular fluid compartments. Alterations in flux rates are therefore monitored and adjusted by changes in plasma calcium which are induced. This homeostatic system can operate with the plasma calcium set at any number of different values, with the relative rates of entry and exit of calcium to and from the extracellular fluid being altered as drift occurs from this set point. Thus, in hypo or hyperparathyroidism fluxes of calcium across the gut and in and out of bone may not be greatly different from normal, and external calcium balance can be maintained even though the plasma calcium is set at a markedly abnormal level. The plasma calcium thus provides the point around which adjustments or error correction are made (4). The major mechanisms which determine the set point include the renal threshold for tubular reabsorption of calcium and the exchange of calcium with the extracellular fluid across the quiescent surfaces of bone (3,5).

With respect to the ECF concentration of ionised calcium, a steady state denotes that the rate of entry (influx) of calcium into the ECF pool equals its rate of exit. At this point serum calcium will be at a value determined by the set point. In practice, man is probably never in a steady state since, for example, feeding and hence the calcium influx from gut is erratic and moreover, involves a variety of homeostatic responses which may take many hours to be complete. Nevertheless, the maintenance of plasma calcium within narrow limits in health and many hypercalcaemic states implies that the integrated fluxes approximate steady state conditions, particularly when fasting.

When considering the mechanisms by which hypercalcaemia is maintained in various disorders the steady state is often more relevant than the transient state. In contrast, a consideration of steady states is commonly less relevant to the treatment of hypercalcaemic disorders, since the responses to treatment must be judged by the ability to induce transient changes in pre-existing steady states.

In man, the most important regulator of acute changes in the concentration of calcium is parathyroid hormone, the secretion of which increases within seconds of a fall in plasma calcium and decreases as the ionised concentration of calcium rises. The rapid control of plasma calcium by PTH is mainly due to its ability to regulate renal tubular reabsorption of calcium and possibly by its effects on calcium exchange between ECF and bone. After parathyroidectomy the fall in plasma calcium can be largely accounted for by a continued loss of calcium into urine, until a new steady state is achieved in which calcium excretion is the same as its starting value, but takes place at a much reduced filtered load of calcium.

A further example of a disruption of the steady state is seen during an infusion of calcium. During a calcium infusion, plasma calcium concentration will begin to rise. If the rate of calcium infusion is constant, levels of plasma calcium will not rise indefinately but only until the rate of efflux of calcium from the ECF (to bone, kidney, gut and other tissues) matches the rate of influx. At this point plasma calcium levels will not rise further despite continuing the infusion and a new steady state prevails. In practice the infusion of calcium will result in the suppression of secretion of PTH and a decrease in renal tubular reabsorption of calcium. This will tend to increase the rate at which a new steady state is achieved. It is notable that the rise in plasma calcium during a calcium infusion is to some extent buffered by the exchange of calcium in bone. The response to prolonged perturbations brings in contributions from changes in vitamin D metabolism and from intestine and bone turnover. An example analogous to calcium infusion is the adaptation that occurs with a change in the dietary intake of calcium. If intake is increased this will induce a small increase in serum calcium and therefore decrease the secretion of PTH. Apart from its effects on renal tubular reabsorption of calcium, a sustained decrease in PTH will decrease osteoclastic resorption of bone and decrease the synthesis of calcitriol. This in turn will reduce intestinal absorption of calcium and resorption of calcium from bone. If the increase in dietary calcium continues these homeostatic changes will act to restore plasma calcium towards its previous value and bone formation rate will decrease to match the rate of decreased bone resorption. The new steady state will consist of a decreased efficiency of intestinal absorption of calcium and a decreased rate of entry and removal of calcium from bone so that net balance can be maintained.

Pathophysiological investigation of hypercalcaemia
The kidney is a major site for calcium losses and provided that plasma calcium is steady, the urinary loss of calcium reflects the net fluxes across bone and gut. The estimation of urinary calcium excretion provides, therefore, an index of these movemements. If bone turnover is normal then the 24 hour urinary excretion of calcium reflects the net intestinal absorption of calcium.

When the urinary excretion of calcium is measured in the post-absorptive state (after fasting), the losses reflect to a greater extent the net skeletal efflux of calcium to the ECF (5,6). Thus, high values of calcium excretion under fasting conditions is due to increased calcium release from bone, depressed calcium entry into bone or both. Concurrent measurement of urinary hydroxyproline excretion may help resolve these possibilities.

Renal tubular reabsorption of calcium in the kidney is a complex process and takes place at several different sites in the nephron. The total amount of calcium reabsorbed can, however, be estimated by subtracting the filtered load of calcium from the renal excretion. The filterable calcium is approximately 60% of total plasma calcium and the filtered load represents the product of the glomerular filtration rate and the filtrable calcium (approximately 250mM daily).

In health there is a curvilinear relationship between plasma calcium concentration (an index of filtered load, assuming no change in GFR) and the renal excretion of calcium (Figs 2 and 3), so that renal tubular reabsorption cannot be assessed simply from the calcium clearance. To take account of variations in glomerular filtration rate, the renal excretion is commonly expressed as a fraction of glomerular filtration rate (Fig 2). Any value below the lines depicting the normal relationship indicates an increase in net renal tubular reabsorption of calcium, and values above and to the left denote decreased net reabsorption. Any value for renal excretion above normal, but within the normal range for the relationship between plasma and urine calcium would indicate an increase in filtered load (gut or bone derived) or a low glomerular filtration rate, but with normal renal tubular reabsorption of calcium. Furthermore, it is possible to use this normal relationship to quantitate the contribution of each of these mechanisms (impaired renal function, increased bone resorption and increased renal tubular reabsorption of calcium) to the increment in serum calcium observed in various hypercalcaemic states (7; Fig 3).

Thus, despite a number of limitations (4,6) the measurement of calcium excretion together with plasma calcium can help provide information about the mechanisms of hypercalcaemia under relatively steady state conditions.

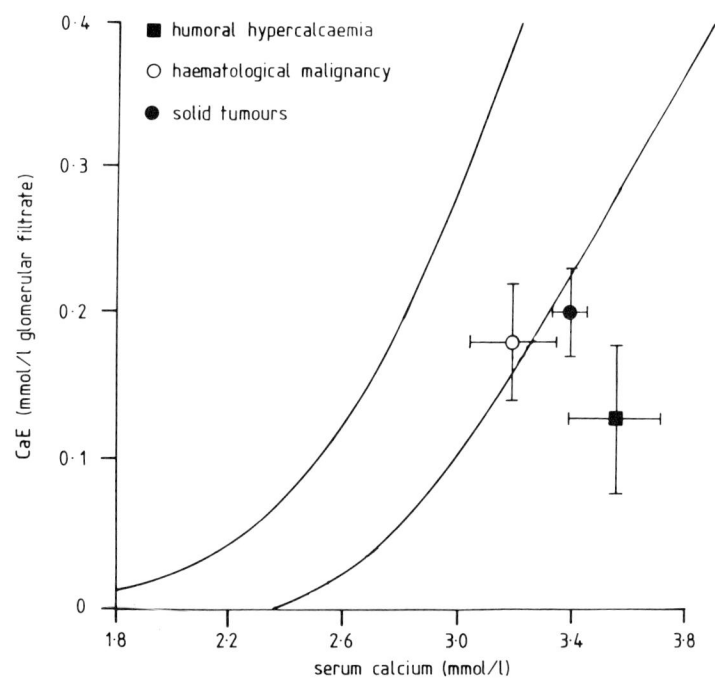

Figure 2.
Relationship between fasting urinary calcium excretion (CaE expressed per unit of glomerular filtrate) and plasma calcium. The solid lines denote the normal range of the relationship in healthy subjects. Symbols denote values found in patients with haematological malignancies or solid tumours with and without metastases. Note that most patients with myelomatosis lie within the reference range. In contrast, patients with humoral hypercalcaemia of malignancy lie to the right of the normal relationship indicating increased renal tubular reabsorption of calcium (mean ± SEM).

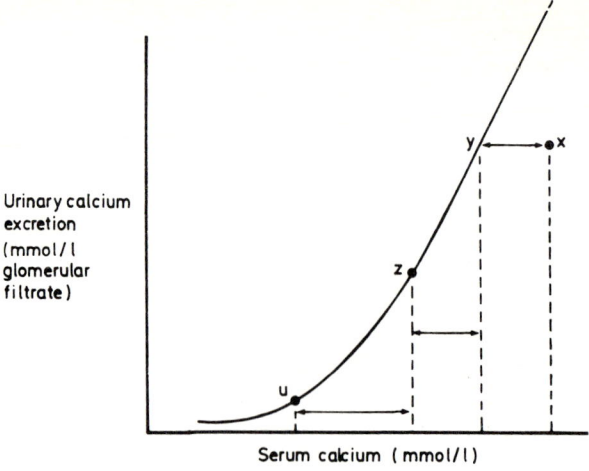

Figure 3.
Diagram to illustrate methods of analyzing the components of hypercalcaemia. Deviations of the plasma calcium from the curvilinear relationship found in normal subjects are attributable to changes in renal tubular reabsorption of calcium (increment = x-y mmol/l). In patients with impaired renal glomerular function, excretion of calcium is recomputed using the mean plasma creatinine concentration in normal subjects (increment due to abnormal glomerular filtration = y-z mmol/l). Any residual increment in plasma calcium concentration is attributed to increased bone resorption (increment = z-u mmol/l).

This can be illustrated in primary hyperparathyroidism. 24 hour urinary excretion of calcium is commonly increased in primary hyperparathyroidism. In contrast, fasting urinary excretion of calcium is normal, particularly in patients with mild primary hyperparathyroidism. The disparity between the non-fasting and fasting calcium excretion reflects the increase in calcitriol-mediated intestinal absorption of calcium. The normal fasting urinary excretion of calcium suggests that the net efflux of calcium from bone to the ECF is normal. Since the majority of patients with primary hyperparathyroidism have increased rates of bone resorption, this finding implies an increase in bone formation sufficient to match the increased bone resorption. This illustrates that when considering factors which give rise to hypercalcaemia the size of the uni-directional flux of calcium (eg bone resorption) is not necessarily important, but rather the difference between influx and efflux from the ECF under steady state conditions. The observation that fasting calcium excretion is normal in the majority of hyperparathyroid patients despite the increase in serum calcium (filtered load) indicates that a major mechanism for the maintenance of hypercalcaemia in this disorder is increased renal tubular reaborption of calcium.

An example of the complex interplay between primary pathology and calcium fluxes at other sites is seen in sarcoidosis. The underlying abnormality of calcium metabolism in this disorder is increased vitamin D-like activity related to excessive production of calcitriol. This increases intestinal absorption of calcium and net influx of calcium from gut to ECF. In addition, calcitriol increases bone resorption and abnormal skeletal fluxes also contribute to the hypercalcaemia. In contrast to primary hyperparathyroidism, hypercalcaemia will suppress the secretion of PTH which decreases renal tubular reabsorption of calcium. The decrease in renal tubular reabsorption of calcium is an important mechanism for ameliorating the hypercalcaemic challenge (6). However, sarcoidosis and many other causes of hypercalcaemia induce secondary changes in renal function. These include a decrease in glomerular filtration rate and increased renal tubular reabsorption of calcium due to extracellular volume depletion. In the case of sarcoidosis, hypercalcaemia is rarely found in the absence of renal impairment and the impairment in GFR decreases the ability to withstand a hypercalcaemic challenge.

The relative importance of disturbed calcium fluxes across bone, gut and kidney can be assessed in all hypercalcaemic states in terms of the influence of changes in:
- net intestinal absorption
- net calcium efflux from bone
- renal tubular reabsorption of calcium
- glomerular filtration rate

Such estimations can be made from simple urine and plasma determinations of calcium and creatinine (7,8).

Application to hypercalcaemia of malignancy

In assessing the mechanisms for hypercalcaemia in malignancy it is useful to distinguish the initiating events from those factors which contribute to the maintenance of hypercalcaemia. Hypercalcaemia has both structural and functional effects on the kidney, including impaired ability to conserve water and sodium. Resultant intravascular volume depletion as well as decreasing GFR, decreases sodium delivery to tubular sites and may be responsible for increased renal tubular reabsorption of calcium. Thus, when assessing the mechanisms for hypercalcaemia more accurate information of the primary disturbances will be gained after adequate rehydration and sodium repletion. Where assessment in malignant hypercalcaemia from various causes has been undertaken following volume expansion until a new steady state has been achieved, it has been shown that the mechanisms for the maintenance of hypercalcaemia are heterogeneous (6-8). The hypercalcaemia of myelomatosis is mainly attributable to an increase in bone resorption, though hypercalcaemia is significantly aggravated by the concurrent impairment of GFR (Table 1). Increased renal tubular reabsorption of calcium in rehydrated patients plays an insignificant role and the relationship between serum calcium and calcium excretion lies within the normal range (Fig 2; 8).

In contrast, in humoral hypercalcaemia of malignancy increased renal tubular reabsorption of calcium appears to be the predominant mechanism (Table 1). Thus, even after extracellular volume repletion serum calcium is higher than would be predicted from the normal relationship between serum calcium and calcium excretion (Fig 2), a situation analogous to that seen in primary hyperparathyroidism. Two mechanisms have been proposed for this marked stimulation of tubular reabsorption of calcium. It has been suggested that this is secondary to a stimulation of sodium reabsorption resulting from dehydration and contraction of the extracellular compartments. This mechanism appears unlikely, at least in our studies (8) since patients were rehydrated before such analysis and renal tubular reabsorption of sodium was not different from that in

	Total serum calcium (mmol/l)	Increment (%) attributable to		
		BR	GFR	RTR
Solid with mets. n=13	3.34	36	23	41
HHM n=4	3.56	28	7	65
Myeloma n=10	3.14	51	29	20

Table 1.
Mechanisms for the maintenance of hypercalcaemia in patients with malignant disease. Values shown are the contribution (expressed as a percentage) of each mechanism to the increment in serum calcium over a normal value of 2.3 mmol/l (BR, increased bone resorption; GFR, decreased GFR; RTR, increased renal tubular reabsorption).

myelomatosis where increased renal tubular reabsorption of calcium was not found. Indeed, increased renal tubular reabsorption of calcium has been clearly demonstrated in the Leydig cell tumour model of hypercalcaemia of malignancy, an effect which is completely dissociable from that of sodium. More recently it has been shown that several tumour types are capable of secreting a protein sharing many homologies with PTH (PTH related protein; PTHRP). The similarities in the pathophysiology between primary hyperparathyroidism and humoral hypercalcaemia of malignancy suggests that PTHRP may be of major aetiological significance.

In patients with skeletal metastases the mechanism of hypercalcaemia is usually presumed to be due to osteolytic bone destruction at the site of metastases. The most common tumour giving rise to this syndrome is carcinoma of the breast. In some patients with breast cancer both bone and kidney appear to contribute equally to the maintenance of hypercalcaemia (Table 1), and about a third of patients show increased renal tubular reabsorption of calcium in addition to increased bone resorption (7,8; Fig 2). It is of interest that the PTH related protein may also be expressed in carcinoma of the breast and thus humoral as well as focal factors are likely to be important in a significant minority of patients.

Therapeutic implications

Because hypercalcaemia due to malignancy is almost invariably multifactorial, it is not surprising that many treatments which affect fluxes at one site have beneficial effects, even if treatment does not influence the primary site responsible for the induction of hypercalcaemia. A good example is the beneficial effect of intravenous saline in most patients with hypercalcaemia due to malignancy. Such treatment decreases pre-renal uraemia and also decreases renal tubular reabsorption of calcium. The corollary is that in malignant hypercalcaemia the use of inhibitors of bone resorption alone (eg the diphosphonates and calcitonins) are unlikely to restore serum calcium to normal unless concurrent treatment with saline is given. However, even in patients following the restoration of intravascular volume depletion, the response to inhibitors of bone resorption is likely to be heterogeneous. Indeed, several studies indicate that the response to the diphosphonate, dichloromethylene diphosphonate (Cl_2MDP), varies according to the nature of the prevailing hypercalcaemic process. When increases in bone resorption appear to be the major mechanism, the response of plasma calcium to Cl_2MDP is complete. In contrast, when increased renal tubular reabsorption of calcium is marked, the response of plasma calcium is incomplete despite the normalisation of bone resorption (8). This incomplete reponse is similar to the incomplete response in serum calcium to clodronate observed both in patients with primary hyperparathyroidism and in animals bearing the Leydig cell tumour and presumably reflects the lack of effect of diphosphonate on renal transport of calcium. Since the effect of clodronate to inhibit tumour mediated bone resorption is nearly complete, the assessment of renal tubular reabsorption of calcium before treatment can predict the final serum calcium attained following treatment with clodronate (Fig 4).

Conclusions

The many causes of hypercalcaemia are each characterised by various abnormalities in the transport of calcium across gut, bone, kidney or a combination of these. It is now possible to assess the relative importance of these factors in the development and maintenance of hypercalcaemia in individual patients, and thereby help in diagnosis and in deciding the therapeutic priorities.

Acknowledgements

We are grateful to the Medical Research Council and the Yorkshire Cancer Research Campaign for the support of our work in hypercalcaemia.

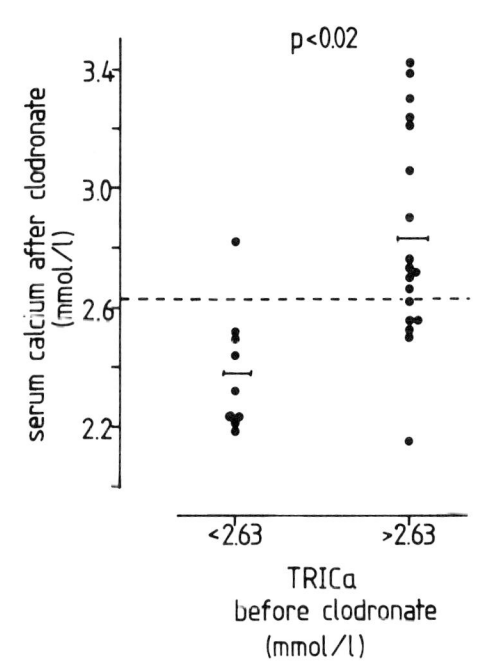

Figure 4.
The relationship between renal tubular reabsorption of calcium assessed before treatment and the serum calcium attained following treatment with the diphosphonate, clodronate. Note the incomplete response in serum calcium in those patients with preexisting increases in renal tubular reabsorption of calcium.

References

1. Kanis, J.A. and Yates, A.J.P. (1985) Br. Med. J. **290**, 728-729.
2. Kanis, J.A., Urwin, G.H., Gray, R.E.S., Beneton, M.N.C., McCloskey, E.V., Hamdy, N.A.T. and Murray, S.A. (1987) Am. J. Med. **82**, (suppl 2A) 55-70.
3. Parfitt, A.M. (1987) Bone **8**, (suppl 1) S1-S8.
4. Kanis, J.A., Paterson, A.D. and Russell, R.G.G. (1983) Scientific Foundations of Clinical Biochemistry, volume 2 (Ed: V Marks & DL Williams) Wm Heinemann, London. pp 299-325.
5. Nordin, B.E.C. (1976) Calcium, phosphate and magnesium metabolism. Churchill Livingstone, London & New York.
6. Kanis, J.A., Cundy, T., Heynen, G. and Russell, R.G.G. (1980) Metab. Bone Dis. Rel. Res. **2**, 151-159.
7. Percival, R.C., Yates, A.J.P., Gray, R.E.S., Galloway, J., Rodgers, K., Neil, F.E. and Kanis, J.A. (1985) Br. Med. J. **291**, 776-779.
8. Bonjour, J.P., Philippe, J., Guelpa, G., Bisetti, A., Rizzoli, R., Jung, A., Rosini, S. and Kanis, J.A. (1988) Bone **9**, in press.

Discussion:

DR. OGATA (Tokyo): I really enjoyed your presentation. I'd like to know, if you treat your patients with hypercalcemia of malignancy with diphosphonate so the cause of hypercalcemia depends only on renal factors, I'm wondering what acid base changes occurred. Because, if PTH or PTH-like substance is only the cause for hypercalcemia, I wonder if the acid base changes should be present?

DR. KANIS (England): I'm not trying to imply that all causes of hypercalcemia malignancy are related to abnormalities in renal tubular reabsorption of calcium. That's not true. In myelomatosis renal tubular reabsorption of calcium is classically low. In many patients with focal skeletal involvement and metastases, renal tubular reabsorption of calcium is normal or low.

In humoral hypercalcemia of malignancy, renal tubular absorption of calcium is usually, but not invariably, increased. But so, too, is bone resorption. This means that a component of the hypercalcemia in HHM will respond very adequately to the diphosphonates, irrespective of the diphosphonate that is used; that in those patients where there is a strong component of increased renal tubular reabsorption of calcium, serum calcium will not be restored to normal in the same way as we don't see a restoration to normal in the vast majority of patients with primary hyperparathyroidism.

So, what I'm saying is that the mechanism will influence the end result. But one can still use inhibitors of bone resorption in patients who have increased bone resorption.

DR. OGATA: My question concerned acid base changes. If only the renal factors remained and suppose PTH-like substance acts exactly the same as PTH metabolically...

DR. KANIS: That's a very good point. And, in fact, I don't know the answer to that. But that would be of interest to look at after long-term treatment.

DR. REEVE (England): John, you haven't said very much about the lining cell and the modulation of the calcemic response. Do you have any views on how it interacts with the kidney in maintaining hypercalcemia or, perhaps, regulating the calcium back to normal?

DR. KANIS: Yes, I purposely avoided entering into the subject of serum calcium homeostasis and the control of serum calcium in order to concentrate on hypercalcemia. Your question relates to whether the lining cells or the fluxes of calcium that occur from the skeleton, particularly from inert surfaces, to the extracellular fluid contribute to serum calcium homoeostasis. I'm sure they do. And they may also respond to changes in the endocrine environment.

Hypercalcemia—Solid Tumors

T.J. MARTIN

University of Melbourne
Department of Medicine
Repatriation General Hospital
Heidelberg, Victoria, Australia

Hypercalcemia is a very common complication of several cancers. Solid tumors give rise to hypercalcemia either in association with their growth as metastases in bone, i.e. metastatic hypercalcemia, or as part of the syndrome of humoral hypercalcemia of malignancy in which the tumor releases into the circulation a substance which acts generally upon the skeleton to promote bone resorption and upon the kidney to restrict calcium excretion.

HYPERCALCEMIA ASSOCIATED WITH METASTATIC BONE DISEASE

This is the most common cause of hypercalcemia in cancer and is found most frequently in patients with carcinoma of the breast, but also with renal cortical carcinoma and some other tumors. Breast cancer is very commonly associated with lytic metastases in bone. The hypercalcemia results from excessive mobilization of calcium from bone due to local tumor cell activity, and the released calcium eventually exceeds the capacity of the normal homeostatic mechanisms. The excessive resorption may be due either to direct effects of the tumor cells themselves or to the production of locally active promoters of bone resorption which act upon bone cells (reviewed in Martin and Mundy, 1987).

The concept that tumor cells can resorb bone directly has some experimental support, but it is by no means certain that this is the major mechanism by which breast cancers erode bone. Current views of mechanisms of cancer metastases are that, in order for tumor cells to grow in a distant organ, they need to have special properties which allow them to do this. In the case of metastases in bone, it would be expected that the tumors should be able to produce enzymes capable of degrading matrix, and this would include lysosomal enzymes, collagenase and neutral proteases. It may also include the property of transporting mineral, and the suggestion has been made that this could be related to the occurrence in the cancers of receptors for 1,25-dihydroxy Vitamin D_3. However there is no direct evidence to the present to support this. A further possible mechanism for resorption in relation to tumor deposits in bone is the capacity of tumors to produce factors capable of stimulating resorption by adjacent cells. An obvious candidate for this is the production of prostaglandins, which occurs commonly in breast and kidney cancers. However it is still not certain how important prostaglandins are for the establishment or progression of tumor deposits in bone. Local production of bone-resorbing cytokines could also be a contributory factor, produced either by the tumor cells, or possibly by lymphocytes or monocytes as a result of a cell-mediated response to the presence of tumor cells. Finally it has not generally been considered that breast cancers produce a parathyroid hormone-like substance, but there is some clinical evidence that this could be so, and furthermore such a protein has been purified recently from a breast cancer cell. This PTH-related protein will be discussed further in relation to humoral hypercalcemia of malignancy. It is possible that it could be a local bone resorbing factor in metastatic cancer in bone.

Understanding the mechanism of tumor-induced bone-resorption is an essential step in approaches to the prevention and treatment of metastatic deposits in bone and hypercalcemia. Indeed, bisphosphanate therapy has been used with success in reducing bone metastases and hypercalcemia in patients with breast cancer, based on the rationale that inhibition of resorption will reduce the ability of tumors to establish in bone (van Holten-Verzantvoort et al, 1987).

HUMORAL HYPERCALCEMIA OF MALIGNANCY

Humoral hypercalcemia of malignancy (HHM) is associated with certain non-metastatic cancers and is caused by tumor products released into the circulation, acting generally to promote bone resorption and upon the kidney to reduce calcium excretion. The condition often occurs in association with squamous cell carcinoma of the lung, with a variety of other squamous carcinomata, with renal cortical carcinoma and less frequently with some other tumors. The biochemical similarity of this syndrome to primary hyperparathyroidism, with a high plasma calcium and a low plasma phosphate, was recognised in the 1920's. It was suggested by Albright (1941) that the cancer syndrome could be due to "ectopic" production of PTH by a non-parathyroid cancer. The idea of an "ectopic" PTH syndrome gained acceptance and was widely applied to patients with cancer who had a high plasma calcium, low phosphate, and minimal or no bony metastases. This was supported with data from the first radioimmunoassay for PTH, which showed that a significant number of unselected patients with lung cancer had elevated PTH levels. Subsequent observations in patients with cancer hypercalcemia provided conflicting data however, and some doubt arose that the syndrome could be explained by ectopic PTH production. In the early 1970's it was reported that circulating immunoreactive PTH in cancer differed from "authentic" PTH. A key study was that of Powell et al (1973) who found that immunoreactive PTH could not be detected in tumor or blood samples of eleven patients with hypercalcemia associated with non-parathyroid cancers in the absence of bony metastases. However tumor extracts promoted bone resorption in vitro in a manner very similar to PTH. Review of all the evidence towards the end of the 1970's resulted in the conclusion that such cancers caused hypercalcemia by producing a factor which was not PTH but which produced PTH-like effects. The close similarity of this syndrome to primary hyperparathyroidism was highlighted even further with the discovery that the patients with cancer had increased renal production of cyclic AMP. This arose out of three independent clinical studies in the early 1980's and led to great interest in identification of a substance capable of acting through the PTH receptor, but chemically diffferent from PTH (Kukreja et al, 1980; Stewart et al, 1980; Rude et al, 1981). Evidence was soon obtained that certain human and animal cancers associated with the HHM syndrome contained a protein which was capable of activating adenylate cyclase in PTH targets, but which was immunochemically distinct from PTH itself (Rodan et al, 1983).

In 1987 we succeeded in purifying such a protein from a human lung cancer cell line and subsequently in cloning of the cDNA encoding the protein (Moseley et al, 1987; Suva et al, 1987). It is a 141-amino acid protein in which 8 of the first 13 residues are identical with human PTH, with no other homology with any known protein in the rest of the molecule. This structure has been confirmed by the cloning and analysis of cDNA from a renal cancer (Mangin et al, 1988). We also synthesized biologically active amino-terminal fragments of this protein, which were assayed in several PTH response systems. The amino-terminal 34 amino acids of the PTH-related protein (PTHrP) contains activity very similar to PTH itself. PTHrP(1-14) is of higher specific biological activity than PTH itself, and PTHrP(1-34) is three to five times more potent than human PTH(1-34) in activating adenylate cyclase in bone and kidney, and in increasing plasminogen activator activity in osteoblasts. However PTHrP(1-34) is less active than PTH(1-34) in promoting bone resorption in fetal rat long bones in vitro (Kemp et al, 1987).

The existence of this protein helps to explain a number of the puzzling features which surround our understanding of the pathogenesis of HHM. The structural similarity about the amino-terminus might be sufficient to explain the PTH-like effects of the protein associated with HHM. On the other hand the differences in the remainder of the molecule can explain the failure of most PTH radioimmunoassays to detect the protein. We have developed radioimmunoassays using synthetic peptides as antigen, based on the amino-terminal sequence of PTHrP. Such assays have the capacity to detect synthetic peptide and tumor protein, but exhibit only weak cross-reactivity or none at all with peptides based on the human PTH sequence. This lack of cross-reactivity is evident not only under conditions of dilute antiserum as used in radioimmunoassay, but also with high concentrations as used in immunohistology. Using an immunoperoxidase method on formalin-fixed, paraffin-embedded sections we have shown that PTHrP immunoreactivity is contained in a range of squamous cell cancers, in samples of renal cortical carcinoma, but only in one of a series of adenocarcinomata (Danks et al, 1988). Pre-incubation of these antisera with PTHrP(1-34) of hPTH(1-34) has no effect. There have been a number of reports over several years of detection of "PTH" by immunohistology in sections of cancers from patients with the HHM syndrome (Mayes et al, 1984; Ilardi and Faro, 1985; Gonzalez et al, 1985). With the high concentrations of polyclonal antibody used in such studies, even low affinity detection of amino-terminal regions could yield such data, and it seems likely that the positive results obtained in these cases were due to production of PTHrP by the tumors.

OTHER POSSIBLE MEDIATORS IN HUMORAL HYPERCALCEMIA OF MALIGNANCY

When prostaglandins were discovered to promote bone resorption, they were considered as possible responsible agents for malignant hypercalcemia, especially since they were produced in substantial amounts by breast and kidney cancers (Greaves et al, 1980) and they were shown to mediate the hypercalcemia in two animal models of malignant hypercalcemia (Voelkel et al, 1975). However subsequent studies (reviewed in Raisz and Martin, 1984) led to the conclusion that prostaglandins were not responsible for the HHM syndrome, but could play a role in the development of bony metastases and the subsequent hypercalcemia.

Several lymphokines and monokines act directly on bone to promote resorption. The term, osteoclast activating factor ("OAF"), introduced originally to describe the bone-resorbing activity in supernatants of lectin-transformed lymphocytes (Horton et al, 1972), undoubtedly encompasses many bone-resorbing cytokines, including interleukin-1 and tumor necrosis factors α and β. These substances are likely to be involved in the mechanisms of hematological hypercalcemia, and possibly also of some solid tumors. Sato et al (1987) have identified interleukin-1^α as a product of a squamous cell carcinoma of the thyroid associated with hypercalcemia and leukocytosis. The same group has produced evidence that both PTH-like and interleukin-1^α-like activities are produced by a cloned esophageal cancer cell line, and interact to increase bone resorption (Sato et al, 1980). The possibility of such interactions needs to be considered in further studies.

Finally, with the discovery of epidermal growth factor (EGF) as a bone-resorbing agent, transforming growth factor $^\alpha$ (TGF$^\alpha$) acting through EGF receptors, was proposed as a mediator of hypercalcemia in the HHM syndrome (Ibbotson et al, 1983; Mundy et al, 1984). Many tumors produce TGF$^\alpha$, and it is a potent bone resorption stimulator (Ibbotson et al, 1985). Although TGFα production cannot explain all the biochemical features of HHM, nevertheless it is also possible that TGF^α might act in concert with the PTH-like protein to result in hypercalcemia.

SIGNIFICANCE OF THE PTH-RELATED PROTEIN IN CANCER

The finding of Kukreja et al (1980) that there is a high frequency of increased nephrogenous cyclic AMP in normocalcemic patients with bronchogenic carcinoma, suggests that production of PTHrP occurs very commonly in squamous cell carcinoma of the lung, and that patients become hypercalcemic only when the capacity of homeostatic mechanisms is exceeded, or when concomitant production of other factors contributes to hypercalcemia. Therefore the application of sensitive assays for PTHrP in plasma would be expected to help in the early diagnosis of squamous cell carcinoma, in the monitoring of treatment and the detection of recurrence. Furthermore, although it has been assumed until recently that the mechanisms of hypercalcemia in breast cancer have little in common with those occurring in HHM (Martin and Atkins, 1979; Stewart et al, 1980; Mundy and Martin, 1982), these views might need to be revised. Two groups have recently reported a number of hypercalcemic patients with breast cancer who have biochemical features similar to those in the HHM syndrome (Kimura et al, 1985; Percival et al, 1985). Additionally, a protein apparently identical with the PTHrP cloned from BEN cells has been purified from human breast cancer by Burtis et al (1987).

It is not known the extent to which the PTHrP contributes to development of hypercalcemia in cancer. It certainly seems likely that it contributes towards the increased nephrogenous cyclic AMP and phosphorus excretion and, by analogy with PTH, probably towards increased bone resorption, especially since we have shown it to have that effect in vitro (Kemp et al, 1987). It is also possible, as has been suggested (Mundy et al, 1985; Martin and Mundy, 1987), that a PTH-like protein might exert a predominant action on the kidney, and in concert with a bone-resorbing transforming growth factor or tumor necrosis factor, lead to hypercalcemia. The fact that this new protein has been characterized provides fascinating new areas for research into the mechanisms of HHM. It also creates new avenues of study in calcium metabolism in general. Quite apart from possible physiological and pathological roles in other organs, for example skin, it now seems that now it will be essential to look afresh at any clinical circumstance in which PTH itself is involved, and consider the possible place of the PTH-related protein. When more is known of its physiological roles and tissue distribution it would be appropriate to devise a name for this new hormone.

ACKNOWLEDGEMENT: Work from the author's laboratory was supported by grants from the NH & MRC, Anti-Cancer Council of Victoria, the Department of Veterans' Affairs, the Wenkart Foundation and the University of Melbourne.

REFERENCES

Albright, F. Case records of the Massachusetts Generl Hospital (case 27401). New Eng. J. Med. 1941, **225:**789-791.

Burtis, W.J., Wu, J., Bunch, C.M., Sysolmerski, J.J., Isogna, K.L., Weir, E.C., Broadus, A.E. & Steward, A.F. Identification of a novel 17,000-dalton parathyroid hormone-like adenylate cyclase-stimulating protein from a tumor associated with humoral hypercalcemia of malignancy. J. Biol. Chem. 1987, **162:**7151-7156

Danks, J.M., Ebeling, P.R., Rodda, C.P., Hayman, J., Chou, S.T., Moseley, J.M., Dunlop, J.M., Kemp, B.E. & Martin, T.J. Immunohistochemical localization of parathyroid hormone-related protein of cancer. J. Bone Min. Res. 1983 (in press).

Gonzalez, R.D., Barrientos, A., Larrodera, L., Rullope, L.M., Leiva, O. & Barobia, V. Squamous cell carcinoma of the renal pelvis associatyed with hypercalcemia and the presence of parathyroid hormone-like substances in the tumor. J. Urol. 1985, **133:**1029-1034.

Greaves, M., Ibbotson, K.J., Atkins, D. & Martin, T.J. Prostaglandins extracted from tumours and produced by cultures of renal cortical carcinoma and benign and malignant breast tumours: relation to bone resorption. Clin. Sci. 1980, **58:**201-210.

Horton, J.E., Raisz, L.G., Simmons, H.A., Oppenheim, J.J. & Mergenhagen, S.E. Bone resorbing activity in supernatants from cultured human peripheral blood leukocytes. Science 1972, **177:**793-795.

Ibbotson, K.J., D'Souza, S.M., Ng, K.W., Osborne, C.K., Niall, M., Martin, T.J. & Mundy, G.R. Tumor-derived growth factor increased bone resorption in a tumour associated with humoral hypercalcemia of malignancy. Science 1983, **221:**1292-1294.

Ibbotson, K.J., Twardzik, D.R., D'Souza, S.M., Hargreaves, W.R., Todaro, G.J. & Mundy, G.R. Stimulation of bone resorption in vitro by synthetic transforming growth factor-alpha. Science 1985, **228:**1007-1008.

Ilardi, C.F. & Faro, J.C. Localization of parathyroid hormone-like substance in squamous cell carcinomas. Arch. path. Lab. Med. 1985, **109:**752-755.

Kemp, B.E., Stapleton, D., Rodda, C.P., Michelangeli, V.P., Ebeling, P.R., Moseley, J.M., Simmons, H.A., Raisz, L.G. & Martin, T.J. Synthesis of biologically active amino-terminal peptide based on sequence of parathyroid hormone-related protein of cancer. Science (in press).

Kimura, S., Adchi, I., Yamaguchi, K., Suzuki, M., Shimada, A., Sato, Y., Nagaoka, K. & Abe, K. Stimulation of calcium reabsorption observed in advanced breast cancer patients with hypercalcemia and multiple bone metastases. Gann 1985, **76:**308-314.

Kukreja, S.C., Shemerdiak, W.P., Lad, T.E. & Johnson, P.A. Elevated nephrogenous cyclic AMP with normal serum parathyroid hormone levels in patients with lung cancer. J. Clin. endocrinol. Metab. 1980, **51:**167-169.

Mangin, M., Webb, A.C., Dreyer, B.E., Posillico, J.T., Ikeda, K., Weir, E.C., Stewart, A.F., Bander, N.H., Milstone, L., Barton, D., Francke, U. & Broadus, A.E. Identification of a cDNA encoding a parathyroid hormone-like peptide from a human tumor associated with humoral hypercalcemia of malignancy. proc. Natl. Acad. Sci. USA 1988, **85:**597-601.

Martin, T.J. & Atkins, D. Biochemical regulators of bone resorption and their significance in cancer. Essays in Medical Biochem. 1979, **4:**49-82.

Martin, T.J. & Mundy, G.R. Hypercalcemia of malignancy. In: "Clinical Endocrinology of Calcium Metabolism" (eds. T.J. Martin & L.G. Raisz), Marcel Dekker, New York, 1987, pp. 171-199.

Mayes, L.C., Kasselberg, A.G., Roloff, J.S. & Lukens, J.N. Hypercalcemia associated with immunoreactive parathyroid hormone in a malignant rhabdoid tumor of the kidney (Rhabdoid Wilms' Tumor). Cancer 1984, **54:**882-884.

Moseley, J.M., Kubota, M., Diefenbach-Jagger, H., Wettenhall, R.E.H., Kemp, B.E., Suva, L.J., Rodda, C.P., Ebeling, P.R., Hudson, P.J., Zajac, J.D. & Martin, T.J. Parathyroid hormone-related protein purified from a human lung cancer cell line. Proc. Natl. Acad. Sci. USA 1987, **84:**5048-5052.

Mundy, G.R. & Martin, T.J. The hypercalcemia of malignancy: pathogenesis and treatment. Metabolism 1982, **31:** 1247-1277.

Mundy, G.R., Ibbotson, K.J., D'Souza, S.M., Simpson, E.L., Jacobs, J.W. & Martin, T.J. The hypercalcemia of cancer. Clinical implications and pathogenic mechanisms. New Engl. J. Med. 1984, **310**:1718-1728.

Mundy, G.R., Ibbotson, K.J. & D'Souza, S.M. Tumor products and the hypercalcemia of malignancy. J. Clin. Invest. 1985, **76**: 391-394.

Percival, R.C., Yates, A.J.P., Gray, R.E.S., Galloway, J., Rogers, K., Neal, F.E. & Kanis, J.A. Mechanisms of malignant hypercalcaemia in carcinoma of the breast. Br. Med. J. 1985, **2**:776-779.

Powell, D., Singer, F.R., Murray, T.M., Minkin, C. & Potts, J.T. Non-parathyroid humoral hypercalcemia in patients with neoplastic disease. New Engl. J. Med. 1973, **289**:176-181.

Raisz, L.G. & Martin, T.J. Prostaglandins in bone and mineral metabolism. In: "Bone and Mineral Research Annuyal 2" (W.A. Peck, ed.) Excerpta Medica, amsterdam, 1984, pp. 286-310.

Rodan, S.B., Insogna, K.L., Vignery, A.M-c., Stewart, A.F., broadus, A.E., D'Souza, S.M., Bertolini, D.R., Mundy, G.R. & Rodan, G.A. Factors associated with humoral hypercalcemia of malignancy stimulate adenylate cyclase in osteoblastic cells. J. Clin. Invest. 1983, **72**:1511-1515.

Rude, R.K., Sharp, C.F. Jr., Fredericks, R.S., Oldham, S.B., Elbaum, N., Link, J., Irvin, L. & Singer, F.R. Urinary and nephhrogenous adenosine 3',5'-monophosphate in the hypercalcaemia of malignancy. J. Clin. Invest. 1981, **52**:765-771.

Sato, K., Ohba, K., Yashiro, T., Fuju, Y., Tsushima, T. & Shizume, K. Production of PTH-like activity and IL-1 -like activity by a clonal esophageal carcinoma line (EC-GI) derived from a patient with hypercalcemia. In: "Calcium Regulation and Bone Metabolism" D.V. Cohn, T.J. Martin & P.J. Meunier (Exc. Med. Amsterdam), Vol. 9, p.555, 1987 a.

Sato, K., Fuju, Y., Ono, M., Nomura, H. & Shizume, K. Production of interleukin- -like factor and colony-stimulating factor by a squamous cell carcinoma of the thyroid (T3M-5) derived from a patient with hypercalcemia and leukocytosis. Cancer Research, 1987 B, **47**:6474-6480.

Steward, A.F., Horst, R., Deftos, L.J., Cadman, E.C., Lang, R. & Broadus, A.E. Biochemical evaluation of patients with cancer-associated hypercalcemia. Evidence for humoral and non-humoral groups. New Engl. J. Med. 1980, **303**:1377-1381.

Suva, L.J., Winslow, G.A., Wettenhall, R.E.H., Kemp, B.E., Hudson, P.J., Diefenbach-Jagger, H., Moseley, J.M., Rodda, C.M., Martin, T.J. & Wood, W.I. Molecular cloning and expression of a novel hormone cDNA encoding a parathyroid hormone-like protein in human lung cancer cells. Science 1987, **237**:893-896.

van Holten-Verzantvoort, A.T., Bijvoet, O.L.M., Hermans, J., Harinck, H., Elte, J., Beex, L., Cleeton, F., Kroon, H., Vermey, P., Neijt, J. & Blijham, G. Reduced morbidity from skeletal metastases in breast cancer patients during long-term bisphosphonate (APD) treatment. Lancet 1987, ii:983-985.

Voelkel, E.F., Tashjian, A.H. Jr., Franklin, R., Wasserman, E. & Levine, L. Hypercalcemia and tumor prostaglandins: The VX_2 carcinoma model in the rabbit. Metabolism, 1975, **24**:973-986.

Discussion:

DR. MUNDY (San Antonio, TX): Could I ask you one question about the recombinant material? There seemed to be a discrepancy between the potency of the recombinant material relative to PTH and the earlier data you showed with the native protein. You showed the native protein was more potent than PTH (1-34) with respect to a cyclase response, and yet, the recombinant protein, on a molar basis, seemed to be equipotent. Is that correct?

DR. MARTIN (Australia): Yes. Well, actually, the PTH-related protein data was not expressed on a molar basis. We calculated it out, but it does work out at about a two to threefold difference on a molar basis.

DR. MUNDY: That would make it more potent.

DR. MARTIN: Yes, the pure material does calculate out to be about two to fourfold -- oh, wait a minute. No, that's right. There is about a five to eightfold difference on a molar basis. So, that is a discrepancy, actually, yes.

Because, certainly, what we've been able to do with the recombinant material has consistently, over about 10 to 12 assays that we've been able to do over the last few weeks, been quite superimposed -- now, that might mean that there is some post-translational modification that takes place. But we don't know that. There's no obvious glycosylation. It's a good point. It may be that there is something different about the native material.

DR. PARFITT (Detroit): Jack, is this material ever produced by normal tissue?

DR. MARTIN: Well, we certainly believe that it's present in normal skin, yes, and normal keratinocytes.

DR. PARFITT: And a parallel question, is there now any situation where authentic PTH is produced by a tumor?

DR. MARTIN: Well, I don't know. I think you can look back at everything that's ever been published and explain it by the presence of this material, including all the immunoassay data, and certainly all the immunohistology data, because in any of the immunohistology data that has ever claimed PTH in tumors, cross-reactivities were quoting immunoassay conditions of cross-reactivity and in those studies where any cross-reactivity is investigated under high concentration that you use in immunohistology. That's why we believe it's important to do the biological assay and to check antisera if you're going to use them for immunohistology.

DR. LANG (New Haven): Two questions. One, the degree of hypercalcemia is more profound than we see with hyperparathyroidism. Second, we biopsied a few patients with HHM and saw very low bone formation, in fact, about the lowest bone formation we've seen in any patients. They were very sick patients, and that may have had something to do with it. Do you know of any other data on bone formation?

DR. MARTIN: Well, Larry Raisz has been doing bone formation studies in vitro with the peptide, and Janet Hock, in vivo, with rats. And in the in vitro data, what Larry Raisz has found at any rate is that, although the materials that he had tested on resorption indicated that the PTH-related protein was less potent, PTH-related protein and PTH were equipotent in inhibiting formation.

If that can be followed up, well, it certainly does appear to be very potent in inhibiting formation. And if you get enough around to be a major promoter of resorption, maybe it's having a bigger effect on inhibiting formation. But, certainly, on Janet Hock's data, it inhibits formation in the in vivo experiments in the rat. And she'll present that at ASBMR. I don't know whether that's the full explanation, but it's all we know at the moment.

DR. LANG: Another quick question. 20 or 30 years ago, breast cancer was far and away the most common cause of hypercalcemia. What's happened to people with breast cancer and why is this so common now?

DR. MARTIN: Well, breast cancer is a very interesting situation. It's not one that we've traditionally thought of being associated with production of this material. However, one of the tumors from which the Yale group has purified this protein was a breast cancer. Two groups, John Kanis' and a Japanese group, have evidence that among breast cancer patients, there are some who biochemically have production of this activity.

I think that we need to look again at breast cancers to see whether the production of this might not necessarily often be a humoral factor, but it could be related to the ability of breast cancers to erode bone. I think that's an open question.

DR. SCHARLA (Heidelberg): I would like to ask you if you have any evidence that your PTH-like peptide stimulates 1-alpha hydroxylase in the kidney. The reason for the question is that we find, in some of our patients, elevated 1,25-dihydroxyvitamin D levels, despite hypercalcemia and suppressed PTH levels. In addition, in our rat model for tumor hypercalcemia we find elevated 1,25 levels, too.

DR. MARTIN: Several people have shown that the 1-34 peptide activates 1-hydroxylase. It's been done by the Merck group. Uli Trechsal has done it, and Toshi Matsumoto's group in Tokyo have.

We don't yet know why it is that the 1,25 levels are commonly low in the patients with HHM. In some of the animal models, the 1,25 levels are high, like they are in hyperparathyroidism. I think it's something that is interesting and will have to be worked out, and I don't know an answer to it at the moment.

DR. SCHARLA: But in some of our patients, we have elevated 1,25 levels, too, so it would fit.

DR. MARTIN: I'm sure you would, yes. I think there will be a mixture. But we don't know why, at the moment.

DR. BERGMANN (Belgium): Is the production of the factor by tumor cells, or also by keratinocytes, completely autonomous or is it possible to modulate this production by some physiological or pharmacological manipulations?

DR. MARTIN: We don't know.

DR. KHOSLA (Rochester, MN): Do you know if the PTH-rP in circulating form is metabolized in any way similar to PTH?

DR. MARTIN: We don't know anything about the circulating form. I don't think anybody else does.

Mechanisms of Hypercalcemia in Hematologic Malignancies

GREGORY R. MUNDY

University of Texas Health Science Center
San Antonio, TX

MECHANISMS OF HYPERCALCEMIA IN HEMATOLOGIC MALIGNANCIES

The mechanisms responsible for hypercalcemia in patients with hematologic malignancies are very different from those in patients with solid tumors. The hematologic malignancies are malignancies of cells normally resident in the bone marrow, and the factors they produce which disrupt calcium homeostasis may also be factors involved in the normal physiologic regulation of bone remodeling at endosteal surfaces, and control of trabecular bone volume. In this review, proposed mechanisms of bone destruction and hypercalcemia in patients with myeloma, various lymphomas and acute and chronic leukemias will be discussed.

Myeloma

Myeloma is a neoplastic disorder of plasma cells characterized by bone pain and skeletal lesions. Bone pain is the most common presenting symptom of patients presenting with this disease (Snapper & Kahn 1971), and occurs as a consequence of bone destruction. In more than 80% of patients with this disease, bone pain is present when the diagnosis is made.

Mechanisms of bone destruction in myeloma

Patients with myeloma usually have extensive destructive bone lesions. These may take the form of discrete osteolytic lesions, or diffuse osteopenia. They almost always involve the axial skeleton, but also occasionally the appendicular skeleton as well. In the majority of patients, these bone lesions are discrete and purely lytic when examined radiologically (Snapper & Kahn 1971). Histologically, the lesions are associated with an intense increase in osteoclast activity (Mundy et al, 1974). Bone forming surfaces and calcification rates are reduced (Valentin-Opran et al, 1982). Bone forming surfaces are covered by thin layers of osteoid (Valentin-Opran et al, 1982). This decrease in the rate of bone formation is characteristic of the bone lesions in myeloma. Patients usually have no or only marginal increases in the serum alkaline phosphatase, a marker enzyme of osteoblast activity, in contrast to patients with solid tumors and osteolytic metastases. Bone scans performed with labeled bisphosphonates often show no increase in activity, since these bone scanning agents highlight sites of active bone formation.

The bone lesions in myeloma occur adjacent to collections of myeloma cells (Mundy et al, 1974; Valentin-Opran et al, 1982). Discrete lytic lesions are associated with increased localized osteoclast activity. When diffuse osteopenia occurs, this represents myeloma cells spread throughout the axial skeleton.

Occasional patients with myeloma have osteosclerotic lesions rather than lytic reasons. The mechanisms are unknown, and this condition has not been studied in any detail. It may be associated with the POEMS syndrome (Bardwick et al, 1980), which is characterized by severe progressive sensory and motor polyneuropathy, organomegaly, endocrine dysfunction including diabetes mellitus, gynecomastia and impotence in males or amenorrhea in females, hyperpigmentation and papilledema with increased cerebrospinal fluid protein. Peripheral neuropathy is frequently associated with this syndrome. The POEMS syndrome or osteosclerosis in myeloma has not been associated with hypercalcemia.

The predominant characteristic of the bone lesions in patients with myeloma is a localized increase in osteoclast activity occurring adjacent to collections of myeloma cells. The mechanism for the increase in osteoclast activity is production by the myeloma cells of factors which stimulate osteoclastic bone resorption. It has been known since 1974 that cultured human myeloma cells produce a stimulator of osteoclast activity (Mundy et al, 1974; Josse et al, 1981; Mundy et al, 1974) which is similar to the bone resorbing activity produced by normal peripheral blood leukocytes when they are activated by a mitogen such as phytohemagglutinin or an antigen to which they have been previously exposed (Horton et al, 1972). Recently, this bone resorbing factor has been identified as lymphotoxin (Garrett et al, 1987), which is also called tumor necrosis factor β and is a potent stimulator of osteoclastic bone resorption (Bertolini et al, 1986). Lymphotoxin is produced by normal activated T-lymphocytes, as well as by certain lymphoid cell lines with B-cell surface characteristics. It causes cytolysis in certain tumor cell lines. It is homologous to tumor necrosis factor, a cytokine produced by activated monocytes, and shares with it the same receptor. Recombinant human lymphotoxin causes hypercalcemia when injected or infused into intact rodents (Garrett et al, 1987).

The evidence that the bone resorbing factor produced by cultured human myeloma cells is lymphotoxin was demonstrated by showing that the bone resorbing activity present in cultured myeloma cell supernatants was neutralized by monoclonal antibodies to this factor (Garrett et al, 1987). In some cell lines derived from patients with myeloma, not all of the bone resorbing activity could be neutralized, but in no case was less than 50% neutralized by these antibodies. Myeloma cells express lymphotoxin messenger RNA. Myeloma cells also express tumor necrosis factor messenger RNA, although tumor necrosis factor biologic activity has not been detected as yet in supernatants harvested from cultured myeloma cells. Interleukin-1 biological activity has also not detected in supernatants harvested from cultured myeloma cells, and neither interleukin-1α nor interleukin-1β messenger RNA has been found in myeloma cell extracts (Garrett et al, 1987).

Mechanisms of hypercalcemia in myeloma

Approximately 20-40% of patients with myeloma develop hypercalcemia (Snapper & Kahn 1971; Mundy & Bertolini 1986). This is usually a bad prognostic sign, and few patients with myeloma live more than 6 months after their first episode of hypercalcemia. In part this may be due to the fact that patients with myeloma who develop hypercalcemia have the largest tumor burdens, and in part because patients with hypercalcemia frequently have impaired renal function (Durie et al, 1981; Harinck et al, 1987).

Hypercalcemia in myeloma occurs predominantly as a consequence of increased osteoclastic bone resorption. This is the mechanism responsible for the increased entry of calcium into the extracellular fluid. However, impaired renal excretion of calcium may also be important in the pathophysiology (Durie et al, 1981). Patients with myeloma develop renal failure as a consequence of chronic infections, uric acid nephropathy and amyloidosis, but most importantly because of Bence Jones nephropathy, due to precipitation of light chain fragments (Bence Jones proteins) in the renal tubules. The combination of increased bone resorption together with impaired capacity to excrete calcium from the kidneys is responsible for the hypercalcemia.

Treatment of hypercalcemia in myeloma

Treatment of hypercalcemia in myeloma may present a difficult therapeutic problem, since the impairment in renal function in these patients may be fixed, and this limits the utility of saline loads to increase calcium excretion. Moreover, many of the drugs currently used in the therapy of hypercalcemia are of limited usefulness in the presence of impaired renal function. For example, plicamycin (mithramycin) is nephrotoxic and is best avoided if renal function is impaired. Similarly, experience with the bisphosphonates is still limited in patients with renal failure. Many patients with myeloma respond well to treatment for the underlying disease, and this may relieve hypercalcemia, particularly if the treatment regimen includes corticosteroids (Mundy & Martin 1982; Binstock & Mundy 1980). The combination of calcitonin and corticosteroids is very effective in patients with myeloma and is not dangerous to use when renal function is impaired. It is essentially always effective in the treatment of hypercalcemia in this particular situation.

Hypercalcemia in lymphomas and leukemias

Hypercalcemia and osteolytic bone lesions are less frequent in patients with lymphoma than they are in patients with myeloma. However, they are still found occasionally, and the mechanisms are probably different from those which are responsible in patients with myeloma or with solid tumors. Hypercalcemia has been reported in Hodgkin's Disease, in adult T-cell lymphomas, in Burkitt's lymphoma and in B-cell lymphomas, as well as in acute and chronic leukemias.

a.   Adult T-cell lymphoma

Certain types of adult T-cell lymphomas are frequently associated with hypercalcemia. Recently, a special type of T-cell lymphoma has been described in patients who are resident in the southern islands of Japan, in the Caribbean and in the southeastern United States (Bunn et al, 1983). These lymphomas are aggressive tumors frequently associated with skin lesions, visceral involvement and hepatosplenomegaly. They tend to run a rapid course and are poorly responsive to chemotherapy. This malignancy is due frequently to infection with an oncogenic Type-C retrovirus, called human T-cell lymphotrophic virus Type-I (HTLV-1). Most of these patients develop hypercalcemia sometime during the course of their disease.

The mechanism of hypercalcemia in these tumors may be due to a combination of increased bone resorption and increased absorption of calcium from the gut. In patients with solid tumors and with myeloma, calcium absorption from the gut is usually suppressed. However, in some patients with this type of lymphoma, not only is calcium absorption from the gut increased, but the patients also have increased circulating concentrations of 1,25 dihydroxyvitamin D (Breslau et al, 1984). The tumor cells are presumably the source of 1,25 dihydroxyvitamin D. Lymphoid cells inoculated with HTLV-I are examined in vitro, have the capacity to metabolize 25 hydroxyvitamin D to 1,25 dihydroxyvitamin D (Fetchick et al, 1986), a function previously thought limited to the renal tubules and certain other specific tissues such as the placenta and sarcoid granulomata. However, these transformed lymphoid cells also produce a myriad of peptide cytokines, and it is likely that these too may be involved in the increased bone resorption.

    b.   Hodgkin's Disease

Hypercalcemia is unusual in Hodgkin's Disease. When it does occur, it is often relatively late in the course of the disease. Frequently these patients have a large tumor bulk, with frequent visceral and retroperitoneal lymph node involvement. Hypercalcemia occurs most frequently in elderly men with Hodgkin's Disease. As with patients with adult T-cell lymphoma, hypercalcemia in Hodgkin's Disease has been described in association with increased 1,25 dihydroxyvitamin D concentrations (Zaloga et al, 1985). However, unlike adult T-cell lymphoma, the majority of patients with Hodgkin's Disease never develop hypercalcemia.

    c.   Other lymphomas and leukemias

Hypercalcemia also occurs occasionally in patients with other types of lymphomas. It has been described in patients with B-cell lymphomas. Again, in this situation there has been a case described with increased production of 1,25 dihydroxyvitamin D (Mudde et al, 1987). We studied a patient with a B-cell lymphoma associated with circulating neoplastic cells 10 years ago (Mundy et al, 1978). This patient had an aggressive malignancy and died following poor response to chemotherapy. The cultured neoplastic cells secreted a macromolecular bone resorbing factor, presumably a lymphokine with elution characteristics from gel filtration columns similar to those of the bone resorbing peptide cytokines. A case of Burkitt's lymphoma has also been described with hypercalcemia (Spiegel et al, 1978). This tumor usually arises in the jaw and is associated with localized increases in osteoclastic bone resorption (Adatia et al, 1968).

Children with either lymphomas or acute leukemias may present with diffuse osteopenia, but rarely with hypercalcemia. Hypercalcemia is occasionally, but infrequently, seen in patients with acute leukemia, chronic lymphocytic leukemia and chronic granulocytic leukemia, particularly during blast transformation (Canellos 1974). It is so unusual in chronic lymphocytic leukemia that when it does occur, another disease such as primary hyperparathyroidism or a second malignancy should be searched for diligently.

Acknowledgements

Some of the work described has been supported by grants AR-28149, CA-40035, and RR-01346. The author is grateful to Nancy Garrett for secretarial assistance.

References

Adatia AK, 'Dental tissues and Burkitt's tumor', Oral Surg (1968) 25: pp. 221-234.

Bardwick PA, Zvaifler NJ, Gill GN, et al, 'Plasma cell dyscrasia with polyneuropathy, organomegaly, endocrinopathy, M protein, and skin changes: The POEMS syndrome', Medicine (1980) 59: pp. 311-322.

Bertolini DR, Nedwin GE, Bringman TS, 'Stimulation of bone resorption and inhibition of bone formation in vitro by human tumour necrosis factors', Nature (1986) 319: pp. 516-518.

Binstock ML, Mundy GR, 'Effects of calcitonin and glucocorticoids in combination in hypercalcemia of malignancy', Ann Intern Med (1980) 93: pp. 269-272.

Bunn PA, Schechter GP, Jaffe E, et al. 'Clinical course of retrovirus associated adult T cell lymphoam in the United States', New Engl J Med (1983) 309: pp. 257-264.

Breslau NA, McGuire JL, Zerwekh JE, Frenkel EP, Pak CY, 'Hypercalcemia associated with increased serum calcitriol levels in three patients with lymphoma', Ann Int Med (1984) 100: pp. 1-7.

Canellos GP, 'Hypercalcemia in malignant lymphoma and leukemia', Ann N Y Acad Sci (1974) 230: pp. 240-246.

Durie BGM, Salmon SE, Mundy GR, 'Relation of osteoclast activating factor production to the extent of bone disease in multiple myeloma', Brit J Haematol (1981) 47: pp. 21-30.

Fetchick DA, Bertolini DR, Sarin PS, Weintraub ST, Mundy GR, Dunn JD, 'Production of 1,25-dihydroxyvitamin D by human T-cell lymphotrophic virus-I transformed lymphocytes', J Clin Invest (1986) 78: pp. 592-596.

Garrett IR, Durie BGM, Nedwin GE, et al. 'Production of the bone resorbing cytokine lymphotoxin by cultured human myeloma cells', New Engl J Med (1987) (in press).

Horton JE, Raisz LG, Simmons HA, et al. 'Bone resorbing activity in supernatant fluid from cultured human peripheral blood leukocytes', Science (1972) 177: pp. 793-795.

Harinck HIJ, Bijvoet OLM, Plantingh AST, 'Role of bone and kidney in tumor-induced hypercalcemia and its treatment with bisphosphonate and sodium chloride', Am J Med (1987) 82: pp. 1133-1142.

Josse RG, Murray TM, Mundy GR, et al, 'Observations on the mechanism of bone resorption induced by multiple myeloma marrow culture fluids and partially purified osteoclast-activating factor', J Clin Invest (1981) 67: pp. 1472-1481.

Mudde AH, van den Berg H, Boshuis PG, et al. 'Ectopic production of 1,25-dihydroxyvitamin D by B-cell lymphoma as a cause of hypercalcemia', Cancer (1987) 59: pp. 1543-1546.

Mundy GR, Luben RA, Raisz LG, et al, 'Bone resorbing activity in supernatants from lymphoid cell lines', New Engl J Med (1974a) 290: pp. 867-871.

Mundy GR, Raisz LG, Cooper RA, et al, 'Evidence for the secretion of an osteoclast stimulating factor in myeloma', New Engl J Med (1974b) 291: pp. 1041-1046.

Mundy GR, Rick ME, Turcotte R, et al, 'Pathogenesis of hypercalcemia in lymphosarcoma cell leukemia - Role of an osteoclast activating factor like substance and mechanism of action for glucocorticoid therapy', Am J Med (1978) 654: pp. 600-606.

Mundy GR, Martin TJ, 'The hypercalcemia of malignancy: Pathogenesis and management', Metabolism (1982) 31: pp. 1247-1277.

Mundy GR, Bertolini DR, 'Bone destruction and hypercalcemia in plasma cell myeloma', Seminars in Oncology (1986) 13: pp. 291-299.

Spiegel A, Greene M, Magrath I, et al. 'Hypercalcemia with suppressed parathyroid hormone in Burkitt's lymphoma', Am J Med (1978) 64: pp. 691-702.

Snapper I, Kahn A, 'Myelomatosis', Karger, Basel, Switzerland. 1971

Valentin-Opran A, Charhon SA, Meunier PJ, et al, 'Quantitative histology of myeloma induced bone changes', Brit J Haematology (1982) 52: pp. 601-610.

Zaloga GP, Eil C, Medbery CA, 'Humoral hypercalcemia in Hodgkin's disease', Arch Int Med (1985) 145: pp. 155-157.

Discussion:

DR. OGATA (Tokyo): You just told that the adult T-cell lymphoma cells produce 1,25 and this might be the only reason for hypercalcemia.

DR. MUNDY (San Antonio, TX): No, no, I didn't say that. At least, I hope I didn't.

DR. OGATA: I think the ATL produced by the HTLV-1 virus is an exception for your statement, for these three reasons. Every patient with ATL due to HTLV-1 infection exhibited exactly the same biochemical profile of HHM with increased cyclic AMP production. Secondly, when we cultured those cells, it produced a protein which is indistinguishable from HHM factor, both biologically and biochemically. and lastly, we clearly could show the presence of messenger RNA's detected by CDNA according to Dr. Martin. So, I think the T-cell lymphoma produced by HTLV-1 virus is different.

DR. MUNDY: Yes. I've seen your data and it's very convincing. I really didn't mean to imply that 1,25 D production was the only mechanism, or even very common in that situation. And I'm sure, as you've shown, that there will be other examples in the future, where there will be overlap between these various syndromes.

DR. HEATH (Rochester, MN): Greg, beautiful presentation. I'd like you to elaborate, if you could, on part of the concept. The present idea is that parathyroid hormone activates bone resorption by acting first on the osteoblast. And in your diagrams you show the cytokines as direct stimulators of activity by an individual osteoclast. Do you believe that cytokines act first on osteoblasts, do they act on the osteoclast progenitor cells, or do they act on osteoclasts already formed, or all of the above?

DR. MUNDY: It's very fashionable at the present time to believe that cytokines act on osteoclasts indirectly. And I think that's grossly oversimplified. I wasn't trying to make any statement with that slide about whether factors are acting directly or indirectly. But my hunch is that some of these cytokines such as interleukin-1 also act directly on osteoclasts. That doesn't mean --

DR. HEATH: On already formed osteoclasts?

DR. MUNDY: Yes. That doesn't mean that they can't also act by sending second signals through other cells. But I'd be willing to bet at least a beer, which is a big bet for me, that we're going to find out a short time from now that cytokines also have direct effects on osteoclasts.

DR. HEATH: But I gather that that's not really been tested yet with pure isolated osteoclasts?

DR. MUNDY: Well, the problem is that nobody has got - well, nobody is really willing to say yet that they've got a pure homogeneous osteoclast population. It's really a problem in the cell biology, and in the techniques.

QUESTIONER: Greg, it seems to be possible to infuse, by mini pump system, the cytokines. Has the opposite test, infusing the molecule antibodies against the cytokines, resulted in some information about their effects in normal mice or rats?

DR. MUNDY: No. No, it hasn't really. And, again, it's probably a technical problem. The only experiments which I know have been done with antibodies and cytokines have been those done by Bruce Beutler and Tony Cerami, in which they've used passive immunization with antibodies to tumor necrosis factor/cachectin, and been able to show that that inhibits the development of endotoxic shock. But they're very short-term experiments. It would be very difficult to do the experiments for long enough duration so that you could determine whether or not there's a physiological role for these cytokines. However, it is conceivable nowadays you could get at that problem in other ways, such as by stimulating endogenous production of antibodies to some of these cytokines.

DR. RAO (Detroit): What is the relationship, if any, between your angry osteoclasts and Michael Parfitt's killer osteoclasts? And the second question is, you put the query mark in the osteoporosis. Many years ago, Dr. Frame showed that there is increased plasma cells in the bone marrow of patients with osteoporosis. Now that you're implying the cytokines, do you think they may have anything - any role in the osteoporosis?

DR. MUNDY: They're just active resorbing osteoclasts. The other issue was plasma cells in osteoporosis and I know of no information there.

Paget's Disease of Bones: Assessment, Therapy, and Secondary Prevention

OLAV L.M. BIJVOET, C.J.L.R. VELLENGA, and H.I.J. HARINCK

*Clinical Investigation Unit of the Department
of Clinical Endocrinology and Metabolism
and Department of Nuclear Medicine
University Hospital
Rijnsburgerweg, Leiden
The Netherlands*

INTRODUCTION

PAGET's disease is not a metabolic bone disorder, but a disorder in the metabolism of one or more bones (1-5). The disease induces local acceleration of bone turnover i.e. of bone-resorption and -formation both, in sundry parts of the skeleton. These bones then change in shape, size and direction, while the remainder of the skeleton remains unaffected. Within the affected bones, there are slowly expanding regions, in which all cells involved in remodeling are increased in number, and where the increase in the rate of tissue breakdown and repair results in bizarre architectural deformation of the hard tissue. The beginning of the disease is probably never noticed. A small "Pagetic" lesion in a large bone, like the pelvis, may remain unobserved or not cause worry, nor are there biochemical changes in blood or urine in the 5 % of the patients in whom less than 2% of the skeleton is affected (Table I). Before the disease becomes symptomatic, the patients are generally well over 35 years of age. By then, relentless progression of the lesion has caused them to become aware of unremitting pains, large deformations, or impairments of function. These cause disability and severe social handicaps in a considerable fraction of patients. Over forty percent amongst a large group from a recent study had to stop work before the age of retirement (3).

Less than two decades ago there was no treatment available (6). The discovery of the therapeutic potential of calcitonin and bisphosphonates has changed this completely (7-13); at present the possibility even emerges that pain, functional impairment and disability have become preventable. The first important observations were that the calcitonins were able to suppress pain, and to achieve some reduction, though incomplete, in biochemical markers of disease activity (7-10,12). Together with this, structural improvement was seen in radiographs of some of the lesions (11). This therapy was mainly efficacious in the symptomatic sense; it had a disadvantage of producing unpredictable results in the individual and it did not contribute to making patients medically independent (2,14). With the bisphosphonates however, one has obtained effects, that are not only more complete, but that are are sustained over prolonged therapy free intervals (15-17). There has been concern about side effects with the earlier drugs. Recent developments are however good enough to justify the expectation that third generation bisphosphonates will in a predictable fashion achieve complete and durable remission of the disease with simple means.

If indeed, this is possible, there is no reason why Paget's disease should be allowed any more to develop into a stage that is associated with pain, deformity or handicap. The transition of therapy from a period in which the major aim was the suppression of activity in symptomatic patients, to one that aims at early treatment and prevention is an important one. It requires not only standards for diagnosis but also the ability to assess the likelihood that the disease will cause complications. Apart from that, criteria should be established for the evaluation of drug efficacy with respect to long term preventive potential, and safety and simplicity of treatment.

ASSESSMENT

The following section concerns methods to evaluate the extent and severity of Paget's disease and to estimate the prognosis. These data should provide guide-lines for subsequent therapy. We will first discuss the parameters that are used to provide material for this evaluation. Next, these findings will be evaluated in the perspective of available epidemiologic information on the population of the patients in general. This then will help in providing a prognostic judgement for the individual.

The parameters of disease

Histology and pathogenesis

The radiographic image is often pathognomonic, but when in doubt, the conclusive element in diagnosing Paget's disease is the bone biopsy. Normal cortical bone is composed of osteon systems, having regular concentric lamellae, and the spongious bone tissue of superimposed flat layers of lamellar bone. In Paget's disease the structure of the two types of tissue is completely disorganized. The calcified matrix now consists of a pattern-less mosaïc of primitive, woven bone, interspersed with older rests of lamellar bone; the trabecules are irregular and have a wild arrangement, and the bone as a whole has poor architectural value. The numbers of osteoclasts and osteoblasts is ten-fold increased on the average, but this can even increase to a hundred-fold. The osteoclasts are impressively enlarged and contain an excessive number of nuclei and cell constituents. The adjacent bone marrow is hypervascular and interspersed with fibrosis and infiltrations of mononuclear cells (18-20).

Many of the abnormalities of the osteoclasts are aspecific, in that they can be seen in other pathological conditions, and in other cells, secondary to disturbances of cell metabolism. André Rebel however, has made the fascinating observation that all osteoclasts in the diseased tissue, but not the osteoclasts in the normal tissue of the same patients, contain nuclear inclusions (21,22). Different aspects of these suggest an evolution in organization of constituent filaments from a scattered group, through parallel bundles, to a paracrystalline array. These inclusions can be compared to the glial cell nuclear inclusions in progressive multifocal leuko-encephalopathy, a disease probably due to a virus. Subacute sclerosing encephalitis demonstrates the presence of intranuclear and cytoplasmic viral material with remarkable similarity to these findings. Comparable structures have been described in virus-infected cell nuclei. The presence in these osteoclasts of antigens belonging to the family of paramyxovirus, but also to both, respiratory syncytial virus and measles virus, has now been demonstrated. It has therefore been suggested that that the disease could be a late manifestation of an infection with a "slow-virus" of the measles group, incurred at an early age (23-24).

The bone cells are considered to belong to two distinct cell lines, the stromal cell line and the hemopoietic system. Stromal cells include osteoblasts, reticular and endothelial cells of the sinusoidal vessels in the marrow cavity, and the adipocytes of marrow which are a sub-line of fibroblastic cells (25,26). The osteoclast is a product of one of the cell lines of the hemopoietic system and is derived from a hemopoietic stem cell. These two cell families depend on each other in their proliferation and differentiation (27). There is concurrent participation of many different cells and structures in the excessive activity in "Pagetic" bone. This could result from transmission of abnormal information originating in the sick osteoclasts, through the cytokines that are otherwise responsible for the maintenance of a normal "ecological" equilibrium in bone (28). The disease could be a self-amplifying process that starts from a single abnormal osteoclast but slowly extends over all cell families and over an increasing portion of the affected bone. It is surmised that osteoclasts can perpetuate themselves through cyclic loss of older nuclear material and fusion with new pre-osteoclasts (27). Despite rapid turnover of nuclear material, the cell would constitute a permanent reservoir of pathogenetic material, and the virus would be transmitted by continuity over ever larger osteoclast populations. The importance of cell-cell interaction for the maintenance of functional equilibrium within the bone ecosystem, could also explain why therapies, specifically directed against osteoclasts, may succeed in gradual spontaneous restoration of normal activity in all other cell systems as well.

Radiodiagnostics: scintigraphy and radiography

Paget's disease can be detected in the course of a radiological evaluation for bone pain, or by accident, during radiologic examinations for other reasons, or in the course of an attempt to explain an ill understood elevation of the serum alkaline phosphatase level. Patients who are referred to specialist centres however, generally have symptoms (3). The first step is then to identify other bones that may be affected. This is best done with scintigraphy. Paget's disease may involve any bone, even the metatarsals and phalanges, the patella, and avulsed bone fragments, but it has a predilection for the axial skeleton. The pelvis (65%), spine (42%), mainly lumbar(33%), sacrum (30%), femur (37%), tibia (37%) and skull (29%) are commonly affected, followed by the humerus (13%), scapula (12%), foot (9%), rib (8%), sternum (7%), forearm/hand (5%) and clavicle (5%) (29,30). The scintigraphic technique not only obviates the necessity of making multiple radiographs, it is also a more sensitive method: 16 to 31% of lesions are only visible on the scintigram and not on radiographs (30). The greater sensitivity is only partly connected with the problem of correct radiographic evaluation of bones like scapula, sternum, clavicles or ribs. More important is an essential difference between the two techniques: radiology reflects morphological, and scintigraphy dynamic changes in the bone. There is confirmation that abnormalities which are only demonstrable on a scintigram, are associated with microscopic anomalies in the bone marrow biopsy (30,32); such areas were also demonstrated peripheral to macroscopically involved bone (34,35). Scintigraphic lesions, only visible on scintigrams may therefore be early lesions. The fraction of positive lesions that are not visible on radiographs, is considerably higher for bones that are not commonly affected (30) and these could represent slowly developing lesions. This might depend on local factors in the bone like the proportion of bone marrow and osteoclasts available for propagation of the disease.

TABLE I: *Number of affected bones and percentage of the skeleton affected by the disease in patients with Paget's disease of bones, and the relation with Serum Alkaline Phosphatase (AP), Urine Hydroxyprolin (OHP), and Turnover of Radiolabelled Calcium (A5). From: Harinck et al, 1986 (3).*

Percentage of patients (in percentiles)	Number of bones	Percentage of skeleton	AP (Bessey U)	OHP (μmol/day)	A5 (mmol/day)
0	0	0	45	150	10
5	1	2	90	300	20
10	1	4	130	400	22
25	1	5	160	500	25
50	2	10	270	800	50
75	3	20	350	1200	100
90	5	30	800	3000	150
95	75	50	1500	4000	250

* Normal values: AP < 60 U ; OHP < 250 μmol/day ; A5 < 15 mmol/day

The intensity of radionuclide uptake in a lesion can be measured. It is interesting that there is a significant correlation between the result of this measurement and the degree of radiological involvement of the same lesion (30). The correlation is intriguing because uptake of the scanning agent Tc-99m-Sn-EHDP would be a function of local bone turnover rather than of microscopic texture. The answer is provided by the results of efficacious treatment (30,36-38). Such treatment can reduce uptake by some 80%, a fraction that is therefore due to metabolic activity. The remaining 20% excessive uptake in lesions that are in remission can be ascribed to a persistent anomaly of the structure of the hard tissue. The major source of activity in untreated patients however is due to cellular activity. This is also reflected in quantitative variations in isotopic uptake within single lesions. Maldague and Malghem (39) and Nagant (40) described an area of subtle radiologic changes ahead of areas of advanced Paget's disease in long bones, calling the respective lesions the primary and secondary fronts. Vellenga et al (29,30) demonstrated the scintigraphic counterpart of the secondary front as a band of intensive uptake, and the region of beginning transformation in the primary front, as only slight elevation of uptake, but with a sharply defined boundary.

The scintigraphic technique has not only been used to identify and count affected bones. The technique was also applied to measure the diseased fraction of a bone and to multiply this fraction with the fraction of the whole skeleton occupied by that bone. The result evaluates the fractional, or the percentage spread of disease over the skeleton. Such data are useful for comparison with biochemical abnormalities, which also represent integrals. We found that in one quarter of the patients with Paget's disease, less than 5 percent of the total bone is affected, in half of the patients 10 percent at most, and in one quarter more than 20 percent. Involvement of more than 50 % of the skeleton is extremely rare (3,30) (Table I). The table "translates" the data into biochemical measurements and gives a feeling for the meaning of the latter.

The cornerstone for diagnosis and for the assessment of prognosis are radiographs of the affected bones. Many early and more recent reports and textbooks have been dedicated to reviewing the radiological descriptions of Paget's disease (2,39,42-48).The first cellular event in the disease takes place in the osteoclast (22,42); just so, the earliest radiological change is a decrease in the density of bone (35,42,44.50). In older lesions, local disturbances in the equilibrium between bone formation and bone resorption become apparent as a mixture of "osteosclerotic" and "osteolytic" lesions, and mixed lesions with very irregular patterns. Transitions from one to another pattern have often been described (42,45,46,50,52) and the generally accepted view that these radiological patterns represent stages in the evolution of the disease (53) may not invariably be true. In 107 patients we found no differences in metabolic activity between the different radiological types, and in particular, the sclerotic lesions that are sometimes considered as "burned out" (52,53), possessed the same activity as lytic and mixed lesions (30). Often the pattern of distribution may remain quite stable, while the deformation of the bone as a whole progresses (39,48). This becomes enlarged and deformed. The cortical bone can be dense and thickened but is usually permeated by lamellar or cyst-like spaces, that blur the endosteal margin (35). The condition does not pass from one bone to an adjacent one, unless there is already a bony bridge.

Two of these radiologic phenomena are of particular importance because these in particular, are associated with an increased fracture risk. These are cyst like lytic lesions that may interrupt the continuity of cortical bone, and Looser's zones, often in and perpendicular to the convex side of the cortex of tubular bones (54). The perpendicular nature of the pseudo fracture heralds the typical transverse fractures that occur in "Pagetic" long bones.

Details of the changes in bone morphology are characteristic for the particular bone that is affected and explain much of the specific symptoms of individuals. The details of the morphology should be studied in the relevant reviews.

Calcium metabolism, and serum and urine chemistry

Although only a small fraction of the skeleton is affected, this has unexpectedly large consequences for calcium metabolism. The serum calcium level is normal, but the constancy of this level can be likened to the constancy of a river level, despite an increased current. Bone-turnover, that is the in- and output of calcium in the bone, is for healthy persons in the order of 400 mg (10 mmoles) per day (55). Quantitative scintigraphy of lesions in Paget's disease does already suggest that the local turnover of calcium is largely increased, occasionally more than a hundred-fold (30). The contribution from a small diseased fraction of the skeleton to the total calcium turnover may therefore be large. Table I shows that the total turnover of calcium in patients with Paget's disease, measured with a radioactive isotope of calcium, may already be more than doubled when only 10 percent of the skeleton is affected (3,56). This makes patients more vulnerable by conditions that affect bone metabolism. In more severe Paget's disease, immobilisation hypercalcemia may develop to an excessive degree (2,4). Bone formation and resorption may roughly be in equilibrium, this equilibrium is not absolute. Local lesions in bone may show either excess formation or excess resorption. Urine calcium shows wider variations than normal and there is a greater than normal incidence of renal stone disease and of normo- and hypercalcemic hyperparathyroidism (3,4,57,59).

The increase in bone turnover may not be readable in the serum calcium level, it is in the serum alkaline phosphatase (AP) and in the urinary excretion of hydroxyproline (OHP). Part of the alkaline phosphatase in the serum is produced by bone-forming cells (60), and urine hydroxyproline comes partly from bone collagen (61). These are parameters of the rate of bone formation and bone resorption, respectively. They are increased in Paget's disease, in direct proportion to each other and to the increase in calcium turnover (2,3,4). They are also increased in proportion to the amount of skeletal tissue affected by the disease, but in addition to that, variations in intensity of bone disease per unit volume of bone tissue, will influence their levels (3,18). Individual values may therefore largely deviate from the averages given in Table I.

The value of AP and OHP in the assessment of the severity of the disease is only relative in that they mainly reflect the extent of involvement of the skeleton. Even so, some lesions, like those in the skull, seem to be associated with higher values than others (3,4,60,62). The large value of AP and OHP reside in that they are the means par excellence for the objective monitoring of the effects of therapy. The observation that AP and OHP are elevated in proportion pertains to their use in assessment of bone turnover in a *steady state*. The rates of bone formation and bone resorption may change differently when manipulated by drugs or altered by disease. This is particularly pertinent to the *transient state* that is obtained while Paget's disease is still reacting to drug treatment. The rates of change of OHP and AP are then so different, that AP cannot replace OHP in the initial assessment of the degree of response to treatment (3,14,15,63).

Osteocalcin (or bone Gla protein) is a non-collagenous protein of bone which is bound to the bone mineral through the carboxyl residues contained in Gla (64). A fraction of it, believed to be derived from new protein synthesis (65), is found in the circulation and can be measured in the serum. Serum osteocalcin levels may therefore provide a sensitive marker of bone metabolic activity. These levels have indeed been found elevated in conditions with increased bone turnover and a close relation between osteocalcin and the rate of bone formation has been reported (64,66,67). In Paget's disease however, serum osteocalcin is increased, but the levels do not vary in proportion to the variation of AP and OHP - they do indeed lag behind, suggesting defective production (68,69). They recuperate upon effective treatment and may initially rise, when OHP and AP decline (69). It appears that the functions of osteocalcin and AP as well as their initial expression by osteoblasts are different, and that this difference may reflect the failing quality of new bone formed in Paget's disease.

Epidemiological aspects

The prevalence of Paget's disease is 3 to 4 percent in Great Britain as estimated by radiology (2). This recent estimate is quite similar to a German estimate from 1932, which was based on post mortem examinations (34). There is however a wide geographical variation as well as a relation with age in the reported prevalence (2). Symptomatic patients are as a rule over 35 years of age and from then on the prevalence, corrected for population density, doubles every decade, with a male to female ratio of 3:2 at all ages (2,3).

The numbers given in Table I do not pertain to gradations of severity of the disease *within* patients, but stress the large dissimilarity in severity that is found *between* patients. The patient whom sir James Paget described (70), the man with curved, foreshortened stature, bowed legs, slightly waggling gait, arms long relative to the shortened rump, and a large skull with deep eyes, but with an intelligent look that remained unaffected until the end - belongs to the 5 % of very rare cases. The fear of some patients with only one or two lesions, that their disease might develop in that direction, is entirely unfounded. The anatomical distribution of the disease remains largely unchanged throughout life. The handicap that may threaten the individual is solely determined by the damage caused by the relentless, predictable progression of the lesions within those bones that are affected at the time of diagnosis, and the particular number and combination of lesions in that patient (4,41,42).

TABLE II: *Occurrence of pain, neurological symptoms or fractures according to location of Paget's disease. From ref.: (3).*

Skeletal Region	Bones with symptoms as fraction and (%) of affected bones	
Tibia	33/56	(59)
Mandibula	2/4	(50)
Lumbar spine	26/56	(46)
Radius	5/12	(42)
Hemipelvis	58/149	(39)
Skull	19/51	(37)
Femur	29/85	(34)
Humerus	6/35	(17)
Scapula	4/31	(13)
Sacrum	6/46	(13)
Thoracic spine	6/49	(12)
Other bones	2/106	(2)
Counted in 180 patients		

There is an interesting aspect to that number of lesions, compatible with the hypothesis that Paget's disease is caused by a fortuitous capture of a virus in an osteoclast during a period of exposure to the infectious agent. Of all patients, 65 percent have more than one lesion. Of all those who have at least two lesions, only 65 percent have more than two, and so on. If the chance that an osteoclast is hit during a period of exposure is 65%, hitting an osteoclast will not reduce the chance for other osteoclasts to be affected, this will remain 65 %. These data also mean that the real incidence of exposure to the pathogenic agent will have been 1.5 times as high as the prevalence of the disease suggests (3). Table I ranges patients in percentiles according to the number of affected bones per patient.

Data on the fractional probability that a bone is affected also support the hypothesis (22,71) of a single exposure in time to a circulating virus. There is an interesting problem here. Usually investigators count relative numbers of patients with affection of a given bone, but not all patients have the same number of lesions. To get the fractional probability, one should divide the frequency per bone by the sum-total of affected bones in all patients, not by the number of patients. The fractional distribution so obtained by Harinck *et al* accords well with the fractional volume of the given bone, but some bones were over-represented (3). These were the vertebral column, the pelvis and the sacrum, all bones with an exceptionally high proportion of spongious tissue (In a long bone Paget's disease starts much more often in the spongious metaphysis, than in the cortical diaphyseal bone). It is interesting that the resulting fractional probability is similar to the relative probability of a bone being affected from hematogenous bacterial osteomyelitis (72). All of this supports the hypothesis of a viral origin. As one would now expect, there is no difference between right and left side of the body, neither do age or sex influence the distribution. An information that seems not to accord with the previous is, that within individuals progression of disease in similar bones on the right and left side of the body is generally dissimilar (3).

The tendency to pathological fracture has already been mentioned. The fracture rate is estimated at 6.6 per 100 patient years, and fractures occur generally in femur, tibia, humerus or spine (73). Typical is that the fractures are often transverse. Fracturing is usually preceded by local pain and tenderness, probably due to transverse pseudo-fractures, but such pseudo-fractures may long remain symptom-less. Pathological fractures are usually associated with poor prognosis, unless proper treatment is instituted for the disease (2).

The incidence and nature of osteosarcoma complicating Paget's disease has been reviewed by Hamdy (2). The incidence, 1-3 %, of osteosarcoma is more than ten fold higher than the incidence of osteosarcoma in the population in general, although the incidence of Paget's disease in osteosarcoma, 5 %, does not seem larger. A rapidly enlarging, excruciating painful lytic lesion must be suspect. The prognosis is poor; one half of the patients have lung metastases at the time of discovery (29,74,76).

TABLE III: *Relationship between percentage involvement of bones and occurrence of pain, deformity, or fracture. From: Harinck et al, 1986 (3).*

| | \multicolumn{6}{c}{Percentage of bones with pain, deformity, or fracture} |
	Long bones		Skull		Hemipelvis	
Percentage involvement	≤50	>50	≤50	>50	≤75	>75
No. of affected bones	90	101	24	27	32	117
Pain †	8	*** 61	12	* 37	6	** 24
Severe deformity	3	*** 38		*** 41	--	--
Fracture	1	** 11	--	--	3	2

† Pain associated with arthritis is not included, $*p≤0.05$; $**p≤0.01$; $***p≤0.001$

Symptoms and prognosis in the individual

In the past, fracture was the major symptom for which patients could get help. It is only since the advent of effective therapy that attention can be given to the less sudden complications of Paget's disease. In our own population, fracture counted as the presenting symptom in only about 8 %, a figure that is not significantly different from the yearly fracture rate per 100 patients. Like others, we found pain to be the presenting symptom in 80 to 90 percent of patients (3,4,60,62,77,78). In half this was bone pain attributable to the disease, in the other half it was probably linked with complications due to deformity or complicating osteoarthritis. Only 8 percent had neurological complications; in the largest majority this was deafness, associated with Paget's disease of the skull. We have already mentioned that the complaints often had a disastrous effect on the professional abilities of untreated patients (3).

Metabolic complications are rare. We have by now seen several hundreds of patients, but only once a clinically relevant high-output heart failure. The most interesting general complications are still those of calcium metabolism, mentioned in the previous paragraph. These metabolic complications are seldom severe in relation to the handicap caused by the local bone disease. We should therefore call this a disease of bones, like Paget did, and not of bone, as has become use.

The particular anatomical distribution of the disease is one significant determinant of morbidity, the extent of involvement the other (Tables II & III). Table II shows how often a particular bone is affected, but also how often affection of a particular bone occasions symptoms. These two are quite different elements. Involvement of the yaw is for instance rare, but two of the four mandibular lesions we have seen caused severe complaints. Lesions in the long bones that are weight bearing, but also those in the radius, which is important for finely tuned manipulation, caused disability. Lumbar vertebral lesions are particularly important when multiple, and cause low back pain in half of the affected patients. Pelvic lesions are mainly important for the definite association with secondary arthritis of the hip joint in one quarter of the cases (3,62,77). One should not forget the consequences for the knee joint of the bowing of femur or tibia. Irreversible hearing loss (in 20%) and headache are typical for skull involvement, much less frequent are cranial nerve palsies and affection of the base of the skull. Hypervascularity of affected bones may cause the relative ischemia of the steel syndrome. When this occurs in a leg, it can affect walking distance. In the skull this can cause headache, and also, but rarely, mental dys-function. All of the vascular symptoms are reversible with effective therapy. Joint damage and neurological damage are irreversible. It is however possible that acute nerve compression develops, caused by edema associated with vertebral disease, compressing vertebral nerve roots (16,78). This is sensitive to medical treatment, but if one can risk delaying early decompression is a difficult decision. Finally, one should not underestimate the cosmetic effects of enlargement of the skull or of the antecurvation of the tibia, the skin problems associated with the latter, and the typical gait associated with the outwards bowing of the femur (70).

The magnificent radiological studies of Maldague have shown how insistent and relentless the slow progression is of Paget's disease in affected bones (41). The slowness of the process makes it difficult to decide when a lesion becomes a risk. It will probably be too late, when this is evident. Once adequate therapy will be available, the extent of the lesion, and the knowledge of the particular risk associated with the presence of disease or deformation in a given bone, will have to determine if one interferes or not. Therapy directed against the disease will be unable to affect complications. Lost gross quality of bone and large deformations cannot be undone. Late therapies will merely affect the pain due to the local inflammatory process and the associated edema, but never the incurred damage. Prevention will prevent both, further extension and development of the process, and the complications.

TREATMENT

Treatment recommendations should be formulated by comparing the risk of the untreated disease with the efficacy, safety, cost and convenience of therapy or prevention. The best that the generally available calcitonin and bisphosphonate treatments can achieve is a significant reduction in the severity of symptomatic disease. These treatments can often significantly alter the biochemical parameters of disease, but it has not nearly been so clear that uniform and more permanent clinical benefit resulted. Indications have hitherto been restricted to symptomatic bone pain, neurologic complications, impending orthopedic surgery and active disease in young patients. The objectives of the generally available therapies are therefore similar and a discussion of treatment usually centres around comparing the properties, advantages and disadvantages of calcitonin and etidronate (80). Clinical research has however advanced beyond the boundaries of mere suppression of symptoms. We should therefore, in the future interest of patients, not organize this section around available means alone, but rather structure it around the various possible aims that have now come into scope. The present discussion is limited to the three bone resorption inhibitory drug families, the calcitonins, mithramycin and the bisphosphonates. Older treatments with fluoride, aspirin, steroids or radiotherapy can be considered obsolete.

Short-term efficacy

The common denominator of the three drugs is their ability to inhibit osteoclastic bone resorption (81-84). Inhibition of osteoclastic bone resorption in Paget's disease is invariably followed by secondary abatement of the associated hyperactivity of all other cell systems. It is interesting that local hyperemia and edema seem even to react quite early. Within days or weeks the hyperthermia above a bone lesion resolves. The suppressive effect on hypervascularity of bone justifies treatment in advance of orthopedic surgery; improvement in nerve palsy, ataxia, myelopathy with spastic paralysis, and paraplegia have been noted with calcitonin as well as with bisphosphonate therapy, and may be due to the resolution of local edema (16,95,86). Unless the therapeutic agent has in itself a direct action on mineralizing bone, the histological structure of the bone that is formed following the start of treatment, changes from a woven to a more normal, lamellar pattern. This is true for calcitonin as well as for bisphosphonates (15,87,88). This improvement of structure can be visible in special radiographs of details of the skeletal structure, especially in lytic areas (11,39,41). The effects of calcitonin and bisphosphonates on bone pain are somewhat different. Calcitonin may cause an immediate and dramatic reduction of intractable bone pain (7), but more usually pain relief starts within two to six weeks; if it is not relieved by eight weeks, it is unlikely to remit (2). With the bisphosphonates, the reduction of pain is delayed for a few days to weeks and there may even be a slight, initial pain increase, a few days after the beginning of treatment (13,15,90). The rapid action of calcitonin could be a direct one at the level of the central nervous system.

The calcitonins

Calcitonin was first used in Paget's disease two decades ago (7,8). Many studies have since shown early biochemical and clinical improvement of treated patients (7-11,14,91-98). The biochemical response is on the whole incomplete. On the average the excess of serum AP and urine OHP decreases by 50 %; this maximum suppression is reached after several months. There is an interesting difference between calcitonin and the bisphosphonates, with respect to the kinetics of these changes. With calcitonin there is an early decrease of serum AP, of bone uptake of radio-labeled calcium, and type I procollagen also shows an early decrease, together with OHP, while with the bisphosphonates, when not applied in extreme doses, AP, calcium uptake and procollagen remain initially unaffected (15,16,63,99-101). This suggests a direct inhibitory effect on osteoblastic activity, particular to calcitonin. Calcitonin can dramatically decrease the clinical symptoms, but they seldom disappear. In about half of the patients AP and OHP tend to drift back during treatment. Although antibodies against calcitonin appear, the presence of antibodies is not correlated with biochemical or clinical resistance (102). In those in whom partial suppression of biochemical values is maintained, these will return to pre-treatment levels within a few months after arrest of treatment, though the clinical effect can be maintained for many months longer (97). High quality radiographs of lytic areas in Pagetic bone show an impressive tendency to improve and the lytic lesions sometimes disappear during the treatment, but they recur after calcitonin arrest (41,103).

On the whole, calcitonin treatment might seem indicated when one desires a rapid clinical effect to be obtained within days. The response varies between patients and the longer the duration of treatment, the more difficult it becomes to monitor the therapy, and the greater the likelihood of resistance. In many cases the treating physician and the patient are left in a state of considerable uncertainty. The drug is administered in doses between 50 - 200 MRC units daily, along the subcutaneous route. Side effects, nausea and flushing, can be cumbersome in a minority. The reduction in bone turnover achieved with calcitonin varies considerably between individuals although it seems not to depend on initial disease activity (104). As a consequence it is difficult to define the optimum dose schedule for this agent (105). Very small doses, in the region of 50 MRC units per week, are clearly insufficient (106) and although 50 MRC units thrice weekly was found to be the minimum effective dose in one study, others have suggested that twice this dose is more appropriate (10,96). A choice of 100 MRC units thrice weekly combines a large, but generally well tolerated dose, with the convenience of relatively infrequent injections. It achieves a 40 to 50 % reduction in AP and OHP comparable to that reported from most large series, some of which used higher or more frequent doses (10, 94-96,102,104). Clinical efficacy has recently been reported with nasal inhalation of calcitonin. In the United States calcitonin is still widely used for this indication (107). In countries where the newer bisphosphonates are available, like in the Netherlands, its use has become rare.

Mithramycin

The antibiotic drug mithramycin has cytotoxic properties (108). It binds to DNA and prevents RNA synthesis (109). Short 10 day intravenous courses of 15 - 25 µg per day cause a rapid inhibition of bone resorption, but also of serum alkaline phosphatase, presumably due to bone toxicity. It gives pain relief, sometimes within 4 - 5 days (78). There should be real concern about the possibility of kidney, liver and thrombocyte toxicity after repeat administration. Remissions have however been prolonged for many months (109,110). The use of mithramycin should only be considered when a rapid suppression of acute symptoms is needed in a very short time, and when this cannot be achieved with other means. This situation should hardly ever occur.

Bisphosphonates

The bisphosphonates have now been around in clinical medicine for one and a half decade (84). They may well develop into one of the major therapeutic agents in metabolic bone disease. Paget's disease is the indication in which the longest and most detailed experience has been obtained, but their bone resorption inhibitory potency is now also profitably used in the treatment of hypercalcemia of malignancy and in paraneoplastic bone disease (111-119).

Three bisphosphonates are currently used for the treatment of bone disease: Disodium Etidronate (EHDP), Disodium Clodronate (Cl_2MDP), developed by Fleisch and Francis (84), who discovered the therapeutic potential of the bisphosphonates, and APD, an analogue which was developed in our unit (120-128). APD is disodium,(3-amino-1-hydroxy-propylidene)-1,1-bisphosphonate. The inhibitory action of the bisphosphonates on bone resorption requires prior chemisorption to the calcified bone matrix (124-186). This chemisorption is achieved through the P-C-P bond, which these bisphosphonates have in common, the two phosphonate groups of which join in forming complexes with free calcium or in the chemisorption to the hydroxyl-apatite of the matrix (84). The high affinity of bisphosphonates for the bone calcium is exploited in scintigraphy to localize bisphosphonate bound tracer in bone areas with increased calcium uptake. Phosphonate bonds are not hydrolyzable.

The other two valencies of the carbon molecule are occupied by chlorine in Cl_2MDP. Both, EHDP and APD, on the other hand, have one OH-group that participates in the chemisorption to mineral. The fourth residue varies between the bisphosphonates, of which there are now many. This residue is probably more important for biological properties, specific to particular bisphosphonates, than the P-C-P group itself (124,129). When one adds for instance, different bisphosphonates to cell culture media, their biological effects vary unpredictably(129). When these bisphosphonates are however given to a live animal, they all cause the serum calcium to decrease and histological as well as radiological studies, combined with metabolic balance studies, have shown that this is due to an inhibition of bone resorption (84,121). The bisphosphonates differ in molar potency, but studies *in-vivo* as well as in *in-vitro* model systems have also discovered qualitative differences. Etidronate, the bisphosphonate for which the inhibitory action on bone resorption was first established, does for instance at the same time exert a significant inhibitory effect on the mineralization of newly formed bone matrix (88,90,130-134). APD and clodronate don't share the last property (84,121,122).

The differences between the bisphosphonates may even extend to the mechanism by which these substances inhibit bone resorption (124). This mechanism is not well understood. There are indications that clodronate is cytotoxic for osteoclasts that ingest it together with the resorbed mineral. APD on the other hand seems to act merely by preventing the recognition of the bone matrix by osteoclast precursors, as well as by the mature osteoclasts (124-126). This may in part explain the paradox that soon after the initiation of resorption inhibition, when there is also a secondary rise of parathyroid hormone levels in the serum, the number of osteoclasts is in-, rather than decreased (121). Relative to the two other bisphosphonates, APD has also an increased potency against bone resorption. Analogues of APD with longer side chains have been made, aminobutane and aminohexane, which have comparable properties. Aminobutane is definitely more potent than APD, but clinical information on the newer compounds is scarce (129,135). The properties of the amino-bisphosphonates can be again improved considerably by retaining the nitrogen but replacing its hydrogens with carbon. The simplest of such substances, (3-dimethylamino-1-hydroxypropylidene)-1,1-bisposphonate, Me_2APD, is almost completely non-toxic in *in-vitro* cell cultures, while its anti resorption potency and its specificity against bone recognition by osteoclasts is considerably increased (125). The substance is mentioned because results of its clinical application will be cited, to indicate a possible direction in which future bisphosphonate therapy in Paget's disease develops.

Etidronate

The bisphosphonate etidronate is widely available. It is usually administered orally; the recommended dose is between 5 and 10 mg/kg/day. As with calcitonin, treatment induces significant suppression of both symptoms and biochemical indices of disease activity, which may be sustained for many months after stopping treatment (16,17). Also similar is the considerable variation in the reduction of disease activity which can be achieved with a given dose of etidronate (105,131,132,136-141). This may reflect variations in susceptibility of bone cells and in drug absorption, although the major determinant of local uptake in bone is the local turnover, as is evident from bisphosphonate scintigraphy. Early studies suggested that there was a dose related reduction in bone turnover, but subsequent experience suggested that all doses between 5 and 20 mg/kg/day produce similar reductions in disease activity if results are assessed after 3 to 6 months, although doses of 20 mg work more rapidly (16,17,102,104,139). In contrast with calcitonin the biochemical response, once it is obtained, continues after arrest of treatment for periods up to two years in 50 % of patients. The duration of this biochemical response is significantly related to the measure of suppression of the biochemical indices.

Doses, higher than those recommended, but also smaller doses, commonly impair mineralization of bone, may be associated with increased bone pain, and may increase the risk of pathological fractures. The proportion of patients responding however, that is with a larger than 25 % reduction in total AP, decreases markedly from 95 to 70 % with reduction of the six monthly dose from 20 to 10 mg (16,17). Prolongation of treatment with etidronate may induce a time dependent further fall in disease activity, but this too increases the risk of defective mineralization and the bone pain syndrome. Because of this, there is interest in short intravenous treatments with higher doses (140,141), but there are yet insufficient long term data on this mode. The effect of etidronate induced osteomalacia on fracture risk has been disputed, because the incidence of fracture seems not to be less than in untreated patients. Fractures do however continue to occur, even in patients treated with low dose (73,138,142). The absence of fracture after treatment with the second generation bisphosphonates APD and clodronate should settle the dispute (15,143).

Both, radiological healing and deterioration of lytic lesions, have been seen with etidronate. Deterioration was seen in one study in half of the lytic areas, and healing in only one fifth. These radiological phenomena were unrelated with the biochemical response, but their development was usually arrested when the treatment was stopped; healing was often delayed. Deterioration did mainly occur in pre-existing Pagetic lesions, but blade like lytic lesions also appeared in normal cortical bone (39,40,89). Etidronate therefore has roughly the same biochemical efficacy as calcitonin. It has the two advantages of oral administration and prolonged biochemical response, but the disadvantages for the quality of bone are considerable and etidronate may sometimes worsen, rather than improve the condition of the patient.

The failure to control disease activity, even with large doses of etidronate, together with the high incidence of serious side effects led to the use of calcitonin and etidronate in combination. The use in combination has consistently produced significantly greater suppression than etidronate or calcitonin singly, and has recently been confirmed in a controlled study. Once combination therapy is withdrawn the combination retains the advantage obtained during treatment (56,105). Combination with calcitonin seems not to prevent the radiologic deterioration typical for etidronate (41).

Predictability and completeness of response and remission

The "second generation" bisphosphonates

The introduction to this section mentioned two bisphosphonates, APD and clodronate that do not affect mineralization. Clodronate has a potency against bone resorption, roughly equivalent to that of etidronate, but the clinical dose response relation has not yet been studied adequately (143,148). APD has a tenfold higher anti-resorptive potency (15,121,124). In animals it has been shown to impair mineralization, but at doses higher than those needed to obtain the anti-osteoclastic effect (121). Both drugs have been investigated in Paget's disease for more than a decade. APD is the one that has been the most extensively investigated in Paget's disease (15,38,41,59,63,69,89,101,117,120,128,137,146). This drug will soon become more generally available; it is desirable to summarize the data, because the importance of these second generation bisphosphonates does not reside in a mere increase in potency. They offer a fundamental change of the therapeutic perspective, justifying discussion under the the heading predictability and completeness of response and remission.

One can now achieve a complete biochemical and clinical response in over 90 percent of the patients, together with a full suppression of disease activity (15,128,146). This response is associated with disappearance of hyperemia and edema in and around lesions within weeks, and a gradual, but marked loss of bone pain, in so far as pain is due to the disease and not to secondary arthritis. These results are obtained with treatments of very short duration (146). With adequate initial monitoring, on an out-patient basis, the patient can be treatment free within a few weeks. Unlike etidronate these effects are obtained without disturbing bone mineralization, but together with improvement of bone structure. This has been documented with histological, radiological, and with biochemical observations.

Bone biopsies document normalization of cell numbers, together with a reduction, rather than an increase in osteoid (15,63). Radiology has established for APD, that improvement in bone structure is obtained as seen with calcitonin, especially in lytic lesions, and with absence of the deterioration of structure that has been found with etidronate. In contrast to calcitonin, the improvements with APD are sustained after treatment arrest (29,41,89,128). The third evidence is that early suppression of bone resorption, without direct suppression of mineralization, causes bone balance to become initially positive to values around 400 mg per day, roughly equal to the calcium absorbed from the gut (63). This is associated with a decrease in serum and urine calcium, and a rise in serum concentrations of parathyroid hormone and of 1.25 dihydroxy-vitamin D (59,147). The phenomenon is significantly less or quasi absent when etidronate is given intravenously in doses high enough to mimic the effects of the third generation bisphosphonates on bone resorption (148).

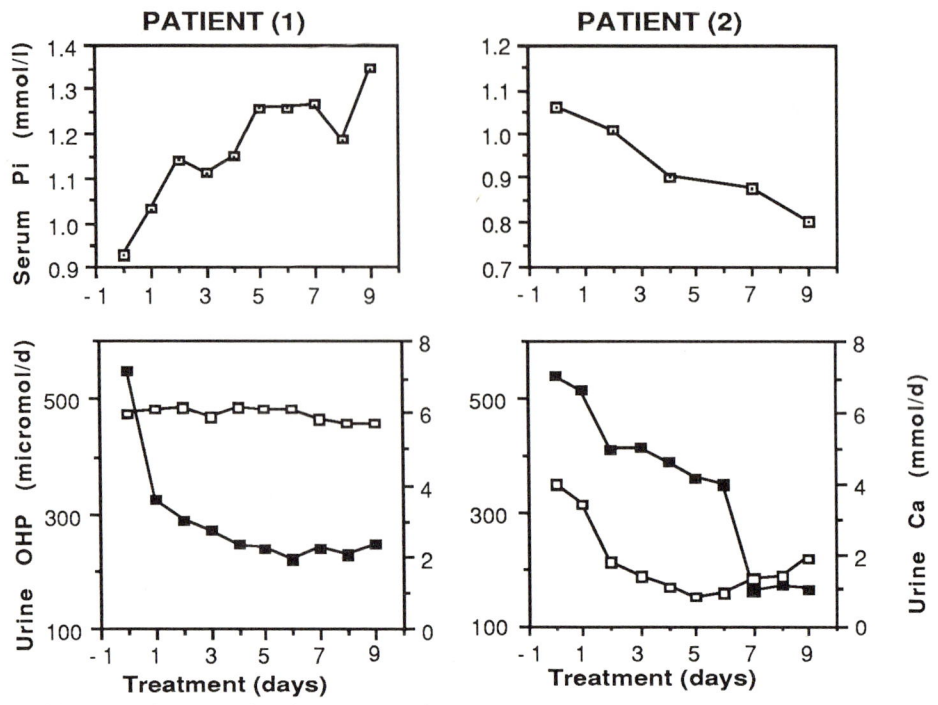

FIG. 1. Sequential changes in serum phosphate concentration and in the urinary excretion of hydroxyproline (closed squares) and calcium (open squares) in two patients with Paget's disease, receiving slow daily infusions of 30 mg APD.

We should at this point caution against infusing patients with extreme doses of APD (116,117). We have found in Paget's disease, that the rate of decrease of urine calcium decreased considerably, while the rate of decrease of urine OHP was maintained, in some but not in all patients, when APD was intravenously infused at daily doses of 30 mg (fig. 1). In addition to that, the usual decrease in serum phosphate as a sign of parathyroid stimulation was replaced by an increase in serum phosphate. These signs, which are in evidence within 48 hours, are quite similar to effects of intravenous etidronate, and like Kanis' group we attribute them to an impairment of mineralization (148). Obviously the phenomenon was not further investigated since this may start a dose range that causes damaging actions on bone. In patients with hypercalcemia of malignancy in whom bone formation is not increased the phenomenon is probably less clear.

The definition of remission is again different from that used for the calcitonins or etidronate. Remission means here a complete absence of clinical and biochemical disease activity together with arrest of radiological progression in the absence of further therapy. The end of remission is defined as any sustained increase in AP or OHP, of whatever small degree. Actuarial analysis has shown that 50 % of patients are still in complete remission after 18 months and in 30 % the remission lasts for four years or more (15,146). Recurrence is always slow and can be monitored by a single yearly determination of serum AP, or by the patient when he feels that pain tends to recur. The duration of remission is definitely associated with the degree of the suppression of OHP *into* the normal range that has been achieved at the end of the initial treatment phase. This means that care in initial monitoring will not be wasted (15,146).

Measurement of OHP, rather than of AP, should be used for monitoring the necessary duration of treatment. Reitsma *et al* have shown in animal studies, and Frijlinck *et al* in patients, that the first event after inhibition of bone resorption is a decrease in urine OHP, while AP remains unchanged (121,15,63). Normalization of bone formation is an entirely secondary event and it takes 3 to 6 months before the equilibrium between bone formation and resorption is again established at the lower, now normal rate. In the transient intervening period the bone balance is strongly positive. The enlarged consumption of calcium by the bone drains calcium from the circulation and secondary elevation of parathyroid hormone and 1.25 dihydroxy vitamin D levels mediate an associated increase of calcium absorption from the gut (59,147). It is interesting that symptomatic hypocalcemia is extremely rare. We have found that PTH may partly reverse the effect of APD on osteoclasts (126). This may perhaps account for this protection against hypocalcemia.

Scintigraphy can register effects of treatment, although quantitative evaluation, which is cumbersome, should then be applied. It is important to mention the technique because effective treatment is not associated with disappearance of all excessive uptake into lesions. On the average around 20 % of the initial excess uptake persists, which may be due to structural abnormalities in the calcified matrix (38). These 20 % may be enough to cause confusion between activity and remission.

The effect of the bisphosphonate on osteoclasts is the only one needed for therapeutic efficacy. It has been demonstrated that the short and long term effects of treatment are not different, wether treatment is continued for months, until AP has normalized, or only for weeks, until after OHP has decreased into the mid normal range (15,146). Monitoring the degree of suppression of OHP will allow assessing efficacy of treatment on the one hand, and prevent many months of superfluous drug administration, on the other.

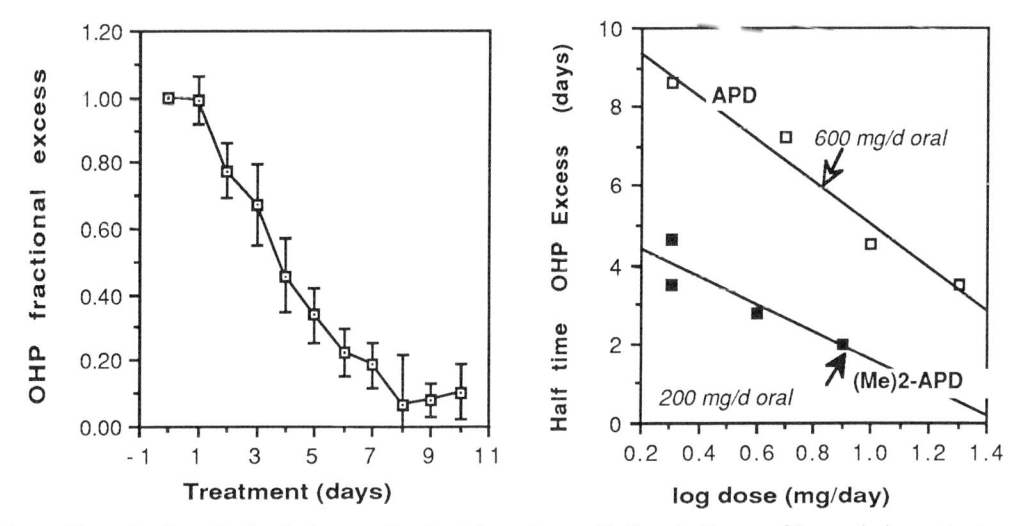

FIG. 2. LEFT: Normalization of urine hydroxyproline in eight patients with Paget's disease of bones during a short course of oral Dimethyl-APD (200 mg/day). Squares represent means ± s.e.m.
RIGHT: Log-dose effect relation for APD and Dimethyl APD, given intravenously. The effect is measured as the time needed to reduce the excess urine hydroxyproline with 50%. Effects of one oral dose level is also given for each of the bisphosphonates.

This importance of monitoring requires some methodological discussion. Monitoring early and late effects of oral and intravenous APD has shown that the rapidity of its effect on OHP is dose dependent (15). We have given ADP orally in enteric coated tablets of 150 mg at doses between 300 and 900 mg per day, and intravenous as slow, two to four hour infusions at doses between 0.5 and 30 mg daily. The slow infusion rate is a safety measure to prevent eventual formation of large calcium-bisphosphonate complexes at high concentrations that may cause organ damage. Low doses require longer treatment to achieve normalization. The first 24 hours after initiating treatment there is a small rise of OHP, but thereafter the fractional decrease of the excess bone resorption is constant for around one to two weeks, and at a given dose of bisphosphonate, the rate of decrease is the same, regardless the initial height of OHP. This implies that patients with a greatly raised OHP will require longer time to normalize (15).

This phenomenon has allowed designing a patient and observer independent model to assess drug efficacy (15,146). Efficacy can be measured as the number of days required for the excess of OHP above the mean normal value, to decrease with 50%. This is 3.5 days with 20 mg APD daily and decreases in a log-dose dependent fashion to 8.6 days at 2 mg (Fig. 2.). Oral treatment with 600 mg has an efficacy equal to 6 mg iv, confirming the low, 1% absorption found in animal studies. Oral doses of 600 mg and higher can cause gastric complaints and still higher doses, damage to the gastric mucosa. The short- and long-term effects of various treatment regimes were compared. A useful schedule is a daily infusion of 20 mg for 10 days,eventually followed by oral treatment with 300 to 600 mg daily, until urine OHP has decreased into the mid normal range (146).

Still unexplained is a series of immunologic phenomena that appear and disappear in the first treatment week with amino bisphosphonates (100,128,146). These occur only at first treatment and never with re-treatment. Half of the patients have a transient increase in body temperature exceeding 0.5 degree C. This is associated with mild flu-like symptoms and with transient hematological changes. There is a rise in granulocyte count at 24 h and a decrease in the lymphocyte count to a minimum of 68% of initial values at 3 days. All changes have reverted to baseline at 9 days. APD interferes with the accession of osteoclast precursors to bone. Since the immune cell system has an important role in the modulation of cell-cell interactions in bone, the symptoms, that look like if they represent local trapping of lymphocytes and stimulation of interleukin 1, might be due to a disturbance of steady state in cell to cell interaction, due to prevention of normal accession of osteoclast precursors to bone (124,125,128,149). Obviously they require further investigation. We have mentioned the paradoxical increase in osteoclasts during the early phase of bisphosphonate treatment. It has yet to be established if this too is a local effect, or a general one, associated with the secondary increase in PTH.

Primary and secondary resistance to bisphosphonate have occurred, although this is rare. Amongst the 5% non responders in our studies (15) are mostly patients with partial, but two with complete resistance to the drug. After relapse patients respond completely to re-treatment, although the rate of the initial decrease of OHP has occasionally tended to be somewhat reduced. The patients with primary resistance had not been previously treated with other bisphosphonates or with calcitonin.

Side effects of oral APD on the gastro-intestinal mucosa are due to irritation of the gastric mucosa due to a high local concentration. They prevent effective use of oral preparations as the sole treatment in this disease (115). It is not impossible that modification of the Galenic form of the oral drug might circumvent the problem. The problem did induce us to choose intravenous therapy as the treatment of choice. Treatment schedules have been proposed to replace the ten-day infusion course with 20 mg daily. One modification has been the use of repeated weekly APD infusions, often at doses higher than 20 mg, up to 120 mg weekly (145). It is of course possible that there are practical advantages to such an approach, although the total time needed to monitor therapy seems to in- rather than decrease. It was already mentioned that there should be concern about a possible loss with too high doses, of one of the large advantages of the second generation bisphosphonates, to improve and not to damage bone structure through the induction of osteomalacia. Carefully collected data supporting an equal benefit of these alternative approaches, over the more conservative one, have as yet to be generated.

TABLE IV: *Improvement of pain after treatment of 156 patients with Paget's disease of bone with APD. From: Harinck et al, 1986 (15).*

Nature of complaints	Number of patients with pain	Numbers according to treatment results			
		+++	++	+	0
Spontaneous pain	79	17	48	11	4
		82%		18%	
Low back pain	34	-	13	6	15
		38%		62%	
Pain with arthritis (hip/knee)	30	-	8	6	16
		27%		73%	
Pain with deformity (femur/tibia)	25	3	10	4	8
		52%		48%	

Ten out of 156 patients suffered from pain in more than one site.
+++ : disappearance of pain; ++ : marked improvement; + : moderate improvement; 0 : no change

Towards prevention

At the outset of this section it was stated that recommendations for therapy or prevention should be formulated by comparing the risk of the untreated disease with the efficacy, safety, cost and convenience of treatment. This review has shown that much has been achieved with respect to efficacy and safety since the first calcitonin treatment, only twenty years ago. There is at present no medical reason why symptomatic patients should be untreated. There are however still patients who are resistant, be it a few, and therapy is perhaps still not entirely convenient. Until more is known about mechanisms of action, pharmaco-kinetics and long term effects on normal bone is available, some prudence with respect to preventive treatment appears justified. The necessity of prevention is illustrated by table IV. The necessity of prevention is evident from the inability of treatment to undo deformations and the complications these have caused.

Developments have not stopped. Figure 2 is probably only one illustration of the on-going efforts. The Me$_2$APD, which we mentioned earlier (125) does not only deploy full efficacy along the intravenous route at doses as low as 2 to 4 mg per day. The result shows that it seems at present possible to achieve full treatment efficacy, obtaining complete remission with a short oral treatment using 200 mg daily for two weeks. Another promising feature is that the drug shows uninhibited activity in all patients with prior complete and incomplete resistance to APD. At present the knowledge of the potential risks associated with disease in particular locations, rather than the development of symptomatic disease should guide recommendations for treatment.

REFERENCES

1. Altman RD, Singer F, ed. Proceedings of the Kroc foundation symposium on Paget's disease of bone. *Arthritis Rheumatism* 1980; 23:1073-1234.
2. Hamdy RC. Paget's Disease of bone. Assessment and Management. *Endocrin Metab Series*, vol 1. Eastbourne, Great Britain, Praeger, 1981.

3. Harinck HIJ, Bijvoet OLM, Vellenga CJLR, Blanksma HJ, Frijlink WB. Relation between signs and symptoms in Paget's disease of bone. *Q J Med* 1986; 58: 133-51.
4. Nagant de Deuxchaisnes CN, Krane S. Paget's disease of bone: clinical and metabolic observations. *Medicine* 1964; 43: 233-266.
5. Rebel A, ed. Symposium Paget's disease. *Clin Orthop Rel Res*. 1987; 217: 1-170.
6. Barry HC. Paget's disease of bone. Edinburgh, Livingstone, 1969.
7. Bijvoet OLM, Jansen A. Thyrocalcitonin in Paget's disease. *Lancet* 1967; ii: 472.
8. Bijvoet OLM, Sluys Veer JD, Jansen AP. Effects of calcitonin on patients with Paget's disease, thyrotoxicosis or hypercalcemia. *Lancet* 1968; i: 876-881.
9. Woodhouse NJY, Bordier Ph, Fisher M, Joplin G, Reiner M, Kalu D, Foster J, MacIntyre I. Human calcitonin in the treatment of Paget's bone disease. *Lancet* 1971; i: 1139-1143.
10. DeRose J, Singer F, Avramides A, Flores A, Dziadiw R, Baker R, Wallach S. Response of Paget's disease to porcine and salmon calcitonins-effects of long term treatment. *Am J Med* 1974; 56 : 858-866.
11. Doyle FH, Pennock J, Greenberg PB, Joplin GF, MacIntyre I. Radiological evidence of a dose related response to long-term treatment of Paget's disease with human calcitonin. *Brit J Radiol* 1974; 47: 9-15.
12. Smith R, Russell RGG, Bishop M. Diphosphonates and Paget's disease of bone. *Lancet* 1971; i: 945-957.
13. Altman RD, Johnston CC, Khairi MRA, Willman H, Serafini AN, Sankey RR. Influence of disodium etidronate on clinical and laboratory manifestations of Paget's disease of bone (osteitis deformans). *New Engl J Med* 1973; 289: 1379-1384.
14. Hosking DJ, Bijvoet OLM. Therapeutic uses of calcitonin. In: *Endocrinology of calcium metabolism*, JA Parsons ed. New York. Raven Press. 1982; pp. 485-535.
15. Harinck HIJ, Bijvoet OLM, Blanksma HJ, Dahlinghaus-Nienhuis PJ. Efficaceous management with aminobisphosphonate (APD) in Paget's disease of bone. *Clin Orthop* 1987; 217: 79-98.
16. Kanis JA, Gray RES. Long-term follow-up observations on treatment in Paget's disease of bone. *Clin Orthop Rel Res* 1987; 217: 99-125.
17. Gray RES, Yates AJP, Preston CJ, Smith R, Russell RGG, Kanis JA. Duration of effect of oral diphosphonate therapy in Paget's disease of bone. *Quart J Med* 1987; 64: 755- 767.
18. Rasmussen H, Bordier Ph. The physiological and cellular basis of metabolic bone disease. Baltimore, Williams and Wilkins, 1974.
19. Rebel A, Basle M, Pouplard A, Malkani K, Filmon R, Lepatezour A. Bone tissue in Paget's disease of bone. *Arthritis Rheumatism* 1980; 23: 1104-1114.
20. Meunier P, Coindre J, Edouard CM, Arlot ME. Bone histomorphometry in Paget's disease. *Arthritis Rheumatism* 1980; 23: 1095-1103.
21. Rebel A, Malkini K, Baslé M. Anomalies nucléaires des osteoclastes de la maladie osseuse de Paget. *Nouv Presse Méd* 1974; 3: 1299-1301.
22. Rebel A, Malkani K, Baslé M, Bregeon Ch. Osteoclast ultrastructure in Paget's disease. *Calcif Tiss Res* 1976; 20: 187-199.
23. Baslé MF, Rebel A, Fournier JG, Russell WC, Malkani K. On the trail of paramyxoviruses in Paget's disease of bone. *Clin Orthop Rel Res* 1987; 217: 9-15.
24. Mills BG, Singer FR. Critical evaluation of viral antigen data in Paget's disease of bone. *Arthritis Rheum* 1986; 217: 16-25.
25. Owen M. Lineage of osteogenic cells and their relationship to the stromal system. In: *Bone and Mineral Research*, Annual 3. WA Peck ed. Amsterdam, Elseviers science publ. 1985 pp. 1-25
26. Nijweide PJ, Burger EH, Feyen JHM. The cells of bone: proliferation, differentiation and hormonal regulation. *Physiological Reviews* 1986; 66: 855-886.
27. Baron R, Vignery A, Horowitz M. Lymphocytes, macrophages and the regulation of bone remodelling. In: *Bone and Mineral Research*, Annual 2. WA Peck ed. Amsterdam, Elseviers science publ. 1984. pp. 175-243.
28. Raisz LG. Local and systemic factors in the pathogenesis of osteoporosis. *New Engl J Med* 1988; 318: 818 - 828.
29. Vellenga CJLR, Bijvoet OLM, Pauwels EKJ. Bone scintigraphy and radiology in Paget's disease of bone. *Amer J Physiol Imaging* 1988, in press.
30. Vellenga CJLR, Pauwels EKJ, Bijvoet OLM, Frijlink WB, Mulder JD, Hermans J. Untreated Paget's disease of bone studied by scintigraphy. *Radiology* 1984; 153: 799-805.
31. Fogelman I, Carr D. A comparison of bone scanning and radiology in the assessment of patients with symptomatic Paget's disease. *Radiology* 1974; 121: 177-183.
32. Maziéres B, Jung-Rosenfarb M, Bouteiller G, Fourine A, Arlet J. La scintigraphie osseuse dans la maladie de Paget. *Rev Rhumat* 1978; 45:311-316.
33. Wellman HN, Schauwecker D, Robb JA, Khairi MR, Johnston CC. Skeletal scintimaging and radiography in the diagnosis and management of Paget's disease. *Clin Orthop Rel Res* 1977; 127: 55-62.
34. Schmorl G. Über osteitis deformans Paget. *Virchows Arch Pathol Anat* 1932; 283: 694-751.

35. Milgram JW. Radiological and pathological assessment of the activity of Paget's disease of bone. *Clin Orthop Rel Res* 1977; 127: 43-54.
36. Vellenga CJLR. Paget's disease. In: *Bone Scintigraphy*, EKJ Pauwels, HE Schütte, WK Taconis eds. The Hague/Boston/London, Martinus Nijhoff publ. 1981 pp. 127-158.
37. Vellenga CJLR, Pauwels EKJ, Bijvoet OLM, Hosking DJ, Frijlink WB. Bone scintigraphy in Paget's disease treated with combined calcitonin and diphosphonate (EHDP). *Metab Bone Dis Rel Res* 1982; 4: 103-111.
38. Vellenga CJLR, Pauwels EKJ, Bijvoet OLM, Harinck HIJ, Frijlink WB. Quantitative bone scintigraphy in Paget's disease treated with APD. *Brit J Radiol* 1985; 58: 1165-1172.
39. Maldague B, Malghem J. Aspects radiologiques de la maladie de Paget. *J Belge Rhum Méd Phys* 1974; 29: 293-321.
40. Nagant de Deuxchaisnes Ch, Rombouts-Lindemans C, Huaux JP, Malghem J, Maldague B. Roentgenologic evaluation of the efficacy of calcitonin in Paget's disease of bone. in: *Molecular Endocrinology*. I MacIntyre, J Szelke eds. Amsterdam, Elsevier/North Holland Biomedical Press 1977; pp. 213-233.
41. Maldague B, Malghem J. Dynamic radiologic patterns of Paget's disease of bone. *Clin orthop Rel Res* 1987; 217: 126-151.
42. Brailsford JF. Paget's disease of bone; its frequency, diagnosis and complications. Brit J Radiol 1938; 11: 507-532.
43. Brailsford JF. Paget's disease of bone. *Brit J Radiol* 1954; 27: 435-442.
44. Collins DH. Paget's disease of bone: incidence and subclinical forms. *Lancet* 1956; ii: 51-57.
45. Dickson DD, Camp JD, Ghormley RK. Osteitis Deformans: Paget's disease of bone. *Radiology* 1945; 44: 449-470.
46. Gutman AB, Kasabach H. Paget's disease (osteitis deformans): analysis of 116 cases. *Am J Med Sci* 1936; 191: 361-380.
47. Edeiken J, Hodes PJ. Roentgen diagnosis of diseases of bone. In: *Golden's diagnostic radiology* (2nd ed). LL Robbins ed. Baltimore, Williams and Wilkins Cy. 1973; pp. 523-542.
48. Murray RO, Jacobson HG. The radiology of skeletal disorders. Edinburg/London, Churchill Livingstone. 1971; pp. 697-707.
49. Edelstyn GA, Gillespie PJ, Grebbell FS. The radiological demonstration of osseous metastases: experimental observations. *Clin Radiol* 1967; 18: 158-162.
50. Seaman WB. The Roentgen appearance of early Paget's disease. *J Roentg* 1951; 66: 587-594.
51. Moore S. Observations on osteitis deformans. *Am J Roentg* 1923; 10: 507-518.
52. Grainger RG, Laws JW. Paget's disease - active or quiescent? *Brit J Radiol* 1957; 30: 120-124.
53. Jaffe HL. Paget's disease of bone. *Arch Pathol* 1933; 15: 83-131.
54. Allen ML, Rutherford LJ. Osteitis deformans-fissure fractures-their aetiology and clinical significance. *Am J Roentgenol* 11937; 38: 109-115.
55. Marshall JH. Measurements and models of skeletal metabolism. In: *Mineral Metabolism*, Vol. III, Calcium physiology. New York, Academic Press 1969; pp. 1-122.
56. Bijvoet OLM, Hosking DJ, Frijlink WB, TeVelde J, Vellenga CJLR. Treatment of Paget's disease with combined calcitonin and diphosphonate (EHDP). *Metab Bone Dis Rel Res* 1978; 1: 251-261.
57. Chapuy MC, Zucchelli PM, Meunier PJ. La fonction Parathyroïdienne dans la maladie osseuse de Paget. *Rev Rhum Mal Osteoartic* 1982; 49: 99-102.
58. Posen S, Clifton-Bligh P, Wilkinson M. Paget's disease of bone and hyperparathyroidism; coincidence or causal relationship. *Calc Tiss Res* 1978; 26: 107-109.
59. Adami S, Frijlink WB, Bijvoet OLM, O'Riordan JLH, Clemens TL, Papapoulos SE. Regulation of calcium absorption by 1.25 dihydroxy vitamin D3. Studies of the effect of bisphophonate treatment. *Calc Tiss Int* 1983; 35: 357-361.
60. Gutman AB, Tyson TL, Gutman EB. Serum calcium, inorganic phosphorus and phosphatase activity in hyperparathyroidism, Paget's disease, multiple myeloma and neoplastic disease of bones. *Arch Int Med* 1936; 57: 379-413.
61. Krane SM, Kantrowitz FG, Byrne M, Pinnell SR, Singer FR. Urinary excretion of hydroxylysine and its glucosides as an index of collagen degradation. *J Clin Invest* 1977; 59: 819-827.
62. Franck WA, Bress NM, Singer FR, Krane SM. Rheumatic manifestations of Paget's disease of bone. *Am J Med* 1974; 56: 592-603.
63. Frijlink WB, TeVelde J, Bijvoet OLM, Heynen G. Treatment of Paget's disease of bone with (3-amino-1-hydroxypropylidene)-1,1- bisphosphonate (APD). *Lancet* 11979; i: 799-803.
64. Price P. Osteocalcin. In: *Bone and Mineral Research*, Annual 1. Amsterdam, Excerpta Medica 1982; pp. 157-
65. Price PA, Williamson MK, Lothringer JW. Origin of the vitamin K-dependent bone protein found in plasma and its clearance by kidney and bone. *J Biol Chem* 1981; 256: 12760-
66. Price PA, Parthemore JG, Deftos LJ. New biochemical marker for bone metabolism. *J Clin Invest* 1980; 66: 878-

67. Delmas PD, Demiaux B, Malaval L, Chapuy MC, Edouard C, Meunier PJ. Serum bone gamma carboxyglutamic acid-containing protein in primary hyperparathyroidism and in malignant hypercalcaemia. *J Clin Invest* 1986; 77: 985-
68. Delmas PD, Demiaux B, Malaval L, Chapuy MC, Meunier PJ. Serum bone GLA-protein is not a sensitive marker of bone turnover in Paget's disease of bone. *Calc Tiss Int* 1986; 38: 60-
69. Papapoulos SE, Frölich M, Mudde AH, Harinck HIJ, vdBerg H, Bijvoet OLM. Serum osteocalcin in Paget's disease of bone: Basal concentrations and response to bisphosphonate treatment. *J Clin Endocrinol Metab* 1987; 65: 89-94.
70. Paget J. On a form of chronic inflammation of bones. *Medico-chirurgical transactions* 1877; 60: 37-63.
71. Editorial. Virus and Paget's disease of bone. *Lancet* 1982; ii: 1199.
72. Waldvogel FA, Medoff G, Swartz MN. Osteomyelitis: a review of clinical features, therapeutic considerations and unusual aspects (first of three parts). *New Engl J Med* 1970; 282: 198-206.
73. Johnston CC, Altman RD, Canfield RE, Finerman GAM, Taubee JD, Ebert ML. Review of fracture experience during treatment of Paget's disease of bone with etidronate disodium (EHDP). *Clin Orthop* 1983; 172: 186-
74. Porretta ChA, Dahlin DC, Janes M. Sarcoma in Paget's disease of bone. *J Bone Joint Surg* 1957; 39A: 1314-1329.
75. Michel D, Filzmayer P, Wiegmann T. Sarkomatöse Entartung bei Osteopathia deformans (M Paget). *Internist Prax* 1980; 20: 289-300.
76. Greditzer HG, McLeod RA, Unni KK, Beabout JW. Bone sarcomas in Paget's disease. *Radiology* 1983; 146: 327-333.
77. Altman RD, Collins B. Musculoskeletal manifestations of Paget's disease of bone. *Arthritis Rheum* 1980; 23: 1121-1127.
78. Ryan WG. Paget's disease of bone. *Ann Rev Med* 1977; 28: 143-152.
79. Douglas DL, Kanis JA, Duckworth T, Beard DJ, Paterson AD, Russell RGG. Paget's disease: Improvement of spinal cord dysfunction with diphosphonates and calcitonin. *Metab Bone Dis Rel Res* 1981; 3: 327-
80. Freeman DA. Southwestern Internal Medicine Conference: Paget's disease of Bone. *Amer J Med Sci* 1988; 295: 144-158.
81. Milhaud G, Perault AM, Moukhtar MS. Étude du mécanisme de l'action hypocalcemiante de la thyrocalcitonine. *C R Acad Sci (Paris)* 1965; 261: 813-816.
82. Chambers TJ, Athanasou NA, Fuller K. Effect of parathyroid hormone, calcitonin and prostaglandins on osteoclastic spreading and motility. *J Endocrinol* 1983; 102: 281-
83. Kiang DT, Loken MK, Kennedy BJ. Mechanism of the hypocalcaemic effect of mithramycin. *J Clin Endocr Metab* 1979; 48: 341-344.
84. Fleisch H. Bisphosphonates: Mechanism of action and clinical application. In: *Bone and mineral research*. Annual 1. WA Peck ed. Amsterdam. Excerpta Medica. 1983; pp. 319-357.
85. Wooton R, Reeve J, Spellacy E, Tellez-Yudelvich M. Skeletal blood flow in Paget's disease of bone and its response to calcitonin therapy. *Clin Sci Mol Med* 1984; 54: 69-74.
86. Melick RA, Ebeling P, Hjorth RJ. Improvement in paraplegia in vertebral Paget's disease treated with calcitonin. *Brit Med J* 1976; i: 627-628.
87. Fornasier VL, Stapleton K, Williams CC. Histologic changes in Paget's disease treated with calcitonin. *Human pathology* 1978; 9: 455-461.
88. Alexandre C, Meunier PJ. Le traitement de la maladie osseuse de Paget par l'éthane-1-hydroxy-1,1-diphosphonate (EHDP). Lyon, Association Corporative des Étudiants en Medicine de Lyon. 1977; pp. 1-302.
89. Dodd GW, Ibbertson HK, Fraser TR, Holdaway IM, Wattie D. Radiological assessment of Paget's disease of bone after treatment with the bisphosphonates EHDP and APD. *Br J Radiol* 1987; 60: 849-860.
90. Johnston CC, Khairi MRA, Meunier PJ. Use of etidronate (EHDP) in Paget's disease of bone. *Arthritis Rheum* 1980; 23: 1172-1176.
91. Bell NH, Avery S, Johnston CC. Effects of calcitonin in Paget's disease and polyostotic fibrous dysplasia. *J Clin Endocrinol Metab* 1970; 31: 283-290.
92. Haddad JG, Birge SJ, Avioli LV. Effect of prolonged thyrocalcitonin administration on Paget's disease of bone. *New Engl J Med* 1070; 285: 549-555.
93. Shai F, Baker RK, Wallach S. The clinical and metabolic effects of porcine calcitonin on Paget's disease of bone. *J Clin Invest* 1971; 5): 1927-1940.
94. Hamilton CR. Effects of synthetic salmon calcitonin in patients with Paget's disease of bone. *Am J Med* 1974; 56: 315-322.
95. Kanis JA, Horn DB, Scott RDM, Strong JA. Treatment of Paget's disease of bone with synthetic salmon calcitonin. *Brit Med J* 1974; 3: 727-731.
96. Martin TJ. Treatment of Paget's disease with calcitonins. *Aust N Z J Med* 1979; 9: 36-43.

97. MacIntyre I, Evans IMA, Hobitz HHG, Joplin GF, Stevenson JC. Chemistry, physiology, and therapeutic applications of calcitonin. *Arthritis Rheum* 1980; 23: 1139-1147.
98. Singer FR, Fredericks RS, Minkin C. Salmon calcitonin therapy for Paget's disease of bone. The problem of acquired clinical resistance. *Arthritis Rheum* 1980; 23: 1148-1154.
99. Simon LS, Krane SM, Wortman PD, Krane IM, Kovitz KL. Serum levels of type I and III procollagen fragments in Paget's disease of bone. *J Clin Endocrinol Metab* 1984; 58: 110-120.
100. Bijvoet OLM, Hosking DJ, van Aken J, Will EJ. The treatment of Paget's disease. Combination of calcitonin and diphosphonate. In; *Bone disease and calcitonin.* JA Kanis ed. Eastbourne, Armour Pharm Comp LTD publ, 1976; pp. 25-36.
101. Bijvoet OLM, Hosking DJ, Lemkes HHPJ, Reitsma PH, Frijlink W. Development in the treatment of Paget's disease. In: *Endocrinology of calcium metabolism*. Proceedings of the Sixth Parathyroid Conference, Amsterdam, Excerpta Medica. 1977; pp. 48-54.
102. Hosking DJ. Paget's disease of bone. An update on management. *Drugs* 1985; 30: 156-173.
103. Doyle FH, Banks LM, Pennock JM. Radiologic observations on bone resorption in Paget's disease. *Arthritis Rheum* 1980; 23: 1205-1214.
104. Hosking DJ. Calcitonin and diphosphonate in the treatment of Paget's disease of bone. *Metab Bone Dis Rel Res* 1981; 4/5: 317-326.
105. O'Donoghue DJ, Hosking DJ Biochemical response to combination of disodium etidronate with calcitonin in Paget's disease. *Bone* 1987; 8: 219-225
106. Avramides A, Flores A, DeRose J, Wallach S. Treatment of Paget's disease of bone with once a week injections of salmon calcitonin. *Brit Med J* 1975; 3: 632.
107. Nagant de Deuxchaisnes C, Devogelaere JP, Huaux JP, Dufour JP, Esselinckx W, Engelbeen JP, Stasse P, Hermans P, de Buisseret JP. New modes of administration of salmon calcitonin in Paget's disease. Nasal spray and suppository. *Clin Orthop Rel Res* 1987; 217; 56-71.
108. Kofman S, Eisenstein R. Mithramycin in treatment of disseminated cancer. *Cancer Chemotherap Reports* 1963; 32: 77-96.
109. Yarbro JW, Kennedy BJ, Barnum CP. Mithramycin inhibition of ribonucleic acid synthesis. *Cancer Res* 1966; 26: 36-39.
110. Kennedy BJ. Metabolic and toxic effects of mithramycin during tumor therapy. *Am J Med* 1970; 48: 494-503.
111. van Breukelen FJM, Bijvoet OLM, van Oosterom AT. Inhibition of osteolytic bone lesions by (3-amino-1-hydroxypropylidene)-1,1-bisphosphonate (APD). *Lancet* 1979; i: 803-805.
112. van Breukelen FJM, Bijvoet OLM, Frijlink WB, Sleeboom HP, Mulder H, van Oosterom AT. Efficacy of aminohydroxypropylidene bisphosphonate in hypercalcemia: Observations on regulation of serum calcium. *Calcif Tissue Int* 1982; 34: 321-327.
113. Sleeboom HP, Bijvoet OLM, van Oosterom AT, Gleed JH, O'Riordan JLH. Comparison of intravenous APD and volume repletion in tumor-induced hypercalcemia. *Lancet* 1983; ii: 239-243.
114. Harinck HIJ, Bijvoet OLM, Plantingh AST, Body J, Elte JWF, Sleeboom HP, Wildring J, Neyt JP. The role of bone and kidney in tumour hypercalcaemia and its treatment with bisphosphonate and sodium chloride. *Am J Med* 1987; 82:1133-1142.
115. Van Holten-Verzandvoort ATh, Bijvoet OLM, Cleton FJ, et al. Reduced morbidity from skeletal metastases in breast cancer patients during long-term bisphosphonate (APD) treatment. *Lancet* 1987; ii: 983-85.
116. Thiebaud D, Jager P, Jaqet AF, Burckhardt P. A single-day treatment of tumour-induced hypercalcaemia by intravenous aminohydroxypropylidene-bisphosphonate. *J Bone Mineral Res 1986;* 1: 555-562.
117. Morton AR, Cantrill JA, Craig AE, Howell A, Davies M, Anderson DC. Single dose versus daily intravenous aminohydroxypropylidene bisphosphonate (APD) for the hypercalcaemia of malignancy. *Brit Med J* 1988; 296: 811-1814.
118. Canfield RE, Ed. Etidronate disodium: a new therapy for hypercalcemia of malignancy. *Am J Med* 1987; 82: suppl 2A pp. 1-78.
119. Kanis JA, ed. Clodronate-a new perspective in the treatment of neoplastic bone disease. Lemkes HPJJ, Reitsma PH, Frijlink WB, Verlinden-Ooms H, Bijvoet OLM. A new diphosphonate: dissociation between effects on cells and mineral in rates and a preliminary trial in Paget's disease. *Adv Exp Med Biol* 1978; 103: 459-469.
121. Reitsma PH, Bijvoet OLM, Verlinden-Ooms H, van der Wee-Pals L. Kinetic studies of bone and mineral metabolism during treatment with (3-amino-1-hydroxypropylidene)-1,1-bisphosphonate (APD) in rats. *Calcif Tissue Int* 1980; 32: 145-157.
122. Reitsma PH, Bijvoet OLM, Potokar M, van der Wee-Pals LJA, van Wijk-van Lennep M. Apposition and resorption of bone during oral treatment with (3-amino-1-hydroxypropylidene)-1,1-bisphosphonate (APD). *Calcif Tissue Int* 1983; 35: 357-361.
123. Reitsma PH, Teitelbaum ST, Bijvoet OLM, Kahn AJ. Differential action of the bisphosphonates (3-

amino-1-hydroxypropylidene)-1,1-bisphosphonate (APD) and disodium dichloromethylene bisphosphonate (Cl2MDP) on rat macrophage mediated bone resorption in-vitro. *J Clin Invest* 1982; 70: 927-933.
124. Boonekamp PM, van der Wee-Pals LJA, van Wijk-van Lennep M, Thesingh CW, Bijvoet OLM. Two modes of action of bisphosphonates on osteoclastic resorption of mineralized matrix. *Bone Mineral* 1986; 1: 27-40.
125. Boonekamp PM, Löwik CWGM, van der Wee-Pals LJA, van Wijk-van Lennep M, Bijvoet OLM. Bone Mineral 1987; 2: 29-42.
126. Löwik CWGM, van der Pluym G, van der Wee-Pals LJA, Bloys van Treslong-de Groot H, Bijvoet OLM. Migration and phenotypic transformation of osteoclast precursors into mature osteoclasts: the effects of a bisphosphonate. *J Bone Mineral Res* 1988; 2: 185-192.
127. Radl J, Croese JW, Zürcher C, van der Enden-Vieveen MHU, Brondijk RJ, Kazil U, Haayman JJ, Reitsma PH, Bijvoet OLM. Influence of treatment with APD-bisphosphonate on the bone lesions in the mouse 5T2 multiple myeloma. *Cancer* 1985; 55: 1030-1040.
128. Bijvoet OLM, Frijlink WB, Jie K, van der Linden H, Meyer CJLN, Mulder H, van Paassen HC, Reitsma PH, te Velde J, de Vries E, van der Wey JP. APD in Paget's disease of bone. Role of the mononuclear phagocyte system? *Arthr Rheum* 1980; 23: 1193-1204.
129. Shinoda H, Adamek G, Felix R, Fleisch H, Schenk R, Hagan P. Structure-activity relationships of various bisphosphonates. *Calcif Tiss Int* 1983; 35: 87-99.
130. Jowsey J, Holley KE, Cinman JW. Effect of sodium etidronate in adult cats. *J Lab Clin Med* 1970; 76 : 126-133.
131. Russell RGG, Smith R, Preston CJ, Walton RJ, Woods CG. Diphosphonates in Paget's disease. *Lancet* 1974; i: 894-898.
133. Krane SM. Etidronate disodium in the treatment of Paget's disease of bone. *Ann Int Med* 1982; 96: 619-
134. Boyce BF, Fogelman I, Ralston S, Smith L, Johnston E, Boyle IT. Focal osteomalacia due to low-dose diphosphonate therapy in Paget's disease. *Lancet* 1984; i: 821-
135. Attardo-Parrinello G, Merlini G, Pavesi F, Crema F, Fiorentini ML, Ascari E. Effects of a new aminodiphosphonate (aminohydroxybutylidene-diphosphonate) in patients with osteolytic lesions from metastases and myelomatosis. *Arch Int Med* 1987; 147: 1629-1633.
136. Khairi MRA, Johnston CC, Altman RD, Wellman HN, Serafini AN, Sankey RR. Treatment of Paget's disease of bone (osteitis deformans). Results of a one year study with disodium etidronate. *J A M A* 1974; 230: 562-567.
137. Fromm G, Schajowicz E, Mautalen CA. Disodium ethane-1hydroxy-1,1-diphosphonate (EHDP) in Paget's disease. *Lancet* 1975; ii: 666.
138. Canfield R, Rosner W, Skinner J, McWorther J, Resnick L, Feldman F, Kammerman S, Ryan K, Kunigonis M, Bohne W. Diphosphonate therapy of Paget's disease of bone. *J Clin Endocrinol Metab* 1977, 44: 96-106.
139. Khairi MRA, Altman RD, DeRosa GP, Zimmerman J, Schenk RK, Johnston CC. Sodium etidronate in the treatment of Paget's disease of bone. A study of long-term results. *Ann Int Med* 1977; 87: 656-663.
140. Kanis JA, Urwin GH, Gray RES, Beneton MNC, McCloskey EV, Hamdy NAT, Murray SA.. Effects of intravenous etidronate disodium on skeletal and calcium metabolism. In: *Etidronate disodium: a new therapy for hypercalcaemia of malignancy*. JA Kanis ed, *Am J Med* 1987; 82: Suppl 2A pp. 55-70.
141. Meunier PJ, Chapuy M-C, Delmas P, Charhon S, Edouard C, Arlot M. Intravenous disodium etidronate therapy in Paget's disease of bone and hypercalcemia of malignancy: effects on biochemical parameters and on bone histomorphometry. In: *Etidronate disodium: a new therapy for hypercalcaemia of malignancy*. JA Kanis ed, *Am J Med* 1987; 82: Suppl 2A pp. 71-78.
142. Evans RA, Dunstan CR, Hills E, Wong SYP. Pathological fracture due to severe osteomalacia following low-dose diphosphonate treatment, *Aust N Z J Med* 1983; 13: 277-
143. Douglas DL, Duckworth T, Kanis JA, et al. Biochemical and clinical responses to dichloromethylene diphosphonate (Cl2MDP) in Paget's disease of bone. *Arthritis Rheum* 1980; 23: 1185-1192.
144. Mautalen CA, Gonzalez D, Ghiringhelli G. Efficacy of the bisphosphonate APD in the control of Paget's bone disease. *Bone* 1985; 6: 429-432.
145. Cantrill JA, Buckler HM, Anderson DC. Low dose intravenous 3-amino-1-hydroxypropylidene-1,1-bisphosphonate (APD) for the treatment of Paget's disease of bone. *Ann Rheum Dis* 1986; 45: 1012-1018.
146. Harinck HIJ, Papapoulos SE, Blanksma HJ, Moolenaar BAJ, Vermey P, Bijvoet OLM.. Paget's disease of bone: early and late responses to three different modes of treatment with aminohydroxypropylidene bisphosphonate (APD). *Brit Med J* 1987; 295: 1301-1305.
147. Papapoulos SE, Harinck HIJ, Bijvoet OLM, Gleed JH, Fraher LJ, O'Riordan JLH. Effects of decreasing serum calcium on circulating parathyroid hormone and vitamin D metabolites in normocalcaemic and hypercalcaemic patients, treated with APD. *Bone Mineral* 1986; 1: 59-78.
148. McCloskey EV, Yates AJP, Beneton MNC, Galloway J, Harris S, Kanis JA. Comparative effects of in-

travenous diphosphonates on calcium and skeletal metabolism in man. In: *Clodronate-a new perspective in the treatment of neoplastic bone disease.* JA Kanis ed. *Bone* 1987; 8: suppl 1 pp. 35-41.
149. Dinarello CA. Interleukin-1 and the pathogenesis of the acute phase response. *N Engl J Med* 1984; 311: 1413-1418.

Renal Calculi: Update

CHARLES Y.C. PAK

Center in Mineral Metabolism and Clinical Research
University of Texas Southwestern Medical Center at Dallas
Dallas, TX

Nephrolithiasis is a disease of high probability of recurrence. Patients with recurrent nephrolithiasis often present with "metabolic" derangements. Many of these metabolic disturbances reflect abnormalities in calcium or vitamin D metabolism. The correction of these disturbances has sometimes resulted in inhibition of stone formation, a finding suggesting that these disturbances are pathogenetically important in stone formation. Thus, a major effort has been directed toward elucidation of metabolic derangements, formulation of diagnostic protocols based on these disturbances, and development of selective treatments directed at the correction of these metabolic derangements.

It is the purpose of this discussion to review and update salient progress made in the following areas: pathophysiologic elucidation with a particular emphasis on hypercalciuria, hypocitraturia and gouty diathesis; diagnostic assessment entailing both an extensive and simplified protocol; and a refinement of selective treatment approach taking into consideration the potential broad application of potassium citrate.

PATHOPHYSIOLOGY

Hypercalciuria (Table 1)[1]

There is considerable evidence for the heterogeneity of hypercalciuria.

In absorptive hypercalciuria, the primary defect is the increase in intestinal calcium absorption, occurring independently of vitamin D. The hyperabsorption of calcium accounts for relative parathyroid suppression and hypercalciuria. The primacy of intestinal hyperabsorption of calcium is shown by independence from 1,25-dihydroxyvitamin D action, a lack of correction by thiazide diuretic and localization of exaggerated calcium transport to the jejunum. There is some evidence that it may be a genetically inherited defect. In a kindred in which nephrolithiasis was encountered in members from three generations, the biochemical evidence of absorptive hypercalciuria was shown to display an autosomal dominant mode of inheritance. Biochemical characteristics of this syndrome have also been uncovered in genetically inbred rats.

In <u>renal hypercalciuria</u>, the primary defect is the impaired renal tubular reabsorption of calcium (i.e., renal calcium leak). This disturbance causes secondary hyperparathyroidism and compensatory intestinal hyperabsorption of calcium from the stimulation of PTH-dependent renal synthesis of 1,25-dihydroxyvitamin D. Renal hypercalciuria is characterized by fasting hypercalciuria and secondary hyperparathyroidism (shown by high serum immunoreactive PTH and/or urinary cyclic AMP). The intestinal calcium absorption is secondarily stimulated, as it is dependent on 1,25-dihydroxyvitamin D action. Treatment with thiazide restores normal serum 1,25-dihydroxyvitamin D and intestinal calcium absorption, by correcting the renal calcium leak and preventing secondary hyperparathyroidism. There may be a more generalized disturbance in renal tubular function, as shown by an exaggerated natriuretic response to thiazide and exaggerated calciuric response to carbohydrate load.

Resorption hypercalciuria, characterized by increased skeletal resorption, is represented principally by primary hyperparathyroidism. Other causes of resorptive hypercalciuria are uncommonly associated with nephrolithiasis. Hypercalcemia and high serum immunoreactive PTH are invariably present. Hypophosphatemia, low radial (shaft) bone density and hypercalciuria often accompany this syndrome. The intestinal calcium absorption may be elevated from the PTH-dependent stimulation of the renal synthesis of 1,25-dihydroxyvitamin D. Stones are composed predominantly of calcium phosphate, whereas calcium oxalate is the main component of stones in other forms of hypercalciuria. The exact cause for renal stone formation in primary hyperparathyroidism is not known. It was previously suggested that the occurrence of intestinal hyperabsorption may predispose patients to the formation of renal calculi, since the prevalence of renal stone disease was higher in those who showed an exaggerated calciuric response to the oral calcium load, than in those who did not. Recently, it was reported that patients with primary hyperparathyroidism presenting with bone disease had a lower renal mass and a more pronounced secondary hyperparathyroidism. However, in our hands, we were unable to show any distinction between the group with stones and those with bone disease with respect to serum calcium, 1,25-dihydroxyvitamin D, PTH, urinary calcium or in intestinal calcium absorption.

In <u>renal phosphate leak</u>, the ensuing hypophosphatemia provides stimulus to the renal synthesis of 1,25-dihydroxyvitamin D which then causes hyperabsorption of calcium and intestinal hyperabsorption of calcium and hypercalciuria. This condition differs from the classic absorptive hypercalciuria in its occurrence of hypophosphatemia and the frequent accompaniment of fasting hypercalciuria in the setting of normocalcemia (due to hypophosphatemia-dependent enhanced mobilization of calcium from the skeleton). In our experience, renal phosphate leak is an uncommon cause of hypercalciuria among patients with renal stones. Even when hypophosphatemia is present, orthophosphate therapy may not correct the intestinal hyperabsorption of calcium.

In <u>primary 1,25-dihydroxyvitamin D excess</u>, the enhanced renal synthesis of 1,25-dihydroxyvitamin D accounts for the hyperabsorption of calcium, and may stimulate bone resorption. The synthetic rate for labeled-1,25-dihydroxy-

Table 1. Classification of Hypercalciuria

Absorptive hypercalciuria Type I and Type II
Renal hypercalciuria
Renal phosphate leak
Primary 1,25-(OH)$_2$D excess
Combined renal tubular disturbances
Prostaglandin excess

vitamin D has been shown to be increased. These patients may represent the severest cases of hyperabsorption of calcium and hypercalciuria. They may be candidates for management by inhibitors of 1,25-dihydroxyvitamin D.

In <u>combined renal tubular disturbances</u>, it is presumed that the same patient may have more than 1 of 3 defects, -phosphate leak, calcium leak or increased 1,25-dihydroxyvitamin D synthesis. For example, the concurrent presence of renal calcium leak and primary increase in 1,25-dihydroxyvitamin D synthesis could cause the picture of fasting hypercalciuria with normal parathyroid function, since secondary hyperparathyroidism of renal calcium leak could be compensated by the increased intestinal calcium absorption from the accelerated 1,25-dihydroxyvitamin D synthesis. The final cause of hypercalciuria is <u>prostaglandin excess</u>. The enhanced production of PGE_2, for example, may cause renal calcium leak from alteration in renal blood flow and filtration rate, or it may produce an excessive skeletal mobilization of calcium by stimulating bone resorption. This syndrome may be responsive to treatment by inhibitors of prostaglandin synthesis. In our experience, it is an uncommon cause of hypercalciuria in nephrolithiasis.

Hypocitraturia

Hypocitraturia often results from acidosis, due to a variety of disturbances, including distal renal tubular acidosis, acquired acidosis of chronic diarrheal states, lactic acidosis from physical exercise, and potassium loss occurring from thiazide therapy.[2] Hypocitraturia is also encountered in patients with active urinary tract infection, presumably from the degradation of citrate by bacterial enzymes. In many patients, hypocitraturia may be present despite lack of evidence for above-mentioned conditions. In such patients, the urinary citrate excretion bears a strong relationship with the calculated net intestinal absorption of alkali. The findings suggest that hypocitraturia may have been the result of the consumption of a diet rich in acid-ash content.

While citrate has long been recognized to play a role in nephrolithiasis, it has received an enormous interest in recent years as an important inhibitor of stone formation. This excitement is due in part to the relative ease of assay for citrate in urine, frequent detection of hypocitraturia, and the availability of an effective drug (potassium citrate)[3] for the correction of this derangement. This emphasis on citrate is not meant to disparage the importance of other inhibitors. For example, exciting work has recently emerged, suggesting that the urinary glycoprotein inhibitor (nephrocalcin) from patients with calcium oxalate nephrolithiasis may be structurally different and functionally defective.[4] However, neither an easy assay for nephrocalcin nor a maneuver to manipulate its renal excretion is currently available.

Gouty Diathesis[5]

The entity is characterized by low urinary pH of less than 5.5 of largely unknown etiology, occurring independently of excessive alkali loss or consumption of a diet rich in acid-ash content. Stones formed by the patients are composed of uric acid alone, calcium stones alone or both types of stones. Some patients, but not necessarily all, present with hyperuricemia, hypertriglyceridemia, frank gouty arthritis, or family history of gout. This condition may include patients with classic gout, presenting with gouty arthritis and hyperuricemia. A majority of these patients, however, may have an early phase of classic gout, manifested biochemically by unusually acid urine, but not with hyperuricemia or gouty arthritis. This conclusion is supported by the finding that stone disease may precede the onset of articular symptoms in many gouty patients. This condition should be distinguished from hyperuricosuric calcium nephrolithiasis in which urinary pH is typically greater than 5.5.

The uric acid stone formation in gouty diathesis could be explained by the unusually acid urinary environment, enhancing the amount of undissociated uric acid in urine. Calcium stones could occur by heterogeneous nucleation or binding of inhibitors by uric acid itself or by an intermediary role of sodium urate which might have formed from a transient rise in urinary pH.

DIAGNOSIS

The nature of diagnostic assessment depends on the severity of stone disease. In patients with inactive stone disease or who present with a stone episode for the first time without obvious predisposing factors, the evaluation may be simple, comprising routine urinalysis and culture, serum calcium, phosphorus, uric acid, and electrolytes, appropriate x-rays of the urinary tract, and analysis of the stone if available. A more extensive evaluation is recommended[6], however, for patients with an active recurrent stone disease, as well as single-stone-formers who are considered to be at risk for further stone formation (for example, a family history of stones). The evaluation generally comprises of the determination of urinary risk factors in a random 24-hour urine sample collected on a random diet, as well as on a sample obtained after maintenance on a diet restricted in calcium, sodium, and oxalate. Risk factors identified in urine include total volume, pH, calcium, phosphorus, sodium, citrate, magnesium, uric acid, and oxalate. Additional procedures might include the test of "fast and oral calcium load" and serum immunoreactive PTH, in order to derive a measure of renal calcium leak and of intestinal calcium absorption. This procedure is critical for the differentiation of hypercalciurias. Some laboratories omit this test.

Using available protocol, it is now possible to discern metabolic or environmental disturbances in virtually every patient with recurrent nephrolithiasis. These disturbances are presumed to contribute to stone formation, although a clear-cut evidence may sometimes be lacking. As discussed before, hypercalciuria consists of absorptive, renal, resorptive, renal phosphate leak, 1,25-dihydroxyvitamin D excess and combined renal tubular disturbances. Other major causes of stone formation are hyperuricosuric calcium nephrolithiasis, hyperoxaluric calcium nephrolithiasis, and hypocitraturic calcium nephrolithiasis, gouty diathesis, infection stones, cystinuria and low urine volume. Miscellaneous causes, seldom encountered, would include 2,8-dihydroxyadeninuria, xanthinuria, non-hyperparathyroid hypercalcemic states and stones secondary to carbonic anhydrase inhibitors. Many patients present with more than one disturbance.

MEDICAL PREVENTION OF RECURRENT NEPHROLITHIASIS (Table 2)

We have long advocated a selective treatment approach, whereby a specific treatment is chosen for each disorder based on its ability to correct the underlying derangement[7]. However, a refinement of this selective treatment approach may be necessary, because of the lack of a suitable drug for absorptive hypercalciuria, problems with the use of sodium cellulose phosphate and thiazide, and the potential wide applicability in usage of potassium citrate.

Problems in the Use of Sodium Cellulose Phosphate

Sodium cellulose phosphate is capable of correcting intestinal hyperabsorption of calcium and hypercalciuria in absorptive hypercalciuria. However, it does so by limiting the amount of available calcium in the intestinal tract. There is currently no drug known to correct the basic transport defect responsible for the increased absorption of calcium in this condition. Thus, sodium cellulose phosphate usage is associated with hyper-

Table 2. Medical Prevention

Condition	Treatment
Absorptive hypercalciuria Type I	
Severe or thiazide-resistant	Sodium cellulose phosphate
Mild-to-moderate or at risk for bone disease	Thiazide & potassium citrate
Absorptive hypercalciuria	Dietary calcium restriction
Renal hypercalciuria	Thiazide & potassium citrate
Renal phosphate leak	Orthophosphate
Hypocitraturic Ca nephrolithiasis	
Distal renal tubular acidosis	Potassium citrate
Enteric hyperoxaluria	Potassium-sodium citrate
Thiazide induced hypokalemia	Potassium citrate
Idiopathic	Potassium citrate
Gouty diathesis	Potassium citrate

oxaluria and hypomagnesiuria. Moreover, an overaggressive or an inappropriate usage of this drug may cause parathyroid stimulation and bone disease. For these reasons, sodium cellulose phosphate is becoming more of a secondary drug, to be utilized when the first line drug (thiazide) is ineffective. Parathyroid function and skeletal status should be monitored using cellulose phosphate therapy.

New Perspectives in the Use of Thiazide

Thiazide is ideally indicated for renal hypercalciuria, since it can correct the renal calcium leak, and thereby avert secondary hyperparathyroidism and restore normal 1,25-dihydroxyvitamin D synthesis and intestinal calcium absorption. In so doing, thiazide causes long-term correction of hypercalciuria in patients with renal leak of calcium.[8]

Unlike in renal hypercalciuria, thiazide causes only a transient decline in urinary calcium excretion in patients with absorptive hypercalciuria.[8] Whereas urinary calcium generally falls during early thiazide therapy, it rebounds to the pre-treatment level in many patients with continued thiazide therapy beyond two years. This attenuation of hypocalciuric response (or the loss of hypocalciuric action of thiazide) may be due to the failure of thiazide to restore normal calcium absorption. Unlike in patients with renal hypercalciuria, patients with absorptive hypercalciuria continued to show intestinal hyperabsorption of calcium during thiazide therapy.

Another problem with thiazide therapy is its induction of hypocitraturia, probably due to renal potassium loss and ensuing hypokalemia.[9]

Potential problems with thiazide in the management of hypercalciuric nephrolithiasis include: (1) a persistent intestinal hyperabsorption of calcium and an eventual loss of hypocalciuric action during long-term thiazide therapy in absorptive hypercalciuria, and (2) an induction of hypokalemia and hypocitraturia in both absorptive and renal hypercalciurias.

Emerging Therapeutic Importance of Potassium Citrate

Citrate therapy has long been known to be useful in the management of uric acid lithiasis and renal tubular acidosis. Our metabolic studies indicated that potassium citrate might be advantageous over sodium citrate in the control of stone formation. Both alkali therapy are effective in the prevention of uric acid stone formation. However, sodium alkali may sometimes exaggerate or cause calcium stone formation whereas potassium citrate has been shown to inhibit calcium stone formation.

Potassium citrate has been approved by the Food and Drug Administration in 1985 for the control of stone formation in patients with distal renal tubular acidosis, hypocitraturic calcium oxalate nephrolithiasis (due to chronic diarrheal syndrome, thiazide-induced hypokalemia and idiopathic hypocitraturia), and in uric acid lithiasis with and without calcium stones (gouty diathesis).[3] Subsequently, it was shown that this treatment may be useful in the control of stone formation in patients with calcium nephrolithiasis due to mild-to-moderate hyperuricosuria.

The physiological and physicochemical actions of potassium citrate are well known. Potassium citrate, by providing an alkali load, reduces renal tubular resorption of citrate and increases citrate excretion. Induced hypercitraturia then enhances the inhibitor activity against the crystallization of calcium oxalate in calcium phosphate, as well as possibly retards urate-induced crystallization of calcium oxalate. Moreover, potassium citrate increases urinary pH by producing an alkali load. In so doing, it lowers the amount of undissociated uric acid, making uric acid crystallization less likely.

Work elsewhere has confirmed our finding of the effectiveness of potassium citrate in the prevention of new stone formation. Moreover, none of our patients maintained on potassium citrate has required surgery for the removal of newly formed stones. Approximately 40% of patients showed a reduction in stone mass, often not accountable by stone passage. In patients with distal renal tubular acidosis, potassium citrate therapy has shown to improve calcium balance and skeletal status.

Refinement of Selective Treatment Approach

From above discussion, it is clear that a modification of selective medical approach would be advisable.

In absorptive hypercalciuria Type I, sodium cellulose phosphate might be used in patients with severe hypercalciuria or those who are resistant to or intolerant of thiazide. Thiazide might be offered to those with mild-moderate hypercalciuria or those who are at risk for the development of bone disease (such as growing children and postmenopausal women). Urinary calcium should be monitored in order to detect loss of hypocalciuric action of thiazide. Potassium citrate should be provided to avert hypokalemia and hypocitraturia.

In hyperuricosuric calcium nephrolithiasis, allopurinol may be used, especially in the setting of marked hyperuricosuria or hyperuricemia. If hypocitraturia co-exists or in the presence of mild-moderate hyperuricosuria, potassium citrate alone may be effective.

A practical approach gaining some acceptance is to use thiazide with potassium citrate in all normocalcemic patients with hypercalciuria regardless of etiology. In such patients, thiazide therapy may be temporarily substituted by sodium cellulose phosphate or orthophosphate if attenuation of thiazide-induced hypocalciuria occurs. In patients with normocalciuria with either calcium stones or uric acid stones (without urinary tract infection), the use of potassium citrate alone has been suggested.

CURRENT ROLE OF MEDICAL THERAPY

Recent introduction of extracorporeal shock wave lithotripsy and other innovative procedures have revolutionalized the surgical treatment of nephrolithiasis. The marked facility with which most stones can now be removed has inevitably led to the reappraisal of the need for medical diagnosis and treatment.

Despite the dramatic progress made in the surgical area, a continued application of medical preventive program would seem justified. First, the goal of medical therapy is a prevention of recurrent renal stone formation, whereas that of surgical treatment is the removal of existing stones. The removal of stones alone does not assure prevention of new stone formation. Second, most renal stone episodes are resolved spontaneously, and do not require "surgical" removal. However, all episodes might be accompanied by considerable morbidity. Such episodes are potentially preventable by appropriate medical treatment. Third, medical treatment may correct extrarenal manifestations of the stone disease, whereas the surgical approach cannot. Finally, for the management of moderate-to-severe stone disease, medical treatment is clearly more cost-effective than the surgical approach.

SUMMARY

Using appropriate medical treatment programs, recurrent new stone formation may be controlled in the vast majority of patients with nephrolithiasis. Moreover, an effective prophylactic program may dramatically reduce the need for stone removal, cause dissolution in vivo of certain stones (including those containing calcium), and overcome non-renal mainfestations under certain circumstances.

Despite these advantages, it is clear that medical treatment cannot provide a total control of the disease. There is no cure, only prophylaxis. Some patients may be recalcitrant to medical treatment no matter how heroic. A satisfactory response to medical treatment requires continued compliance by the patient to the recommended treatment program, and a commitment by the physician to provide long-term follow-up care.

REFERENCES

1. Pak, C.Y.C. Pathogenesis of hypercalciuria. IN: Bone and Mineral Research/4. Ed. W.A. Peck. Elsevier, New York. 1986, pp. 303-334.

2. Nicar, M.J., C. Skurla, K. Sakhaee and C.Y.C. Pak. Low urinary citrate excretion in nephrolithiasis. Urol. 21:8-14, 1983.

3. Pak, C.Y.C., C. Fuller, K. Sakhaee, G. Preminger and F. Britton. Long term treatment of calcium nephrolithiasis with potassium citrate. J. Urol. 134:11-19, 1985.

4. Worcester, E.M., Y. Nakagawa and F.L. Coe. Glycoprotein calcium oxalate crystal growth inhibitor in urine. Min. Elec. Metab. 13:267-272, 1987.

5. Pak, C.Y.C., K. Sakhaee and C. Fuller. Successful management of uric acid nephrolithiasis with potassium citrate. Kid. Int. 30:422-428, 1986.

6. Pak, C.Y.C., et al. Ambulatory evaluation of nephrolithiasis: Classification, clinical presentation and diagnostic criteria. Am. J. Med. 69:19-30, 1980.

7. Pak, C.Y.C., et al. Is selective therapy of recurrent nephrolithiasis possible? Am. J. Med. 71:615-622, 1981.

8. Preminger, G.M. and C.Y.C. Pak. Eventual attenuation of hypocalciuric response to hydrochlorothiazide in absorptive hypercalciuria. J. Urol. 137:1104-1109, 1987.

9. Nicar, M.J., R. Peterson and C.Y.C. Pak. Use of potassium citrate as potassium supplement during thiazide therapy of calcium nephrolithiasis. J. Urol. 131:430-433, 1984.

Discussion:

DR. PARFITT (Detroit): Charles, the calcium balance data that you inferred in response to potassium citrate would amount to a retention of approximately 100 grams of calcium over a two-year period. That ought to be detectable by the various methods for measuring bone mass. Have you verified your calcium balance calculations by attempting to check whether the calcium is retained in the long term in that amount?

DR. PAK (Dallas): Yes, both for thiazides in absorptive hypercalciuria, as well as for potassium citrate. I didn't show them to you. With thiazide, we showed several years ago that radial bone density increases during the first two years in absorptive hypercalciuria and is maintained thereafter. This would be commensurate with the short-term hypocalciuric effect of the thiazide.

In renal leak, we were not able to show any change in radial bone density. In the case of distal renal tubular acidosis, we have only two-year data. Radial as well as lumbar bone density increases.

DR. MALLUCHE (Lexington, KY): Did you follow patients for extraosseous calcification?

DR. PAK: Dr. Malluche, I did not purposely go around looking for extraosseous calcification. But on routine x-ray, we could not find any evidence of aortic calcification. Renal function remained quite normal. In fact, in general, it improved somewhat, for example on potassium citrate therapy. But I have not done very careful scans or so on.

DR. MALLUCHE: How would you explain the improvement in GFR in these patients?

DR. PAK: Improvement in GFR? I think it may correlate to removal of some of the existing stone mass.

DR. ETTINGER (San Francisco): Thank you for a lucid presentation and for kind remarks about our research. I have a question about the survey you did across the United States. First, a comment. In California, an epidemiologic survey we did showed that people from the southeast United States, who live in California, are more likely to develop stone disease while living in California, the initial stone disease developing there. So, our sense is that these people bring with them some habit that makes them more likely to have stone disease.

My question has to do with the survey. Was this a survey of only stone-formers, or of the whole population in these areas?

DR. PAK: That's an excellent point. What I've shown you is a selected population. These data are random from physicians throughout the country obtaining samples from patients with stones and submitting them to the laboratory for analysis. What is interesting, however, is that the number of samples we obtained from five regions, are fairly similar.

The other point which I didn't show because of time is that the percentage of patients with abnormalities were the same in the five regions. But, in addition, among those with the abnormalities, if you just take those with abnormal calcium, for example, and take the mean of their calcium, they were also identical in the five regions.

I sometimes think that it's perhaps the mobile society that no longer allows for special predilection in certain regions. As an anecdote, when I decided to leave NIH in 1972, my colleagues said, "You're going to commit professional suicide. You're not going to see anybody with stones in Texas." But I have more stones than ever.

DR. ARNSTEIN: I'm interested to know whether citrate has a role in patients who have normal urinary citrate levels?

DR. PAK: That's a question repeated oftentimes. I, personally, have not pursued that. I do have preliminary data, however. Some patients were inadvertently admitted to the program, even though they had normal urinary citrate. Those patients did not do as well with respect to stone disease. They did fairly well, but not as well as those with hypocitraturia.

The explanation is fairly obvious. Those with normal citraturia with stones had other abnormalities, like hypercalciuria and so on. I think if you take care of everything, your patients probably would do well.

Current Problems in Renal Osteodystrophy

BRENDAN F. BOYCE,[1] ZIYA MOCAN,[2] DAVID J. HALLS,[3] and
BRIAN J.R. JUNOR[2]

University Departments of [1]Pathology and [3]Clinical Biochemistry
Royal Infirmary
Glasgow, Scotland
and [2]Renal Unit
Western Infirmary
Glasgow, Scotland

BACKGROUND

Renal osteodystrophy is a term used to describe a variety of disorders of bone turnover that can occur in patients with end-stage renal disease. There are three major forms: osteitis fibrosa (secondary hyperparathyroidism); osteomalacia (responsive to vitamin D metabolites) and aluminum bone disease. One bone biopsy study[1] has shown that approximately 60% of patients have osteitis fibrosa at the time they first begin regular dialysis treatment, 30% have osteomalacia which in most cases responds to treatment with vitamin D metabolites and regular dialysis and the remainder have normal bone turnover. Review of bone biopsy specimens taken from 94 patients in Glasgow at the time of their first hemodialysis revealed that 70 (75%) had osteitis fibrosa and 24 (25%) had osteomalacia. In all these cases stains for aluminum were negative.

Osteitis fibrosa is characterized by the presence of increased osteoclastic bone resorption - and increased new bone formation (Fig. 1). These changes represent a PTH-driven response to hypocalcemia that follows the increased phosphate retention of chronic renal failure. Altered vitamin D metabolism and decreased calcium absorption can lead to impaired mineralization of the new bone and thus to osteomalacia. This is typically accompanied by mild osteitis fibrosa and is characterized by the presence of thickened osteoid seams along most of the bone surface (Fig. 2), a reduced rate of mineralization measured after double tetracycline labeling and negative aluminum staining.

Regular dialysis and treatment with vitamin D metabolites have been shown to result in marked clinical, biochemical and histologic improvement of the osteodystrophy in many patients, although the response is variable[2,3]. In the study by Pierides et al.[2] patients with osteitis fibrosa ± osteomalacia benefitted from treatment whereas some patients who had "pure" osteomalacia without osteitis fibrosa developed hypercalcemia and this was usually associated with bone pain and an increased risk of fracture. Later studies have demonstrated that these abnormalities are related predominantly to the toxic effects of aluminum present in the water used during dialysis[4]. Removal of aluminum from the dialysis water by reverse osmosis or deionization has prevented the serious complications of aluminum toxicity such as

---

*Present address: University of Texas Health Science Center, Department of Medicine, Division of Endocrinology and Metabolism, 7703 Floyd Curl Drive, San Antonio, TX 78284-7877

encephalopathy and fracturing osteodystrophy in most centers in which water aluminum levels are high. Subsequently, it has become evident that bone disease and, especially in children, encephalopathy could result from the effects of aluminum taken orally in phosphate binders to reduce intestinal absorption of phosphate[5]. Although alternative phosphate binders such as calcium carbonate have been proposed by some, aluminum hydroxide remains the most widely used form of therapy and thus aluminum toxicity has persisted and remains the major cause of troublesome renal osteodystrophy in long-term dialysis patients.

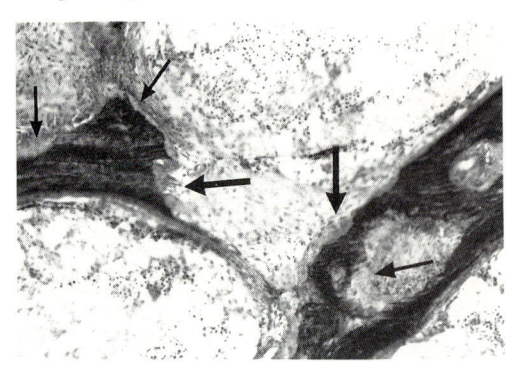

Fig. 1. Moderate osteitis fibrosa. There is increased osteoclastic resorption (large arrows) associated with marrow fibrosis and increased bone formation (small arrows) (1% Toluidine blue).

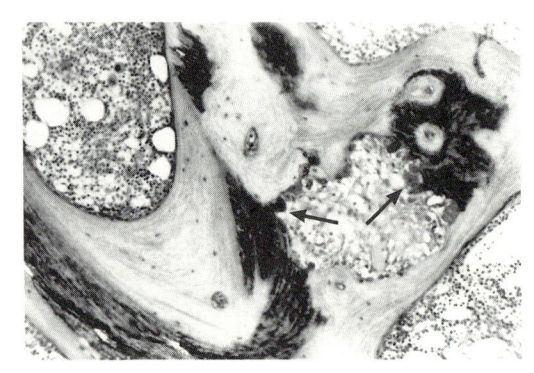

Fig. 2. Severe osteomalacia. Thickened osteoid seams (pale staining) cover most of the bone surface. A focus of active resorption (arrowed) and marrow fibrosis is present (1% Toluidine blue).

In this paper the effects of aluminum on bone metabolism will be reviewed and some of the associated clinical problems will be discussed.

ALUMINUM-RELATED BONE DISEASE

Histologic Features

Two main forms of aluminum bone disease can be recognized histologically[3,6,7]: osteomalacia in which there is focal or widespread distribution of thickened osteoid seams along bone surfaces (Fig. 3) and so-called aplastic bone disease in which osteoid seams are increased in extent but are not increased in thickness (Fig. 4). In both types of osteodystrophy

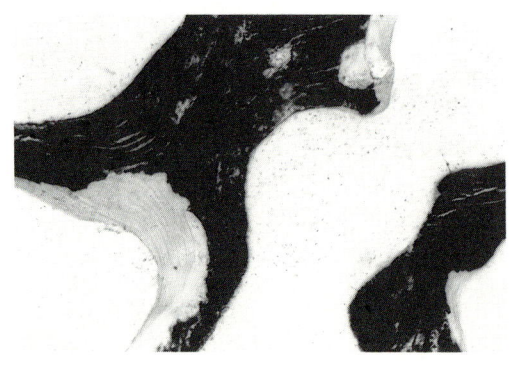

Fig. 3. Aluminum-related osteomalacia. Thickened osteoid seams (pale staining) are focally distributed along the trabecular surfaces. Bone resorption is absent. (1% toluidine blue).

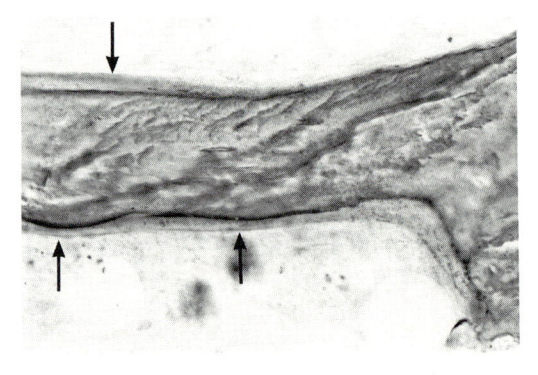

Fig. 4. Aplastic bone disease. High magnification showing thin osteoid seams (arrowed) and aluminum (dark line) present along the interface between osteoid and calcified bone. (Aluminon stain).

aluminum is present along the calcification front at the interface between osteoid and calcified bone, where it is ideally situated to inhibit mineralization. In many cases aluminum is also present along cement lines which have become embedded within fully calcified bone matrix indicating that osteoid may eventually calcify despite the presence of aluminum along the calcification front. The osteomalacic form may be slightly more common than the aplastic variety. In a review of 275 aluminum-positive biopsy specimens from 219 patients Ott et al.[3] found osteomalacia in 108 and mild or aplastic bone disease in 76. However, we reviewed biopsy specimens from 78 patients in Glasgow with aluminum bone disease and found osteomalacia in 35 and aplastic bone disease in 43.

In most cases of aluminum-related osteomalacia histologic indices of bone resorption are within the normal range or only mildly elevated but in some cases these may be increased and give rise to the so-called mixed picture of osteomalacia and osteitis fibrosa[3]. It is likely that in such cases active bone resorption indicates recovery from the effects of aluminum toxicity following withdrawal from exposure to aluminum. An alternative explanation is that exposure to high levels of aluminum occurred in the recent past before the biopsy was taken and that bone resorption had not yet been suppressed. However, in biopsy specimens from patients in Glasgow with this mixed picture osteoclasts can typically be seen resorbing through aluminum lines within calcified bone indicating that the aluminum had been present within bone for a long period of time and that the former explanation is likely to pertain in most cases. Active bone resorption and bone formation are rarely seen in cases of aplastic bone disease and, thus, the term aplastic seems appropriate.

It is not clear why osteoid seams are thickened (osteomalacia) in some patients with aluminum bone disease and thin in others (aplastic). The presence of thick osteoid seams implies that the amount of matrix formed has been normal or increased but mineralization has been inhibited whereas thin osteoid in aplastic cases suggests that both matrix formation and mineralization have been impaired. A possible explanation is that patients with aplastic bone disease have been exposed to very high concentrations of aluminum which consequently inhibit both formation and resorption whereas in patients with osteomalacia aluminum exposure is less severe and leads only to inhibition of mineralization. Charhon et al. reported higher PTH concentrations in plasma from patients with osteomalacia than in patients with the aplastic lesion. However, these findings were not confirmed by others[3,7]. Furthermore, in Glasgow we found no difference in PTH, alkaline phosphatase, calcium or aluminum levels in blood between patients with either type of aluminum bone disease. It is not yet clear whether the type of renal disease may influence the pattern of aluminum-related osteodystrophy although a recent study has indicated a high prevalence of aplastic bone disease among patients with diabetic nephropathy[8].

PATIENTS AT RISK

<u>'Hyperabsorbers' of Aluminum</u>

It appears likely that while receiving similar amounts of aluminum containing phosphate binders and being exposed to similar dialysis conditions some patients absorb aluminum more avidly from the gastrointestinal tract than others and thus have an increased risk of developing aluminum-related bone disease[5]. Children may be at greater risk than adults because they receive a higher dose of aluminum per kilogram of body weight. However, identification of these hyperabsorbers by measurement of aluminum absorption following an oral load of aluminum is not straightforward. Direct measurement is not possible since there is no harmless isotopic form of aluminum. Although measurement of urinary excretion of aluminum provides the best indirect estimate of absorption in normal subjects it is impractical in renal patients who have little or no urinary output. Measurement of changes in blood levels of aluminum after an oral load may be difficult to interpret.

The difficulties associated with indirect tests of aluminum absorption can be illustrated by a study carried out in Glasgow. We studied 4 patients with biopsy proven aluminum-related osteomalacia and 4 patients with osteitis fibrosa and no stainable aluminum in their biopsy specimens. All had been dialyzed for between 2 and 7 years with use of dialysates that were low in aluminum (<30 µg/liter). During this time the patients with aluminum osteomalacia had taken 1.8 to 2.3 kg aluminum as phosphate binders while those with osteitis fibrosa had taken 2.6 to 12.8 kg aluminum. To determine whether the patients with aluminum bone disease absorbed more aluminum than the patients with osteitis fibrosa, aluminum therapy was stopped for one week and each patient was then given 2 Alucaps 3 times daily (2.8 g aluminum hydroxide per day) for two weeks. Serum aluminum concentrations were measured before, during and one week after taking aluminum. The results of this study are shown in the Table.

Table: Changes in serum aluminum concentrations in hemodialysis patients during treatment with 2.8 g aluminum hydroxide per day for 2 weeks.

	Patients	Serum Aluminum Concentration (µg/liter)		
		Before	During Study	Increase
Aluminum-related osteomalacia	1	16	35	19
	2	59	76	17
	3	54	111	57
	4	57	108	51
	Mean ±SE	46 ± 10	82 ± 17	36 ± 10
Osteitis fibrosa	1	30	73	43
	2	24	19	− 5
	3	54	59	5
	4	35	35	0
	Mean ±SE	36 ± 6	46 ± 12	11 ± 11

Serum aluminum concentrations rose during the study in all 4 patients with osteomalacia and in only 1 of the patients with osteitis fibrosa. However, the increase in 2 of the patients with osteomalacia was small and mean values during the study were not significantly higher than pre-study values using Student's paired t-test. The mean increase in serum aluminum concentration in the osteomalacic group was higher than the mean increase in the osteitis fibrosa group but in this small number of subjects the difference did not reach statistical significance. Nevertheless, the findings suggests that patients with biopsy-proven aluminum-related osteomalacia may absorb more aluminum from their gastrointestinal tract than patients without aluminum bone disease. However, it is also possible that there was no difference in absorption in the two groups and that serum aluminum levels rose in the osteomalacic group because the absorbed aluminum could not be transferred to their bones since these were already loaded with aluminum. In contrast, absorbed aluminum may have been taken up avidly by bone in the patients with osteitis fibrosa thus preventing a rise in serum concentrations. Although this explanation is possible it does not account for the lack of osteomalacia and stainable aluminum in the biopsy specimens of the osteitis fibrosa patients who had taken large quantities of aluminum orally for up to 7 years.

It is likely that aluminum hydroxide will continue to be the most widely used phosphate binder for several years and that patients who "hyperabsorb" aluminum will remain at risk of developing aluminum toxicity. It may be possible to identify some of these by demonstrating labile serum aluminum concentrations, particularly if they rise above 100-150 µg/liter[5]. Until a more widely accepted aluminum-free therapy is developed, it is suggested that aluminum hydroxide intake should be reduced to the minimum required to maintain control of hyperphosphatemia and that its use should be restricted to those meals with a high phosphate content.

Failure of Water Treatment Units

Reverse osmosis (RO) and deionization are the two most commonly used techniques to lower dialysate aluminum concentrations. Aluminum can exist in ionic, cationic and colloidal forms in solution and deionization removes anionic and cationic forms while reverse osmosis removes all three. The use of these techniques has all but eliminated aluminum bone disease in Newcastle, England[9] where water aluminum concentrations were high and aluminum toxicity was a major clinical problem in the 1970's. However, in other centers such as Edinburgh, Scotland[10] where water aluminum levels are high the effects of RO water treatment for a minimum of 3 years have been variable with some patients having no change in the severity of the bone disease and others having reversal of the mineralization defect.

In areas where aluminum levels in public water supplies are high there may be considerable variation in water aluminum concentrations from month to month, as illustrated in Fig. 5.

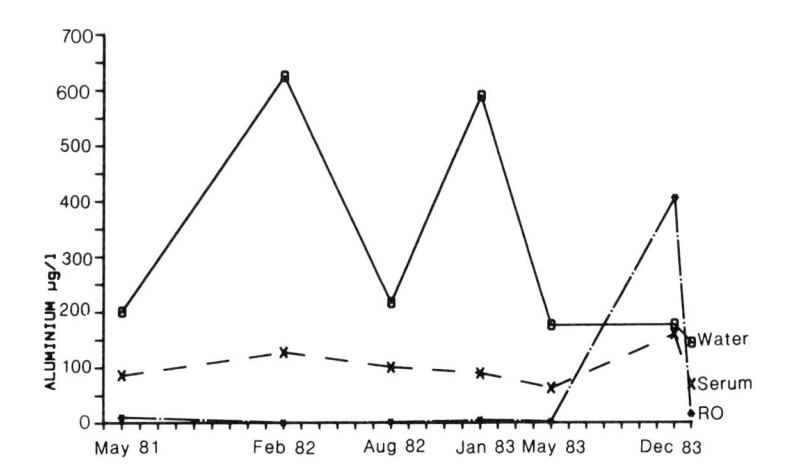

Fig. 5. Concentrations of aluminum in dialysis water before (water) and after (RO) reverse osmosis treatment and in serum from a home dialysis patient measured on 7 occasions in 32 months. Failure of the reverse osmosis unit in December 1983 was associated with only a small rise in serum aluminum concentration.

This can lead to periodic overloading of membranes in reverse osmosis units with the result that the concentration of aluminum in water coming out of the unit may quickly rise above the level in the water going in (Fig. 5) and so place the patient at great risk of acute aluminum intoxication. Regular measurement of serum aluminum concentrations cannot be relied upon to give an indication of RO failure as illustrated by the following study carried out in the West of Scotland. Serum and post RO water aluminum levels measured two months before and at the time of 13 RO failures in 10 home dialysis patients were examined retrospectively. Serum concentration rose at the time of RO failure in only 3 out of the 13 episodes (increases ranged from 57-97 µg/liter) while the mean (±SE) increase in aluminum concentration for all RO-treated water samples was 576 (±130) µg/liter. Reverse osmosis membrane failure can only be detected by regular monitoring of the RO water aluminum concentration. In areas where aluminum levels in the water supply are high monitoring should be carried out at least every 3 months but preferably once a month, RO units should be serviced 6 monthly and RO membranes should be changed every 12 to 18 months.

Patients with Hypercalcemia

Hypercalcemia is a common finding in patients with aluminum bone disease[11] and is a useful diagnostic marker of aluminum toxicity. The accumulation of aluminum along the mineralization front appears to block the uptake of calcium into bone. Hypercalcemia may develop as a result of this and the increased availability of calcium due to treatment with vitamin D metabolites and the addition of calcium to the dialysis fluid. Hypercalcemia can also occur in renal patients as a result of autonomous function of one or more hyperplastic parathyroid glands - so called tertiary hyperparathyroidism - and this usually requires to be treated by subtotal parathyroidectomy. Thus, if hypercalcemia develops in a patient with chronic renal failure it is important that aluminum toxicity be excluded as the cause to prevent unnecessary exposure to the risks associated with parathyroidectomy.

Bone biopsy provides the only reliable means of identifying all patients with aluminum bone disease and of distinguishing them from hyperparathyroid patients without aluminum toxicity. However, recent studies have indicated that a desferoxamine infusion test may be used as a noninvasive procedure to screen patients who are suspected on clinical and biochemical findings to have aluminum bone disease before the instigation of long-term corrective therapy. Milliner et al.[12] have suggested that at 24 hours after a 2 hour intravenous infusion of 40 mg desferoxamine/kg body weight the plasma aluminum concentration will rise by more than 200 µg/liter in most patients with aluminum bone disease. Although this test has a low specificity for aluminum osteodystrophy (50%) its sensitivity is high (94%). However, the sensitivity of the test may be lower in patients with aplastic bone disease[7,8] (T. Drueke; S. Charhon, personal communications). Nevertheless, it should be helpful in the management of patients with hypercalcemia in whom parathyroidectomy is being considered since a positive test should obviate the immediate need for bone biopsy and indicate treatment of aluminum bone disease and postponement of parathyroidectomy. The test should be repeated after appropriate therapy and, if doubt about the diagnosis persists, a further bone biopsy should be taken before parathyroidectomy is performed.

Aluminum Accumulation After Parathyroidectomy

It has been suggested that the high PTH secretion of secondary hyperparathyroidism might protect against the development of aluminum bone disease. The following mechanism has been proposed: increased PTH secretion leads to an absolute increase in the extent of mineralizing surfaces on bone and to an increase in the rate of bone mineralization. Since aluminum is deposited in bone predominantly at sites of bone mineralization, patients with moderate or severe secondary hyperparathyroidism have a greater capacity to take up a given load of aluminum into bone than others with mild secondary hyperparathyroidism or with low mineralization rates. Thus, the aluminum can be dispersed widely in the skeleton without the concentration at sites of uptake rising sufficiently high to inhibit calcification.

Recent studies have indicated that there may be increased staining of aluminum on bone surfaces and increased aluminum-related osteomalacia in patients who have undergone parathyroidectomy. The reason for the increase in aluminum staining remains unclear but it has been suggested by Andress et al.[13] that it might result from the effects of decreased bone formation and mineralization secondary to low PTH secretion after parathyroidectomy. Thus, if aluminum exposure remains unchanged after parathyroidectomy there will be fewer mineralizing surfaces available to take up the same load of aluminum and each surface would then be exposed to concentrations of aluminum sufficiently high to inhibit mineralization and to be stainable histochemically. However, in a similar study by De Vernejoul et al.[14] increased stainable aluminum was seen on bone surfaces post-parathyroidectomy in 4 out of 6 patients whose plasma PTH concentrations remained significantly elevated above the normal range and whose serum calcium levels did not fall significantly. These findings suggest that the surgery had been unsuccessful in these patients and that increased PTH secretion may not protect all patients from aluminum bone disease.

The numbers of patients reported in the above studies[13,14] were samll. In a large study of 36 patients who underwent parathyroidectomy in Newcastle[15], only 2 (5%) developed aluminum-related osteomalacia after surgery. One of these patients had aluminum staining before operation and the other may have been dialyzed with aluminum-contaminated water. Sections were stained for aluminum in 28 of the 36 cases and 12 (43%) of these were positive for aluminum. However, at least 4 had been positive before surgery indicating that a maxiumum of 8 (28%) of these patients may have had increased deposition of aluminum after parathyroidectomy. The post-parathyroidectomy biopsy specimens were taken from 5 of these patients between 17 and 52 months after the first biopsy during which time some of them may have been exposed to high dialysate aluminum concentrations. Thus, increased aluminum staining in bone after parathyroidectomy may occur in only a relatively small percentage (up to 28%) of patients undergoing surgery and may be only partly related to the decreased rate of bone formation associated with lower PTH secretion.

REFERENCES

1. Ellis HA, Peart KM. Azotaemic renal osteodystrophy: A quantitative study on iliac bone. J Clin Pathol 1973; 26:83-101.
2. Pierides AM, Ellis HA, Simpson W, et al. Variable response to long-term 1α hydroxycholecalciferol in haemodialysis osteodystrophy. Lancet 1976; i:1092-95.
3. Ott SM, Maloney NA, Coburn JW, et al. The prevalence of bone aluminum deposition in renal osteodystrophy and its relation to the response to calcitriol therapy. N Engl J Med 1982; 307:709-713.
4. Ward MK, Feest TG, Ellis HA, et al. Osteomalacic dialysis osteodystrophy: evidence for a water-borne aetiological agent, probably aluminium. Lancet 1978; i:841-45.
5. Alfrey AC. Aluminum intoxication. N Engl J Med 1984; 310:1113-15.
6. Charhon SA, Chavassieux PM, Chapuy MC, et al. Low rate of bone formation with or without histologic appearance of osteomalacia in patients with aluminum intoxication. J Lab Clin Med 1985; 106:123-131.
7. Andress DL, Maloney NA, Coburn JW, et al. Osteomalacia and aplastic bone disease in aluminum-related bone disease. J Clin Endocrinol Metab 1987; 65:11-16.
8. Andress DL, Kopp JB, Maloney NA, et al. Early deposition of aluminum in bone in diabetic patients on hemodialysis. N Engl J Med 1987; 316:292-96.

9. Kerr DNS, Ward MK, Arze RS, et al. Aluminum-induced osteodystrophy: The demise of "Newcastle bone disease"? Kidney Int 1986; 29:S58-S64.
10. Smith GD, Winney RJ, McLean A, Robson JS. Aluminium-related osteomalacia: Response to reverse osmosis water treatment. Kidney Int 1987; 32:96-101.
11. Boyce BF, Fell GS, Elder HY, et al. Hypercalcaemic osteomalacia due to aluminium toxicity. Lancet 1982; ii:1009-13.
12. Milliner DS, Nebeker HG, Ott SM, et al. Use of the desferoxamine infusion test in the diagnosis of aluminum-related osteodystrophy. Ann Intern Med 1984; 101:775-80.
13. Andress DL, Ott SM, Maloney NA, et al. Effect of parathyroidectomy on bone aluminum accumulation in chronic renal failure. N Engl J Med 1985; 312:468-73.
14. De Vernejoul MC, Marchais S, London G, et al. Increased bone aluminum deposition after subtotal parathyroidectomy in dialyzed patients. Kideny Int 1985; 27:785-791.
15. De Francisco AM, Ellis HA, Owen JP, et al. Parathyroidectomy in chronic renal failure. Quart J Med 1985; 55:289-315.

ACKNOWLEDGEMENTS

This work was partly supported by a grant to Brendan F. Boyce from the Scottish Hospital Endowments Research Trust.

We thank Thelma Barrios for typing the manuscript.

Discussion:

DR. ITTEL (Germany): I thought it was very difficult to interpret your aluminum absorption test since an increase in serum aluminum after an overload of aluminum might reflect the deposition of aluminum in bone rather than absorption. So, I found it interesting that the patients in your tests which already had osteomalacia had a more marked increase in serum aluminum, since this might reflect the fact that they cannot accumulate aluminum at a faster rate in bone because they don't have any mineralization front anymore. So, I think the only way to make a valid interpretation of your test would be, either to infuse aluminum and to see how high the rate of tissue uptake is in these patients, or to perform a prospective study.

DR. BOYCE (San Antonio, TX): Yes, I understand the point you're making about the bones of these patients already being loaded with aluminum so that they're likely to have a higher increase in the serum aluminum. But this doesn't explain the absence of aluminum in the four patients who had been on dialysis, taking large amounts of aluminum orally. But, I agree, this is not the best way to do it. To be honest, I think the best way to identify these patients is when they still have urinary output, give them an aluminum load and see if urinary aluminum levels increase significantly. We would then need to follow these patients up for a couple of years and biopsy them and see if these patients, rather than those who don't have this increase, are the ones who develop aluminum bone disease.

DR. ITTEL: Second question. Those patients who had a marked increase in serum aluminum after being exposed to aluminum orally, did they differ with respect to parathyroid hormone or 1,25 vitamin D3 to the other patients?

DR. BOYCE: At the time of doing the study.

DR. ITTEL: Yes.

DR. BOYCE: Some of them had increased - two out of the four had detectable and increased level of parathyroid hormone and two of them did not. Three of the patients with osteitis fibrosa had high aluminum, high PTH levels, and one of them didn't.

DR. MALLUCHE (Lexington, KY): I enjoyed your presentation. I would like to offer a slightly different view of the problem. We feel that there is renal osteodystrophy even without aluminum. If you remove aluminum, there is still renal osteodystrophy. The scope of renal osteodystrophy consists of predominant hyperparathyroid bone disease, mixed renal osteodystrophy, and low turnover osteomalacia, even without aluminum.

And we feel that aluminum, then, is superimposed on those abnormalities. It might change the histologic picture from one type to the other. The patient who had predominant hyperparathyroid bone disease before being exposed to aluminum, might then decrease bone turnover and eventually wind up having low turnover osteomalacia and vice versa. If you remove aluminum, you can see that patients change the histologic picture from low turnover osteomalacia to mixed renal osteodystrophy or predominant hyperparathyroid bone disease. I think we have to keep in mind that aluminum certainly is not responsible for everything and there's a lot of other pathologic features involved.

DR. BOYCE: I agree with you. And there was a short time available for the presentation. I did say at the beginning that I was talking about troublesome renal osteodystrophy. And I think, today, the aluminum bone disease is the most troublesome form, particularly when we have 1,25 and other agents available to control the types of bone disease you've spoken about.

DR. MALLUCHE: It's just a short additional comment since you're a pathologist. I think the old pathologists coined the misnomer osteitis fibrosa. There is no inflammation here. And we are now coining another misnomer, which is aplastic bone disease. Bone is not aplastic. Bone is there, it's just adynamic. It doesn't turn over.

DR. FORBES (New York): I'd like to comment on the use of the aluminum stain to reach conclusions about whether parathyroidectomy enhances the content of aluminum in bone. In fact, Alfrey has shown that parathyroid hormone increases the content of aluminum in both bone and other tissues. I'd like to suggest that parathyroidectomy may allow for the rearrangement of aluminum in bone or the denser accumulation of aluminum at mineralization fronts. But I doubt that it increases the uptake of aluminum in bone.

In that regard, I believe that all of the data you cited showed increased aluminum staining at mineralization fronts after parathyroidectomy. But they don't show that aluminum uptake is increased after parathyroidectomy. Could you comment on that?

DR. BOYCE: You mean, increased uptake in the bone as a whole, measured using atomic absorption as opposed to a stain?

DR. FORBES: Correct.

DR. BOYCE: I think the problem with looking at this question of aluminum uptake in bone is that there have been few studies that are really controlled. And we've had reports of increased aluminum in selected patients. The study I cited from Newcastle reported the largest number of patients I'm aware of. And it would seem to me that, from their study, aluminum staining is not all that prevalent. And there's a good correlation between in some studies anyway, the extent of staining and the amount of aluminum in the bone. But I think more work needs to be done on that. I think it's still unclear.

DR. PAK (Dallas): Your comment that orange juice augments aluminum absorption is intriguing to me because it has bearing on the type or form of aluminum which is absorbed. If it were aluminum ion that were absorbed, citrate, theoretically, could reduce it by complexing the aluminum. On the other hand, if it is a complex that's absorbed, one would envision citrate would augment the aluminum absorption. My question is, how secure is the evidence that fruit juice or citrate augment aluminum absorption?

DR. BOYCE: Okay. I think the evidence is fairly good that citrate can enhance the absorption of some of the species of aluminum. You are right. There are different species of aluminum which exist in different forms. What I cannot say is, which of these is preferentially absorbed.

The Pathogenesis and Clinical Course of Multiple Endocrine Neoplasia, Type 2A

ROBERT F. GAGEL

*Departments of Medicine and Cell Biology
VA Medical Center and Baylor College of Medicine
Houston, TX*

Multiple Endocrine Neoplasia, Type 2a (MEN 2a) is a heritable syndrome characterized by the association of medullary thyroid carcinoma, parathyroid hyperplasia and pheochromocytoma. Since the description of this syndrome in 1961 by Sipple (1) there have been 3 phases in development of understanding of this syndrome. The **descriptive phase** (from 1961-69) emphasized the autosomal dominant form of inheritance and the mode of presentation of each of the three manifestations of the syndrome and culminated in the classic article by Steiner et al. in 1968 (2) summarizing the clinical features of the syndrome. The discovery during the late 1960's that medullary thyroid carcinoma produced calcitonin and that calcitonin measurements could be used to diagnose early C-cell abnormalities ushered in the **second phase** of progress for this syndrome. Subsequent studies from several groups defined the natural history of this syndrome (3,4,5) and demonstrated that early thyroidectomy appeared to be curative (6). Study of the syndrome is now entering the **third phase**, the elucidation of the genetic and molecular basis for the syndrome. This report will focus on recent advances in mapping of the MEN II gene and studies defining the long-term natural history of the syndrome.

A Deletional Model for Hereditary Malignancy

There is increasing evidence that multiple endocrine neoplasia belongs to a group of heritable malignancies caused by **deletion of a regulatory gene on a specific chromosome**. The prototype heritable malignancy caused by deletion of a specific gene is retinoblastoma. From an analysis of age of onset data comparing hereditary (bilateral) to nonhereditary (unilateral) retinoblastoma, Knudson proposed a "two hit" theory for development of retinoblastoma (7). He postulated that the "first hit" (or mutation) was inherited whereas the "second hit" (mutation) occurred in somatic cells. Knudson's theory has been confirmed for retinoblastoma. Studies from several groups have now convincingly demonstrated that retinoblastoma in both its hereditary and nonhereditary form results from deletion of genetic information from chromosome 13 (13 q14.1q14.2). These observations were initially made by observing cytogenetic deletions in peripheral blood chromosomes from affected individuals. Studies of tumors from affected individuals have shown deletion of the second allele at this same site presumably from a somatic cell mutation (Figure 1). Additional studies have resulted in the cloning and sequencing of the retinoblastoma gene (8,9,10) which encodes a phosphoprotein. Although direct evidence is still lacking, this phosphoprotein appears to serve an inhibitory regulatory role in the growth of certain retinal cells. Exactly which recessive gene is released from suppression is currently not known.

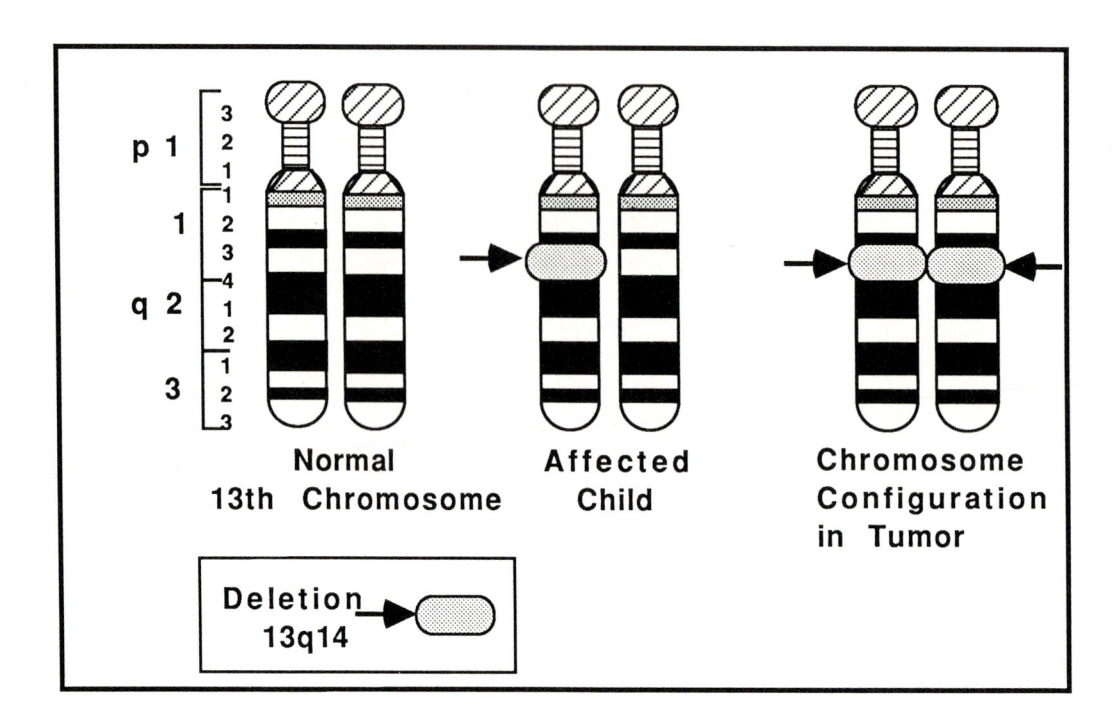

Figure 1. Proposed mechanism for transformation in hereditary retinoblastoma. A deletion of the retinoblastoma gene at 13 q14.1 is inherited. A second somatic mutation results in the deletion of the other retinoblastoma gene allele.

A number of different mechanisms including non-disjunction loss, nondisjunction reduplication, mitotic recombination, gene conversion and point mutation-deletion (11) have been demonstrated to be possible mechanisms by which the second somatic mutation occurs.

Relevance of this Model to Multiple Endocrine Neoplasia Syndromes

Can this model explain the events which occur in the multiple endocrine neoplasia syndromes? The multiple endocrine neoplasia syndromes share many features with the retinoblastoma syndrome. MEN is inherited as an autosomal dominant trait, the tumors which develop in MEN 2, like hereditary retinoblastoma, are known to be polyclonal (12), and the age of onset data for hereditary versus non-hereditary medullary thyroid carcinoma are very similar to that observed for retinoblastoma (13,14). There is convincing evidence in a limited number of **MEN 1** families that a deletional mechanism is the basis for the syndrome. Recent studies have linked **MEN 1** to the centromeric area on the long arm of chromosome 11 and studies in 2 insulinomas from family members utilizing probes mapped to chromosome 11 have demonstrated a deletion of a second allele (15).

Linkage of MEN 2a to Chromosome 10

Progress toward identification of a specific genetic abnormality in **MEN 2a** has been slow because there is no specific cytogenetic abnormality such as is observed for retinoblastoma. Through linkage analysis studies utilizing restriction fragment length polymorphism, Mathew et al. (16) and Simpson et al. (17) have demonstrated linkage to an area near the centromere of chromosome 10 (Figure 2) in a total of 6 families. Subsequent reports from other investigators have confirmed these findings in an additional 5 families of diverse geographic origin (18). It, therefore, seems reasonable to believe that the MEN 2a gene is located on chromosome 10. A paucity of informative markers in this region, presumably because of low recombination near the centromere, has made further efforts at localization of the gene difficult and there has been no demonstration of a specific deletion on chromosome 10 in patients with MEN 2a analagous to the deletion demonstrated in retinoblastoma or MEN 1.

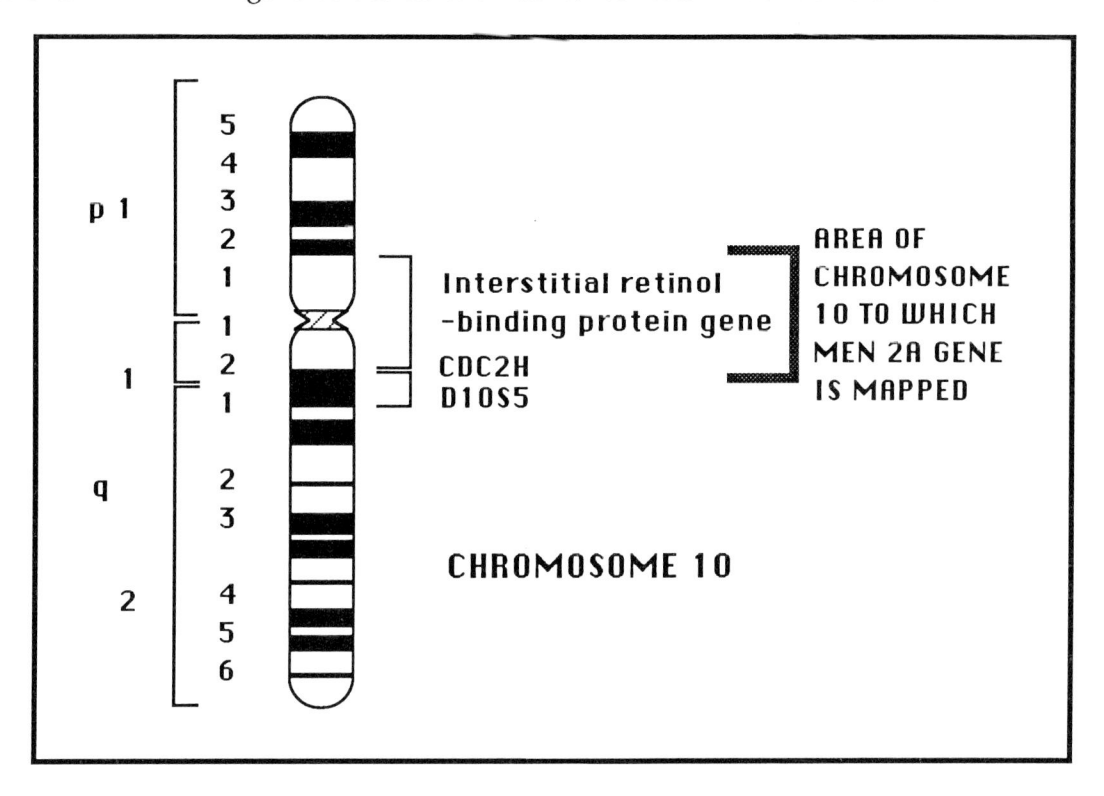

Figure 2. MEN 2a has been linked to a centromeric region of chromosome ten (16,17,18).

Despite these present gaps in knowledge, a deletional mutation in an area near the centromere of chromosome 11 causing the MEN 2A syndrome remains the favored hypothesis and progress is likely to be forthcoming. There is currently no information about the genetic defect in MEN 2b.

Clinical Course of Medullary Thyroid Carcinoma in Multiple Endocrine Neoplasia, Type 2a.

It seems likely that identification of specific MEN 2a gene carriers at or shortly after birth will soon be possible. How will this information be used? Should all individuals be thyroidectomized at or shortly after birth or should gene carriers be intensively screened with removal of the thyroid at the time of first detection of an abnormalitiy? To answer these questions requires information about natural history of the disease and the impact of current techniques for detecting the disease on the clinical course of the disease. Data from several groups studying this disease indicate that annual screening of family members at risk for the disease detects C-cell abnormalities at a very early stage, usually before the development of metastatic disease (3,4,5). Followup data from patients thyroidectomized 10 or more years ago are now becoming available. In the J-kindred* we have followed 22 prospectively screened patients after thyroidectomy for a mean period of 11 years (13 patients with C-cell hyperplasia and 9 with microscopic medullary thyroid carcinoma). None of these individuals had demonstrable metastasis at the time of surgery. Nineteen of these 22 patients are now considered to be disease free by all criteria (normal clinical exam and normal calcitonin values after provocative pentagastrin tests measured in 3 different calcitonin radioimmunoassays) (6). Three patients had abnormal calcitonin values on more than one occasion when the samples were measured in the standard calcitonin assay, but were low or nondetectable when measured in two other more sensitive radioimmunoassays (6). Results of early thyroidectomy from the Mayo Clinic experience (19) indicate that 14 children thyroidectomized for early, occult C-cell abnormalities remain disease free whereas 3 children with clinically apparent disease at the time of surgery have persistent calcitonin elevations. Combining our results with the Mayo Clinic experience (19) it would appear that 33 patients (85%) with early thyroidectomy remain disease free, 3 patients (7.5%) are in an equivocal status and 3 patients (7.5%) have evidence of metastatic disease. These results indicate that most patients with early C-cell disease can be detected and cured by currently available screening techniques, but there is a minority who may have more aggressive disease or early metastasis.

That some children should develop early malignancy is not surprising. If the average age for development of the second mutation is below the age of 10 and is a random event, then it is reasonable to believe that the C-cells in some children will undergo the second mutation at an early age, possibly even in utero as has been described in MEN 2b. If this logic proves to be correct, then the only reasonable course of therapy, if a high cure rate is to be expected, is to remove all C-cells at the earliest possible age. The decision to perform thyroidectomy in the first year of life should balance several factors including the belief that early thyroidectomy will more likely result in a cure, the age at which a safe and **total** thyroidectomy can be performed and family acceptance of such surgery. There is little data or experience currently available to provide answers for these issues. Prenatal diagnosis and termination of pregnancy will be another alternative, but one which will probably not be utilized because of the knowledge that most individuals born with this syndrome can be successfully managed and live normal lives utilizing currently available treatment techniques.

The results obtained utilizing currently available screening techniques, which have resulted in an 85% or greater cure rate, provide optimism that a shift in the age of diagnosis from 10 years of age to birth can only lead to an improved cure rate. It is reasonable to believe most patients with a genetic propensity to develop the disease can be cured by early thyroidectomy.

Management of Adrenal Medullary Disease

Diagnosis and management of adrenal medullary disease remains the most challenging aspect of managing the MEN 2a syndrome. Several facts have emerged in recent years to help guide the clinician. The first is the observation that proven adrenal medullary malignancy in the MEN 2a syndrome is rare [less than 10 reported cases (20)] with most of the cases clustering in a few families. Second, almost all of

---

* These studies were supported by grants (AM-31307, M01-RR-00054, and AR-10206) from the National Institutes of Health and by merit review and clinical investigator awards from the Veterans Administration.

these tumors are intraadrenal with only rare periadrenal rests reported (21). Third, because these tumors are intraadrenal and well differentiated they produce primarily epinephrine (6). The increased production of epinephrine accounts for early symptoms of palpitations, tachycardia, jitteriness and anxiety. The fact that there is not a large amount of norepinephrine production early in the course of the disease probably accounts for the lack of hypertension in early cases of the disease. With large tumors later in the course of the disease norepinephrine production and hypertension may develop.

Current techniques for diagnosis include measurement of fractionated urine catecholamines or metanephrine, scanning with [^{125}I] metaiodobenzylguanidine (MIBG), and computerized tomography or magnetic resonance imaging of the adrenal gland. The high radiation dosage associated with computerized tomography or MIBG scanning make these techniques unsuitable for repeated screening. In a prospective analysis of 11 MEN 2a patients with surgically proven adrenal pheochromocytoma, we found that 10 of the 11 patients had abnormal 24 hour urine epinephrine excretion (6). The one exception was a young woman with symptoms consistent with a pheochromocytoma with normal urine epinephrine values and a small pheochromocytoma demonstrated by radiographic techniques and surgical exploration. We have found that yearly screening of patients at risk for development of pheochromocytoma routinely identified individuals with pheochromocytoma before development of life-threatening manifestations. These studies, however, have not allowed us to routinely detect adrenal medullary hyperplasia and there have been difficulties obtaining urine collections in an outpatient setting. Despite generally cooperative family members, the compliance rate for urine collection in our studies was not greater than 60%, making it possible that a pheochromocytoma could reach life-threatening size before identification. Better techniques for identification of pheochromocytoma in its early stages are clearly needed.

The approach to management of pheochromocytoma in this syndrome varies. In a family in which there is no history of adrenal medullary malignancy, we have attempted to balance the risks of adrenal insufficiency with those associated with pheochromocytoma and remove only adrenal glands with demonstrable pheochromocytoma or enlargement consistent with adrenal medullary hyperplasia. The radiologic findings are confirmed by exploration of the apparently unaffected gland at the time of primary surgery. Our experience indicates that about one-half of these patients will develop a pheochromocytoma in the contralateral adrenal within 10-12 years (6), but close followup has resulted in a satisfactory outcome in each case. An alternative is to perform bilateral adrenalectomy at the time of primary surgery, an approach routinely employed in a few centers (4,20).

Parathyroid Disease

Parathyroid disease is rarely observed in prospectively screened MEN 2a patients (6). The quoted 10-20% incidence of parathyroid disease (2) occurred in family members diagnosed before the onset of prospective screening. Even family members followed for up to 10 years following primary thyroidectomy for C-cell disease have not developed parathyroid abnormalities [Figure 3 (6)].
Several explanations for the lack of parathyroid involvement in patients thyroidectomized early can be suggested. First, the average age of patients prospectively screened and thyroidectomized is likely to be below the average age for development of parathyroid disease in this syndrome. It is possible these patient will develop parathyroid disease as they age. Second, at the time of thyroidectomy inferior parathyroid glands are frequently removed, resulting in a decreased mass of

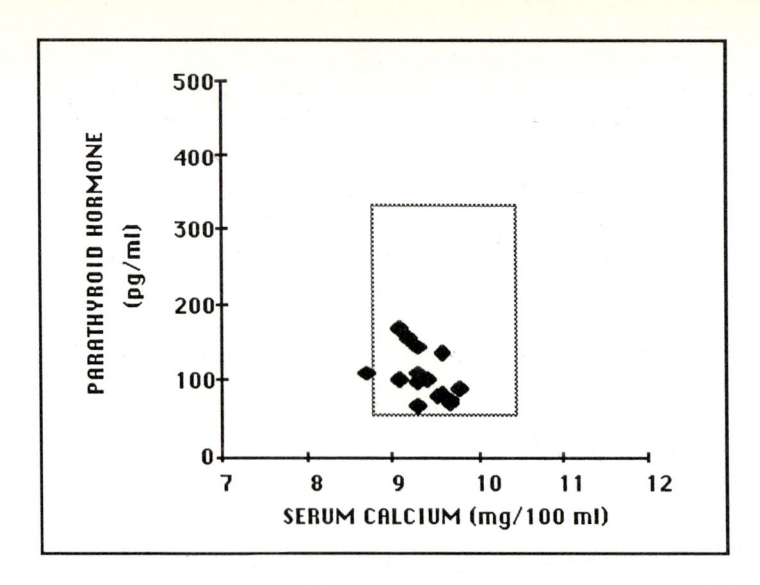

Figure 3. Normal serum calcium and parathyroid hormone values in 15 patients thyroidectomized for early C-cell abnormalities a mean of 10 years earlier. Data presented in reference (6). The box shows the normal range for serum calcium and parathyroid hormone in unaffected family members.

parathyroid tissue, with the possibility of a delayed onset of parathyroid disease. Finally, it is possible that removal of the thyroid gland eliminates a growth factor for parathyroid tissue analogous to the parathyroid growth factor described in MEN I. Additional followup and study over the next two decades should provide insight into the mechanism for development of parathyroid hyperplasia.

The fact that MEN 1 has been linked to chromosome 11 and MEN 2 to chromosome 10 indicates there must be at least two mechanisms for causing parathyroid hyperplasia, a condition observed in both syndromes. For MEN 1 a reasonable hypothesis might be that deletion of a gene regulating a parathyroid growth factor [as has been described by Brandi et al. (22)] results in parathyroid hyperplasia. The absence of such a growth factor in MEN 2 suggests another mechanism may be operative.

Conclusion

A final question. Is MEN 2 a single syndrome or 3 distinct syndromes consisting of medullary thyroid carcinoma, pheochromocytoma and parathyroid disease? The observation that certain families express only one or two components of the syndrome in a reproducible pattern raises the possibility that MEN II is caused by 3 distinct genes which are contiguously located so that a large deletion of genetic information results in the development of all 3 manifestations, whereas a small deletion results in only one or two manifestations. Answers to these and other important questions as well as improved diagnostic accuracy necessary for successful management of this should become available as this story unfolds.

References

1. Sipple JH. (1961) Am J Med **31**, 163-6.
2. Steiner AL, Goodman AD, Powers SR. (1968) Medicine **47**, 371-409.
3. Graze K, Spiler I, Tashjian AH Jr, et al. (1978) N Engl J Med **299**, 980-5.

4. Sizemore GW, Heath H III, Carney JA. (1980) Clinic Endocrine Metab **9**, 299-315.
5. Wells, SA Jr., Dilley-W-G, Farndon-J-A et al. (1985) Arch Int Med **145**, 1248-52.
6. Gagel RF, Tashjian AH, Cummings T, et al. (1988) N Eng J Med **318**, 478-484.
7. Knudson AG Jr. (1986) Ann Rev Genet **20**, 231-51.
8. Friend SH, Bernards R, Rogel J, et al. (1986) Nature **323**, 643-646.
9. Lee WH, Brookstein R, Hong F, et al. (1987) Science **235**, 1394-99.
10. Fung Y-KT, Murphree AL, T'Ang A, et al. (1987) Science **236**, 1657-61.
11. Cavenee, WK. (1987) Birth Defects: Original Article Series 23:93-107.
12. Baylin SB, Hsu SH, Gann DS et al. (1978) Science **199**, 429-31.
13. Jackson CE, Block MA, Greenawald KA, et al.. Am J Hum Genet 31:704-10, 1979.
14. Block, MA, Jackson CE, Greenawald, KA, et al. (1980) Surgery **115**, 142-148.
15. Larsson C, Skogseid B, Oberg K, et al. (1988) Nature **332**, 85-87.
16. Mathew CGP, Chin KS, Easton DF et al. (1987) Nature **328**, 527-528.
17. Simpson, NE, Kidd KK, Goodfellow PJ, et al. (1987) Nature **328**, 528-530.
18. Sobol H, Salvetti A, Bonnardel C, Lenoir GM. (1988) Lancet **1**:8575-6, 62.
19. Telander RL, Zimmerman D, vanHeerden JA, Sizemore G. Abstracts of the 2nd International Workshop on Multiple Endocrine Neoplasia, Type 2, Cambridge, England, September 17- 20, 1986, Abstract 5.2.
20. Sisson JC, Shapiro B, Beierwaltes WH. (1984) Henry Ford Hospital Med J **32**, 254-60.
21. Lips CJM, Minder WH, Leo JR et al. (1978) Am J Med **64**, 569-78.
22. Brandi ML, Aurbach GD, Fitzpatrick LA et al. (1986) N Engl J Med **314**, 1278-93.

Discussion:

DR. WOODHOUSE (Saudi Arabia): In the children in whom you've performed total thyroidectomy, have you done thyroid scans afterwards, how complete has been the surgery, and might failure of removal of some thyroid tissue be responsible for those people who relapse a few years later?

DR. GAGEL (Houston): We have not routinely done postoperative scans in our patients. And, in large part because most of them had normal or nondetectable calcitonin values afterwards, we did not feel that it was necessary to do so.

My feeling is that residual tissue could be an important cause of development of subsequent abnormalities. In other words, every C-cell that you leave behind, whether it's normal or abnormal, has the potential for developing a mutation. And, as a result of that, it seems quite likely that in residual thyroid tissue one could develop recurrent or newly-formed tumors. So, I think that if there is any evidence of abnormalities, then it's very reasonable to look for additional thyroid tissue.

DR. WOODHOUSE: We routinely ablate ours, but even in the best surgical hands (and we're fortunate to have an expert thyroidectomist), there is still residual tissue which you can see a month later in a proportion of his cases. It's worth ablating them, I think.

DR. ZIEGLER (Heidelberg): My question is in the same direction. Wouldn't this mean that you should consider, again, radioiodine treatment, as we do in differentiated thyroid carcinoma because even there we don't think that tumor is present at the time of operation, but we think that the risk of recurrence decreases. And, so, as mostly C-cells are adhering to the thyroid follicular cells, is it worth performing radioiodine treatment afterwards?

DR. GAGEL: Well, Professor Ziegler, as you know, we have not done that. I think, as you've pointed out, there are some good reasons to consider that. One concern that I would have, though, is that the C-cell is not particularly radio-sensitive. And unlike the thyroid follicular cells you may kill the thyroid cells, but not kill the C-cells.

I think the only way to address that is probably for someone to do it in a prospective, controlled fashion. I think it would be worthy of consideration.

DR. BONE (Detroit): I'm glad to see you addressing this difficult problem of diagnosing the pheochromocytomas. I have a question. You mentioned that you saw the elevation in epinephrine and epinephrine/norepinephrine ratios at about the time of diagnosis, which, I suspect, was one of the means of diagnosis. In how many of your cases did you have clinical findings highly suggestive of pheochromocytoma with or without radiographic findings of pheochromocytoma and no distinct elevation of even the epinephrine? How good a test is that?

DR. GAGEL: From the data that I showed you, there was one patient, a young woman, who at the time of the diagnosis of her first pheo, had no elevation or no abnormalities in catacholamine that we could detect.

But, also, when she later developed a pheo on the opposite side, again she had no abnormalities that we could detect on several urine collections. And, so, there is a false/negative rate in our series at slightly less than ten percent. So, it's not perfect, by any means.

DR. SANTORA (Detroit): Do you know whether the form of calcitonin secreted by the medullary carcinoma of the thyroid is detected by the standard two-site IRMA? I mention that because some of the calcitonin forms in small cell carcinoma of the lung are not identical to the native sequence.

DR. GAGEL: Our assay certainly detects that higher molecular weight species. The Nichols assay also detects the higher molecular weight species. Other assays do not, but detect only monomeric calcitonin. And there are other assays which are specific for only the higher molecular weight forms, or are directed against the precursor portion of the molecule.

DR. SIZEMORE (Maywood, IL): Bob, I enjoyed the paper very much. I think, first, a question, and then maybe a comment, in view of the I131 thoughts. I hear you saying that if we have genetic positivity, then we're going to operate on all those patients rather early. Are you willing to say that we should operate them all at age one, age two? Did you look at your data? Most of those patients, I think, are older than that when they are first operated. And, we've shown that if you operate within the first decade for the MEN IIA, there's uniform cure rate, at least with the follow-up we have. Would that be your thought? And are we going to do calcitonins on those patients, or are we just going to operate to be cost-effective?

DR. GAGEL: I have not gone back to look at the age at which the patients who had abnormalities were operated upon. And that's something that I need to do.

I firmly believe that we should be operating upon these children at the earliest reasonable age at which we can do a thyroidectomy. And my reasons for that are very specific. Number one, there is a statistical chance of developing a second mutation. And that could occur before birth, in utero, or it could occur in the first year of life. And because of that, I think we're playing with a loaded gun not to be operating upon these children at the earliest reasonable age at which a thyroidectomy could be done. I don't have an answer to what that age might be, but I think that it will emerge in collaboration with our surgical colleagues.

DR. SIZEMORE: I agree. Thank you. That comment was in light of the questions from Dr. Woodhouse and Dr. Ziegler. I have, anecdotally, given I131 to five patients postoperatively with high CT, with the hope of "sterilizing" the neck. It does not work.

XI
Therapeutic Advances in Metabolic Bone Disease

Overview: Newer Therapies in Hypercalcemia and Metabolic Bone Disease

HUNTER HEATH III

General Clinical Research Center
Mayo Foundation
Endocrine Research Unit
Division of Endocrinology and Metabolism
Department of Medicine
Mayo Clinic
Rochester, MN

The decade of the '80s has been an exciting one for all investigators in the area of calcium and bone metabolism, because a remarkable convergence of technology, basic science applications, and clinical interest has led to major advances in understanding. The physiology of calcium-regulating hormone secretion and action, mechanisms of plasma calcium homeostasis, the cellular basis of metabolic bone disease--all have yielded to concerted attack. However, the practicing physician has seen much of this advance somewhat from the sidelines, asking legitimately when this new information was going to be translated into practical measures for care of patients. The session I chaired was intended to address this justified query, and to point out several important therapeutic maneuvers that are available now, are about to see general use, or represent promising first approaches to new agents. We focused on three important areas: the life-threatening hypercalcemia frequently accompanying malignant tumors, aluminum-related renal osteodystrophy, and osteoporosis.

Hypercalcemia of malignancy

The pathogenesis of hypercalcemia in malignancy is complex, and varies among tumor types. The older classification as "ectopic parathyroid hormone (PTH)-secreting" versus that caused by direct tumor destruction of bone was based on indirect and largely mistaken premises. Secretion of authentic PTH by non-parathyroid tumors has never been convincingly demonstrated, and tumor metastases are now known to destroy bone indirectly, by stimulating generation and activity of osteoclasts.

It is now clear that almost all non-parathyroidal malignant tumors causing hypercalcemia do so by secreting or inducing the formation of factors that in turn stimulate osteoclasts. One such tumor product is a 141-amino acid peptide with some PTH-like structure and bioactivities. This PTH-related peptide (PTHrP) lyses bone, but also stimulates renal tubular reabsorption of calcium; these two actions may account for the viciousness of the ensuing hypercalcemia. Other direct or indirect tumor hypercalcemic substances may include 1,25-dihydroxyvitamin D, prostaglandins, transforming growth factors, and other peptide cytokines.

Dr. Heath's work is supported in part by grants from the NIH (RR-0585, AR-32526, DK-38855, and AG-04875).

Aside from various antitumor measures, there are no effective ways to inhibit secretion of hypercalcemic factors. Thus, treatment of the hypercalcemia has focused on first, inhibition of osteoclasts, and second, enhancing renal excretion of calcium. Dr. Jean Jacques Body (Brussels) reviewed agents currently available, then concentrated on the bisphosphonates (diphosphonates). These synthetic analogs of pyrophosphate are potent inhibitors of bone resorption, but with varying potencies and mechanisms of action. They are effective against the osteolytic component of hypercalcemia, but do not alter renal tubular reabsorption of calcium and therefore are relatively ineffective when the latter is a major causative factor.

The only bisphosphonate currently approved and on sale in the U.S. is also the least useful in hypercalcemia: etidronate (EHDP) or Didronel.℗ It is quite ineffective against hypercalcemia when given orally, but is effective intravenously. Several other bisphosphonates have seen considerable testing in Europe, and seem generally to be more effective than etidronate. For example, clodronate (dichloromethylene bisphosphonate) at 100-300 mg/d for up to 10 d can restore normocalcemia in up to 90% of cases. However, relapse may occur rapidly after discontinuance of clodronate. Amidronate (APD) (or AHPr BP) is very effective when given as 2 hr infusions of 15 mg daily for up to 10 d. Doses less than 0.25 mg/kg/d are ineffective. This drug is efficacious whether or not skeletal metastases are present. Importantly, normocalcemia may last for several weeks after stopping amidronate, and its toxicity is low, including transient fever and lymphopenia.

Still newer bisphosphonates of even greater potency than amidronate are being tested abroad, and some of them are entering clinical trials in the U.S. It seems very likely that, within a few years, we shall have available extremely potent bisphosphonates capable of inducing prolonged normocalcemia in cancer patients, and some of these agents may be active orally. It is possible that these agents could also reverse or prevent skeletal destruction by metastases.

Dr. Jean-Philippe Bonjour (Geneva) discussed two anti-hypercalcemic agents that are much further from general use than the bisphosphonates: gallium nitrate and WR-2721 (an organic thiophosphate).

Gallium nitrate has been used for scanning bone and tumors, but because of its localization in non-skeletal malignancies, it saw further development as a chemotherapeutic agent. During initial human studies, investigators occasionally saw transient hypocalcemia, apparently caused by gallium nitrate. In vitro studies indicated a direct effect of the compound on PTH- or lymphokine-stimulated bone resorption, and further clinical investigations suggested that it might be an effective antihypercalcemic agent in various types of malignancies. A recent randomized, double-blind study suggests that gallium nitrate is effective in lowering the hypercalcemia of malignancy, and that it may be superior to maximally effective doses of calcitonin. The clinical use of gallium nitrate is not yet at hand, because proper comparative studies versus other agents, such as methramycin and the bisphosphonates are not yet available. Further studies are also needed to better understand gallium nitrate's mechanisms of action. The existing data suggest that gallium nitrate or compounds derived therefrom may be very effective in the acute treatment of humoral hypercalcemia of malignancy.

WR-2721 was also developed as a potential cancer therapeutic agent, to increase the resistance of normal tissues to ionizing radiation and alkylating chemotherapeutic agents. Just as for gallium nitrate, the hypocalcemic action of WR-2721 was noted incidentally during phase I clinical trials. WR-2721 is a remarkable compound, in that it both decreases the secretion of PTH in vitro and in vivo, and directly inhibits renal tubular reabsorption of calcium. Furthermore, WR-2721 may directly inhibit osteoclastic bone resorption. Some evidence suggests that WR-2721 is less potent than bisphosphonates or gallium nitrate, but more clinical studies are indicated. It is not yet clear whether WR-2721 can inhibit secretion of the PTH-related peptide from tumors, but if it did, then it would have remarkable triple efficacy in treating the humoral hypercalcemia of malignancy. Just as for gallium nitrate, the very fact that WR-2721 has its known effects greatly encourages the search for related compounds that may be highly effective in treating hypercalcemia of multiple causes.

Aluminum-associated renal osteodystrophy

Dr. Hartmut H. Malluche (Lexington, KY) described the syndromes of bone disease related to skeletal aluminum accumulation that can occur in patients undergoing chronic hemodialysis. The aluminum is ingested as aluminum hydroxide-containing phosphate-binding antacid gels, or enters from contaminated dialysis solutions. Excess bone aluminum may be demonstrable in nearly half of patients on chronic dialysis, and can occur even in mild to moderate renal failure. In particular, stainable aluminum gathers at the interface between unmineralized bone matrix (osteoid) and mineralized bone, and it appears to impair the mineralization process. Clinical manifestations of aluminum-associated bone disease include bone pain, fractures, and hypercalcemia. The latter must be carefully differentiated from the hypercalcemia of "tertiary" hyperparathyroidism, because parathyroidectomy may only aggravate aluminum-associated bone disease.

Dr. Malluche discussed chelation therapy with the iron-binder, deferoxamine (Desferal®), which also binds aluminum. Deferoxamine binds circulating aluminum ion, which is then removed during dialysis. The lowered plasma aluminum level reverses the blood-bone concentration gradient, and thus allows aluminum to diffuse out of bone. Important reductions in bone aluminum can follow several months of treatment.

The histologic manifestations of aluminum-associated bone disease vary from so-called "aplastic" or adynamic bone (no active bone formation or resorption, and no excess osteoid) to florid osteomalacia. In all cases he has treated, Dr. Malluche felt that aluminum chelation yielded improvement, although reminding us that whatever other type of renal osteodystrophy preceded or accompanied the aluminum accumulation would remain or emerge.

Deferoxamine therapy has serious side effects, potentially including hypotension, angina, and ocular damage. Because of this and the difficulties in selecting cases for chelation therapy, the treatment is best undertaken only after appropriate studies on iliac crest bone biopsies and consultation with a nephrologist experienced in use of the drug. Dr. Malluche stated that more long-term studies are needed to firmly establish the safety and effectiveness of deferoxamine in renal osteodystrophy.

Osteoporosis

Of all problems related to bone and calcium metabolism, the clinical and economic impact of late-life and postmenopausal osteoporosis is the greatest. Acute care of hip fracture alone costs several billion dollars per year in the U.S., the worldwide cost in human suffering and national resources is incalculable. While we have made dramatic progress toward understanding the causes of bone loss, physicians have been frustrated by the few treatment options available. In particular, they are impatient with the lack of treatments to increase bone mass, rather than just slow its loss. In this part of the session, we focused on new ways to deliver old treatments (transdermal estrogen), and preliminary reports on efficacy of two methods to increase bone mass (fluoride and PTH).

Dr. Robert Lindsay (West Haverstraw, NY) outlined trends in estrogen prescription over recent years, and highlighted controversies over risks and benefits of estrogen treatment after the menopause. Estrogen clearly retards or even stops bone loss after the menopause, but increases bone mass little if at all. Estrogen therapy may also decrease the risk of cardiovascular disease, but on the other hand, the risk of endometrial carcinoma is increased. While simultaneous use of a progestin, with endometrial shedding, seems to eliminate that risk, the relative effects on cardiovascular risk and bone mass remain unclear.

Similarly, delivery of estrogen transdermally bypasses the liver, and reduces certain estrogen effects mediated by the liver (e.g., increased plasma binding proteins and clotting factors). It is not yet known if transdermal estrogen is cardioprotective, or if its salutary effect on bone equals that of oral estrogen. Trials in osteoporosis are underway, but it will be a long time before all the answers are in on how best to give estrogen, to whom, and for how long. The transdermal route for estrogen is likely to be available soon as a treatment alternative, in any case.

Current studies with sodium fluoride (NaF) were summarized by Dr. Richard Eastell (Rochester, MN), on behalf of Dr. B. Lawrence Riggs. It has been known for many years that skeletal fluorosis can result in sclerotic bones, but only over the last 5 years have there been two long-term, placebo-controlled trials of NaF in established osteoporosis, one at the Mayo Clinic, and one at Henry Ford Hospital. Dr. Eastell described preliminary data from the Mayo study, which is nearing completion. In brief, more than half of the patients taking NaF have had increased lumbar spine bone mineral density, but NaF had no effect at all on appendicular (cortical) bone mass. The drug therefore may be of benefit only to those primarily suffering from the crush fracture syndrome. Furthermore, there was a significant minority who did not respond to NaF, and the treatment was associated with a fairly high incidence of various side effects, including gastric irritation and bleeding, anemia, and lower-extremity pain from stress fractures. Data on fracture rates are still being obtained. Obviously, antifracture efficacy of NaF must be determined before it can be approved for general use. Because the bone generated during NaF treatment is structurally abnormal, it is possible (but unlikely) that the increased bone mass would not stop fracturing. The bone community eagerly awaits definitive reports from both of the large trials, to see if NaF will find a major role in treatment of osteoporosis.

Dr. Jonathan Reeve (Harrow, U.K.) updated us on clinical trials with a seemingly paradoxical treatment for osteoporosis: parenteral synthetic PTH fragment 1-34 [hPTH-(1-34)]. In hyperparathyroid diseases, endogenous PTH generally causes bone loss, but intermittent elevation of PTH in animals by injection sometimes causes osteosclerosis. Dr. Reeve and colleagues have taken advantage of the fact that PTH can increase bone formation as well as resorption. They have administered hPTH-(1-34) as once-daily injections alone, or in combination with 1,25-dihydroxyvitamin D or estrogen. The latter compounds were given to enhance calcium absorption, which does not reliably follow intermittent elevations of plasma PTH.

When daily hPTH-(1-34) was given alone, they saw increased trabecular volume in iliac crest biopsies, but neutral calcium balance and decreased femoral bone mass! In early studies, alternating hPTH-(1-34) for 6 weeks with 1,25-dihydroxyvitamin D for 6 weeks appeared to increase spinal bone mass, as did combination of hPTH-(1-34) with estrogen.

This work is important for what it teaches about physiology of bone, but application of hPTH-(1-34) to clinical practice in these complex regimens is problematic. The peptide is very expensive, and must be given parenterally. Further, the difficulty in finding a simple, safe, and effective regimen is somewhat discouraging. At a minimum, this work shows that bone formation can be increased by something other than fluoride, and certainly will encourage continued research.

In conclusion, our speakers showed that safe, effective acute therapy for life-threatening hypercalcemia is now available, and will soon be even better; that alternative methods for administering estrogen will soon be out; and that effective treatments to increase bone mass (at least in the spine) are feasible and may reach clinical use within the next 5 years. If advances in the coming decade match those of the last, it may not be too much to hope that death and morbidity from several major bone and calcium disorders could be virtually eliminated before the end of the century.

Bisphosphonate Treatment of Severe Hypercalcemia

J.J. BODY

Service de Médecine et Laboratoire d' Investigation Clinique H.J. Tagnon
Unité d' Endocrinologie
Centre des Tumeurs de l' Université Libre de Bruxelles
Institut Jules Bordet
Brussels, Belgium

Bisphosphonates: general considerations for human use

Bisphosphonates (also called diphosphonates) are synthetic analogues of the naturally occurring pyrophosphate that keep a high binding affinity for hydroxylapatite crystals without being degraded by pyrophosphatase. They are extremely potent inhibitors of bone resorption although their exact mechanism of action is still unclear and probably varies from one bisphosphonate to another. Their first recognized activity, namely the capacity to inhibit hydroxylapatite crystals dissolution, does not correlate with their inhibitory power on bone resorption and it is now clear that they act mainly by causing various metabolic inhibitory effects on the osteoclasts, notably a decrease of lysosomal enzyme release[1]. In vitro cytotoxicity is function of the bisphosphonate concentration and the type of derivative, but amino-compounds can inhibit osteoclast- or macrophage-mediated bone resorption at dose levels not causing any evident cellular toxic effects. Contrasting with the rapid inhibitory effect of calcitonin on bone resorption which leads to a fall of serum calcium within a few hours, the inhibitory activity of bisphosphonates becomes evident only after 1 or even 2 days. This observation is consistent with the hypothesis that bisphosphonates progressively enter the osteoclasts during the process of active bone lysis.

Bisphosphonates, at least the amino-compounds, could also inhibit bone resorption by acting on osteoclast precursors. It has thus recently been demonstrated that they can inhibit macrophage proliferation from bone marrow precursors[2] and limit the accession of osteoclast precursors to the bone matrix[3]. Such an action on the precursors of the bone-resorbing cells would be entirely consistent with the prolonged clinical activity of bisphosphonates. Lastly, an action on the immune cells would explain the occasional "acute-phase response" observed in vivo[4], but an action on the production of osteolytic cytokines has not been demonstrated so far.

Whatever the mechanism, bisphosphonates lower serum calcium by inhibiting bone resorption and it is then rational to administer them for hypercalcemic conditions resulting from a pathological increase in bone resorption. It is therefore not surprising that bisphosphonates are only partly effective for hypercalcemia of primary hyperparathyroidism, since increase of bone resorption, stimulation of intestinal calcium absorption, and of kidney calcium reabsorption contribute to a variable extent to the hypercalcemic status of that condition. Similarly, one could even more expect a poor response to bisphosphonate treatment in severe hypercalcemia resulting from vitamin D intoxication. On the contrary, immobilization hypercalcemia has been successfully treated with bisphosphonate administration(5) and, not surprisingly, bisphosphonates have been used primarily for the treatment of tumor-associated hypercalcemia. As developed elsewhere in this symposium, cancer hypercalcemia mainly results from a marked stimulation of bone resorption unmatched by an increase in bone formation. Although the kidneys have a major contributing role in some cases of tumor-associated hypercalcemia, it remains a fact that osteoclastic activation, whether locally by metastatic tumor cells or systemically by humoral mechanisms, is the main pathogenic mechanism leading to an increase of serum calcium in cancer patients. This explains why bisphosphonates are so successful for treating tumoral hypercalcemia. In addition, their enthusiastic use for the treatment of this condition is justified by the relative inefficacy of the currently available therapeutic means.

Treatment of tumor-associated hypercalcemia: a short review of currently available means

Treatment of cancer hypercalcemia remains unsatisfactory, the available drugs being either toxic or insufficiently active, and of short-term efficacy(6,7). The only current way of obtaining a long-term control of serum calcium is indeed to markedly reduce the tumor burden which most of the time is not feasible when hypercalcemia complicates advanced cancer.

Rehydration with intravenous saline should always be part of the initial therapy, since hypovolemia is almost invariably present in hypercalcemic cancer patients. This depletion of extracellular fluid volume should be promptly corrected because it further increases serum calcium and contributes to the symptomatology of hypercalcemia. From the few available controlled studies, one can estimate that rehydration with 3 liters per day of intravenous saline will on the average lower serum calcium by 1.0 to 2.0 mg/dl. It is of course not recommended to systematically prescribe loop diuretics such as furosemide, since they will aggravate the volume depletion. On the other hand, forced saline diuresis with 6 liters or more per 24 hours is no longer advisable: the results probably are not really better than those obtained with a simple rehydration protocol, and, more importantly, the procedure is often dangerous, difficult to conduct and of course leaves unchanged the increased calcium load from bone.

Priority must therefore be given to agents that potently decrease bone resorption. Calcitonin is a non-toxic drug that acts very rapidly by inhibiting osteoclast activity and promoting calciuresis. Calcitonin can thus be very useful for patients presenting severe life-threatening hypercalcemia and recommended doses vary from 2 to 8 U/kg/day 2 to 4 times daily. Unfortunately, the hypocalcemic activity of calcitonin is variable, and most often is only partial and transient. Serum calcium usually increases again after a few days, and there will be no further response to dose escalation. Glucocorticoids can prevent this escape from calcitonin effect in vitro, but the in vivo efficacy of the combination calcitonin-corticoids remains unproven beyond 4 days. I prefer short and repeated therapeutic cycles of calcitonin, the treatment being rapidly stopped when the level of hypercalcemia is no longer dangerous, and repeated when serum calcium starts to rise again. Mithramycin is another active agent, but its use is much limited by major potential toxicities when the drug is administered repeatedly. Corticosteroids alone are still frequently prescribed, even though their reported efficacy is much variable and is probably mainly limited to patients with lymphoproliferative malignancies. Their delayed efficacy, their immunosuppressive and catabolic effects are other major drawbacks. Prostaglandin synthetase inhibitors have not been adequately studied, but the consensus is that they are ineffective. Phosphate administration supposedly causes skeletal calcium precipitation by raising the serum calcium-phosphorus ion product and could also inhibit bone resorption. However, intravenous phosphates can lead to major toxicities by causing extraskeletal calcium precipitation; they must be given very cautiously and only when serum phosphorus is low. Oral administration is preferable and the equivalent of 1 to 3 g of elemental phosphorus per day can still be considered a good treatment for chronic moderate hypercalcemia; the use of oral phosphates is however limited by the digestive secondary effects and the potential risk of diffuse extraskeletal deposition of calcium phosphate salts.

Given these generally unsatisfactory effects of currently available hypocalcemic drugs, numerous trials with various bisphosphonates have already been carried out in tumor-associated hypercalcemia.

Use of bisphosphonates for tumor-associated hypercalcemia

Three bisphosphonates mainly have been studied for the treatment of cancer hypercalcemia: 1-hydroxyethylidene-1,1-bisphosphonate (HEBP or EHDP, etidronate), dichloromethylenebisphonate (Cl_2MBP or Cl_2MDP, clodronate), and 3-amino-1-hydroxypropylidene-1,1-bisphosphonate (AHPrBP or APD, amidronate).

Etidronate

Etidronate is the only commercially available bisphosphonate, but it is also unfortunately the least potent of the clinically evaluated derivatives. Given its poor digestive absorption, which is a characteristic of all bisphosphonates, it is therefore not surprising that oral etidronate is inefficient for treating tumor-associated hypercalcemia. It is only recently that the intravenous form of etidronate has been extensively studied(7,8). These and other studies have shown that intravenous etidronate can normalize serum calcium in at least 75% of hypercalcemic cancer patients. The commonly employed dosage has been 7.5 mg/kg/day infused daily over 2 hours for 3 to 5 days. The success rate seems to increase with treatment duration and recent data suggest that administration for 7 days could normalize serum calcium as frequently as more potent bisphosphonates. Intravenous etidronate appears to be very well tolerated and the deleterious consequences of the inhibition of mineralisation caused by this bisphosphonate are not observed with such a short-term administration. A large multicenter double-blind trial comparing intravenous etidronate with placebo has recently demonstrated the superiority of the bisphosphonate, which is not surprising given the relentless nature of cancer hypercalcemia and the already known efficacy of the more potent bisphosphonates.

Clodronate

Intravenous clodronate can normalize serum calcium in almost 90% of hypercalcemic cancer patients with a therapeutic scheme consisting in the daily administration of 100-300 mg for 3 to 10 days(9). Solid tumors and hematological malignancies respond as well, but patients with a high renal tubular reabsorption of calcium, probably of paraneoplastic origin, are less likely to respond(9). Intravenous clodronate has been given without evident side effects besides a slight fall of serum phosphorus, but it has been noted that hypercalcemia often recurs rapidly after stopping clodronate administration.

Oral clodronate can also correct cancer hypercalcemia but, despite the absence of comparative studies, available data seem to indicate that it is much inferior to the intravenous form(9,10).

Amidronate

Initial clinical studies with amidronate have been carried out by Bijvoet and collaborators, who have demonstrated the considerable efficacy of this bisphosphonate for the treatment of tumor-associated hypercalcemia. Twenty-nine out of 30 patients became thus normocalcemic with daily 2-hour infusions given for up to 10 days, most of the patients receiving 15 mg per day(11). It was also shown in this study that amidronate treatment corrected the other metabolic abnormalities associated with hypercalcemia, such as reduced glomerular filtration rate and hypomagnesemia, whereas no toxic effects were observed(11).

We confirmed these excellent results in 24 hypercalcemic cancer patients who were treated by daily 15-mg two-hour IV infusions of amidronate: serum calcium was normalized in all patients after a mean of 3 daily doses [range, 1 to 6 days](12). As shown in Fig 1, amidronate was as effective in hypercalcemia resulting from bone metastases as in humoral hypercalcemia. This incidentally confirms the essential role of osteoclastic activation in the pathogenesis of hypercalcemia resulting from bone metastases.

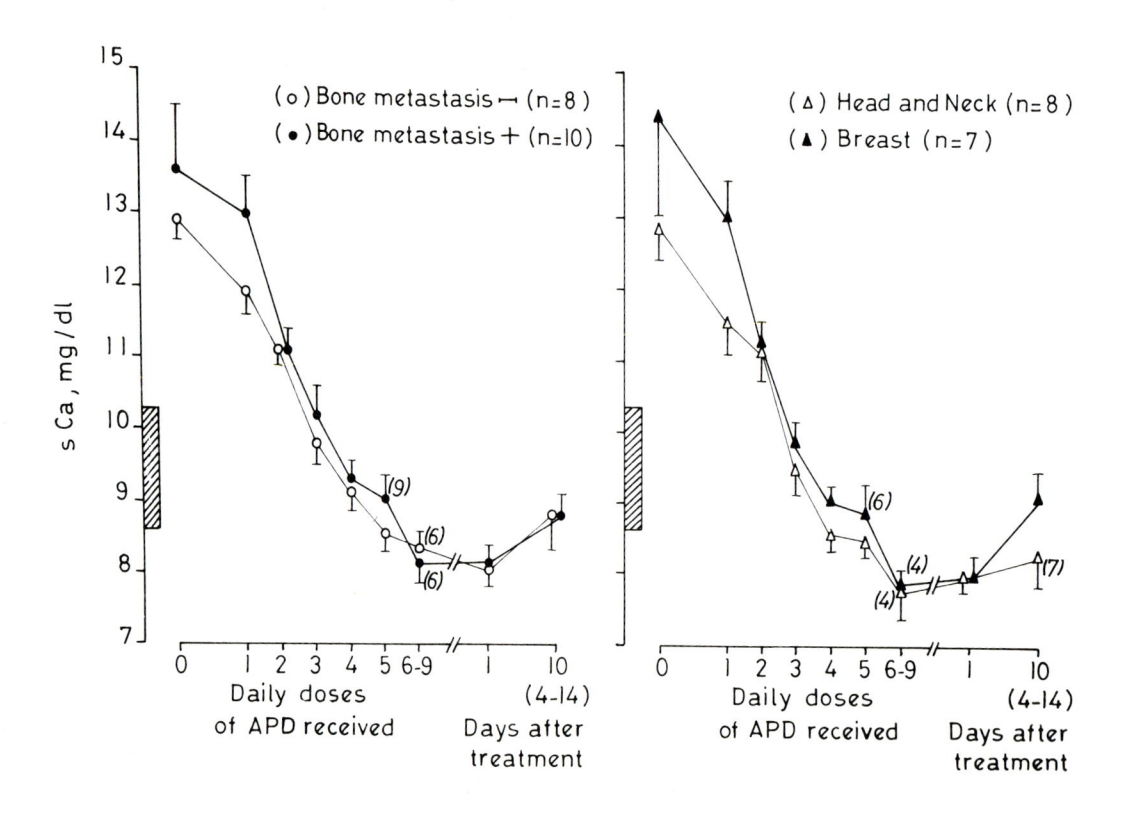

Fig.1. Effects of intravenous amidronate on serum calcium before, during, and after treatment. Patients were divided according to the presence or the absence of bone metastases (A), or according to the primary tumor site (B).

The fall in serum calcium resulted from decreased bone resorption, as evidenced by the dramatic decrease of the urinary excretion of calcium and hydroxyproline. The drug was tolerated without side effects, except for a decrease in serum phosphorus from a mean baseline of 2.9 ± 0.2 to

2.0 ± 0.1 mg/dl after treatment. This hypophosphatemia can probably be attributed to the inhibition of bone resorption and has been confirmed by other investigators. We also demonstrated in this trial the prolonged efficacy of amidronate which constitutes another major advantage of the drug: serum calcium indeed remained normal during 3+ weeks (1+ to 8+) in 17 evaluable patients for that matter, i.e. patients who did not receive or did not respond to general antitumoral treatment.

Amidronate or other new analogues are potentially very useful for diseases characterized by an increased bone lysis, such as bone metastatic involvement, osteoporosis, Paget's disease, and rheumatoid arthritis. Because available information on adequate therapeutic doses and potential toxicity of high doses was insufficient, we carried out a dose-response trial of amidronate in tumor-associated hypercalcemia which can be considered as a human model for diseases characterized by an excessive bone resorption. Only patients remaining hypercalcemic after 48 hours of rehydration were included in this study and antineoplastic therapy was delayed at least until normocalcemia was reached. Amidronate was given as two-hour daily infusions for 3 days, and 3 different patients were treated at each of the 6 following dose levels: 0.01, 0.05, 0.25, 0.75, 1.5, and 3.0 mg/kg/day(13). If the two lowest dose levels were found to be insufficient to normalize serum and urinary calcium concentrations, the efficacy of the four other dosages was however very similar (Fig. 2).

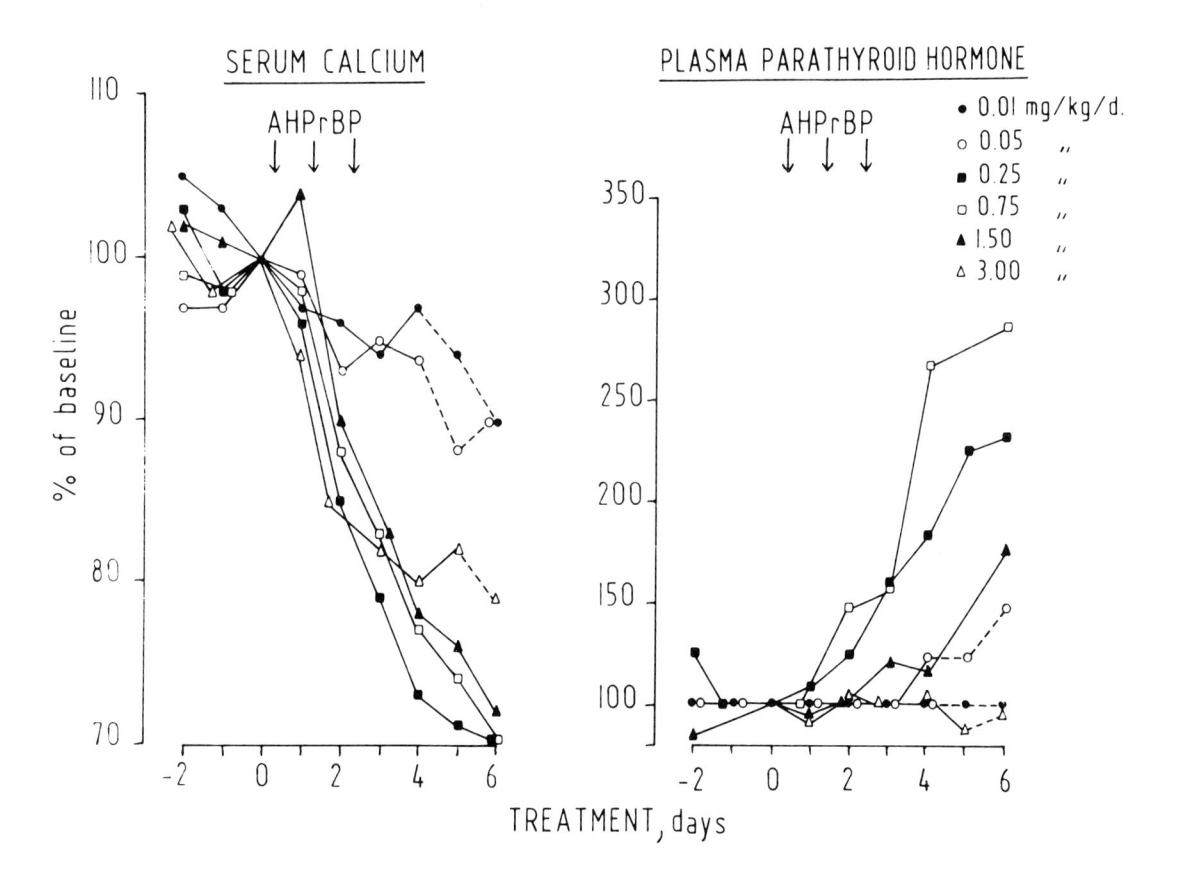

Fig. 2. Changes in corrected serum calcium (left) and plasma PTH (right) levels for the 6 indicated dosages of amidronate (AHPrBP). Data shown are median values and are expressed as percentages of baseline. Dashed lines indicate that patients had been retreated at that time.

The increase of immunoreactive PTH concentrations was more related to serum calcium than to amidronate dosage, but was clearly observed before a possible hypocalcemia. The decrease of fasting urinary calcium excretion paralleled the decrease of serum calcium, but the magnitude of the fall was about three time larger and fasting urinary calcium should be the most reliable and easily measured parameter to follow bisphosphonate inhibition of bone resorption in normocalcemic patients. Possible toxic effects were very closely monitored during this dose-escalation study and we confirmed that the drug was generally very well tolerated: only 6 patients had transient fever and/or decrease in lymphocyte counts possibly due to amidronate but not related to the dose administered. The only important problem was observed at the very high dose of 3.0 mg/kg in one obese woman who developed transient high fever and hypotension. We could thus define that the therapeutic range of amidronate, when given for 3 days as 2-hour daily infusion, lies between 0.25 and 1.5 mg/kg/day. Incidentally, we and other investigators have shown appropriate responses of $1,25(OH)_2$ vitamin D levels to the increase of circulating PTH concentrations.

Thiébaud et al have recently shown that a single 24-hour infusion of amidronate was also very effective for the treatment of tumor-associated hypercalcemia: whereas 60 mg corrected serum calcium in all 10 treated patients, only 6/10 patients were made normocalcemic with a unique dose of 30 mg(14). No toxic effects were observed, except again a slight elevation of body temperature in 2/20 patients. This dose dependency of the 24-hour treatment has recently been confirmed by the same investigators. We are currently performing a trial comparing daily 2-hour infusions for 3 days with a single 24-hour administration.

Intravenous amidronate thus constitutes a very efficient and well tolerated treatment for tumor-associated hypercalcemia which has most importantly a lasting efficacy. We have also shown that amidronate can be efficiently and safely administered to dehydrated patients at the same time as intravenous rehydration(13). Lastly, preliminary results obtained with oral amidronate, 1200 mg daily for 6 days, suggest that this simpler form of administration could be very efficient too(15); better absorbed oral forms of amidronate are however under preparation and should be awaited before oral administration is to be recommended.

Newer derivatives and conclusions

Several groups are working on bisphosphonates derivatives more potent than amidronate which should be active in humans at even lower doses(16). Whereas it has been demonstrated that clodronate acted more rapidly than etidronate, the place of such new derivatives compared to amidronate or even clodronate must still be defined in controlled studies.

There are also very few comparative studies between bisphosphonates and "classical" therapies of cancer hypercalcemia such as calcitonin. However, it seems obvious from the existing data that the overall efficacy of new bisphosphonates such as amidronate is much superior to generally available therapies. The rapid action of calcitonin could nevertheless complement the somewhat delayed but prolonged action of bisphosphonates, and such a combination could thus be particularly useful for severe life-threatening hypercalcemia.

The place of oral bisphosphonates also remains to be defined, particularly for the maintenance of normocalcemia achieved with a short intravenous course of amidronate for example. There are some preliminary data favoring this approach, although retreatment with intravenous bisphosphonates when hypercalcemia recurs is a perfectly valid choice.

In conclusion, the introduction in the near future of the new bisphosphonates for routine clinical care will completely change the current therapeutic approach of tumor-associated hypercalcemia. These new compounds are indeed very potent, well tolerated and have a prolonged efficacy. They also offer the exciting prospect of inhibiting or even preventing the progressive bone destruction associated with skeletal metastases.

Acknowledgements

The author wishes to thank the "Fondation Lefèvre" (Belgium) for their generous support, Drs A. Borkowski and S. Levin for their critical review of the manuscript, and Mrs N. Verhelle for secretarial assistance.

References

1. Lerner UH, Larsson A. Effects of four bisphosphonates on bone resorption, lysosomal enzyme release, protein syntesis and mitotic activities in mouse calvarial bones in vitro. Bone, 8:179-189, 1987.
2. Cecchini MG, Felix R, Fleisch H, Cooper PH. Effect of bisphosphonates on proliferation and viability of mouse bone marrow-derived macrophages. J. Bone Miner. Res., 2:135-142, 1987.
3. Boonekamp PM, van der Wee-Pals LJA, van Wijk-van Lennep MML, Thesing CW, Bijvoet OLM. Two modes of action of bisphosphonates on osteoclastic resorption of mineralized matrix. Bone Miner., 1:27-39, 1986.
4. Adami S, Bhalla AK, Dorizzi R et al. The acute-phase response after bisphosphonate administration. Calcif. Tissue Int., 41:326-331, 1987.
5. Merli GJ, McElwain GE, Adler AG et al. Immobilization hypercalcemia in acute spinal cord injury treated with etidronate. Arch. Intern. Med., 144:1286-1288, 1984.
6. Body JJ. Cancer hypercalcemia: recent advances in understanding and treatment. Eur. J. Cancer Clin. Oncol., 20:865-869, 1984.
7. Singer FR, Fernandez M. Therapy of hypercalcemia of malignancy. Am. J. Med., 82 (Suppl. 2A):34-41, 1987.
8. Ryzen E, Martodam RR, Troxell M et al. Intravenous etidronate in the management of malignant hypercalcemia. Arch. Intern. Med., 145:449-452, 1985.
9. Urwin GH, Yates AJP, Gray RES et al. Treatment of the hypercalcaemia of malignancy with intravenous clodronate. Bone, 8 :S43-S51, 1987.
10. Percival RC, Paterson AD, Yates AJP et al. Treatment of malignant hypercalcaemia with clodronate. Br. J. Cancer, 51:665-669, 1985.
11. Sleeboom HP, Bijvoet OLM, van Oosterom AT, Gleed JH, O'Riordan JLH. Comparison of intravenous (3-amino-1-hydroxypropylidene)-1, 1-bisphosphonate and volume repletion in tumour-induced hypercalcaemia. Lancet II:239-243, 1983.
12. Body JJ, Borkowski A, Cleeren A, Bijvoet OLM. Treatment of malignancy-associated hypercalcemia with intravenous aminohydroxypropylidene diphosphonate. J. Clin. Oncol. 4:1177-1183, 1986.
13. Body JJ, Pot M, Borkowski A, Sculier JP, Klastersky J. Dose/response study of aminohydroxypropylidene bisphosphonate in tumor-associated hypercalcemia. Am. J. Med., 82:957-963, 1987.
14. Thiébaud D, Jaeger P, Jacquet AF, Burckhardt P. A single-day treatment of tumor-induced hypercalcemia by intravenous amino-hydroxypropylidene bisphosphonate. J. Bone Miner. Res., 1:555-562, 1986.
15. Thiébaud D, Portmann L, Jaeger P, Jacquet AF, Burckhardt P. Oral versus intravenous AHPrBP (APD) in the treatment of hypercalcemia of malignancy. Bone 7:247-253, 1986.
16. Boonekamp PM, Löwik CWGM, van der Wee-Pals LJA, van Wijk-van Lennep MLL, Bijvoet OLM. Enhancement of the inhibitory action of APD on the transformation of osteoclast precursors into resorbing cells after dimethylation of the amino group. Bone Miner., 2:29-42, 1987.

Potential Use of Gallium Nitrate and WR-2721 in the Treatment of Hypercalcemia and Hyperparathyroidism

JEAN-PHILIPPE BONJOUR, RENÉ RIZZOLI, and
JOSEPH CAVERZASIO

Division of Clinical Pathophysiology
Department of Medicine
University Hospital
Geneva, Switzerland

Introduction:

The overproduction of different factors, particularly calciotropic hormones and cytokines from various tumoral or non tumoral origins can cause hypercalcemia (1). These factors increase the extracellular concentration of calcium (Ca) by disturbing the fluxes of Ca at the intestinal, skeletal and/or renal tubular sites (2). Therapeutically, the first and most logical approach should be aimed at normalizing or abolishing the excessive production of the hypercalcemic molecule(s) by either surgical or pharmacological means. If such a direct action on the source of hypercalcemic factors is not possible or fails the next most rational therapeutical strategy is to correct the flux(es) of Ca which are abnormally increased. Finally, the least desirable approach consists in modifying a flux of Ca that is not implicated in the hypercalcemic process, as for instance by completely blocking bone resorption when hypercalcemia essentially results from an increased tubular reabsorption of Ca.

Several pharmacological tools or manoeuvres can influence the fluxes of Ca and thereby the level of Ca in the extracellular compartment. At the gut level, glucocorticoids can reduce the capacity of the small intestine to absorb Ca. This property may contribute to the antihypercalcemic effect of glucocorticoids that is observed in presence of an excessive production of 1,25 dihydroxyvitamin D3. At the bone level, two antihypercalcemic manoeuvres could be theoretically envisaged: promoting Ca deposition into bone and/or inhibiting bone resorption. At the present time, there is no efficacious agent capable of rapidly enhancing the process of bone formation and thereby Ca deposition into the skeletal tissue. The only manoeuvre that may affect this process is to maintain a mechanical stress on the skeleton. In contrast, several agents such as mithramycin, calcitonin or diphosphonates have been used for reducing the release of Ca from bone. Because of their great efficacy and low toxicity, diphosphonates are certainly today the drugs of choice for correcting an elevation of plasma Ca due to an increased osteolysis, as observed in numerous cases of malignant hypercalcemia (2). At the kidney level, an increase in the tubular reabsorption of Ca plays an important role not only in primary hyperparathyroidism, but also in several types of malignant hypercalcemia (2,3,4). Until now, most therapeutical attempts aimed at correcting an increase in the tubular reabsorption of Ca have been indirect, ie by interfering with the renal reabsorption and urinary excretion of sodium. Thus, powerful loop diuretics, such as furosemide, were administered with isotonic saline solution given in excess to the amount required for correcting and maintaining the fluid balance. This manoeuvre can, at least initially, increase the urinary excretion of Ca. However, in hypercalcemia of malignancy, the mechanism which maintains an elevated tubular reabsorption of Ca after adequate rehydration and extracellular volume expansion is probably directly related to the secretion by the tumor of a parathyroid hormone-related peptide (PTHrP) (5). Therefore the use of natriuretic agents combined with massive saline infusion for reducing a PTH or PTHrP-mediated increase in the tubular reabsorption of Ca appears to be an inappropriate therapeutical approach. In addition, such treatment can have dangerous consequences on electrolyte and fluid balance.

These basic pathophysiological and therapeutical considerations should be kept in mind in the following discussion regarding the mechanism of action and the potential usefulness of two new comers into the antihypercalcemic arsenal, namely gallium nitrate and the organic thiophosphate WR-2721.

Gallium nitrate:

This anhydrate salt of gallium, a group IIIa heavy metal, has been recently shown to be efficacious as an antihypercalcemic agent. Until 1970, Gallium nitrate (GaNO3) was used for diagnostic purposes as a bone and tumor scanning agent (6). Because of its localization in non-osseous malignancies, GaNO3 was then developped as a potential chemotherapeutic agent. In preclinical studies, GaNO3 was shown to inhibit the growth of various types of tumors, including Walker carcinoma 253, Mammary carcinoma YMC and Osteosarcoma 124F (6). GaNO3 also increased the median survival time of tumor-bearing animals (6). Its dose-limiting toxicity was shown to be renal. During initial human studies aimed at testing the antitumor efficacy of GaNO3, transient hypocalcemia was occasionally observed (7). In vitro experiments indicated a direct effect of GaNO3 on PTH- or lymphokine-stimulated bone resorption (7). Further clinical investigations suggested that GaNO3 was an effective antihypercalcemic agent in various types of malignancies. Very recently a randomized double-blind study indicated that GaNO3 was effective and superior to maximally approved doses of calcitonin for acute control of cancer related hypercalcemia (8). To our knowledge, the efficacy of GaNO3 has not been yet compared to that of available diphosphonates, at least in clinical investigation. In animal experiments, we have recently compared GaNO3 to several diphosphonates, particularly to 3-Amino-1-hydroxypropane-1, 1-diphosphonic acid (APD). The results indicated that in rats, GaNO3 was 2-3 orders of magnitude less potent on a molar basis than APD for inhibiting retinoid-induced bone resorption. Other investigators observed that in rats GaNO3 impaired the calcemic response to PTH (9). They concluded that the GaNO3-induced hypocalcemia seems to be related to skeletal resistance to PTH and increased renal Ca loss (9). Further studies are needed to understand better the mechanism of action of GaNO3 on Ca and bone metabolism. Furthermore, clinical investigations aimed at comparing GaNO3 to diphosphonates of the first, such as Clodronate or APD, or the new generation, such as Aminobutane diphosphonate are required.

WR-2721

Like gallium nitrate, the organic thiophosphate WR-2721 (S-,2-(3-aminopropylamino)- ethyl-phosphorotioic acid) has been mainly developed for its potential use in cancer therapy. The main interest in this compound originated from its remarkable property of increasing the resistance of normal tissues to both ionizing radiation and alkylating chemotherapeutical agents (10). Like for GaNO3, the hypocalcemic action of WR-2721 was serendipitously observed during a phase I clinical trial aimed at testing its radioprotective efficacy (11). Several studies were then conducted in order to elucidate by which mechanism(s) WR-2721 can lower blood Ca, as well as the possible clinical use of this "side-effect" in disorders of Ca metabolism. In vivo, it was clearly shown that WR-2721 rapidly decreased the plasma level of PTH (11,12). In vitro a direct inhibitory action on PTH secretion was observed in both bovine and human parathyroid cells (13,14).

This action appears to occur via a Ca-independent cAMP-dependent mechanism (13). The inhibition of PTH secretion appears to contribute extensively to the acute hypocalcemic response to WR-2721 administration (15). However, strong evidence for a PTH-independent inhibition of the tubular reabsorption of Ca has also been presented (15). This renal tubular effect may well contribute to the rapid hypocalcemic response. Furthermore, WR-2721 is still able to inhibit, at least in vitro, osteoclastic mediated bone resorption (16). To what extent this direct skeletal action contribute to the rapid fall in plasma Ca remains to be documented. In our hands, WR-2721 appears to be much less potent that diphosphonates, or even GaNO3 for inhibiting retinoid-induced bone resorption in TPTX rats. At this stage of our knowledge, it is not known whether the effect of WR-2721 on PTH secretion and Ca metabolism might be related to the action of this sulfhydryl containing compound on the cellular redox potential.

An effective inhibitor of PTH secretion such as WR-2721 could be useful in the treatment of primary hyperparathyroidsm in cases where surgery has failed or is contra-indicated. In this regard, WR-2721 was able to reduce the plasma level of both PTH and Ca in cases of parathyroid carcinoma (17,18). Further clinical trials are needed to evaluate the efficacy of WR-2721 in the long-term management of primary hyperparathyroidism. As far as secondary hyperparathyroidism is concerned, no clinical data from controlled trials are yet available to our knowledge. In experimental animals, however, WR-2721 was quite effective in protecting the kidneys against the deleterious effects of increased PTH secretion. Thus, PTH-dependent nephrocalcinosis was shown to be markedly reduced by chronic administration of WR-2721 (19). Furthermore, in a rat model of chronic renal failure, we observed that WR-2721 reduced the elevated plasma PTH level, prevented secondary kidney calcifications and the progressive decrease in glomerular filtration rate. In addition WR-2721 significantly reduced the effect of severe secondary hyperparathyroidism on osteoclast number and resorption surfaces (20). Here too, further studies are needed to evaluate whether WR-2721 could be useful clinically in the prevention of renal osteodystrophy and other deleterious consequences of excessive PTH secretion.

In hypercalcemia of malignancy WR-2721 may also be useful, particularly in cases where the elevation of plasma Ca results from the tumoral secretion of PTH related peptides. WR-2721 has been tested in Leydig cell tumor-bearing rats, a condition wherein the development of hypercalcemia is probably due to an increase in both bone resorption and tubular Ca reabsorption (21). In this animal model, WR-2721 normalized the plasma Ca level within a couple of hours and corrected the increased tubular Ca reabsorption (22). This observation suggests that WR-2721 may be efficacious in the management of hypercalcemia of malignancy, particularly in those tumors where enhanced renal Ca reabsorption contributes to the elevation of the plasma Ca level and where even powerful antiosteolytic agents such as diphosphonates are not very effective (4). In addition, WR-2721 could exert an additional inhibitory effect on tumor-induced bone resorption, as suggested from in-vitro experiments (23) using conditioned medium from Walker mammary carcinosarcoma cells, another tumor-inducing hypercalcemia in rats.

When tested clinically as a radio- and chemoprotector agent, WR-2721 was usually well tolerated except for mild to moderate nausea and emesis observed in a certain number of patients (24,25). A transitory and asymptomatic decrease in systolic blood pressure has also been recorded following acute infusions of WR-2721. Other minor toxic effects were somnolence and sneezing. These side-effects appeared to be dependent upon the dose and the infusion times (24,25). The importance of these untoward effects will have to be reevaluated during future clinical trials in disorders of Ca metabolism. Indeed, the mode of administration of WR-2721 or its analogs will probably differ from that applied sofar for radio- and chemoprotection in cancer therapy. In this perspective, preclinical informations in various pathophysiological models of hypercalcemia and hyperparathyroidism should still be obtained in order to understand better how WR-2721 and its derivatives exert their action on Ca metabolism.

In conclusion, both gallium nitrate and WR-2721 can influence bone and Ca metabolism. The mechanisms of action of these two agents appear to differ markedly. The antihypercalcemic action of gallium nitrate seems to be mainly due to an inhibition of bone resorption. Therefore, gallium nitrate should be classified as an antiosteolytic drug and compared to compounds such as calcitonin and diphosphonates. In sharp contrast, the antihypercalcemic activity of WR-2721 can mainly be explained by an inhibition of PTH secretion with an additional PTH-independent effect on the tubular reabsorption of Ca. As compared to diphosphonates, WR-2721 appears to be a very weak direct inhibitor of bone resorption. These important differences in the mode of action should be kept in mind for designing clinical trials aimed at determining the actual place of gallium nitrate and WR-2721 in the treatment of hypercalcemia and hyperparathyroidism.

Acknowledgements

All mentioned works of the authors were supported by the Swiss National Science Foundation (Grant 3.806.0.82 and 3.954.0.85), the Elsie and Carlos de Reuter Foundation and the League against Cancer of Geneva (Switzerland).

References

1. Mundy, G.R., Ibbotson, K.J., and D'Souza, S. (1985) J.Clin.Invest. 76, 391-394

2. Bonjour, J.-P., Rizzoli, R., Hirschel-Scholz, S., and Caverzasio, J. (1987) Bone 8, Supp. 1, S29-S33
3. Ralston, S.H., Fogelman, I., Gardner, M.D., Dryburgh, F.J., Cowan, R.A., and Boyle, J.T. (1984) Clin.Sci. 66, 187-191
4. Bonjour, J.-P., Philippe, J., Guelpa, G., Bisetti, A., Rizzoli, R., Jung, A., Rosini, S., and Kanis, J.A. (1988) Bone, in press
5. Suva, L.J., Winslow, G.A., Wettenhall, R.E.H., Hammonds, R.G., Moseley, J.M., Dieffenbach-Jagger, H., Rodda, C.P., Kemp, B.E., Rodriguez, H., Chen, E.Y., Hudson, P.J., Martin, T.J., and Wood, W.I. (1987) Science 237, 893-896
6. Foster, B.J., Clagett-Carr, K., Hoth, D., and Leyland-Jones, B. (1986) Cancer Treat. Rep. 70, 1311-1319
7. Warrell, R.P. Jr, Bockman, R.S., Coonley, C.J., Isaacs, M., and Staszewski, H. (1984) J.Clin.Invest. 73, 1487-1490
8. Warrell, R.P. Jr, Israel R., Frisone, M., Snyder, T., Gaynor, J.J., and Bockman, R.S. (1988) Annals Intern. Med., in press
9. Cournot-Witmer, G., Bourdeau, A., Lieberherr, M., Thil, C.L., Plachot, J.J., Enault, G., Bourdon, R., and Balsan, S. (1987) Calcif.Tissue Int. 40, 270-275
10. Yuhas, J.M. (1982) Int.Radiat.Oncol.Biol.Phys. 8, 513-517
11. Glover, D., Riley, L., Carmichael, K., Spar, B., Glick, J., Kligerman, M.M., Agus, Z.S., Slatopolsky, E., Attie, M., and Goldfarb, S. (1983) N.Engl.J.Med. 309, 1137-1141
12. Hirschel-Scholz, S., and Bonjour, J.-P. (1987) Trends in Pharmacol. Sciences 8, 246-247
13. Weaver, M.E., Morrissey, J., McConkey, C. Jr, Goldfarb, S., Slatopolsky, E., and Martin, K.J. (1987) Am.J.Physiol. 252, E197-E201
14. Larsson, R., Nygren, P., Wallfelt, C., Akerstrom, G., Rastad, J., Ljunghall, S., and Gylfe, E. (1986) Biochem.Pharmacol. 35, 4237-4241
15. Hirschel-Scholz, S., Caverzasio, J., and Bonjour, J.-P. (1985) J.Clin.Invest. 76, 1851-1856
16. Attie, M.F., Fallon, D., Spar, B., Wolf, J.S., Slatopolsky, E., and Goldfarb, S. (1985) J.Clin.Invest. 75, 1191-1197
17. Glover, D.J., Shaw, L., Glick, J.H., Slatopolsky, E., Weiler, C., Attie, M., and Goldfarb, S. (1985) Ann.Int.Med. 103, 55-57
18. Hirschel-Scholz, S., Jung, A., Fischer, J.A., Trechsel, U., and Bonjour, J.P. (1985) Clin.Endocrinol. 23, 313-318
19. Hirschel-Scholz, S., Caverzasio, J., and Bonjour, J.-P. (1987) Calcif.Tissue Int. 40, 103-108
20. Hirschel-Scholz, S., Charhon, S., Rizzoli, R., Caverzasio, J., Paunier, L., and Bonjour, J.-P. (1988) Kidney Int. 33, 934-941
21. Rizzoli, R., Caverzasio, J., Fleisch, H., and Bonjour, J.-P. (1986) Endocrinology 119, 1004-1009
22. Hirschel-Scholz, S., Caverzasio, J., Rizzoli, R., and Bonjour, J.-P. (1986) J.Clin.Invest. 78, 319-322
23. Weiss, J., Walker, S.T., Fallon, M., and Goldfarb, S. (1986) J.Pharmacol.Experim.Therap. 238, 969-973
24. Turrisi, A.T., Glover, D.J., Hurwitz, S., Glick, J., Norfleet, A.L., Weiler, C., Yuhas, J.M., and Kligerman, M.M. (1986) Cancer Treat.Rep. 70, 1389-1393
25. Glover, D., Glick, J.H., Weiler C., Fox, K., Turrisi, A., and Kligerman, M.M. (1986) J.Radiat.Oncol.Biol.Phys. 12, 1509-1512

Discussion:

DR. HEATH (Rochester, MN): Thank you very much. I especially appreciate the pathophysiologic approach you've taken in explaining how these agents work.

DR. BOCKMAN (New York): The stars told me to be here today. I think your presentation of Dr. Waral's and my work is very fair, and I think you did a very good job in presenting it. And I appreciate that you presented that last slide; this double-blind study that Dr. Waral completed is the first published double-blind randomized trial in hypercalcemia. It just came out today in the Annals of Internal Medicine.

The thing I'd like to say is, I think it is probably not fair to make the comparison on the dose basis that you did. You're really comparing apples and oranges. If you actually measure, by x-ray microscopy or various techniques that we've used, the amounts of gallium that are in the bone after treatment with rather high doses, the amounts are there in the same level that trace elements are there; they're extremely small.

So, the problem of how much gallium you actually get and deliver to the bone is probably not going to be very far off from the total amounts, for example, of the newer diphosphonates that accumulate in bone. And the problem of comparing blood levels is probably not a legitimate way to compare drug potencies.

I would just comment further that gallium is unique, in that it has a number of other effects on bone. It clearly affects the physical parameters of bone in terms of crystal perfection, carbonate contamination. But more interestingly, if you treat animals in vivo, you'll find that you'll increase calcium content, and that you actually increase osteocalcin as well as collagen synthesis in the bone. So, I think that it's a unique agent and it really needs to be explored much further.

With regards to WR-2721, I think one thing that the audience ought to be made aware of is that the compound is extremely unstable. And that might have a tremendous drawback to clinical applicability.

DR. KLEEREKOPER (Detroit): I need a consultation on a patient we currently have with a carcinoma of the parathyroid in her mediastinum, who is asymptomatic with a serum calcium of 12.5 or 13 mg/dl. If we operate on her, we will make her probably hypoparathyroid until she gets a recurrence. Can I treat her repeatedly with either of the drugs that either of the two of you have talked about?

DR. BONJOUR (Switzerland): You mean with diphosphonate?

DR. KLEEREKOPER: Or WR-2721 or gallium. Can I get her calcium down with medication, now, and then wait till she gets hypercalcemic again, and get her calcium down again, and then wait till she gets hypercalcemic again, do it again and again?

DR. BONJOUR: Well, I think there are several examples in hypercalcemia of malignancy where you see a patient, you treat with diphosphonate, you normalize the calcemia, calcemia goes up and again you get the same response to treatment after a variable interval. It could be one week later, it could be one month later.

DR. BODY (Belgium): I have the same thing to say. I have treated probably now at least 10 or 15 patients two or three times, and they responded as well to the second treatment as to the first treatment. So, I think you can give a second course without any trouble.

DR. PARFITT (Detroit): What is the contribution of treating

hypercalcemia, by whatever means, to the long-term outcome in patients with cancer-associated hypercalcemia?

DR. BODY: I think that is right. I think that the problem is not to know with what drug you have to treat the patients. The problem is to know if you have to treat the patients at all. I agree with you that in some cases it's probably better not to treat the cancer -- hypercalcemia. But still, in some cases it is very, very useful for the patients.

DR. PARFITT: Are there studies looking specifically at that issue in terms of long-term outcome? Are patients treated in different ways?

DR. BODY: I do not know of any studies that have shown that treatment of cancer hypercalcemia with these drugs will increase the survival of these patients. These are very difficult studies to do, I think.

DR. HEATH: It obviously increases the short-term survival.

DR. BODY: Yes, but for the long-term I have no idea.

DR. BIJVOET (Leiden): I can answer the questions. First, we published in the *Lancet* the study of APD and metastatic breast cancer where we have long-term treatment, and the intake in that trial has by now been finished. There is no effect on survival, whereas we reduced the morbidity due to breast cancer in bone by 50 percent. And the results are even better than in that paper as we are getting more cases. But there is no effect on survival.

Then, the second thing is that we have used APD in hyperparathyroidism or parathyroid carcinoma. We published the first data on diphosphonate in hyperparathyroidism in 1977, and we showed nicely that there is an interference with increased renal tubular reabsorption of calcium.

But there's another point. There is, at the bone level, a competition between an effect of PTH and the diphosphonate. And what you see in the treatment of hyperparathyroidism with diphosphonate is that bone resorption starts to increase despite continued diphosphonate. So, it's not good treatment and the effect on the bone does not persist. And it is a funny question, that in tumors, and even in squamous cell carcinoma, where there is definitely an increase in renal tubular reabsorption of calcium, and in that I agree, that there is no escape of the bone effect, whereas in hyperparathyroidism and in breast cancer there is an escape. And we are invariably unsuccessful.

I can add to that, you will never read any paper on diphosphonate and renal failure. Why not? Because there also, bone resorption in the presences of a high PTH is fairly unresponsive. There is an exception in that it's Dichloral, but Dichloral acts by cell toxicity to the osteoclast. So, that's the answer.

DR. HEATH: Dr. Bijvoet makes an excellent point. And I think that any medical therapy for primary or secondary hyperparathyroidism is always going to be limited if it fails to suppress parathyroid hormone secretion itself.

DR. MAUTALEN (Buenos Aires): Our experience with APD intravenously in patients with parathyroid carcinoma is a little different from what has been said by Dr. Bijvoet. We have a poster here -- we treated three patients, with an excellent response to APD, but it was short-lived. They responded quite well to the second course of APD administration. And perhaps, since I'm here, I could ask a question about any experience of the long-term or prolonged use of WR-2721 in parathyroid carcinoma?

DR. BONJOUR: Not that I know.

Therapy of Aluminum Related Bone Disease

HARTMUT H. MALLUCHE and MARIE-CLAUDE FAUGERE

*Division of Nephrology
Bone and Mineral Metabolism
University of Kentucky Medical Center
Lexington, KY*

Accumulation of aluminum in bone has been shown to be a relatively frequent complication in patients with end-stage renal failure. Our group found stainable aluminum at the mineralization front in 47% of 87 non-selected patients on chronic maintenance dialysis.[1] Bone aluminum content was elevated in almost all patients. In mild to moderate renal failure, 5 out of 100 patients studied had stainable aluminum and bone aluminum content was elevated in more than 20%. These data show that accumulation of aluminum at the mineralization front and throughout bone are a common clinical complication deserving attention and possibly therapeutic intervention.

Who should be treated?

Given the high prevalence of aluminum accumulation in bone, it is important to address the question whether this accumulation of aluminum has undesirable effects on bone or whether it merely represents an epiphenomenon. The latter has been postulated based on experiments done in young growing Beagle dogs with normal renal function.[2] The dogs were rendered vitamin D deficient and given aluminum which resulted in accumulation of aluminum in bone evidenced by increased bone aluminum content and appearance of stainable aluminum. Administration of vitamin D produced healing of osteomalacia and reduction in stainable aluminum despite continued aluminum administration. In addition to the interpretation of the authors[2] that stainable aluminum represents an epiphenomenon, it is conceivable that vitamin D might affect the distribution of aluminum within bone and, thus, is associated with less stainable aluminum at the osteoid-bone interface. We could show that the known histopathology of "aluminum osteomalacia" i.e., osteoblastic dysfunction resulting in abnormal mineralization and accumulation of osteoid correlates very well with the extent of stainable aluminum, whereas, total bone aluminum content correlates with osteoid only (See Table I). These findings indicate that presence of stainable aluminum and not necessarily increased bone aluminum content is associated with bone pathology. Therefore, redistribution of aluminum within bone resulting from Vitamin D administration might avoid histopathologic derangements. Based on these findings and our results in experimental dogs[3] that Vitamin D deficiency is an important factor for accumulation of aluminum in bone and maintenance of normal Vitamin D status prevents aluminum accumulation in bone, we deem it reasonable that patients receive supplementation of Vitamin D to avoid aluminum bone disease or specific chelation therapy aimed at removing aluminum from their bones when significant amounts of stainable aluminum (over 30% of trabecular surface) are present. It is of note that aluminum accumulation might occur in all different subgroups of renal osteodystrophy and, therefore, removal of aluminum from bone cannot necessarily be expected to heal the underlying renal osteodystrophy, rather, only the aluminum related component of the histologic abnormalities.

Considering the formidable intestinal hindrance for absorption of aluminum, contamination of water used for dialysis which bypasses the intestinal barrier should be carefully avoided. Even routine use of reverse osmosis does not prevent sporadic severe aluminum loading in patients on chronic dialysis which might result from glitches in the RO system. Long-term intake of high doses of aluminum containing phosphate binders represents a major risk factor for non endemic aluminum intoxication. Aluminum contained in medications, such as Heparin and other intravenous fluids, may add up to the other sources of aluminum and, thus, may contribute to accumulation of aluminum in individual dialysis patients.

What can therapy accomplish?

Several methods are available for removal of aluminum from bone. In general, any maneuver that will lower blood aluminum levels should create a concentration gradient across the bone-extracellular fluid membrane and, therefore, result in translocation of aluminum from bone to blood. This gradient may remove aluminum from dialysis patients with aluminum overload. Due to the binding of aluminum to proteins only approximately 20% of aluminum in blood is ultrafiltrable. Dialysate may contain 5-10 µg/l of aluminum even after reverse osmosis. Therefore, an osmotic gradient exists only at plasma aluminum levels exceeding 50 µl[4-6]. This explains the findings that aluminum clearances vary during hemodialysis from 4-50 ml/min at plasma levels between 50-200 µg/l. Aluminum clearances achieved by peritoneal dialysis may exceed those of hemodialysis[7]. This might be ascribable to protein losses during peritoneal dialysis or less likely to active aluminum transport or convective aluminum transfer during ultrafiltration. It awaits further studies whether CAPD is preferable for removal of aluminum over HD in patients not amenable to chelation therapy. Certain hemodialysis membranes may have higher aluminum clearance than others. However, based on the discussed calculable removal of ultrafiltrable aluminum, it is apparent that neither alteration of dialysis membranes nor hemofiltration without dialysis will be sufficient for removal of larger amounts of aluminum. Trials utilizing plasma exchange for removal of aluminum have been unsatisfactory. Sorbent hemoperfusion may remove both protein bound and ultrafiltrable aluminum, however, our experience with sorbent hemoperfusion and no additional chelator therapy is rather disappointing. The added expense, technical requirements and logistic problems readily explain why both plasma exchange and sorbent hemoperfusion are not widely used as method of choice for aluminum removal.

Because of the problems existing with methods capable to remove total aluminum, it is advisable to increase the complex bound fraction by administration of a chelator which will allow removal of aluminum through dialysis. An optimal chelating agent should have a high specificity for the substance to be removed and little or no toxicity. Clearly, no such chelator is available at this time. EDTA lacks specificity for aluminum and binds other physiologic ions such as calcium. Deferoxamine (Desferal[R]; CIBA Geigy, Summit, NJ) has been used for years for removal of iron. It is preferable over other chelators because of its relatively low toxicity, however, it is not specific for aluminum and may bind iron, lead, copper, zinc, cobalt, magnesium and others. Careful documentation of aluminum overload is therefore required before long-term deferoxamine (DFO) therapy is instituted. DFO is a by-product of the mold Streptomyces; it acts as a siderophore in the metabolism of the organism. Its chemical structure is similar to the heme molecule, explaining its specificity for trivalent ions of the ferric type. The trivalent aluminum ion is chemically similar to the ferric ion and aluminum is known to interact with iron dependent biologic systems such as hemoglobin synthesis and iron transport proteins. This explains the high affinity of DFO for aluminum. Since gut absorption of DFO is marginal, DFO has to be administered parenterally. Its molecular weight is approximately 600 and it is excreted by renal filtration and tubular secretion

with partial tubular reabsorption. Bile secretion is relatively small. Even though DFO has been employed for removal of iron in patients with normal and reduced kidney function, at this time there is no FDA approval for the use of DFO in patients with aluminum related bone disease. After initiation of DFO therapy, rises in serum aluminum are observed indicating the translocation of aluminum from organs into the blood compartment. With continuation of chronic intermittent chelation therapy in dialysis patients, a saw tooth pattern of blood aluminum levels before and after infusion is customarily observed with a trend towards baseline values after three to twelve months. When rises are no longer observed, removal through dialysis equals translocation from organ into the blood compartment. No rises in serum aluminum and zero dialysance of aluminum calls for discontinuation of therapy to avoid removal of other substances than aluminum from organs. At this point, bone biopsies are helpful for documentation of successful removal of aluminum from bone and information on underlying renal osteodystrophy. Histologically, an increase in bone turnover is usually seen after long-term DFO therapy, low turnover osteomalacia might be converted to mixed uremic osteodystrophy and mixed uremic osteodystrophy might change to predominant hyperparathyroid bone disease. This is usually associated with a rise in serum levels of parathyroid hormone and high alkaline phosphatase levels. Serum calcium levels might fall during therapy necessitating administration of the active Vitamin D metabolite $1,25(OH)_2D_3$. Bone pain, muscle pain, and "bone strength" might improve between four to twelve months after initiation of therapy. Improvement in histologic findings of bone requires usually six to eighteen months. Changes in histomorphometric parameters of bone observed with long term DFO therapy are shown in Table II. Further experience with the use of the drug is necessary to answer the following important questions:
1. Does aluminum reaccumulate after successful chelation therapy when patients continue to take low doses of aluminum containing phosphate binders and, thus, are non aluminum containing phosphate binders mandatory for prevention of aluminum accumulation in bone?
2. Does chelation therapy remove other essential substances during well monitored intermittent therapy requiring supplementation to avoid deficiency in these substances?

The best know side effect of DFO is related to its vasodilatory effect causing a drop in blood pressure. This is believed to be a histamine mediated event though antihistamines are not helpful for prevention of this side effect. It is not known whether iron overload, impaired myocardial function (which might be associate with aluminum overload) or other factors contribute to this side effect. Sometimes the drop in blood pressure is attributable to an infusion rate exceeding the recommended ceiling of 15 mg/kg/bw/hr. Slowing of infusion rate or temporary discontinuation of the infusion will correct the hypotension. In our experience, approximately 2% of patients develop severe hypotension which may be associated with angina, even at doses and infusion rates at or below the recommended maximum level. Short of a practical alternative for DFO in these patients, they have to be managed employing sorbent hemoperfusion and/or frequent dialysis. Another potential serious side effect of chronic DFO therapy is development of cataracts, altered color vision, night blindness, or scotoma. None of these problems were seen during our six years of experience with DFO in more than 120 patients. The occurrence of cataracts was mainly described in patients receiving long-term DFO therapy for iron removal. Minor side effects including neuromuscular irritability, nausea and vomiting are usually transient. A frequently observed side effect is the development of pruritus which appears to be related to increased parathryoid gland activity. The association between chronic DFO therapy and occurrence of thrombophlebitis or infections caused by rare organisms[8] awaits further studies. Side effects observed with DFO therapy in individual patients are difficult to interpret since it is not clear whether aluminum accumulation per se might render the patient susceptible to the side effects. Results of long term prospective and controlled studies are needed before a final assessment can be given on the safety of DFO in the management of chronic dialysis patients.

The observed prevalence of aluminum related bone disease in approximately half of the unselected patients on dialysis[1] and the high rate of morbidity associated with this abnormality ascribes an important role to long-term chelation therapy in the overall maintenance of quality of life and longevity of patients on dialysis.

TABLE I

CORRELATION COEFFICIENTS BETWEEN HISTOMORPHOMETRIC PARAMETERS OF BONE AND STAINABLE BONE ALUMINUM (sBA) AND BONE ALUMINUM CONTENT (BAC)

	sBA	BAC
Lamellar osteoid volume	0.71*	0.77*
Osteoid-osteoblast interface	-0.80*	0.06
Mineralized bone-osteoclast interface	-0.86*	0.30
Mineral apposition rate	-0.79*	0.10
Bone formation rate (osteon level)	-0.75*	0.20

* $p < 0.01$.

TABLE II

STATIC AND DYNAMIC PARAMETERS OF BONE STRUCTURE, FORMATION AND RESORPTION IN PATIENTS BEFORE AND AFTER DEFEROXAMINE THERAPY

	Before	After
Parameters of bone structure		
Cancellous bone mass (%)	21.5 ± 3.41	26.5 ± 3.81*
Mean trabecular diameter (μm)	282 ± 33.97	334 ± 50.32*
Parameters of bone formation		
Lamellar osteoid volume (mm³/cm³)	24.5 ± 9.28	5.75 ± 2.13*
Lamellar osteoid thickness (μm)	13.6 ± 2.94	10.8 ± 1.73*
Lamellar osteoid surface (%)	49.0 ± 9.02	16.8 ± 5.56*
Woven osteoid volume (mm³/cm³)	9.60 ± 2.51	20.1 ± 7.58*
Woven osteoid seam thickness (μm)	17.8 ± 3.73	16.8 ± 3.39
Woven Osteoid Surface (%)	17.1 ± 5.07	33.0 ± 7.76*
Osteoid-osteoblast interface (%)	14.5 ± 7.50	48.9 ± 13.49*
Peritrabecular fibrosis (%)	19.3 ± 15.17	25.1 ± 13.46*
Parameters of bone resorption		
Bone-osteoclast interface (%)	2.07 ± 1.29	4.70 ± 1.71*
Total resorption lacunae (%)	9.74 ± 5.28	14.0 ± 3.55*
Parameters of bone dynamics		
Mineralization rate (μm/day)	0.66 ± 0.29	1.14 ± 0.25*
Doubly labelled osteoid seam (%)	13.3 ± 8.58	38.6 ± 12.63*
Mineralization lag time (days)	35.6 ± 11.59	11.2 ± 3.24*
Stainable bone aluminum		
% of osteoid surface	50.8 ± 18.18	4.18 ± 2.73*

Results are given as means ± SEM $p < 0.05$

BIBLIOGRAPHY

1. Smith, A.J., Faugere, M.C., Abreo, K., Fanti, P., Julian, B., and Malluche, H.H.: Aluminum related bone disease in mild and advanced renal failure. Am. J. Nephrol. 6:275-283, 1986.

2. Quarles, L.D., Dennis, V.W., Gitelman, H.J., Harrelson, J. and Drezner, M.K.: Aluminum deposition at the osteoid-bone interface. An epiphenomenon of the osteomalacia state in vitamin D-deficient dogs. J. Clinc. Invest. 75:1441-1447, 1985.

3. Malluche, H.H., Faugere, M.C., Fanti, P., and Friedler, R.M.: Calcitriol, parathyroid hormone and the accumulation of aluminum in bone in dogs with renal failure. J. Clin. Invest. 79:754-761, 1987.

4. Chang, T.and Barre, P.: Effect of desferrioxamine on removal of aluminum and iron by coated charcoal hemoperfusion and hemodialysis. Lancet ii: 1051-1053, 1983.

5. Simon, P., Ang, K.S., Cam, G., Allain, P. and Mavras, Y.: Desferrioxamine, aluminum and dialysis. Lancet ii. 1489-1490, 1983.

6. Smith, A.J., Faugere, M.C., Fanti, P. and Malluche, H.H.: Trade in and trade off of deferoxamine therapy in hemodialyzed patients (Abstract). Kidney Int. 31:246, 1987.

7. Rottembourg, J., Gallego, J.L., Jaudon, M.C. and Clavel, J.P.: Serum concentration and peritoneal transfer of aluminum during treatment by continuous ambulatory peritoneal dialysis. Kidney Int. 25:919-924, 1984.

8. Segal, R., Zoller, K.A., Sherrard, D.J. and Coburn, J.W.: Mucormycosis: A life threatening complication of deferoxamine therapy in long-term dialysis patients (Abstract). Kidney Int. 33:238, 1988.

Discussion:

DR. HEATH (Rochester, MN): I was a little surprised by your statement that patients with low turnover bone disease improved markedly after deferoxamine therapy. Were those patients who had had prior parathyroid surgery? My impression would be that, if the patients were hypoparathyroid to begin with, you would just continue to see a very low turnover state, even after removal of aluminum.

DR. MALLUCHE (Lexington, KY): Well, our experience is not exactly the same as was published by two other groups. I know what you're referring to. We have the feeling that, if a patient has a very low turnover such as aplastic or adynamic bone disease, that it takes longer to remove the aluminum. But if you keep on treating them, they will respond.

To answer your question, two of our patients had prior parathyroidectomy, the others not. So, I would think that if you're patient enough, the patient might respond. But I agree with you, parathyroidectomy makes things more difficult and it takes longer and the response is somewhat blunted. But it's not zero.

DR. ITTEL (Germany): I'm interested in the improved muscle strength you have reported. Did you actually check whether your patients experienced a change in the vitamin D status in terms of 1,25 vitamin D concentration, since this might have improved muscle strength, as well?

DR. MALLUCHE: Yes, that's a very good question. We found, in six patients who initially had very low 1,25 levels, a significant rise in plasma 1,25(OH)2D. But some others did not have the same rise, and still we could observe some improvement in myopathy. So, I'm not sure whether that can be just simply ascribed to changes in vitamin D.

DR. PHELPS (Brooklyn, NY): Could you comment on what you're doing presently to prevent the emergence of hyperparathyroidism when you treat with deferoxamine?

DR. MALLUCHE: I think that this is not a hyperparathyroidism related to the deferoxamine therapy. I think these patients would have had the hyperparathyroidism if they didn't get aluminum in the first place. So, I think it is just the ordinary renal osteodystrophy that I'm seeing. And your question is, obviously, very well taken.

I think, at this point, careful monitoring of serum phosphorus levels at early times, during the initial stages of dialysis, may help. And we have a study going on where we look into the value of early therapy with 1,25(OH)2D. That means maintenance of normal mineralization status and supplementation of the deficient hormone. And we'll see whether that will prevent the hyperparathyroidism in the long run.

DR. PHELPS: One further remark. Perhaps you'd like to comment on the very interesting complication of mucormycosis in patients who are receiving deferoxamine.

DR. MALLUCHE: I expected that question, and I tried to mention that parenthetically during my presentation. We did not observe any kind of rare infection. I'm aware of the incidence of mucormycosis, but I'm also aware of a study published by an Italian group, where they found a relatively high incidence of mucormycosis in unselected dialysis patients not treated with deferoxamine.

Let me give you a little story. When we started out with DFO therapy, we were kind of scared because we didn't know how it was going to work in these dialysis patients. When the second patient, a child, was called in to the hospital she didn't show up. I called the parents and they told me, "She died last night." If I had started therapy one day earlier, I'm sure I would have attributed that death to aluminum.

I think there are a lot of complications in patients with end stage renal failure. And I could ascribe something to deferoxamine if I had a controlled study that told me that mucormycosis occurs significantly higher in treated patients versus nontreated patients.

DR. OGATA (Tokyo): How often have you had to stop deferoxamine due to the eye complications?

DR. MALLUCHE: We did not have any ocular complications.

DR. BOYCE (San Antonio, TX): Just one question of the differential effects of deferoxamine in different types of aluminum bone disease. I wasn't really sure how many of your patients may have had what has been described as "aplastic bone disease" as opposed to "mixed bone disease," given that your parathyroid hormone level, as a mean, was about 1900 and therefore elevated, if your normal range, I think, is 70. Did you look at the differential effects and response in those who had low PTH against those who clearly must have had very high parathyroid hormone levels?

DR. MALLUCHE: By and large, I think I can say that the patients with a higher turnover to begin with have a better response. They are more rapid, I should say, in their response. I didn't sort out adynamic bone disease from low-turnover osteomalacia because they both responded almost the same way. That means they needed more prolonged deferoxamine therapy and they notably had less decrease in stainable aluminum than other patients, let's say with predominant hyperparathyroid bone disease, given the same amount of deferoxamine over an equal period of time.

DR. BOYCE: We certainly have treated some patients in Glasgow with deferoxamine. And patients with aplastic bone disease, certainly one of them, treated for 18 months, still had no difference in the staining of aluminum or the content of aluminum in their bone. So, you know, I'm just concerned that these patients are not going to respond nearly so well as certain of the ones who have got osteoclasts already present within their bone.

DR. MALLUCHE: I think we need to keep in mind the possible contribution of iron, here. We find, for example, that our false-negative deferoxamine test patients (in other words, those patients who have received deferoxamine and do not have a clear rise in serum aluminum) have a lot of iron. It might be that iron inhibits or impairs the removal of aluminum. It might not be related only to the fact that they have low bone turnover. So, I think that deserves further studies.

DR. HEATH: I think I took your point to be that you got good evidence that you eliminated the aluminum, and nonetheless turnover stayed very low and --

DR. MALLUCHE: No.

DR. BOYCE: The exact opposite. The aluminum stayed in the biopsy specimens and there was no response.

DR. HEATH: At 18 months?

DR. BOYCE: Yes.

DR. HEATH: All right.

DR. BOYCE: Furthermore, there was lots of iron and macrophages within bone marrow, and it wasn't eluted from macrophages. But there was no iron stainable along the calcification fronts, which can be confounding, as you say.

DR. MALLUCHE: But we also have to keep in mind that there is still a kind of enigma, to me at least, there are the patients who have low-turnover osteomalacia or adynamic bone disease without stainable aluminum. So, we certainly don't have all the answers in at this point.

The Role of Sodium Fluoride in the Treatment of Osteoporosis

B. LAWRENCE RIGGS, STEPHEN F. HODGSON, and
RICHARD EASTELL

Endocrine Research Unit
Mayo Clinic and Foundation
Rochester, MN

Osteoporosis is defined as an absolute decrease in the amount of bone to a level at which fractures occur after minimal or no trauma. Bone loss implies a relative or absolute increase in bone resorption over bone formation. Normally, these two components of bone remodeling are tightly coupled, so that bone formation increases in parallel with increases in bone resorption, thereby preventing or eliminating bone loss. In osteoporosis, bone formation and bone resorption are uncoupled so that progressive bone loss occurs.

The effects of estrogens, calcitonin, and calcium on bone mass are mainly due to inhibition of bone resorption. Small transient increases in bone mass may occur in the first few months after initiation of treatment when the resorption phase is depressed while the formation phase in bone remodeling units that were initiated prior to therapy is being completed. After about 6 months, however, bone formation also decreases, and no further increase in bone mass occurs. Thus, the best that can be expected with anti-resorptive therapy is to stabilize bone mass and prevent further loss.

The ideal therapeutic agent for osteoporosis, however, should increase bone mass to a level above the fracture threshold (Fig. 1). In order to accomplish this, bone formation should be stimulated to a level that is substantially higher than bone resorption. Several therapeutic regimens to accomplish this have been suggested and are currently under evaluation. These include selective manipulation of separate bone cell populations (ADFR), chronic low-dose treatment with parathyroid hormone (1-34), and chronic calcitonin treatment combined with oral phosphate. At present, however, these newer approaches must be considered experimental. The only therapeutic agent that has been widely evaluated and has given consistent results in stimulating bone formation is sodium fluoride. In contrast to other experimental programs, moreover, therapy with sodium fluoride is inexpensive, and the drug can be administered orally.

Historical Background

In areas where fluoride concentration in drinking water is only moderately high (5 to 10 ppm) such as Bartlett, Texas, osteosclerosis is the sole skeletal manifestation. There is a lower prevalence of osteoporosis in these areas than in low-fluoride (<2 ppm) regions. Even with higher fluoride intakes (10 to 40 ppm), such as occur in the Punjab area of India, asymptomatic osteosclerosis is a much more common manifestation than is crippling fluorisis.

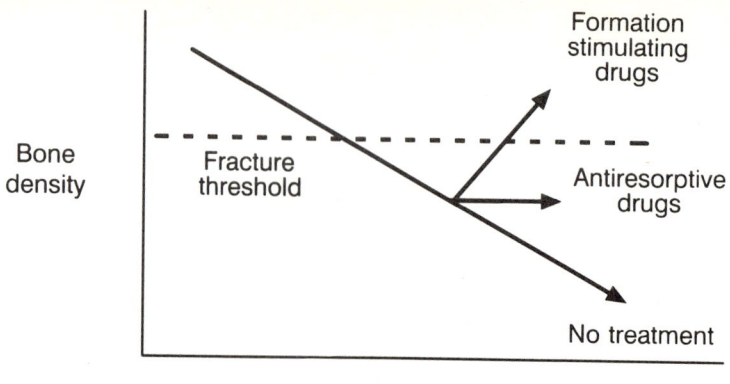

Fig. 1. Model for the effect of treatment on bone loss. As bone loss ensues, bone mineral density (BMD) falls below the fracture threshold, and fractures begin to occur. If the patient receives no treatment or ineffectual treatment, there is continued bone loss, and as bone density levels become progressively lower, there is an increased number of fractures. If an antiresorptive drug is given, bone mass is maintained. Because BMD remains below the fracture threshold, the patient will remain at risk for fractures, although at a lower rate because further bone loss is prevented. A formation-stimulating drug, however, will increase bone mass to above the fracture threshold, thereby preventing further fractures. From Cecil Textbook of Medicine, 18th Edition, with permission from W. B. Saunders Co., Philadelphia, PA.

In 1961, Rich and Ensinck used sodium fluoride to treat patients with osteoporosis in the hope that inducing subclinical fluorosis might strengthen the skeleton. They found that treatment induced calcium retention by metabolic balance studies. Encouraged by these observations, a number of other investigators studied the effect of administering sodium fluoride to patients with primary osteoporosis (see Riggs (1) for review). The initial results from these studies were conflicting and were not uniformly reproducible. Moreover, bone biopsy studies showed that the administration of sodium fluoride alone to osteoporotic subjects increased bone formation but also increased bone resorption and impaired mineralization resulting in histologic osteomalacia. These unfavorable findings led to a waning of interest in fluoride therapy for osteoporosis.

As a result of new studies in the 1970's, however, it became clear that these untoward results were influenced by three controllable factors: 1) the dosage of sodium fluoride employed, 2) the use of supplementary calcium, and 3) the duration of treatment. First, there is a narrow therapeutic window: dosages of 30 mg/day or lower have a variable effect on stimulating bone formation, whereas dosages of 75 mg/day and higher result in impaired mineralization with excessive osteoid tissue and the formation of woven bone (2). Moreover, because fluoride is excreted from the body largely by the kidney, the presence of moderate to several renal failure results in higher serum fluoride levels, and the dosage must be reduced accordingly. Therefore, the optimal dosage in a patient with normal renal function is about 50 mg/day. Second, supplementary calcium in dosages of 1 to 2 g/day offsets, in part, the effect of fluoride on impairing mineralization (2). The mechanism of this effect is as yet not well understood. The supplementary calcium also prevents the increase in bone resorption that occurs when sodium fluoride is given alone, an event that may be mediated by secondary hyperparathyroidism, possibly stemming from an increased demand for calcium as a result of accelerated bone formation (3). Third, with continued treatment, the mineralization defect worsens despite the continued administration of fluoride, thereby, increasing the risk of new fractures. Thus, it is generally agreed, therefore, that fluoride therapy should not be continued for longer than about 5 years.

Fluoride in the Skeleton

Effects on bone formation. The predominant effect of fluoride on bone is to stimulate bone formation (1,2). Both indirect and direct cellular mechanisms have been suggested as explanations for the observed increase in bone formation during chronic fluoride administration. Bone cells are responsive to changes in electrical currents. Bone crystals may act as transducers for mechanical stress and generate piezoelectric currents in bone that may affect osteoblastic activity. This could explain the more pronounced effect of fluoride on weight-bearing axial skeleton (vertebral column and os ilium) than on nonweight-bearing bone such as the radius. Moreover, Farley et al. (4) demonstrated direct effects of fluoride on osteoblast-like cells *in vitro*: at concentrations of fluoride in the media comparable to therapeutic levels in humans, there was increased proliferation and differentiation of bone cells.

Effects on bone resorption. Some evidence suggests that fluoride may affect bone resorption (1). In vitro, fluoride decreases the solubility of bone mineral, and fluoride pretreatment decreases the bone resorption induced by parathyroid hormone. In osteoporotics treated with fluoride from 2 to 5 years, a decrease in bone resorption has been demonstrated by calcium kinetics and histomorphometric methods (3).

A positive balance between resorption and formation, demonstrated by calcium balance and calcium-kinetic analysis of bone turnover has been found after 2 to 4 years of fluoride treatment (3). The positive balance is attributable to a decrease in resorption rate with a concomitant increase in bone formation rate.

Effects on bone mass. Studies on iliac crest bone have demonstrated that fluoride therapy substantially increased trabecular bone of the axial skeleton, often by over 100% and often into the normal range (5,6). Dual-photon absorptiometry has demonstrated increases in bone density of the lumbar spine of 1% per month after 18 to 24 months of therapy. Densitometric findings in our osteoporotic patient with an excellent response to fluoride therapy are given in Figure 2. Increases in bone density of the central spongiosum, assessed by quantitative computed tomography, have been even greater. About one-half of patients receiving long-term treatment develop radiographically evident osteosclerosis (Fig. 3).

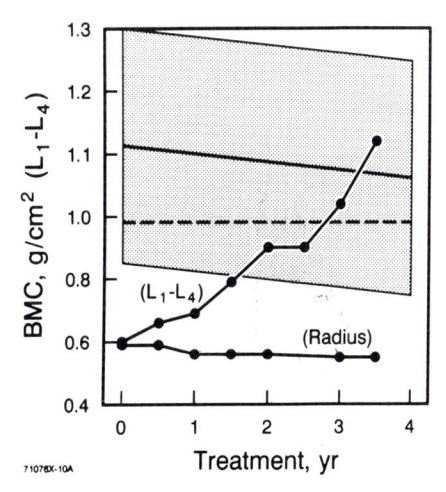

Fig. 2. Dramatic increase in bone density during a $3\frac{1}{2}$-year period in a 63-year-old woman treated with 75 mg/day of sodium fluoride and 1,500 mg/day of calcium supplements. Shaded area represents normal range. Broken line represents fracture threshold. Note doubling of bone density in the lumbar spine after treatment. Bone density of the shaft of radius, however, did not increase.

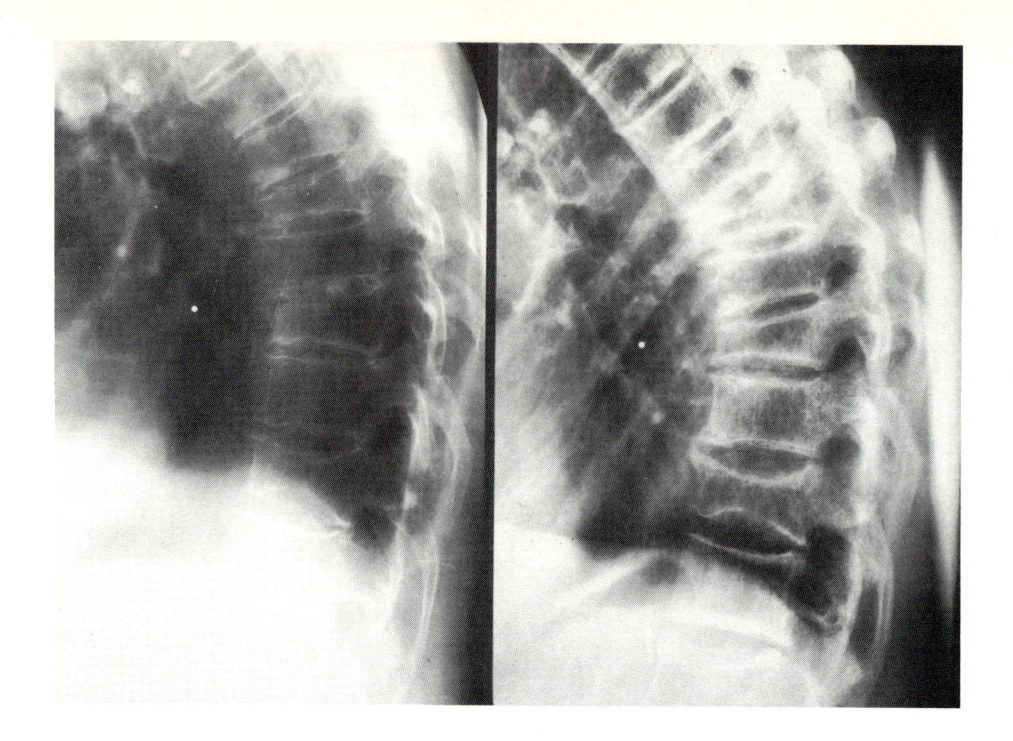

Fig. 3. Radiographic findings in patient whose bone density is shown in Fig. 2. Pretreatment spinal radiograph is given in the left panel and posttreatment in the right panel. Note the evident osteosclerosis. There is thickening of the cortex and remaining trabeculae consistent with fluoride effect.

The dramatic increase in trabecular bone in the vertebrae and iliac crest is not accompanied by a corresponding increase in cortical bone mass of the limb bones (1 and Fig. 2). In cortical bone, formation and resorption remain balanced despite increased turnover, whereas in trabecular bone, the increase in formation exceeds the increase in resorption, leading to an increase in bone mass. Indeed, some, but not all, investigators have found that cortical bone mass decreases with fluoride therapy in the appendicular skeleton. These reports raise the possibility that fluoride therapy may protect against fractures of the vertebral bodies (which consist of predominantly trabecular bone) but may not protect against, and even could increase the risk for, fractures of the proximal femur (which consist of predominantly cortical bone). A recent five-center study involving 416 osteoporotic patients, who were followed more than 1,000 patient years of fluoride therapy, however, did not show an increase in the incidence of hip fracture. In this study, the observed incidence of 1.6%/year was similar to the incidence of 1.9%/year for 120 untreated osteoporotic patients (7).

Variation in Individual Responsiveness

Recent data suggest that responsiveness of individual patients to fluoride therapy varies (1). Although the majority of patients respond with a dramatic increase in bone formation and bone density, four recent studies have found that about 30% of patients have little or no response. The cause of the individual variability in responsiveness is unknown. It does not appear to be due to noncompliance in most instances. Attempts to correlate lack of response to baseline histomorphometric findings on iliac bone biopsy or to clinical features have been unsuccessful (5,6). Possibly, there is a primary defect in osteoblast function that prevents response to therapy. Whatever its cause, individual nonresponsiveness remains a practical problem of management.

Side Effects

Results of several large series reported that significant side effects occur in 30 to 50% of patients (1). These have been of two types: symptoms related to gastric irritation and a lower extremity pain syndrome. The gastric symptoms or epigastric pain, nausea, vomiting, and, occasionally, blood loss anemia. Minor gastric symptoms are even more common. These side effects result from an irritant effect of fluoride ion on gastric mucosa.

The second major side effect is a syndrome of periarticular pain and tenderness about the large joints of the lower extremities or in the feet (8). The symptoms most commonly involve a single region, although two or more regions are sometimes involved. In order of decreasing frequency, the most commonly involved areas are the ankles and lower leg, the feet, the knees and lower femur, and the upper femur. These symptoms disappear within 2 to 6 weeks of discontinuing treatment and usually do not recur when therapy is reinstituted at a lower dosage. If symptoms recur, the same area or another area may be involved.

In about half of the patients with the pain syndrome, it has been possible to demonstrate the presence of trabecular stress fractures in the painful region (8). Because quantitative skeletal uptake of ^{99m}Tc-diphosphonate demonstrate that fluoride-treated osteoporotic patients with the pain syndrome had a greater bone activity than did asymptomatic fluoride-treated patients or calcium-treated osteoporotic patients, some investigators (8) have concluded that the underlying mechanism might be intense skeletal remodeling, which may be complicated by the development of stress fractures. In some patients with skeletal pain, we have demonstrated intense periosteal changes with new bone formation between the cortex and the periosteum visible radiographically.

Thus far, none of the major symptoms of skeletal fluorosis, such as neurological changes, have been observed during fluoride therapy of osteoporosis.

Antifracture Efficacy

Because fluoridic bone has increased crystallinity, decreased elasticity, and sometimes, abnormal structure, a gain in bone mass after therapy does not necessarily equate with a gain in bone strength. Studies in experimental fluorosis in animals and on human skeletal fluorosis, have generally shown that fluoridic bone is less strong that an equivalent amount of normal bone (9). No netheless, the increase in net bone mass may be associated with a net increase in bone strength, particularly in trabecular bone mass, they increase substantially.

Obviously, antifracture efficacy must be established before fluoride therapy can be recommended for wide-spread clinical use. A number of partially controlled studies have suggested that fluoride and calcium therapy decrease vertebral fractures as compared with a control group receiving either placebo or only calcium (10 and Fig. 4). The United States Public Health Service, NIH, has funded two clinical trials at Mayo Clinic and Henry Ford Hospital to assess the effect of fluoride and calcium therapy on fracture rate. The trials, which are randomized, double-blind, prospective, and controlled, are presently underway and should provide an unequivocal answer to this crucial question. Until these are completed, fluoride therapy should continue to be reserved for investigational purposes.

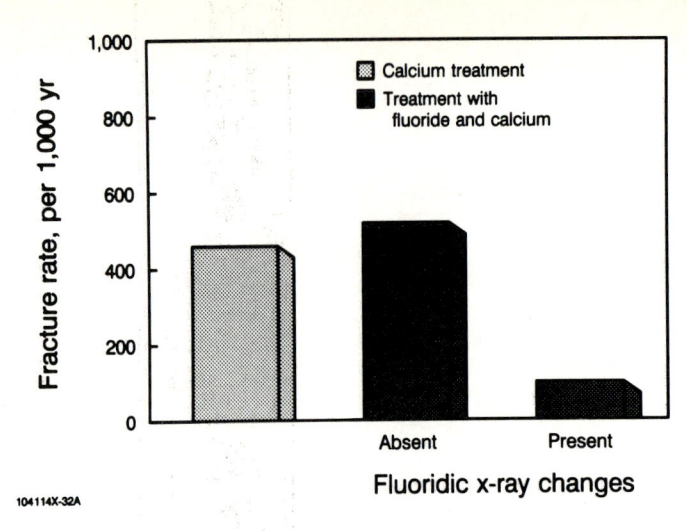

Fig. 4. Among 33 osteoporotic patients treated with fluoride and calcium, those with roentgenographically apparent increases in bone density had a decreased vertebral fracture rate, whereas those without this finding had a fracture rate that was similar to 27 osteoporotic patients treated only with calcium. In <u>Osteoporosis</u>, Proceedings of the International Symposium on Osteoporosis, Denmark, Sept. 27-Oct 2, 1987, edited by Cohn, D.V. Christiansen, C., Johannsen, J.S., and Riis, B.J. with permission.

References

1. Riggs, B.L. (1984) Bone Mineral Res. 2, 366-393
2. Jowsey, J., Riggs, B.L., Kelly, P.J., and Hoffman, D.L. (1972) Am. J. Med. 53, 43-49
3. Eriksen, E.F., Hodgson, S.F., and Riggs, B.L. (1988) in Osteoporosis: Etiology, Diagnosis, and Management (Riggs, B.L., and Melton, J. III, eds) pp 415-432, Raven Press, New York
4. Farley, J.R., Wergedal, J.E., and Baylink, D.J. (1983) Science 222, 330-332
5. Briancon, D., and Meunier, P.J. (1981) Orthop. Clin. N. Am. 12, 629-648
6. Lane, J.M., Healey, J.H., Schartz, E., Vigorita, V.J., Schneider, R., Einhorn, T.A., Suda, M., and Robbins, W.C. (1984) Orthop. Clin. North Am. 15, 729-745
7. Riggs, B.L., Baylink, D.J., Kleerekoper, M., Lane, J.M., Melton, L.J. III, and Meunier, P.J. (1987) J. Bone Min. Res. 2, 1213-126
8. O'Duffy, J.D., Wahner, H.W., O'Fallon, W.M., Johnson, K.A., Muhs, J.M., Beabout, J.W., Hodgson, S.F., and Riggs, B.L. (1986) Am. J. Med. 80, 561-566.
9. Mosekilde, L., Kragstrup, J., and Richards, J. (1987) Calcif. Tissue Int. 40, 318-322
10. Riggs, B.L., Seeman, E., Hodgson, S.F., Taves, D.R., and O'Fallon, W.M. (1982) N. Engl. J. Med. 306, 446-450

Discussion:

DR. MURRAY (Toronto): Very interesting presentation and a very important study. You really have illustrated the importance of having a randomized controlled trial. Lately, our study and others, and most public discussion about fluoride therapy, have focused on the high incidence of side effects. At Toronto we also have just completed a fairly large four-year study. While it was not randomized, we did vary the dose and were able to study the effects of variation in dose. It's clear that for the lower extremities, fractures are related to dose. While we get an inverse relationship between vertebral fractures and dose, we have a direct relationship with non-vertebral fractures and dose. On the other hand, the mean dose in our patients was about 48 mg a day compared to your 75 mg. The incidence of lower extremity pain syndrome was only about 20 percent. So, I think that some things can be done to reduce the side effects. The other thing is that we used an enteric coated preparation of sodium fluoride so that GI side effects were below five percent in our study.

DR. BONE (Detroit): Both your remarks and the previous comment prompt me to ask, have you related both the therapeutic effect and the side effects to some measurable quantity, such as serum or urine fluoride level?

DR. EASTELL (Rochester, MN): Yes, we do have serum fluoride measurements on all these patients. We haven't related them in the whole study. But in a small study that we published a couple of years ago, it appeared that the patients with the lower extremity pain syndrome had exactly the same level of serum fluoride as did those patients who had no side effects and no pain. So, that particular syndrome doesn't seem to be affected by sodium fluoride level.

DR. BONE: If it's dose-related it ought to be --

DR. EASTELL: Well, the majority of patients were on 75 mg per day. We had to reduce it in some because of the side effects. So, we can't answer that.

DR. PARFITT (Detroit): Just a quick comment on the use of the term "microfracture." A microfracture is a histologic abnormality. A stress fracture is a fracture, not a microfracture.

DR. MALLUCHE (Lexington, KY): I wonder whether you can give us some information on bone histology in these patients. In particular, what was the mineralization status and did you observe woven bone?

DR. EASTELL: Yes. Unfortunately, I don't have any of those data. Dr. Baylink may be in the audience and may be able to help us, because he is doing the bone histomorphometry. I don't think he has analyzed the samples after fluoride therapy yet. But, if he's here, he may correct me.

DR. SCHNITZLER (Johannesburg): Just a comment. In addition to analyzing biochemical variables, we had a look at a number of other parameters. The patients who sustained stress fractures, either trabecular or cortical stress fractures, had significantly lower radiogrammetric metacarpal cortical indices, which would support that we should withhold fluoride from patients with severe cortical osteoporosis. We propose that the stress fracture occurs at those particular junctions of cortical and metaphyseal bone, first of all, because the cortical bone seems to be thinner in these patients. Secondly, we biopsied the iliac crest in a number of patients at the time of the stress fracture, and found increased resorption and formation surfaces, but that osteoid was unmineralized. So, there seems to be a critical period where, perhaps, trabecular bone mass is reduced to critically low levels without having the support of cortical bone around it.

DR. SANTORA (Detroit): In the retrospective study of hip fracture incidents you referred to, was there a power calculation done to determine the possibility of type 2 error?

DR. EASTELL: Well, this paper was published six years ago. So, we've not been doing analysis on it recently. And in the paper as it was published, there was no power calculation performed.

DR. KLEEREKOPER (Detroit): I understand the data showed there was no change in bone density, up or down, in the patients treated with placebo and calcium at any of the three sites. I think that's a very important observation.

DR. EASTELL: Yes, I agree. I think it's a very important observation. We would have expected a loss of one or two percent per year in these osteoporotic subjects. We didn't observe it, and the data are looking pretty tight now. There's no change at four years.

DR. STAUFFER (Vermont): I'm aware of the data that have been published with regard to your study on trabecular bone, which was published last year in abstract form at the ASBMR meetings. That work has been done by Dr. Baylink's group, Dr. Lundy. And he did find that there was an increase in trabecular bone volume, these are on static measurements, an increase in osteoid-covered surface and width. The dynamic studies, tetracycline measurements, haven't been analyzed yet.

New Methods of Administration of Estrogens

ROBERT LINDSAY

Regional Bone Center
Helen Hayes Hospital
West Haverstraw, NY
and Department of Medicine
Columbia University
New York, NY

It is now well established that the administration of estrogen to the postmenopausal woman reduces the rate of bone loss and protects against fractures in the aging female population.(1) The effect of estrogen on bone loss has been determined in formal controlled prospective studies that have varied in duration from one year to ten years in duration. Prevention of bone loss appears to occur in all estrogen deficient women and to be independent of the duration of ovarian deficiency, prior to the institution of treatment (2). The maximum beneficial effects on mass are obtained when estrogens are started early, since the initial bone mass is at its maximum at that point. With one exception all the fracture data are retrospective or case control, and in general terms agree well with the prospective bone mass data (1). One prospective study suggested that estrogens might be effective in preventing as many as 90% of the vertebral fractures, while the epidemiological data indicate about a 50% reduction in hip fracture frequency after estrogen exposure.

However, estrogen delivery by the oral route, although it is satisfactory for the majority of postmenopausal women, is subject to a number of potential metabolic effects that in theory at least could produce negative effects in the aging population and perhaps limit the more general acceptance of estrogen treatment for osteoporosis prevention (3). In addition the use of estrogen without the addition of a progestogen has been associated with an increased incidence of carcinoma of the endometrium (4). Over the past few years concern about the potential side effects of estrogen treatment has resulted in both changes in the method by which estrogens are prescribed, and in addition the development of alternate routes of delivery to circumvent the delivery of large doses of estrogen in bolus fashion to the liver as happens with the oral route.

This article will review the changes that have occurred in estrogen prescription over the past few years, dealing principally with the delivery of estrogen by routes other than per oram.

Progestogen Prescription. In the late 1970's, data were presented that the continued stimulation of the endometrium with estrogen would result in hyperplasia, and eventually in some individuals the initiation of carcinoma (4). Biochemical and clinical data have indicated that the processes leading to hyperplasia will be reversed by the addition of a progestogen (5). The usual procedure is to provide the progestogen cyclically, mimicking the luteal phase of the normal ovarian cycle. To obtain complete conversion to a secretory endometrium, the duration of progestogen therapy appears to be as important as the dose. Thus at least 12 days of therapy in each cycle of estrogen therapy has been advocated, determination of the timing of bleeding being suggested as a useful indicator of the adequacy of the prescribed dose. Vaginal bleeding is a regular consequence of such therapy, and this may be unacceptable to many individuals. In an attempt to overcome this problem continuous combination therapy has been suggested, but an effective therapeutic regimen has yet to be described, those that have been used thus far associated with intermittent irregular bleeding during the early treatment phase that is even more of a problem than regular menses. If treatment can be maintained, endometrial hypoplasia results presumably eliminating the risks of endometrial malignancy.

Progestogens given as the single therapeutic agent to postmenopausal patients appear to be capable of reducing the rate of bone loss. Previous studies from our group demonstrated that both depot and oral progestogens can inhibit bone loss without the addition of estrogen (6). The 19-nor testosterone derivative norethindrone is an effective agent in a dose comparable to that often used when prescribed with estrogen. The true progestogens may require to be given in somewhat higher doses. In vitro data suggest that progestogens may stimulate bone formation, and some short term human data indicate that the addition of a progestogen may also stimulate osteoblast function (7). However this requires to be proven in long-term studies, and such data as are currently available suggest that the addition of a progestogen will neither add nor detract from the skeletal effects of estrogen.

The use of progestogens may have a far reaching effect in another area where a beneficial effect has been suggested for estrogen use. Epidemiological data indicate that estrogen therapy may reduce the incidence of ischemic heart disease among the postmenopausal population (8). The effect seems to be dramatic with a 50% reduction in risk reported in several studies. It has been assumed that this effect is directly consequent upon the decrease in total cholesterol and increase in HDL that follows estrogen use. While definitive proof has yet to be obtained, the coincidence of occurrence of biochemical effects likely to produce favorable effects on ischemic heart disease and the reported reduced risk, cannot easily be ignored. If they are indeed cause and effect, then the addition of progestogens, which have the reverse effects on lipoproteins, might conceivably eliminate the beneficial estrogen effect on ischemic heart disease. Should the estrogen effect be mediated by a more direct route, such as on blood vessel walls, where estrogen receptors have been demonstrated, then progestogen addition may have less of a negative effect than feared. Finally, if a progestogen dose can be found, effective in preventing the uterine response to long-term estrogen, and that is lower than that required to reverse the lipoprotein response to estrogen, then clearly the issue would be resolved.

Alternate Routes for Estrogen Administration. The realization that the liver receives a massive dose of estrogen after oral administration, and that this led directly to increased hepatic synthesis of proteins, some of which, at least potentially, may have negative metabolic effects, has resulted in the development of estrogen administration by routes other than the oral (3). Estrogens can be given parenterally, per vaginam, or across the skin. Parenteral estrogen is given as a long acting intramuscular injection, or as a subcutaneous pellet. The disadvantage of that route is the inability to stop the effects of estrogen easily, should the need arise. Data, mostly from the United Kingdom, have demonstrated that estrogen is rapidly absorbed when given as a vaginal cream. However, absorption is variable, and the method of administration less well tolerated by patients, than the oral route.

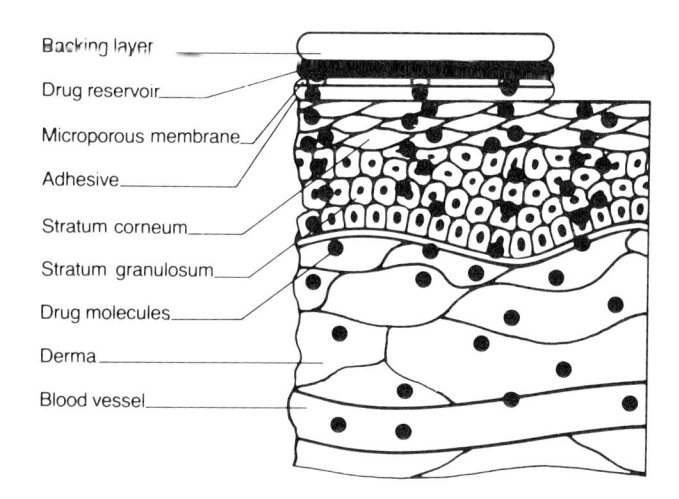

FIGURE 1: Schematic diagram of transdermal estrogen delivery

The administration of estrogens across the skin has been pioneered in the USA by the Alza corporation and marketed by the Ciba-Geigy company. Transdermal estrogen (Estraderm*) or the estrogen patch, releases a small amount of 17-beta estradiol from a reservoir in a continuous fashion (9). The format of the patch is shown in diagrammatic form in figure 1. Application of the patch to the skin results in predictable increments in serum estradiol that last virtually only as long as the patch is applied. The patch is changed twice weekly, giving an acceptable regimen with good patient compliance. Increases in serum estradiol are ~30pcg/l with the smaller 50mcg patch, and ~50pcg/l with the larger 100mcg size. There is no bolus effect, as occurs with other routes of administration, and even blood levels are maintained throughout the application. Preliminary data have shown that the administration of estrogen in this fashion is well tolerated and associated with a high degree of patient compliance. In a short term study of the metabolic effects of transdermal administration, Chetkowski et al (3) demonstrated no adverse hepatic effects from doses up to 200mcg/day, double the maximum currently available. Not surprisingly, the administration of estrogen in this fashion has similar effects on the endometrium to estrogen administered by the oral route. Indeed it might be worrisome if that were not so. Whitehead et al demonstrated that 58% of patients had proliferative endometrium after 3 months of treatment (10). The addition of a progestogen for 12 days per calender month reversed these changes, but of course resulted in withdrawal bleeding.

In larger multi-center studies, good patient compliance and acceptance of the route of administration was also demonstrated. The main problem with this form of estrogen administration is skin irritation, which seems to occur in 24% of patients, although only in 4% of patients in this study did the treatment require to be discontinued and most were on the placebo preparation (11). If skin irritation is a problem, the patch can be removed daily and reapplied. Warming the edges improves the adhesion for reapplication (a hair drier is a useful method of achieving this). Skin reactions and patch loosening are more common in warmer climates.

The use of estrogen in this fashion raises the questions of whether it is only estrogen by the oral route that protects against osteoporosis, and whether the levels of estrogen achieved by this method of administration are sufficient to affect the skeleton. The first question has been answered in part by data from Christiansen et al (12), who demonstrated that percutaneous estrogen (estrogen cream) reduces the rate of bone loss in postmenopausal women. Uncontrolled data have also shown that subcutaneous estrogen implants reduce bone loss. Therefore, it seems likely that the route of administration is not a determinant of the effect of estrogen on the skeleton.

No long term data of significance have yet been published using the transdermal estrogen approach, but short term biochemical data suggest that a skeletal effect will be observed in the large scale studies ongoing (3, 13). In the first of the short term studies, reduction in urinary calcium was observed after application of the 50mcg patch for 3 weeks. The other index of bone resorption, urinary hydroxyproline did not change in that study, but also did not fall after administration of conjugated equine estrogen, even at a daily dose of 1.25mg. In a more recent study, Peacock et al (13) showed reduction in both urinary calcium and hydroxyproline at both the available doses of transdermal estrogen. Similar reductions in the biochemical indicators of bone resorption have preceded retardation of bone resorption in long term studies of oral estrogen, suggesting that transdermal estrogen is likely to be effective. Recently one uncontrolled study has indicated that indeed these short term findings will be predictive of a beneficial effect of transdermal estrogen on bone mass. However completion of the long term carefully controlled studies of bone mass are required before efficacy can be claimed. Rather curiously the second of these biochemical studies also examined changes in plasma and urinary phosphate, which, in studies with oral estrogen, show changes compatible with increased parathyroid function, and failed to find any alteration with transdermal estrogen administration. This requires confirmation in further studies.

More recently preliminary data have been presented suggesting that these biochemical changes will be predictive of skeletal effects. Ribot et al. (14) showed that bone mineral density of the lumbar spine (Table 1) increases by about 8% during 18 months of treatment with transdermal estrogen (50mcg). Although

TABLE 1

Spinal BMD During Treatment with Transdermal
Estrogen in Women Average Age 50.5 Years

Time (months)	0	6	12	18
BMD (mean)	0.98	0.99	1.03	1.01
% Change		1.15	5.12	5.43

these data are uncontrolled they do suggest that the controlled studies now being conducted in the USA and Great Britain will be able to confirm that transdermal estrogen is indeed effective in prevention of bone loss. As determined in the biochemical studies, the likely question is not whether or not transdermal estrogen is effective, but rather whether the dose of estrogen delivered by the smaller of the patch systems is sufficient to effectively reduce the rate of bone loss in postmenopausal women.

As stated previously, recent interest has surrounded the potential reduction in cardiovascular events in postmenopausal patients taking oral estrogens, documented in several epidemiological studies. It has been proposed, although by no means proven that this results from increased circulating HDL and reduced LDL in such patients. It will be important to examine this issue in detail for the transdermal route of administration, since this may be a more potent argument for more general use of estrogen among the postmenopausal population than prevention of osteoporosis, important though that is.

Conclusions. Transdermal estrogen is an alternative to the administration of oral estrogen for the treatment of the postmenopausal woman, and some women may express preferences for one method over the other. While short term data suggest that a bone sparing effect will be evident with this route and dose of administration, long term controlled data are required before absolute confirmation of efficacy can be claimed. Long term uncontrolled data confirm the likelihood of success. It will be important to assess the effects of this route of administration of estrogen on the cardiovascular system, since a cardioprotective effect seems to occur with oral estrogen.

References

1. Lindsay R. Sex steroids in the pathogenesis and prevention of osteoporosis. In: Osteoporosis: Etiology, Diagnosis and Management. Riggs BL, Melton LJ (eds), Raven Press, NY 1988 pp 333-358

2. Lindsay R, Hart DM, Abdalla H, Al-Azzawi F. Inter-relationship of bone loss and its prevention and fracture expression. In: Osteoporosis I. Christiansen C, Johansen JS, Riis BJ (eds), Osteopres, Copenhagen 1987 pp 508-512

3. Chetkowski RJ, Meldrum DR, Sterngold KA et al. Biologic effects of transdermal estradiol. New Engl J Med 1986 314:1615-1620

4. Zeil HK, Finkle WK. Increased risk of endometrial carcinoma among users of conjugated estrogens. New Engl J Med 1975 293:1167-1170

5. Padwick ML, Pryse-Davies J, Whitehead MI. A simple method for determining the optimal dosage of progestogen in postmenopausal women receiving estrogens. New Engl J Med 1986 315:930-934

6. Abdalla H, Hart DM, Lindsay R, Leggate I, Hooke A. Prevention of bone loss in postmenopausal women by norethisterone. Obstet & Gynecol 1985 6:789-792

7. Christiansen C, Riis BJ, Nilas L, Rodbro P, Deftos L. Uncoupling of bone formation and resorption by combined estrogen and progestogen therapy in postmenopausal osteoporosis. Lancet 1985 ii:800-801

8. Bush TL, Cowan LD, Barrett-Connor E, et al. Estrogen use and all cause mortality. Preliminary results from the Lipid Research Clinics Program Follow-up Study. J Amer Med Assoc 1983 249:903-906

9. Lievertz RW. Pharmacology and pharmacokinetics of estrogen. Amer J Obstet Gynecol 1987 156:1289-1293

10. Whitehead MI, Padwick ML, Endacott J, Pryse-Davies J. Endometrial response to transdermal estradiol in postmenopausal women. Amer J Obstet Gynecol 1985 52:1079-1084

11. Utian WH. Transdermal estradiol overall safety profile. Amer J Obstet Gynecol 1987 156:1335-1338

12. Riis B, Thomsen K, Christiansen C. Does calcium supplementation prevent postmenopausal bone loss. N Engl J Med 1987 316:173-177.

13. Peacock M. The effect of transdermal oestrogen on bone, calcium regulating hormones and liver in postmenopausal women. Clin Endocrinol 1986 25:543-547.

14. Ribot C, Tremallieres F, Pouilles JM, Louvet JP, Peyron R. Transdermal administration of 17-beta estradiol in postmenopausal women. Preliminary results of a longitudinal study. In: Osteoporosis I. Christiansen C, Johansen JS, Riis BJ (eds), Osteopres, Copenhagen 1987 pp 546-548

Discussion:

DR. MURRAY (Toronto): I enjoyed your extremely lucid and color-coordinated talk. I have a comment and a question. The comment refers to the effect of estrogen in treating patients with established osteoporosis. And you alluded to the reason for the increase in bone mass in some of these patients being due to an imbalance between formation and resorption. A number of years ago we studied a group of patients like this, comparing them to a calcium-treated group, and showed a similar increase measuring bone mineral mass using partial body neutron activation analysis. The increase was about five percent at two years, very similar to your own data. But when following these patients out for four to five years, the effect pretty well went back to base line. So, it may well be that the effect of estrogen is a temporary one and calls out the need for longer terms of study of this particular problem.

My question has to do with lipoprotein metabolism. There have been some data suggesting that estrogens which don't pass through the liver may not have the beneficial effects of estrogen in elevating HDL. Would you comment on that?

DR. LINDSAY (New York): I take all three points that you raised. I think you very rightly point out the color coordination. And when you don't have data, then color coordination is the next best thing that you can do.

The question of whether or not the effect of estrogen is stable in patients with osteoporosis, you're quite correct, has not been studied to the detail that it needs to be. Our own long-term data in younger individuals suggests that the reduction in rate of cortical bone loss is certainly maintained, at least over a ten-year period. A cross-sectional review of those patients suggests that there is about a 24 percent difference between the placebo-treated patients and the estrogen-treated patients in spinal mineral density after ten years, and a 12 percent difference between femoral neck density in the placebo-treated patients and the estrogen-treated patients after the same period of time, suggesting that it is maintained in the younger individuals.

But your point is very well made that there are very few data that go on beyond that two-year period. And as far as we can see, there is a tendency for those patients to lose bone that is not yet significant when we followed them into the third year of that study.

The question of lipoprotein metabolism is a difficult one. And, really, I think that that section of the talk was meant to point out that we don't have the answers for this, both in terms of the administration of estrogen by alternative routes, but also whether or not the lipoprotein effects really have anything to do with whether or not there is a cardio-protective effect.

The data on transdermal estrogens and data on estrogens that are given are either subcutaneously by pellet or by injection suggests that, yes, there are lipoprotein effects. They're just a bit smaller than they are with the oral estrogens.

DR. MAUTALEN (Buenos Aires): Last night, Dr. Hedlund showed a 25 percent bone loss at the neck of the femur in the first five years after normal menopause. Do you know if there are any prospective data showing that estrogen can protect against this bone loss?

DR. LINDSAY: There are, to my knowledge, no prospective data looking at women immediately after the menopause with introduction of estrogen. There are only our own cross-sectional data on women who are followed prospectively with single-photon absorptiometry. And there, there certainly was protection. You may remember that I asked the question last night related to why there seem to be protective effects in the greater trochanter from estrogen in these cross-sectional data, but no protective effect in the femoral neck. And it's a little worrying that those data differ from other data in the literature on bone mass measurements at other sites, and certainly from our own prospective data. In fact, it was that talk that really stimulated me to show those prospective data today.

DR. MAZESS (Madison, WI): Bob, you're a master of the metacarpal, so I'm surprised you hadn't shown your data on compact bone of the appendicular skeleton in the treated osteoporotic women. Did you see the same kind of difference between the treated and the untreated in looking at either the metacarpal or the radius measurements, which you no doubt did?

DR. LINDSAY: The trends were in the same direction, but they were not significantly different at the end of two years. The changes were very small. And this time it was the mid-shaft of the radius, not the metacarpal. But the changes were very small. They were in the same direction. They were not significant. I should have said there were 20 patients in each group. And the large changes in the spine, I think, demonstrate -- really allow us to show the differences, whereas we just may not be seeing them because of the paucity of individuals with radius measurements.

DR. HEATH (Rochester, MN): Bob, if you dealt with this I didn't hear it. Would you speculate, just a moment, on what you think ought to be the duration of estrogen therapy? If we initiate it at the time of the menopause, we have, on average, many years to go. Give it a quick shot.

DR. LINDSAY: There's an easy way out of that question. I say that the introduction of estrogen is an event that occurs on discussion between a patient and her physician. And my view for the termination of estrogen therapy is the same, that it is an event that must occur as a result of the physician and patient making a determination of whether the benefits outweigh the risks. If at any point the physician and the patient feel that the risks outweigh the benefits, then treatment should be discontinued.

Parathyroid Peptide (hPTH 1–34) in the Treatment of Osteoporosis

J. REEVE, URSULA M. DAVIES, MONIQUE ARLOT,[1]
J.N. BRADBEER, J.R. GREEN, R. HESP, CLAUDE EDOUARD,[1]
PATRICIA HULME, R.D. PODBESEK, D. KATZ,
JOAN M. ZANELLI,[2] and P.J. MEUNIER[1]

*MRC Clinical Research Centre
and Northwick Park Hospital
Harrow, UK
[1]Unité Inserm 234
Faculté Alexis Carrel
Université Claude Bernard
Lyon, France
[2]National Institute for Biological Standards & Control
South Mimms, UK*

Summary

A considerable body of experience in the treatment of idiopathic and postmenopausal (type 1) osteoporosis with daily injections of the human parathyroid peptide hPTH 1-34 is reviewed. Results have been published on 49 patients given daily injections for 12-24 months and on 22 patients given two different alternating regimes of hPTH injections and oral calcitriol (1,25 dihydroxy vitamin D_3). Daily injections given alone markedly increase bone formation, but do not improve calcium absorption in patients, a finding which contrasts with the enhanced absorption found in dogs. Consequently, the just over 50% median improvement in iliac trabecular bone volume was associated with an estimated 5% loss in femoral midshaft cortical bone at 1 year. Attempts to correct this by enhancing calcium absorption with either supplementary calcitriol or (indirectly) with oestrogens are showing early success. The two alternating regimes gave differing results. Seven day course of hPTH repeated every 28 days appeared to depress bone turnover and were not anabolic for trabecular bone. In contrast, ongoing studies with alternating periods of 6 weeks hPTH and 6 weeks calcitriol are reportedly more successful in increasing spinal trabecular bone. Dogs and rats also show the anabolic response to daily injections of hPTH 1-34 in trabecular bone. However this response was lost in both when hPTH was given as a continuous infusion.

Introduction

The architectural derangement in vertebral trabecular bone which precedes crush fractures may have its origin soon after menopause[1,2]. In women with osteoporosis, there is a diminution of trabecular elements with a particularly marked loss of cross-ties between vertical trabeculae. Many remaining trabeculae approximate in shape to rods rather than plates, due to excessive fenestration. According to the Euler formula[3], a strut of circular cross section, which has its unsupported length doubled due to the disappearance of a cross tie, becomes one quarter as resistant to buckling. Trabecular thickness is also important; for an element of circular cross section, an induced 50% increase in diameter will lead to a more than twofold increase in its resistance to buckling.

Treatments which increase the thickness of remaining trabecular elements are attractive in the absence of any means of replacing elements once they have been lost. Since 1974 we have been conducting studies arising from the old observation[4] that low to moderate, daily or alternate day injections of parathyroid hormone increase trabecular bone in experimental animals. We here review our experience with the parathyroid peptide hPTH given alone to patients with crush fracture osteoporosis, or in combination with other agents.

Treatment with daily injections of hPTH 1-34

A multicentre study involving 21 patients was reported in 1980 [5]. Each received 500 units hPTH 1-34 by daily subcutaneous injection for at least one year. There was a highly encouraging increase in trabecular bone volume in the ilium, as estimated by morphometry of 7.5 mm transiliac biopsies (Fig. 1), which correlated with the osteoblastic response determined by ^{47}Ca kinetic studies performed at the end of treatment (Fig. 2). This study was performed before techniques for accurately quantitating spinal trabecular bone had become available. However, a subgroup of patients had serial densitometry of their femurs performed at the 1/3 distal site using single photon ^{241}Am densitometry[6]. This suggested that hPTH 1-34 as a single treatment may have a modest adverse effect on femur cortical bone density amounting to a mean loss of 5.0% (95% confidence interval : 11.9% loss to a 1.9% gain). For that

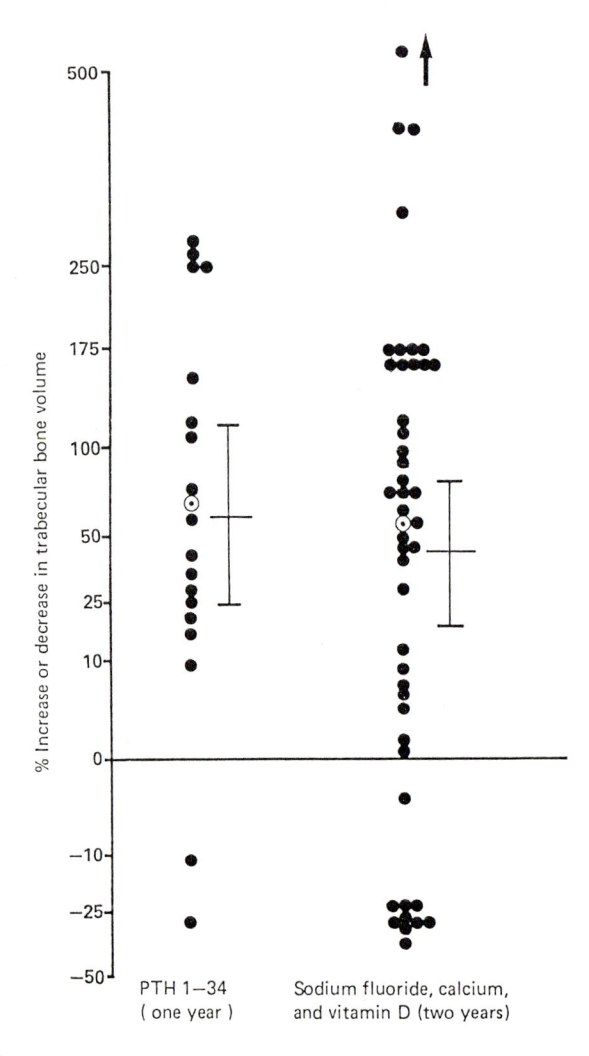

Fig. 1. Changes in iliac trabecular bone volume measurements in response to two treatments for osteoporosis. (Square root scale used to normalise distributions.) Bars indicate mean values and 95% confidence intervals; O = median value.

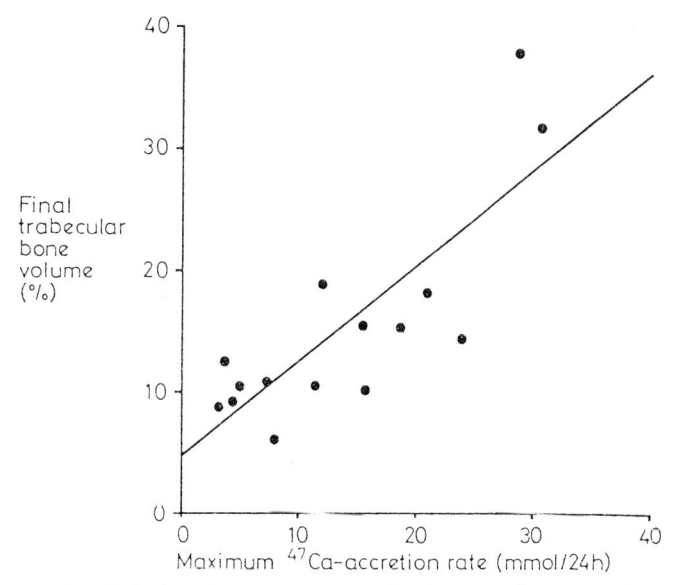

FIG 2—Relation between trabecular bone volume at time of final bone biopsy and maximum recorded ^{47}Ca-accretion rate during period of treatment.

reason, and because no demonstrable improvement in calcium balance or absorption was observed with the regime (Fig. 3 and ref 7) several further studies have now been undertaken in search of a treatment which increases axial bone mineral without adversely affecting the periphery.

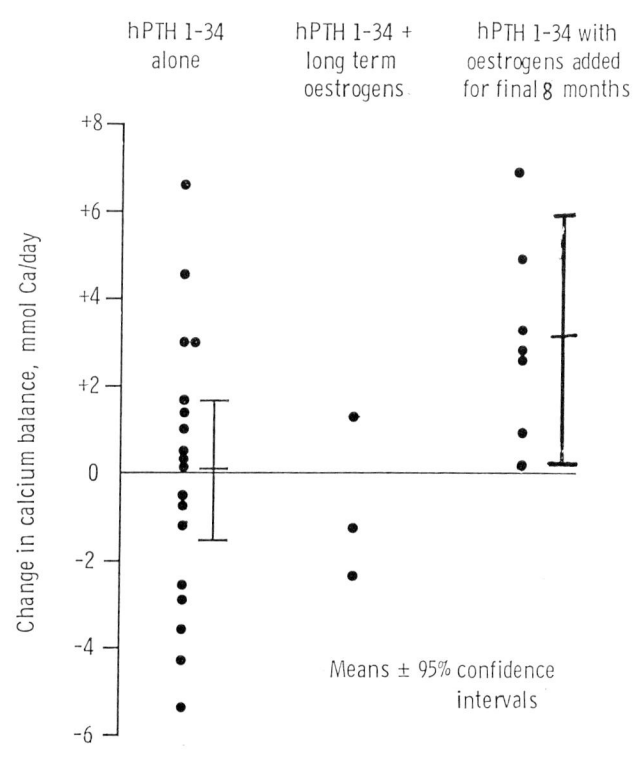

Fig. 3 Calcium balance changes in female patients submitting to balance studies lasting 15-18 days both before and during chronic treatment with daily hPTH 1-34 injections (450-600 Units/day). The middle group had been on hormone replacements for at least 1 year before starting hPTH 1-34.

623

Continuous infusion of hPTH 1-34

Two animal studies have been conducted in which daily injections, which lead to highly discontinuous[8] elevations of plasma PTH-like activity (Fig. 4), have been contrasted with smoother delivery modes. Tam et al[9] showed that at equivalent doses in rats, the infusion regime led to greater increases in bone resorption, loss of the trabecular anabolic response, and hypercalcaemia at a dose which did not cause hypercalcaemia with the injection regime. Podbesek et al[10] found that a lower daily dose in dogs with subcutaneous infusions was needed to produce an equivalent increase in resorption surfaces to their daily injection regime. The daily injections significantly increased iliac trabecular bone volume whereas the infusions did not. Interestingly, radiocalcium absortion tests were performed in this study which demonstrated that dogs[11], unlike patients[5,7], responded with increased radiocalcium absorption indices to daily injections of hPTH 1-34.

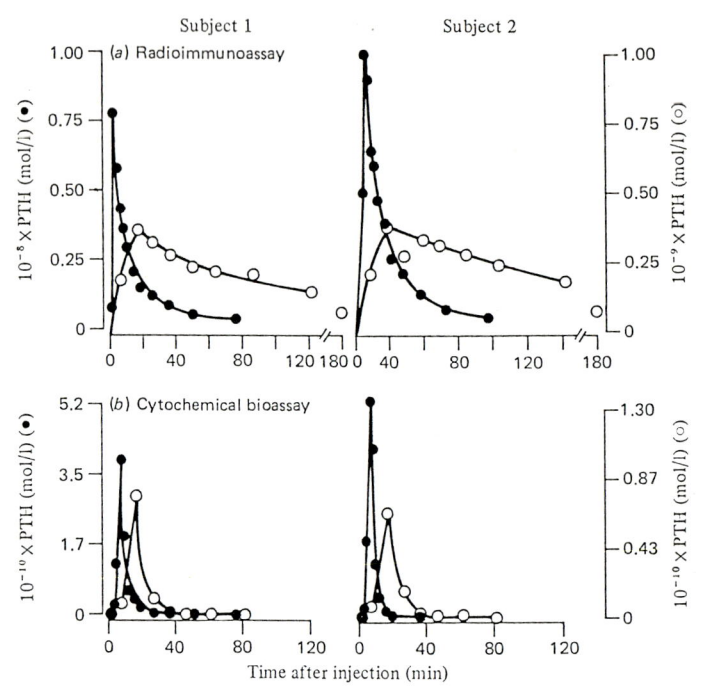

FIG. 4. Plasma concentration of hPTH 1-34 measured by either (a) radioimmunoassay or (b) cytochemical bioassay in the two subjects after intravenous (●) and subcutaneous (○) injection of hPTH 1-34. Note the different scales for the intravenous and subcutaneous results in both assay systems (on the left and right respectively).

Combination of daily injections of hPTH 1-34 with other agents

Two groups have studied combined regimes. In an attempt to conserve peripheral bone by increasing calcium absorption, Neer[12,13] and his colleagues have treated eleven men and six women with daily injections of 400-500 units hPTH 1-34 plus 0.125-0.5 micrograms calcitriol daily. Midshaft measurements of radial bone density using single photon absorptiometry showed no measurable changes, while the trabecular bone density of the remaining intact vertebrae in lumbar spine measured by quantitative computed tomography increased significantly (P<0.01) at both 12 and 18 months into treatment.

We are studying a group of 12 women with osteoporosis treated with hPTH 1-34 plus oestrogens in replacement doses (conjugated equine oestrogens 0.625 mg daily, 3 weeks in 4 plus balancing progestogens, or the equivalent)[14]. Quantitative CT studies on their intact lumbar vertebrae both before treatment and at the end or 1 year after the end of treatment were possible in 9 using a slight modification of Cann & Genant's technique as previously described[15].

The mean improvement in trabecular bone density was 22.6 mg/cm^3 (95% confidence interval 2.2 - 45.0 mg/cm^3). Four other patients were treated with hPTH 1-34 plus nandrolone deconoate 25 mg every 3 weeks with similar results. The combined group of 13 patients showed a mean increase of 23.9 mg/cm^3 (95% CI 9.8 - 38.0 mg/cm^3). The patients on hPTH 1-34 + oestrogens showed a mean improvement in calcium balance (for technique see ref. 5) of 3.1 mmol/day (Fig. 3). An interesting aspect of these bone density results was the tendency in 4 patients for the QCT results to improve further in the first year after cessation of treatment. Perhaps this relates to the tendency of patients with osteoporosis to have prolonged values of σ_F (the lifespan of the osteoblast, including 'resting' periods), allowing a prolonged period of continued osteoblastic activity in already generated BMUs.

Initial results suggest that the regime of hPTH plus oestrogen therapy may improve calcium balance through an increase in calcium absorption. Serial densitometry showed that the mean improvement in distal radial trabecular bone density trend was 4% annually by comparison with the mean pretreatment trends. This change was not statistically significant. Nor was the mean change of -1% annually in radial midshaft cortical bone trend significant.

Intermittent treatments with hPTH 1-34 given by daily injections

The first such study was inspired by the ADFR* concept. The daily injections of hPTH 1-34 were only given for the first week in every 4, 0.25 microgrammes calcitriol being given daily on the other three. It was not strictly an ADFR regime because there was no agent included to positively depress the osteoclasts after the activation phase. The 12 patients, after intensive pre-treatment studies, were treated for over 1 year[16]. Unexpectedly, activation in the sense of an increase in the birthrate of new BMUs did not occur. Instead there appeared to be a depression. There was no evidence of any substantial or consistent improvement in any parameter except calcium absorption. The bulk of the extra calcium absorbed found its way into the urine, except for a subgroup of 3 patients with high turnover initially who might therefore have benefited. Overall, the results were reminiscent of those expected with a simple course of calcitonin injections. The results are of interest for the light they shed on the biology of bone.

Neer and colleagues have had more success with a regime in which the cycles were of longer duration[13]. They treated 10 women with 400-500 units hPTH daily for six weeks followed by 6 weeks therapy with 0.125 - 0.5 microgrammes calcitriol daily. This 3 month cycle was iterated and the provisional results at 18 months reported. These women had similar responses in spinal trabecular bone to women given hPTH and calcitriol simultaneously.

Rittinghaus *et al* have treated 8 patients with daily hPTH 1-38 given subcutaneously in a dose of up to 750 units for the first 70 days of a 104 day cycle[17]. Three 14-day courses of calcitonin were also given by nasal spray, in each cycle; treatment continued for 14 months. Six of the eight patients showed increased spinal trabecular bone mineral content measured by QCT, which were comparable to those observed by Neer and ourselves.

Some interesting animal studies have recently been reported. Takahashi *et al* found that a 3 month cycle, repeated once, in which hPTH was given for the first four weeks only in each cycle to dogs increased plasma alkaline phosphatase and histomorphometrically determined trabecular fractional formation surfaces (using tetracycline + calcein *in vivo* labelling)[18]. Gunness-Hey and colleagues found that in rats the anabolic effect in long bone trabeculae obtained after 12 days therapy with hPTH 1-34 was lost again 12 days after cessation of treatment[19]. This finding is concordant with our suggestion[16] that the anabolic effect of PTH is dependent on the intermittent administration of the hormone sustained for an adequate period.

*ADFR: Activate, Depress, Free, Repeat

Conclusion

That daily injections of parathyroid peptides, given chronically, can increase axial trabecular bone volume in the majority of patients studied now appears well established. Although in young rats this effect is seen in long bones, it has not been demonstrated in similar sites in man. In view of the natural concern that agents given to strengthen the vertebrae should not do so at the expense of fracture resistance at other vulnerable sites, such as the distal radius and proximal femur, recent work has been directed towards stabilizing the endosteal surface of long bones by the addition to hPTH regimes of calcitriol (to provide an adequate supply of mineral) or, more directly, oestrogens or calcitonin.

Further animal work has suggested that the anabolic effect of hPTH on bony trabeculae is independent of oestrogens[20] and of an intact nerve supply to bone[21]. Since hPTH therapy, when successful, increases the number of functioning BMUs, it seems likely that it acts directly or otherwise as a mitogen for bone cells. However, it has been argued elsewhere that the speed of the anabolic response in many patients could only be achieved by holding the bone forming osteoblast in its actively synthetic phase longer than is normal by inhibiting its transformation to the lining cell[22]. This suggestion has received recent support from the observation that hPTH 1-34 treatment substantially increases iliac trabecular mean wall thickness[23] as well as trabecular thickness.

Side effects have been relatively few; one woman developed transient hypoparathyroidism which resolved with treatment withdrawal. She may have generated anti-idiotypic antibodies[24]. Another woman developed a delayed-type hypersensitivity reaction[13]. Three additional patients have developed plasma binding which may have neutralized the effects of therapy. Additionally, about one third of patients failed to respond objectively to hPTH 1-34 for unknown reasons (Fig. 1).

Future research should concentrate on three areas. It is first necessary to obtain additional definitive evidence that combination therapy (e.g. with oestrogens) is not harmful to peripheral bone. Next, a randomized controlled study is required with extended follow up (e.g. 5 years) to determine whether hPTH therapy results in a reduced frequency of further vertebral deformations. Finally, to address the problem of non-response to hPTH therapy, the molecular mechanisms involved in the osteoblastic response to parathyroid peptides requires continued investigation.

There is therefore considerable work required before parathyroid peptides can be recommended in the routine management of established crush fracture disease. Nevertheless, there are new grounds for hope that adverse effects on cortical bone may be avoided with combination therapies. With their relative freedom from side-effects and the ease with which patients adapt to self injection for restricted periods, parathyroid peptides may prove to be of considerable clinical value in the future management of osteoporosis.

Acknowledgement

We thank Rorer Pharmaceuticals for supplies of hPTH 1-34 peptide.

References

1. Parfitt, A.M., Matthews, C.H.E., Villanueva, A.R., Kleerekoper, M., Frame, B., and Rao, D.S., *J. Clin. Invest.*, **72**, 1396 (1983).

2. Reeve, J., *Brit. Med. J.* **295**, 757 (1987).

3. Gibb, A., *Calcif. Tiss. Res.*, **1**, 83 (1967).

4. Parsons, J.A., and Potts, J.T. Jr., *Clinics in Endoc. Metab.*, **1**, 33 (1972).

5. Reeve, J., Meunier, P.J., Parsons, J.A., Bernat, M., Bijovet, O.L.M., Courpron, P., Edouard, C., Klenerman, L., Neer, R.M., Renier, J.C., Slovik, D., Vismans, F.J.F.E., and Potts, J.T. Jr., *Brit. Med. J.*, **280**, 1340 (1980).

6. Hesp, R., Hulme, Patricia, Williams, D., and Reeve, J., *Metab. Bone Dis. & Rel. Res.*, **2**, 331 (1981).

7. Reeve, J., Bijvoet, O.L.M., Neer, R.M., Slovik, D., Tellez, M., Vismans, F.J.F.E., and Zanelli, G.D., *Metab. Bone Dis. & Rel. Res.*, **2**, 233 (1980).

8. Kent, G.N., Loveridge, N., Reeve, J., and Zanelli, J.M., *Clin. Sci.*, **68**, 171 (1985).

9. Tam, C.S., Heersche, J.N.M., Murray, T.M., and Parsons, J.A., *Endocrinol*, **10**, 506 (1982).

10. Podbesek, R., Edouard, C., Meunier, P.J., Parsons, J.A., Reeve, J., Stevenson, R.W., and Zanelli, Joan, M., *Endocrinol*, **112**, 1000 (1983).

11. Podbesek, R.D., Mawer, E.B., Zanelli, G.D., Parsons, J.A., and Reeve, J., *Clin. Sci.*, **67**, 591 (1984).

12. Slovik, D.M., Rosenthal, D.I., Doppelt, S.H., Potts, J.T. Jr., Daly, H.A., Campbell, J.A., and Neer, R.M., *J. Bone & Mineral Res.*, **1**, 377 (1986).

13. Neer, R.M., Slovik, D., Doppelt, S., Daly, M., Rosenthal, D., Lo, C., and Potts, J.T. Jr., in C. Christiansen *et al* (Editors), 'Osteoporosis 1987', Osteopress ApS, Copenhagen, 1987, p.829.

14. Reeve, J., Hesp, R., Audran, M., Renier, J.C., Slovik, D., and Neer, R.M., *Bone* **7**, 160 (1986) Abstract.

15. Sambrook, P.N., Bartlett, C., Evans, R., Hesp, R., Katz, D., and Reeve, J., *Brit. J. Radiol.* **58**, 621 (1985).

16. Reeve, J., Arlot, M.E., Price, T.R., Edouard, C., Hesp, R., Hulme, P., Ashby, J.P., Zanelli, J.M., Green, J.R., Tellez, M., Katz, D., Spinks, T.J., and Meunier, P.J. *Eur. J. Clin. Invest.* **17**, 421 (1987).

17. Rittinghaus, E.F., Busch, U., Prokop, M., Delling, O., and Hesch, R.D., in C. Christiansen *et al* (Editors), Osteoporosis 1987, Osteopress ApS, Copenhagen, 1987, p.888.

18. Takahashi, H., Inone, J., Minato, I., Noda, T., Hora, M., and Uzawa, T., in D.V. Cohn *et al* (Editors), Calcium Regulation and Bone Metabolism, Basic and Clinical Aspects, Excerpta Medica ICS 735, Amsterdam, p.662 (Abstract).

19. Gunness-Hay, M., Fonseca, J., Raisz, L.G., and Hock, J.H., *J. Bone & Mineral Res.*, **2** (suppl. 1) Abstract 58.

20. Gera, I., Fonseca, J., Raisz, L.G., and Hock, J.H., *J. Bone & Mineral Res.*, **2** (suppl. 1) Abstract 55.

21. Steen-Hackett, L., Gera, I., Fonseca, J., Raisz, L.G., and Hock, J.M. *J. Bone & Mineral Res.*, **2** (suppl. 1) Abstract 57.

22. Reeve, J., *Clin. Orthop. & Rel. Res.*, **213**, 264 (1986).

23. Bradbeer, J.N., Arlot, M., Reeve, J., & Meunier, P.J. *J. Bone & Mineral Res.*, **3** (suppl. 1) Abstract (in press).

24. Audran, M., Basle, M-F., Defontaine, A., Jallet, P., Bidet, M.T., Ermias, A., Tanguy, G., Pouplard, A, Reeve, J., Zanelli, J., and Renier, J-C., *J. Clin. Endoc. & Metab.* **64**, 937 (1987).

Discussion:

DR. MALLUCHE (Lexington, KY): Jon, I'm a little bit puzzled. During the last ten years we have heard, first, data on the positive effect of PTH in bone in continuous infusion. Then we were told, no, that's not really so, we might lose bone or that this bone is being rebuilt at the expense of cortical bone. And then we heard data with and without 1,25(OH)2D treatment, and now with and without estrogen. I wonder what do you think are the effects of PTH on bone? What is your rationale to design these studies? How do you see PTH acting on bone, rebuilding bone? What mechanisms do you propose to explain these data?

DR. REEVE (England): Well, that's a complex question, and I can't answer it in great detail. I'll try to answer it, however, in a pithy sort of way to draw out the main points. First of all, this is not hyperparathyroidism. The time course is quite wrong. Secondly, if you expose parathyroid hormone-sensitive cells to continuous levels of parathyroid hormone you down-regulate their receptors, and in this study these are not continuous levels. And as O'Riordan showed some years ago, 24 hours after an injection, the receptors will be back waiting to be hit. So, I don't think one wants to draw analogies between daily injections and hyperparathyroidism. That's the first thing.

The second thing is that the treatment doesn't increase the plasma calcium over the 24 hours, unless it's given in overdose. So, where does that bring us back to? I believe that some patients are able to respond to PTH as a mitogen for some element of the precursor pool for osteoblasts. How this works I don't know; we need cell and molecular studies to further evaluate how this works.

DR. MALLUCHE: How do you think estrogen facilitates this effect, because it appears that PTH alone cannot do it and the addition of estrogen does it?

DR. REEVE: I don't think the estrogen is necessarily having any effect on the axial trabecular response. Where I think the estrogen is having an effect is on the peripheral cortical bone, which we showed without estrogen tended to go into negative balance. So, without estrogen, you've robbed Peter to pay Paul. You've gotten the mineral for the axial skeleton from the peripheral skeleton. And, now, we're able to stop that, and the mineral is coming from the gut, either by controlling bone loss through the urine, or by increasing gastrointestinal absorption.

DR. WUSTER (Heidelberg): Did you actually look quantitatively at the fracture rate of your vertebral fractures? And was there a difference in the responsiveness in patients with only one vertebral fracture or with multiple vertebral fractures?

DR. REEVE: There was one patient in that group with less than two vertebral fractures, but the protocol strictly called for patients with two or more vertebral fractures. And the second point is that the only protocol in which we've observed a fracture, a clinical fracture with pain, or a radiological fracture with a demonstrable further deformity, was the ADFR-type protocol. In the current protocol, we've had no fractures since the start of treatment. I don't claim that means anything because the numbers are too small to evaluate.

DR. KLEEREKOPER: During the course of the week I've heard lots of comments about this symposium. I thought I might just share three with you as we close the meeting. The first comes from Barbara Tilley, who really can't make comments, she just makes statistical statement. She's the head of the Division of Research Statistics and Epidemiology at Henry Ford Hospital. She says that the 180 people in the room at the end of the last day's session is not statistically significantly different from the number at the beginning of the first day's session.

Dr. Rao, my colleague, made the second comment I wanted to pass on. He suggested that we really missed an opportunity to do a good clinical experiment, and that we should have measured bone mineral density on everybody as they walked in on Monday and checked it again on the way out to see the effects of immobilization.

And while I don't want to belabor the humor we've had this week about astrology - I must have missed reading that book - the best comment of the week I think came from Dr. Singh at 2:00 this morning as we -- well, never mind. At 2:00 this morning Dr. Singh said we should have another meeting. We should have a meeting in Detroit, but it must be in May. So, what's so special about May? The zodiac sign for May is Taurus, the bull. I think I've already said too much other than to say, for us who put it on, it's been a tremendous pleasure, really, to have put on a symposium for you. We thank you all for your patience, your forbearance, and for what we think has been a superb set of presentations by all our speakers.

Have a good trip home.

Author Index

Akerstrom, G., 353
Arlot, M., 621
Arnold, A., 311
Aurbach, G.D., 323
Avioli, L.V., 129

Bansal, M., 287
Basile, J., 475
Baylink, D.J., 293
Bell, N.H., 435, 475, 481
Bickerstaff, D., 499
Bijvoet, O.L.M., 525
Bilezikian, J.P., 305, 359
Block, J.E., 153
Body, J.J., 581
Bone, H.G., 129
Bonjour, J.P., 589
Boyce, B.F., 553
Bradbeer, J.N., 621
Brandi, M.L., 323
Brazy, P.C., 469
Brown, E.M., 317
Burkinshaw, L., 253
Byers, P.H., 407

Caverzasio, J., 589
Charles, P., 73
Chen, C.J., 317
Chesney, R.W., 395
Chestnut, C.H., 135, 199
Christiansen, C., 189
Clemens, T.L., 273
Cohn, D.H., 407
Cornell, C.N., 287
Cummings, S.R., 231

Davidai, G.A., 469
Davies, U.M., 621
DeGrange, D., 323
Dekanic, D., 165
Dempster, D.W., 247
Drezner, M.K., 469
Drinkwater, B.L., 173

Eastell, R., 605
Edouard, C., 621
Epstein, S., 481
Eriksen, E.F., 73
Ettinger, B., 153

Faugere, M.C., 597
Frost, H.M., 15

Gagel, R.F., 563
Gallagher, J.C., 205
Genant, H.K., 153
Glorieux, F.H., 425
Glowacki, J.A., 113
Glueer, C.C., 153
Goldsmith, P., 323
Goltzman, D., 341
Green, J.R., 621

Halloran, B.P., 455
Halls, D.J., 553
Hamdy, N., 499
Harinck, H.I.J., 525
Harris, S.T., 153
Haussler, M.R., 439
Heaney, R.P., 59, 181
Heath, H., 575
Hendy, G.N., 341
Hesp, R., 621
Hillman, L.S., 415
Hodgson, S.F., 605
Hordon, L., 265
Horsman, A., 253
Hulme, P., 621

Joborn, C., 353
Junor, B.J.R., 553

Kanis, J.A., 499
Katz, D., 621
Kleerekoper, M., iii
Kraenzlin, M.E., 293
Krane, S.M., iii, 191
Kronenberg, H.M., 311

Lane, J.M., 287
Leboff, M.S., 317
Levine, M.A., 333
Libanati, C.R., 283
Liberman, U.A., 447
Liel, Y., 475
Lindsay, R., 227, 613
Ljunghall, S., 353

Malluche, H.H., 597
Marcus, R., 49
Mariano-Menez, M.R., 293
Martin, T.J., 305, 509
Marx, S.J., 323, 447
Matkovic, V., 165
McCloskey, E., 499
McGuire, M.H., 117
Melsen, F., 73
Melton, L.J., 145
Mitchell, J.A., 341
Mocan, Z., 553
Morris, R.C., 455
Mosekilde, L., 73
Muenier, P.J., 621
Mundy, G.R., 495, 517

Nesbitt, T., 469
Nevitt, M.C., 231

O'Doherty, D., 499

Pak, C.Y.C., 543
Palmer, M., 353
Parfitt, A.M., 7, 45
Peacock, M., 265
Peck, W.A., 141
Podbesek, R.D., 621
Portale, A.A., 455
Potts, J.T., 3

Raisz, L.G., 211
Rastad, J., 353

Recker, R.R., 59
Reeve, J., 621
Riggs, B.L., 145, 605
Riis, B.J., 189
Rizzoli, R., 589
Roodman, G.D., 105
Rowe, D.W., 95

Sakaguchi, K., 323
Schneider, R., 287
Schulz, E.E., 293
Schwartz, S.B., 287
Shane, E., 359
Silverberg, S.J., 359
Sly, W.S., 373
Starman, B.J., 407
Steiger, P., 153
Steinicke, T., 73

Tsipouras, P., 95
Tudtud-Hans, L.A., 293

Vellenga, C.J.L.R., 525

Wahner, H.W., 237
Wallis, G.A., 407
Whyte, M.P., 369, 383
Willing, M.C., 407

Zanelli, J.M., 621
Zimering, M.B., 323

Subject Index

Absorptiometry, single and dual photon, 153-154
Absorption, See Metabolism
Acidosis, renal tubular, 373-382
Acromegaly
    trabecular remodeling, 83 84
    see also Hormonal effects
Activation
    bone mass effects, 22, 24, 27
    and trabecular remodeling, 74
Acute lymphoblastic leukemia, 131
Adenomas
    double, 313
    primary hyperparathyroidism, 353-354
    parathyroid, 311-316
Adenylate cyclase
    in G proteins, 335-336
    hormonal inhibition, 335
    pseudohypoparathyroidism, 344-345
ADFR (activate-depress-free-repeat)
    bone mass and fragility, 32
    parathyroid peptide therapy, 625
Adolescents
    bone development, 165-166
    calcium metabolism, 167-168
    see also Children
ADP (adenosine diphosphate)
    ribosylation factor in G proteins, 334-335
Adrenal medullary disease
    diagnosis and management, 566-567
    multiple endocrine neoplasia, 566
    pheochromocytoma, 567
Adult hypophosphatasia, 384, 386
Age and aging
    biochemical markers, 64
    bone mass, 16
    bone remodeling, 46, 61-65
    chronic disease, 148
    fracture risk, 254, 255
    Gompertzian model, 148-149
    histomorphometry, 61-63
    morphology and geometry, 61
    osteoporosis, 273-285
    plasma levels, 276, 277
    radiocalcium kinetics, 63
    working model, 67
Age-related bone loss
    calcium deficiency, 182
    femoral fractures, 265-266
    hormonal effects, 182
    perimenopausal, 181-183
    risk factors, 182

    senescence, 182
    vertebral fractures, 10-12
    vitamin D, 265-266
AIDS (acquired immunodeficiency syndrome)
    CSF application, 108
    neutropenia with, 108
Albers-Schonberg disease, See Osteopetrosis
Albright's hereditary osteodystrophy, See Pseudohypoparathyroidism
Albumin in hip fractures, 284
Alkaline phosphatase
    age-related changes, 64
    bone formation marker, 52
    hepatic vs. skeletal, 52
    hypophosphatasia, 385, 387
    Paget's disease, 528
    see also TNSALP
Allied disciplines, 91-93
    bone induction, 113-116
    hematopoietic growth factors, 105-112
    molecular genetics, 95-103
    surgical management of skeletal tumors, 117-126
Allograft reconstruction in osteosarcoma, 124
Alopecia (baldness), 447-449
Aluminum
    absorption tests, 556
    bone content, 600
    citrate-augmented absorption, 562
    in dialysis water, 557
    hyperabsorbers, 555-557
    public water supplies, 557
    staining at mineralization, 559, 562
    water treatment units, 557-558
Aluminum-related bone disease, 496, 554-555
    deferoxamine treatment, 577, 598, 599
    in dialysis patients, 597-598
    histology and indications, 554-559
    hypercalcemia, 558
    newer therapies, 577
    osteodystrophy, 459
    patients at risk, 555-559, 597-598
    plasma exchange, 598
    sorbent hemoperfusion, 598
    therapeutic advances, 597-604
Amenorrhea
    in athletes, 136
    bone mass, 174
Amidronate
    hypercalcemia of malignancy, 576

Amidronate (cont)
   metastatic breast cancer, 595
   serum calcium effects, 584-585
   tumor-associated hypercalcemia, 584-586
Angiogenesis in multiple endocrine neoplasia, 326-327
Antacids
   osteomalacia, 458-459
   phosphorus content, 458
Anti-rachitic activity, See Williams syndrome
APD (aminohydroxypropylidene bisphonate)
   osteoporosis, 214
   Paget's disease, 533-534
   pain treatment, 536
   side effects, 536
Aplasia, aluminum-related, 554-555
Appendicular bone remodeling, 7-9
Arthritis, See Rheumatoid arthritis
Asphyxia, calcitonin surges in, 416
Atherosclerotic heart disease, molecular genetics, 95-96
Athletes
   menstrual cycle, 174
   osteoporosis, 136
Atraumatic fractures, 155
Autoimmune theory of multiple endocrine neoplasia, 324
Autosomal bone disorders
   carbonic anhydrase deficiency, 373-382
   Handigodu syndrome, 129
   see also Chromosome
Axial bone remodeling, 7-8

B-cell lymphomas and hypercalcemia mechanisms, 520
Baldness, See Alopecia
BGP (bone GLA-protein)
   age-related changes, 64
   ethnic differences, 490
   sex differences, 65
Bicarbonate transport in renal tubular acidosis, 374
Biochemical markers, 49
   age-related changes, 64
   bone remodeling, 11, 49-57, 61, 64
   functions, 49-50
   hydroxyproline, 45
   resorption, 50-52
   sex differences, 65
Biologic effects on bone mass, 15-19, 30-31
Bisphosphonates
   current treatments, 582-583
   general considerations, 581-582
   malignant hypercalcemia, 589-590
   osteoporosis, 138
   Paget's disease, 530-531
   perimenopausal bone loss, 199-203
   physicochemical effects, 200
   remodeling measurements, 60
   second generation, 533-536
   sex differences, 65
   severe hypercalcemia, 581-587
   tomography measurements, 200
   types of, 532
Bite effects on bone mass, 22, 24

BMU (basic multicellular unit), 59
Bone
   aluminum content, 600
   architecture, 23
   banks, 15-16, 22-24
   biology, 34
   demineralized grafts, 114-115
   destruction (myeloma), 517-518
   development, 165-172
   diseases, 373-382
   fatigue, 26
   growth, 15-16, 142
   induction, 91, 113-116
   loads and resistance, 21
   marrow transplants, 107, 378
   mineral content, 190, 194
   mineral values, 243
   pain, 34
   preservation, 174-177
   reconstruction, 113
   strength, 298
   structure, 247-249, 600
   tumors, 92, 120, 188
   turnover, 249-251
   see also Densitometry; Metabolism; Resorption
Bone biopsy, See Iliac crest biopsy
Bone density
   fluoride effect, 294, 606-608
   lymphoblastic leukemia, 131
   transdermal estrogen, 616-617
   see also Absorptiometry
Bone formation
   alkaline phosphatase marker, 52
   biochemical markers, 52-54
   deferoxamine therapy, 600
   ethnic differences, 66, 490
   fluoride effects, 215, 606
   glucocorticoids, 212-213
   hormonal effects, 74
   measurements, 45
   osteitis fibrosa, 553-554
   postmenopausal, 10-12
   sex differences, 65
   surface-based, 10-12
Bone loss
   age-related, 10-12, 181-183, 265-266
   biochemical markers, 54
   diphosphate inhibitors, 41
   endocortical, 10
   estrogen effects, 182, 613
   fast and slow, 54
   femoral neck, 237-246
   heterogeneity, 145-147
   hip fracture risk, 253-263
   morphology, 146
   noninvasive measurement, 237-246
   osteoblast-mediated, 146
   osteocalcin marker, 54
   osteoclast-mediated, 146
   perimenopausal and postmenopausal, 137, 182
   prednisone-induced, 215
   reversibility in athletes, 174
   stochastic models, 253-263
   thyroid-related, 282
   treatment model, 606
   see also Osteoporosis

Bone mass
    activation effects, 22, 24, 27
    ADFR treatment, 32
    age effects, 16, 182
    amenorrhea, 174
    baseline properties, 30
    biologic effects, 15-19, 30-31
    bite effect, 22, 24
    calcitonin and diphosphonates, 199-203
    calcium and estrogen, 181-197
    clinical therapies, 32-34
    development and preservation, 137
    estrogen replacement, 183
    ethnic differences, 66
    fluoride effects, 32, 606
    and fragility, 32-34
    future research, 141
    genetic factors, 102
    iliac crest biopsy, 247-249
    measurement techniques, 153-154, 157-158
    mechanostat and setpoints, 25-26
    mechanical usage, 15-42
    parathyroid hormone treatment, 32
    pharmacologic therapies, 32
    physical therapy, 32
    positive factors, 173
    postmenopausal and perimenopausal, 181-204
    quantitative measurement, 136
    reversible and irreversible changes, 75
    risk factors, 137, 173
    tissue response modes, 30-31
    transient vs. steady-state, 31
    see also Absorptiometry; Bone density
Bone modeling, 16
    defined, 59-60
    activity effects, 27
    mechanostat and setpoints, 25-26
    special laws, 24-25
Bone remodeling, 17-18, 45-47
    activity effects, 27
    age-related, 46, 61-65, 238-239
    axial and appendicular, 7-9
    biochemical markers, 11, 45, 49-57, 61, 64
    clinical features, 19
    defined, 59-60
    ethnic differences, 66
    femoral, 238-239
    functions, 18
    future research, 141
    histomorphometry, 61-63
    hormonal effects, 46
    known and probable functions, 29
    measurement methods, 60-61
    mechanostat and setpoints, 25-26
    microdamage pathway, 28-29
    vs. modeling, 59-60
    morphology and geometry, 61
    overloads and underloads, 22-24
    pathophysiology, 19
    sex differences, 65
    static measurements, 63
    steroid and peptide hormones, 444
    supracellular organization, 45
    surface-specific, 7-14
    vitamin D receptor, 444-445
    working model, 67
Brain function and cerebral calcification, 377
Breast cancer
    amidronate treatment, 595
    hypercalcemia with, 509
    see also Carcinomas
Brittle bones, See Osteogenesis imperfecta
Bronchogenic carcinoma, 512
Burkitt's lymphoma with hypercalcemia, 520

Cadmium detoxification, 464
Caffey's disease, indomethacin treatment, 42
Calcification, See Cerebral calcification
Calcinosis and renal phosphate transport, 470
Calcitonin
    bone mass, 199-203
    challenge tests, 51
    and diphosphonates, 199-203, 586
    dosage rates, 202
    infant asphyxiation, 416
    nasal spray, 199, 202
    neonatal levels, 421-422
    osteoporosis, 138, 199
    Paget's disease, 530-531
    perimenopausal bone mass, 199-203
    resorption marker, 51
    trabecular remodeling, 74
    Williams syndrome, 399-400
Calcitriol, See 1,25-Dihydroxyvitamin D
Calcitropic hormones, 589
Calcium
    absorption, 185, 266-267
    adequate intake, 185-186
    adolescent retention, 166
    amidronate effect, 584-585
    bone preservation, 175
    deficiency, 182, 419-420
    and estrogen, 181-197
    exchange and excretion sites, 500-501
    and exercise, 175-177
    future research, 142
    infant formula, 419-420
    infusion, 502
    intestinal absorption, 500
    parathyroid inhibition, 305-306
    perimenopausal intervention, 181-197
    pyrophosphate deposition disease, 384
    remodeling measurements, 60
    renal tubular reabsorption, 502, 503
    requirements, 185
    resorption marker, 51
    supplements, 185, 186
    urinary and plasma, 503
    see also Parathyroid secretion; Radiocalcium kinetics
Calcium metabolism
    clinical disorders, 495-497
    diseases related to, 475-476
    genetic disorders, 306-307
    magnesium, 171
    Paget's disease, 528
    primary hyperparathyroidism, 355
    sarcoidosis and related diseases, 475-480

Calcium metabolism (cont)
  teenagers, 167-168
  see also Metabolism
Cancellous bone
  age, 10-12
  remodeling, 7-8
  turnover rate, 249-250
  vertebral fractures, 10-12
  see also Bone remodeling
Cancer, See Breast cancer
Carbonic anhydrase deficiency, 369, 373-382
Carcinomas, staging system, 121
Cardiovascular disease in primary hyperparathyroidism, 356-357
Cerebral calcification
  carbonic anhydrase deficiency, 382
  brain function, 377
  in children, 373-382
  clinical features, 374-375
  osteopetrosis, 373-382
  pathophysiology, 377
CFU (colony forming unit), 105
Children
  acute lymphoblastic leukemia, 131
  aluminum-related bone diseases, 459, 555
  carbonic anhydrase deficiency, 369, 373-382
  cerebral calcification, 373-382
  fractures, 374
  hypophosphatasia, 369-370, 383-393
  mechanical usage effects, 21-22
  metabolic bone disease, 369-371
  neonatal disorders, 371, 415-423
  nutrition surveys, 168
  osteodystrophy, 459
  osteogenesis imperfecta, 370, 407-414
  osteopetrosis, 369, 373-382
  renal insufficiency, 456-457
  renal tubular acidosis, 373-382
  VDRR, 425-432
  Williams syndrome, 370, 395-405
Cholera and G proteins, 337
Chondrocalcinosis, 384
Chromosome
  centromeric region, 565
  multiple endocrine neoplasia, 324, 564
  theory, 564-565
  see also DNA
Chronic disease
  age effects, 148
  Gompertzian model, 148-149
Circulating growth factor in parathyroid cell hyperplasia, 323-332
Clinical cases, 129-132
  calcium deficiency rickets, 130
  childhood acute lymphoblastic leukemia, 131
  1,25-dihydroxyvitamin D3 resistance, 130
  endemic multiple epiphyseal dysplasia, 129
  familial expansive osteolysis, 129
  fluoride for chronic malabsorption, 131
  hypercalcemia and osteopenia, 131
  hypophosphatemic rickets, 130-131
  myelodysplastic syndrome, 131
  Paget's disease, 130
Clodronate
  hypercalcemia of malignancy, 576
  postmenopausal osteoporosis, 200
  tumor-associated hypercalcemia, 583
Clonal tumors
  cytogenetic studies, 311
  DNA analysis, 312
Collagen
  biosynthesis in osteogenesis imperfecta, 407-408
  defects, 97-98
  enzymes and location, 408
  genes, 408, 411
  see also Procollagen
Colles' fracture, 145
  age and sex, 148
  risk heterogeneity, 147-148
Compression fractures
  age effects, 10-12, 41
  bone loss, 10-12
  pathogenesis, 10-12
Computerized tomography, 92, 118-119
Cortical bone
  fracture risk, 297
  mechanical usage effects, 23
  turnover rate, 249-250
Cortical bone remodeling, 8-9, 74
  age-related changes, 61
  formation period, 62
  morphology and geometry, 61
Corticosteroid-induced osteopenia, 138-139
CPRS (comprehensive pathological rating scale), 355
Cranial nerve compression and osteopetrosis, 374
Craniofacial disorders and bone induction, 115, 116
Creatinine
  biochemistry, 268
  bone turnover, 50-51
  clearance with age, 266-267
  vitamin D metabolites, 207
CSF (colony stimulating factor)
  bone marrow transplants, 107-108
  glomerulonephritis, 107-108
  neutropenia and leukemia, 108, 109
  types and sources, 106
Cushing's syndrome, bone densitometry, 156
Cytogenetic analysis of clonal tumors, 311
Cytokines in hypercalcemia, 522, 589

Deafness and carbonic anhydrase deficiency, 381-382
Deferoxamine
  aluminum-related bone disease, 577, 598
  as chelating agent, 598
  histology and side effects, 599
  mucormycosis, 602-603
  ocular complications, 599
  vasodilatory effect, 599
Deflazacort in osteoporosis treatment, 214
Deletional model of hereditary malignancy, 563-564
Demineralized bone
  preparation and clinical use, 114-115
  types of implants, 114-115

Densitometry
    accuracy and appropriate use, 153-163
    clinical applications, 154-158
    estrogen replacement therapy, 156
    future research, 142
    metabolic diseases, 156
    monitoring treatment interventions, 157-158
    new developments, 154, 155
    osteoporosis, 136
    perimenopausal, 156
    sensitivity and precision, 154
    techniques and sites, 153-155
    see also Absorptiometry; Bone density; Bone mass
Dental malocclusion and carbonic anhydrase deficiency, 375
DEXA (dual energy x-ray absorptiometry)
    accuracy and precision, 242
    instrument features, 241
    femoral neck measurements, 237, 240
    proximal femur, 240-245
Diabetes mellitus
    G proteins, 337
    primary hyperparathyroidism, 356
Dialysis patients
    chelation therapy, 599
    with osteitis fibrosa, 553-554
    serum aluminum levels, 556
1,25-Dihydroxyvitamin D
    amino acid sequence, 440-441
    biochemical experiments, 440-441
    clinical and biochemical features, 450, 452
    dermal fibroblast response, 450
    diagnosis and treatment, 447-453
    ethnic differences, 482, 489-490
    hereditary resistance, 447-453
    hormonal effects, 439-440
    hydroxylase transport mechanism, 469
    hypercalcemia, 475
    intracaval calcium infusions, 450
    intracellular defects, 449-450
    kinetic analysis, 477
    metabolic clearance, 477
    molecular cloning, 440-441
    nonrenal production, 478
    osteoporosis therapy, 205-206
    with parathyroid peptide, 624, 625
    pathophysiology, 447-453
    phosphorus modulation, 460-461
    production rates, 477
    receptor defects, 449-450
    receptor function, 436, 439-446
    renal phosphate transport, 469-471
    resistance, 130
    sarcoidosis, 476-478
    serum calcium levels, 449
    therapy and results, 450-453
    tissue defects, 450
    VDRR treatment, 425-427, 430-431
    Williams syndrome, 309
Diphosphonates, See Bisphosphonates
Diuretics and bone resorption, 214
DNA (deoxyribonucleic acid)
    osteoporosis markers, 99
    tumor clonality analysis, 312
    see also Chromosome; Gene
Double adenomas, 313

DPA (dual photon absorptiometry)
    bone loss, 153-154, 237
    femoral neck, 227, 237, 253, 260
    instrument features, 241
    precision and accuracy, 154, 242
    proximal femur, 240-245
    see also Absorptiometry; Bone density; Bone mass
Dwarfism, See Osteogenesis imperfecta

Ectoenzymes, See TNSALP
Ectopic calcification in hypophosphatemic rickets, 130-131
Elasticity, Young's modulus of, 21
Elfin facies, See Williams syndrome
Endemic diseases
    fluorosis, 301
    multiple epiphyseal dysplasia, 129
Endocrine disorders
    G protein related, 337
    trabecular remodeling, 78
    types of, 78
    see also Hormonal effects; Multiple endocrine neoplasia
Endocortical bone loss, 10
Endosteal envelope, 7-8
Epidermal growth factor and bone resorption, 511
Epiphyseal dysplasia, endemic multiple, 129
Erythrocytes in carbonic anhydrase deficiency, 375
Erythropoietin, 106
Estrogen
    bone loss, 138, 189-197
    bone preservation, 174
    deficiency by age, 182
    hip fractures, 235
    lipoprotein metabolism, 619
    percutaneous, 616
    radiocalcium kinetics, 63
    receptors, 442, 444
    trabecular bone remodeling, 82-83
    turnover rate, 29
    vitamin D, 444-445
Estrogen replacement therapy
    alternate routes, 615-617
    biochemical predictors, 54
    bone loss, 54, 183
    cardio-protective effect, 46
    densitometry, 156
    future research, 142
    new methods, 613-620
    oral methods, 613-614, 616
    perimenopausal, 191-193
    transdermal, 615-617
Ethnic differences
    bone mass, 66
    children, 484
    clinical cases, 132
    1,25-dihydroxyvitamin D3, 489-490
    femoral bone loss, 262-263
    remodeling and mineralization, 66, 132
    serum values, 481, 484
    vitamin D metabolism, 481-491
Etidronate
    hypercalcemia of malignancy, 576

637

Etidronate (cont)
    postmenopausal osteoporosis, 200
    tumor-associated hypercalcemia, 583
    see also Bisphosphonates
Exercise
    amenorrhea, 174
    bone preservation, 175-177
    vs. hormone replacement therapy, 176
    special programs, 32
Exotoxin catalysis of G proteins, 334-335

Falls
    age-related, 231-232
    epidemiology, 227, 231-236
    residual energy, 232
    stochastic models, 253-254
    see also Hip fractures
Familial expansile osteolysis, 129
Fanconi's syndrome, 470
Fat in bone measurements, 243
Fatigue
    bone, 26
    see also Microdamage
Femoral bone
    age-related remodeling, 238-239
    developmental changes, 237
    ethnic differences, 262-263
    hip fractures, 253-263
    ilium vs. proximal femur, 249
    mineral measurements, 245
    stochastic models of bone loss, 253-263
Femoral fractures
    age-related, 265-266
    biochemical abnormalities, 268
    histology and histomorphometry, 268-271
    vitamin D, 265-271
Femoral neck
    bone loss, 237-246
    fat in measurements, 244
    fractures, 289
    orthopedic management, 289
    measurement techniques, 239-240
Fibroblast growth factors in multiple endocrine neoplasia, 325-327
Fixed nail in trochanteric fractures, 290
Fluoride
    bone formation, 215, 606, 607
    bone mass, 32, 606
    density and strength, 294, 298
    drinking water, 605
    mitogen enhancer, 298
    in skeleton, 607-608
Fluoride therapy
    antifracture efficacy, 609
    chronic malabsorption, 131
    clinical cases, 131
    hip osteoporosis, 293-295
    historical background, 605-606
    methods and results, 293-294
    pain syndrome, 609
    side effects, 609
    see also Sodium fluoride
Fluorosis, clinically induced, 606
Food, calcium-fortified, 185
Formation markers, 52-54
    alkaline phosphatase, 52
    osteocalcin, 53-54
    procollagen extension peptide, 53
    traditional and potential, 52
Fractures
    age-specific, 254, 255
    childhood, 374
    cortical bone, 297
    genetic factors, 102
    osteoporotic, 374
    postmenopausal, 190
    risk models, 253-254
    see also Hip fractures
Fragility
    ADFR treatment, 32
    clinical therapies, 32-34
    excessive skeletal, 59
    fluoride treatment, 32
    and osteoporosis, 32, 59
    parathyroid hormone therapy, 32
    sports medicine, 32-34

G proteins, 333-339
Gallium nitrate
    vs. bisphosphonates, 590
    dosage and delivery, 594
    hypercalcemia and hyperparathyroidism, 576, 589-595
Gammopathy, benign monoclonal, 311
Gastric irritation in fluoride therapy, 609
Gene
    bone mass factor, 102
    calcium metabolism, 306-307
    carbonic anhydrase deficiency, 377, 382
    cloning and mutations, 377, 382
    chromosome linkage, 564-565
    collagen, 408, 411-412
    expression and tumor clonality, 315
    osteogenesis imperfecta, 411-412
    osteopenic bone disease, 99, 102
    statistical analysis, 99
    vitamin D receptor, 442
Genetic counseling, 378
Gigantism, See Acromegaly
Global bone bank, 15-16, 22-24
Glomerular filtration rate, 267
Glomerulonephritis, 107-108
Glucocorticoids
    assessment and management, 213-215
    bone formation, 212-213
    epidemiology and pathogenesis, 211-213
    hypercalcemia, 589
    inhibitory effects, 213
    receptors, 442
    systemic vs. topical, 211, 214
Glucose tolerance in primary hyperparathyroidism, 356
Gompertzian model of chronic disease, 136, 148-149
Gonadal hormone and bone loss, 182
Gouty diathesis, pathophysiology, 545
Granulocytes, 105
Granulomatous diseases with hypercalcemia, 475, 476
Grave's disease, 311
Growth factors
    bone formation, 222-223
    circulating, 323-332

Growth factors (cont)
    multiple endocrine neoplasia, 324-327
    parathyroid hyperplasia, 323-332
    see also Hematopoietic growth
        factors
Growth retardation
    mechanical usage effects, 21-22
    renal tubular acidosis, 375, 377
Guanyl nucleotide binding protein, 341

Handigodu syndrome, 129
Hearing impairment in osteoporosis, 374
Hematologic disorders, See
    Hypercalcemia; Myeloma
Hematopoietic growth factors, 105-112
    eosinophils and granulocytes, 106
    osteoclast differentiation, 92
    types and sources, 106
    see also Growth factors
Hemiarthroplasty, 229, 289
Hereditary disorders
    deletional model, 563-564
    molecular genetics, 100
    see also Osteoporosis
Hereditary resistance
    clinical and biochemical features,
        447-449
    1,25-dihydroxyvitamin D, 447-453
    intracellular defects, 449-450
    therapy and results, 450-453
    tissue defects, 450
Heterogeneity
    bone loss, 145-147
    clinical implications, 149-150
    fracture risk, 147-148
    osteoporosis syndromes, 145-152
Hip bone
    experimental procedures, 241
    fluoride effect, 294
    mineral measurements, 241
    see also Femoral bone
Hip fractures, 145, 227-230
    age-related, 150, 227, 231, 233
    bone loss, 253-263
    defenses, 233
    densitometry, 155
    epidemiology, 227, 231-236
    estrogen protection, 235, 613
    hemiarthroplasty, 289
    orthopedic management, 287-292
    pathogenesis, 232-233
    physical exercise, 176
    risk factors, 150, 234
    site interrelationships, 228
    stochastic models, 253-263
    types and treatment, 288
    vs. vertebral fractures, 42
    Ward's triangle region, 155
    see also Femoral fractures
Hip osteoporosis, 293-301
    DPA measurements, 293
    fluoride treatment, 293-295
    fractures, 293-301
    medical management, 293-301
    scanning methods, 299-300
Hip replacement, 299
Histomorphometry, 49
    age-related changes, 61-63
    bone remodeling, 60-63
    cell biology, 46-47
    femoral fractures, 270-271
    hormonal effects, 76-77
    iliac crest biopsy, 249
    secular trends, 63
    sex differences, 65
    see also specific disorders
Hodgkin's disease, hypercalcemia
    mechanisms, 520
Hormonal effects
    activation frequency, 74
    bone formation, 74
    histomorphometry, 76-77
    hypothyroidism, 79-80
    osteoid mineralization, 73-87
    remodeling and resorption, 46, 74
    skeletal turnover, 73-87
    stereology, 76
    trabecular remodeling, 73-87
Hormones
    adenylate cyclase inhibition, 335-336
    carbonic anhydrase deficiency, 378-379
    1,25-dihydroxyvitamin D3, 439-440
    vs. exercise therapy, 176
    inhibitors, 378-379
    tetracycline labeling, 73
Human milk, phosphorus-deficient, 418-419
Humoral hypercalcemia of malignancy,
    510-512
    DNA analysis, 510
    parathyroid hormone, 510, 512
    pathogenesis, 511
    radioimmunoassays, 511
Humoral secretagogue theory of multiple
    endocrine neoplasia, 324
Hydroxyproline
    age-related changes, 64
    biochemical marker, 45
    Paget's disease, 528
    resorption marker, 50
    see also Collagen
Hyperabsorbers, aluminum, 555-557
Hypercalcemia
    aluminum-related, 558
    analytical methods, 504
    B-cell lymphomas, 520
    bisphosphonate treatment, 506, 576,
        581-587
    breast cancer, 509
    Burkitt's lymphoma, 520
    calcitropic hormones, 589
    calcium exchange sites, 500-501
    cytokines, 589
    dietary treatment, 404
    1,25-dihydroxyvitamin D, 475
    epidemic, 395
    excretion studies, 502, 576
    granulomatous diseases, 475, 476
    hematologic disorders, 517-523
    Hodgkin's disease, 520
    hyperparathyroidism, 515
    infantile forms, 385, 475
    leukemias and lymphomas, 519-520
    mechanisms, 517-523
    metastatic bone disease, 509-510
    myelodysplastic syndrome, 131
    neonatal form, 415-417
    osteocalcin levels, 53-54

Hypercalcemia (cont)
　　osteoclast inhibition, 576
　　pathophysiology, 499-507
　　primary hyperparathyroidism, 359
　　solid tumors, 509-516
　　steady state mechanisms, 502
　　therapeutic advances, 589-595
　　tumor-associated, 582-586
　　Williams syndrome, 395, 396
Hypercalcemia of malignancy, 575-577
　　amidronate treatment, 576, 584-586
　　clodronate therapy, 576, 583
　　cytokines, 522
　　gallium nitrate, 576, 589-595
　　newer therapies, 575-577
　　WR-2721 treatment, 589-595
Hypercalcinuria
　　absorptive and renal, 543-544
　　classification, 544
　　1,25-dihydroxyvitamin D, 544
　　infantile hypophosphatasia, 385
　　pathophysiology, 496, 543-545
　　phosphorus modulation, 456
　　prostaglandins, 545
　　sodium cellulose phosphate, 546-547
　　thiazide treatment, 547
　　Williams syndrome, 400
Hyperchloremia and renal tubular
　　　acidosis, 374
Hyperparathyroidism
　　calcium set point, 501
　　gallium nitrate and WR-2721, 589-595
　　glucocorticoid-mediated, 212-213
　　hormonal changes, 81-82
　　and hypercalcemia, 504
　　primary form, 8-10, 353-365
　　remodeling inbalance, 9
　　surface-specific remodeling, 8-10
　　surgical management, 353-358
　　therapeutic advances, 589-595
　　trabecular remodeling, 81-82
Hyperplasias, parathyroid cell, 323-332,
　　　353-354
Hypertension, 356
Hyperthyroidism
　　bone volume, 79
　　hormonal changes, 77-79
　　see also Grave's disease
Hypervitaminosis
　　Williams syndrome, 396
　　see also Vitamin D
Hypocalcemia, neonatal, 371
Hypocitraturia, 496
　　pathophysiology, 545
　　renal stones, 545
Hypomagnesemia, 417
Hypomineralization
　　infantile, 417-420
　　periosteocystic lesions, 426
Hypophosphatasia
　　adult form, 384-386
　　alkaline phosphatase activity, 385,
　　　387
　　biochemical markers, 385
　　calcitonin treatment, 392
　　classification, 383
　　clinical features, 383-384
　　cortisone treatment, 388
　　dental manifestations, 383, 387
　　hereditary, 387
　　laboratory studies, 384-385
　　natural substrates, 385
　　orthopedic management, 389
　　pediatric forms, 369-370, 383-393
　　perinatal and infantile, 383-386
　　phospholipid defect, 393
　　prenatal diagnosis, 389
　　radiology and histopathology, 386-387
　　routine assays, 384-385
　　TNSALP treatment, 389-390
　　treatment and diagnosis, 388-389
　　vitamin B6 metabolism, 390, 392
Hypophosphatemia
　　genetic defect, 387
　　molecular basis, 387
　　phosphorus modulation, 457-458
　　see also VDRR
Hypophosphatemic rickets, 130-131
　　ectopic calcification, 130-131
　　phosphorus metabolism, 469
　　see also VDRR
Hypothyroidism
　　bone volume, 80
　　hormonal changes, 79
　　osteoid mineralization, 79-80
　　trabecular remodeling, 77-80
Hypoxanthine phosphoribosyltransferase,
　　　313

Iliac crest biopsy, 49-50
　　bone mass, 247-249
　　vs. noninvasive techniques, 249
　　skeletal sites, 247-252
　　turnover rate, 249-251
Implants, demineralized bone, 114-115
Indomethacin treatment of Caffey's
　　　disease, 42
Induction, See Bone induction
Infantile hypophosphatasia, 383-386
　　calcitonin treatment, 392
　　clinical features, 384
　　genetic defect, 387-388
　　radiologic findings, 386
Infants
　　calcium deficiency, 419-420
　　formula, 419-420
　　hypomineralization, 419
　　phosphorus deficiency, 418-419
　　vitamin D deficiency, 419
　　see also Pediatric patients
Infectious diseases and G proteins, 337
Infusion, calcium, 502
Insulin-like growth factors, 215
Interleukin, 106
Intertrochanteric fractures, orthopedic
　　　management, 289-290
Intestinal absorption of calcium, 500
Intracaval infusions, 450, 452
Intracellular defects and vitamin
　　　deficiency, 449-450
Involutional osteoporosis, 149
Ischemic heart disease, estrogen-mediated,
　　　54, 614
Isoenzymes, thermolability, 52

Jewett nail in trochanteric fractures, 290

Kidney stones, See Renal stones
Knudsen's model of oncogene activation, 324

Leukemia
  acute lymphoblastic, 131
  bone density, 131
  CSF applications, 109
  hypercalcemia mechanisms, 519-520
  and lymphoma, 519-520
Linear stochastic model of bone loss, 254-257
Lipoprotein metabolism
  estrogen effects, 619
  parathyroid-mediated, 356
Lithotripsy, 548-549
Local shock absorbers in hip fractures, 232
Looser's zones in Paget's disease, 528
Lung disease and carbonic anhydrase deficiency, 375
Lymphoblastic leukemia, childhood acute, 131
Lymphokines in bone resorption, 511
Lymphoma, hypercalcemia-associated, 475, 519-520
Lymphotoxin, 518

Macromodeling, 16, 29
Macrophages, 105
Magnesium
  neonatal hypocalcemia, 417
  uptake, 171
Malabsorption and vitamin deficiency, 275
Malnutrition and bone loss, 168
Malignant hypercalcemia
  corticosteroid therapy, 583
  current treatments, 582
  rehydration therapy, 582
Marble bone disease, See Osteoporosis
Mass screening for osteoporosis, 158
Measurement methods
  biochemical markers, 61
  bone remodeling, 60-61
  calcium kinetics, 60
  see also Densitometry; Histomorphometry
Mechanical usage, 19-25
  adult effects, 22
  baseline properties, 30
  bone mass, 15-42
  children, 21-22
  clinical features, 19
  cortical modeling, 23
  and disuse, 22
  growth effects, 21-22
  known and probable functions, 29
  overloads and underloads, 22-24
  pathophysiology, 19, 20, 23
  remodeling functions, 15-42
  strain and stress, 20-21
  tissue response modes, 30-31
Mechanostat
  bone mass, 25-26
  modeling and remodeling, 25-26
Mediator mechanisms in bone biology, 35

Medullary thyroid carcinoma
  clinical features, 565-566
  osteoid mineralization, 83
  trabecular remodeling, 83
Menopause and bone loss, 137, 182-183
Menstrual cycle and bone preservation, 174
Mental retardation in carbonic anhydrase deficiency, 374
Metabolic bone disease
  aging and osteoporosis, 273-285
  allied disciplines, 91-93
  aluminum-related, 597-604
  in children, 369-371
  carbonic anhydrase deficiency, 369, 373-382
  femoral bone, 253-263
  femoral fractures, 265-271
  femoral neck, 237-246
  hematopoietic growth factors, 105-112
  hip fractures, 227-230, 231-236, 253-263
  hip osteoporosis, 293-301
  hypercalcemia and hyperparathyroidism, 589-595
  iliac crest biopsy, 247-252
  induction methods, 113-116
  medical management, 293-301
  neonatal disorders of mineral metabolism, 371, 415-423
  osteogenesis imperfecta, 370, 407-414
  osteopetrosis, 369, 373-382
  osteoporosis, 605-612, 621-630
  pediatric hypophosphatasia, 369, 383-393
  severe hypercalcemia, 581-587
  stochastic models, 253-263
  surgical management of skeletal tumors, 117-126
  therapeutic advances, 575-579
  vitamin D, 265-271, 273-285
  VDRR, 425-432
  Williams syndrome, 370, 395-405
Metabolism
  clinical disorders, 495-497
  hematologic malignancies, 495-496, 517-523
  hypercalcemia, 499-507, 517-523
  multiple endocrine neoplasia, 563-571
  Paget's disease, 525-542
  renal osteodystrophy, 553-562
  solid tumors, 509-516
  see also Mineral metabolism
Metabolites, 205-210
Metacarpal bone loss, 10, 260
Metallothionine, 464
Metaphyseal bone changes, steroid-induced, 222
Metastatic bone disease
  amidronate treatment, 585
  hypercalcemia, 509-510
  mechanisms, 509-510
Microdamage, 29
  bone pain, 34
  drug-induced, 28
  macromodeling, 29
  management, 34
  metabolic bone disease, 33-34
  pathophysiology, 26-29

Microdamage (cont)
  remodeling pathway, 28-29
  repair techniques, 28
Micromodeling, 17, 18
Mineral metabolism
  clinical disorders, 495-497
  hematologic malignancies, 517-523
  hypercalcemia, 499-507, 517-523
  neonatal disorders, 415-423
  renal osteodystrophy, 553-562
  solid tumors, 509-516
  see also Calcium metabolism
Mineralization
  age-related, 62, 190, 194
  apposition rate, 62, 63
  ethnic differences, 132
  lag time, 62
  postmenopausal, 190
  premature infants, 417-420
  surface changes, 62
Minimodeling, 16
Minimum effective strain, 26
Mithramycin
  malignant hypercalcemia, 582
  Paget's disease, 532
Mitochondrial function, phosphate effect, 486-487
Molecular cloning, 440-441
Molecular genetics, 95-103
  atherosclerotic heart disease, 95-96
  hereditary osteoporosis, 100
  hypophosphatemia, 387
  osteopenic bone disease, 91, 95-103
Monoamine metabolism in hyperparathyroidism, 355
Monoclonal antibodies
  osteosarcoma management, 124
  skeletal tumors, 126
Monoclonal tumors, 311, 314
Monokines in bone resorption, 511
Monte Carlo techniques, 253
Morphogenetic proteins and bone formation, 215
Movement disorders, See Carbonic anhydrase deficiency
MRI (magnetic resonance imaging)
  musculoskeletal disorders, 92
  skeletal tumors, 118-119
Mucormycosis, deferoxamine-related, 602-603
Multiple endocrine neoplasia (type 1), 323-332
  angiogenesis, 326-327
  autoimmune theory, 324
  chromosomal theory, 324
  familial form, 323
  fibroblast growth factors, 325-327
  humoral secretagogue theory, 324
  multistage theory, 324
  screening and etiology, 323-324
Multiple endocrine neoplasia (type 2A), 563-572
  adrenal medullary disease, 566-567
  chromosome linkage, 564-565
  deletional model, 563-564
  descriptive phase, 563
  gene mapping, 564-565
  hereditary malignancy, 563-564
  medullary thyroid carcinoma, 565-567
  pathogenesis and indications, 563-571
  see also Parathyroid hormone disorders
Musculoskeletal disorders
  biopsy and staging, 119-124
  MRI techniques, 92
  tumors and sarcomas, 119-124
Myelodysplastic syndrome, clinical cases, 131
Myelogenous leukemia, 109
Myeloma, 517-519
  bone destruction, 517-518
  calcitonin challenge test, 51
  hematologic malignancy, 517-519
  hypercalcemia mechanisms, 495, 518-519
Myelomatosis, See Myeloma

Nasal spray, See Calcitonin
Neck fractures in osteoporosis, 189
Neonatal disorders
  mineral metabolism, 415-423
  see also Children; Infants
Neonatal hypocalcemia
  early and late, 415-417
  hypophosphatemia, 416-417
  magnesium sulfate therapy, 417
  pathophysiology, 415-416
  parathyroid hormone function, 417
  seizures, 416-417
Nephrocalcinosis, 591
Nephrolithiasis, See Renal stones
Nesidioblastosis theory of multiple endocrine neoplasia, 323-324
Neural crest theory of multiple endocrine neoplasia, 323, 324
Neurofibromatosis, See Pheochromocytoma
Neutropenia
  AIDS-related, 108
  CFS applications, 108-109
  see also Leukemia
Nutrition
  aging and osteoporosis, 273-285
  calcium and magnesium, 171
  older patients, 274-275
  surveys of children, 168
  vitamin D, 273-285
Noncollagen proteins, 414
Nongenetic heart disease, 95
Noninvasive measurement of bone loss, 237-246
Nonlinear stochastic model, 256, 257

Obesity
  serum values, 482
  urinary values, 483
  vitamin D metabolism, 481-491
Ocular complications of deferoxamine therapy, 599
Odontohypoohosphatasia, 383, 387
Oligomenorrhea and bone mass, 174
Oncogene
  Knudsen model of activation, 324
  multiple endocrine neoplasia, 324, 327
Optic atrophy in carbonic anhydrase deficiency, 375
Orange juice, calcium-fortified, 185-186
Orthopedics
  hip fractures, 287-292

Orthopedics (cont)
    osteoporotic fractures, 287-288
    see also Sports medicine
Orthopedist, 287-292
Ossification, See Osteogenesis imperfecta
Osteitis fibrosa
    bone formation, 553-554
    dialysis patients, 553-554
    serum aluminum levels, 556
    vitamin D therapy, 553-554
    see also Paget's disease
Osteoarthritis, See Rheumatoid arthritis
Osteoblast-mediated bone loss, 146
Osteocalcin
    bone marker, 53-54
    hypercalcemia, 53-54
    Paget's disease, 528
    radioimmunoassays, 53
Osteoclasts
    activating factor, 511
    bone loss mediator, 146
    CSF applications, 111
    hypercalcemia inhibitor, 576
Osteoconduction, 113
Osteodystrophy
    aluminum-related, 459
    childhood, 459
    induced endochondral, 114
    see also Renal osteodystrophy
Osteogenesis, induced endochondral, 114
Osteogenesis imperfecta
    biochemistry, 408-412
    childhood, 370, 407-414
    clinical heterogeneity, 408-409
    collagen biosynthesis, 97-98, 407-408
    dwarfism, 411
    inherited phenotype, 410
    medical therapies, 412
    mild to severe, 411-412
    molecular basis, 407-414
    molecular genetics, 96-98
    phenotype correlation, 412
    perinatal, 410-411
    point mutations, 411
    procollagen biosynthesis, 407-408
    progressive deforming, 411
    types and features, 409-412
Osteogenic sarcoma, 126
Osteoid mineralization, 75-76
    age-related changes, 63
    acromegaly, 83-84
    estrogen-treated osteoporosis, 82-83
    hormonal effects, 73-87
    hyperthyroidism, 77-79
    hypothyroidism, 79-80
    medullary thyroid carcinoma, 83
    sex differences, 65
    surface thickness, 63
Osteoinduction, 113, 114
Osteolysis, familial expansile, 129
Osteomalacia, 553-554
    alkaline phosphatase, 52
    aluminum-related, 554-555, 597
    antacid-induced, 458-459
    biochemical features, 269
    vs. early renal osteodystrophy, 284-285
    femoral fractures, 265
    histomorphometry, 270-271
    renal phosphate transport, 470
    treatment, 388
    tumor-induced, 470
    vitamin D deficiency, 52, 282
    see also Rickets
Osteomyelitis, See Fractures
Osteopenia
    clinical cases, 131
    corticosteroid-induced, 138-139
    genetic basis, 96, 99, 102
    heterogeneity, 96-97
    mechanical usage effects, 22
    molecular genetics, 91, 95-103
    myelodysplastic syndrome, 131
    osteocalcin levels, 53-54
    single gene disorders, 98-99
    vertebral fractures, 11-12
Osteopetrosis, 373-382
Osteoporosis, 273-285
    ADFR regimen, 142
    age and aging, 273-285
    biochemical features, 269
    bone development, 165-172
    calcitonin therapy, 138, 199-204
    calcium controversy, 137
    deflazacort management, 214
    densitometry, 136, 153-163
    diagnosis and severity, 157
    1,25-dihydroxyvitamin D3, 205-206
    diphosphonate therapy, 138, 199-204
    distal cross section, 189, 192
    fluoride treatment, 578, 605-612
    fractures, 266, 287-288
    fragility, 32, 59
    future research, 142
    gene markers, 99-100
    glucocorticoid-induced, 212-213
    Gompertzian model, 136
    hereditary, 100
    heterogeneity of syndromes, 145-152
    histomorphometry, 270-271
    hydroxyproline marker, 51
    involutional, 149
    mass screening, 158
    neck fractures, 189
    newer therapies, 577-579
    osteocalcin levels, 54
    parathyroid peptide treatment, 578-579, 621-630
    phosphate effects, 277-278
    postmenopausal and perimenopausal, 145, 181-204
    recognition and prevention, 135, 142, 191-193
    remodeling and preservation, 7-14, 173-179
    risk factors, 189-191
    sex hormone deficiency, 214-215
    steroid problem, 211-223
    stochastic models, 253-263
    trabecular remodeling, 82-83, 621
    transdermal estrogen, 578, 616
    treatment model, 606
    vitamin D therapy, 138, 205-210, 273-285, 444-445
Osteosarcoma
    biological features, 92
    surgical management, 124
    see also Paget's disease

Osteosclerosis, See Osteopetrosis
Osteotomy, medial displacement, 290
Osteotropic drugs, See Estrogen
Overloads and underloads, 22-24

Paget's disease, 525-542
    anatomic distribution, 529, 530
    alkaline phosphatase, 52, 528
    APD treatment, 532, 533-534
    assessment and therapy, 525-542
    bones affected, 526-527
    calcitonin and bisphosphonate
        treatments, 530-531
    calcium metabolism, 528
    clinical cases, 130
    clodronate treatment, 532, 533
    cyst-like lesions, 528
    epidemiology, 528-529
    etidronate treatment, 532-533
    hereditary, 130
    histology and pathogenesis, 526
    hydroxyproline measurements, 534-535
    immunologic features, 535-536
    mithramycin treatment, 532
    monitoring methods, 535
    osteogenic sarcoma, 126, 529
    pain and fractures, 529
    radiodiagnostics, 526-527
    response and remission, 533-536
    scintigraphy and radiography, 526-527
    second generation bisphosphonates,
        533-536
    secondary prevention, 525-542
    serum and urine chemistry, 528
    stromal and hemopoietic cells, 526
    symptoms and prognosis, 530
Pain therapy, 536
Parathyroid adenomas
    gene cloning, 313
    methylation patterns, 313-314
    molecular genetics, 313
    vs. primary hyperplasia, 312-313
    tumor clonality, 311-316
Parathyroid hormone
    age and aging, 266-267
    biochemistry, 268
    cancer significance, 512
    circulating markers, 359
    function, 353-354
    inhibitors, 342-343
    plasma levels, 266-267
    radioimmunoassays, 360
    resistance mechanism, 341-342
    serum levels, 277, 280
    surgical effects, 353, 354
Parathyroid hormone disorders, 305-309
    adenomas, 311-316
    C-cell abnormalities, 567, 568
    cell hyperplasia, 323-332
    circulating growth factor, 323-332
    clinical course, 567-568
    G proteins, 333-339
    multiple endocrine neoplasia, 323-332,
        567-568
    primary hyperparathyroidism, 353-365
    pseudohypoparathyroidism, 341-351
    signal transduction, 333-339
    tumor clonality, 311-316

Parathyroid hormone secretion
    calcium-regulated, 317-322
    hypersecretion pathogenesis, 305-306
    physiology and pathophysiology, 317-322
Parathyroid peptide
    ADFR concept, 625
    animal studies, 625
    calcium balance changes, 623
    continuous infusion, 624
    cytochemistry, 624
    daily injections, 622-623
    1,25-dihydroxyvitamin D3, 624, 625
    estrogen-mediated, 624-625
    future research, 626
    intermittent treatment, 625
    multicenter studies, 622-623
    osteoporosis treatment, 621-630
    radioimmunoassays, 624
    side effects, 626
Parathyroid secretion
    abnormal coupling, 320
    cell surface perturbations, 320
    cooperativity, 319
    distal effects, 321
    dysfunctional derangements, 319-320
    intact and permeabilized cells, 317
    mediators stimulating, 318
    receptor-mediated, 318-319
    physiology and pathophysiology, 317-322
Parathyroid surgery, 353-358
    aluminum accumulation, 558-559
    cardiovascular risk, 356
    function effects, 353-354
    serum calcium levels, 353
    subjective symptoms, 354-355
Parathyroidectomy, 466
Patch, estrogen, 615-616
Peak bone mass
    genetic factors, 165
    perimenopausal, 193
Pediatric patients
    hypophosphatasia, 369-370, 383-393
    see also Children; Infants
Peptide hormones in bone remodeling, 444
Periarticular pain from fluoride therapy,
    609
Perimenopausal patients
    age and aging, 181-183
    bone loss, 137, 181-183
    bone mass, 181-204
    calcium intervention, 184
    densitometry, 156
    diphosphonate therapy, 199-203
    genetic factor, 181
    mechanical loading, 181
Perinatal hypophosphatasia, 383-386
    biochemistry, 387-388
    clinical features, 383
    genetic defects, 387-388
    osteogenesis imperfecta, 410-411
    phospholipid defect, 393
    radiologic findings, 386
Periodontitis, 384
Periosteal envelope, 7-8
Pharmacologic therapies, 32-33
Pheochromocytoma
    adrenal medullary disease, 567
    diagnosis and management, 567
    epinephrine levels, 570

Phosphatase, See Alkaline phosphatase
Phosphoethanolaminuria, 385, 389
Phospholipid defect in hypophosphatasia, 393
Phosphorus
    antacid-bearing, 458
    1,25-dihydroxyvitamin D, 460-467
    hypercalcinuria, 456
    hypophosphatemia, 457-458
    metabolism, 469-474
    modulation, 455-467
    normal diet, 466
    vitamin D metabolism, 455-467
Phosphorus deficiency
    human milk, 418-419
    premature infants, 418-419
Physical therapy and bone mass, 32-33
Pituitary adenomas, 337
Polyarthritis, See Rheumatoid arthritis
Polyclonal tumors, gene analysis, 311, 314
Positive feedback theory of multiple endocrine neoplasia, 324
Postmenopausal patients
    bone formation, 10-12
    clodronate therapy, 200
    osteoporosis, 199-200
    therapeutic agents, 199-200
Potassium
    age-related, 190, 193
    body content, 190, 193
    renal stones, 547-548
Potter syndrome, 421
Prednisone in osteoporosis management, 214
Premature infants
    mineralization problems, 417-420
    phosphorus deficiency, 418-419
    vitamin D deficiency, 417-418
Prenatal diagnosis of hypophosphatasia, 389
Primary hyperparathyroidism, 308
    adenomas and hyperplasias, 353-354
    bone remodeling, 8-10
    calcium metabolism, 355
    cardiovascular disease, 356-357
    densitometry, 359, 360
    diabetes mellitus, 356
    estrogen effects, 362
    genetic factors, 305
    glucose tolerance, 356
    histomorphometry, 360
    hypercalcemia, 359
    hypertension, 356
    malignant diseases, 357
    medical management, 359-365
    monoamine metabolism, 355
    pathogenesis, 305
    phosphorus modulation, 456
    postmenopausal, 8-10
    psychiatric symptoms, 354-355
    renal stones, 354
    resorption depth, 9
    serum calcium levels, 353-354
    sex differences, 360
    subjective symptoms, 354-355
    surgical management, 353-358
Procollagen
    biosynthesis, 407-408
    bone formation, 53
    extension profile, 53
    osteogenesis imperfecta, 410-411
Progestogen
    bone loss, 614
    ischemic heart disease, 614
    side effects, 614
    see also Steroid hormones
Prophylactic agents in postmenopausal osteoporosis, 199-200
Prostaglandins
    bone formation, 215, 219
    hypercalcinuria, 545
    malignant hypercalcemia, 511
Protective responses and hip fractures, 232
Proximal femur
    developmental changes, 237
    DPA measurements, 240-245
    mineral content, 240-245
    Singh index patterns, 238
    trabecular structure, 238
Pseudohypoparathyroidism, 306-307
    adenylate cyclase, 344-345
    classification, 342
    G protein-induced, 336
    hypocalcemia, 343, 347
    parathyroid resistance, 341-351
    pathogenesis, 341-351
    receptor resistance, 342-345
    vitamin D therapy, 345, 348-349
Pseudohypophosphatasia, 384
Psychiatric symptoms in primary hyperparathyroidism, 354-355
Public water supplies, aluminum in, 557
Pulmonary alveolar macrophages, 477
Pyridoxal phosphate, plasma levels, 385
Pyridoxine, See Vitamin B6
Pyrophosphate
    accumulation in hypophosphatasia, 385, 390
    calcium deposition disease, 384
    extracellular, 388
    urine and blood samples, 385

Race, See Ethnic differences
Radiocalcium kinetics
    absorption studies, 266-268
    age-related changes, 63, 266
    biochemistry, 268
    estrogen studies, 63
Radiolabeled bone-seeking agents, 64
RAP (regional acceleratory phenomenon), 41
Red blood cells, See Erythrocytes
Rehydration therapy in malignant hypercalcemia, 582
Remodeling, See Bone remodeling
Renal function
    insufficiency, 456, 459, 464
    phosphorus modulation, 456-457
    vitamin D metabolites, 206-207
    Williams syndrome, 403
Renal osteodystrophy
    aluminum-related, 577, 598
    chelation therapy, 577
    current problems, 553-562
    newer therapies, 577

Renal phosphate transport
   animal models, 471-473
   biochemistry, 472
   calcinosis, 470
   1,25-dihydroxyvitamin D, 469-471
   diseases, 469-472
   hypercalcinuria, 544
   vitamin D metabolism, 469-473
Renal stones, 543-552
   diagnosis and prevention, 546-549
   gouty diathesis, 545
   hypercalcinuria, 543-544
   hypocitraturia, 545
   lithotripsy, 548-549
   pathophysiology, 543-545
   potassium citrate, 547-548
   primary hyperparathyroidism, 354
   selective treatment, 548
   sodium cellulose phosphate, 546-547
   thiazide therapy, 547
   vitamin D receptor, 444
Renal tubular acidosis, 373-382
   bicarbonate transport, 374
   calcium reabsorption, 502, 503
   childhood, 373-382
   clinical features, 373-375
   growth retardation, 375, 377
   hypercalcinuria, 545
   hyperchloremia, 374
   osteopetrosis, 373-382
   pathology and pathogenesis, 375
   proximal and distal, 376-377
   type and severity, 374
Resistance and bone loads, 21
Resorption
   bisphosphonate-inhibited, 581-582
   calcium excretion, 501
   deferoxamine therapy, 600
   depth calculation, 9
   diuretic effect, 214
   drifts, 16
   epidermal growth factor, 511
   fluoride effects, 606, 607
   glucocorticoids, 212
   hormonal effects, 74
   lymphokines and monokines, 511
   measurements, 45
   osteopetrosis, 376
   phosphorus-stimulated, 458
   primary hyperparathyroidism, 8-9
   transdermal estrogen, 616-617
   tumor-induced, 509-510
   whole body rate, 45
Resorption markers, 50-52
   calcitonin, 51
   calcium, 51
   hydroxyproline, 50
   urinary calcium, 51
Retinoblastoma, 330
   hereditary, 553-554
   proposed mechanism, 564
   two-hit theory, 553
Retinol, 442
Reverse osmosis treatment of dialysis water, 557
RFLP (restriction fragment length polymorphism)
   atherosclerotic heart disease, 95-96
   single gene disorders, 98
   tumor clonality, 312, 315
Rheumatoid arthritis
   hormone replacement therapy, 214-215
   prednisone treatment, 214
   primary hyperparathyroidism, 363
   steroid management, 219
Rickets
   alkaline phosphatase, 383
   calcium deficiency, 130
   childhood, 384
   clinical cases, 130
   hereditary, 435
   phosphorus-mediated, 460
   treatment, 388
   vitamin D dependent, 435, 444
   see also Hypophosphatemic rickets; VDRR

Sarcoidosis, 475-480
   calcium metabolism, 475-480
   1,25-dihydroxyvitamin D, 476-478
   related diseases, 475-480
   hypercalcemia, 504
   vitamin D metabolism, 475-480
Sarcoma
   local resection, 124
   see also Osteosarcoma
Scintigraphy in Paget's disease, 526-527
Screening, See Mass screening
Second messengers and parathyroid hormone secretion, 317-322
Secretory cells, parathyroid, 305
Senescence, See Age and aging
Serum calcium
   amidronate effect, 584-585
   ethnic differences, 481
   homeostasis, 499-500
   and obesity, 482
   plasma binding, 499-500
   set point and error correction, 501-502
   surgical effects, 353-354
Sex differences
   biochemical markers, 65
   bisphosphonate retention, 65
   bone remodeling, 46, 65
   histomorphometry, 65
   primary hyperparathyroidism, 360
   working model, 67
Sex hormone
   deficiency in osteoporosis, 214-215
   see also Steroid hormones
Shell teeth, 384
Shock absorbers in hip fractures, 232
Signal transducers, See G proteins
Single gene disorders, 95
   identification, 98-99
   see also Osteogenesis imperfecta; Osteopenia
Singh index patterns for proximal femur, 238
Skeletal tumors, 117-126
   biopsy and staging, 119-124
   diagnosis and imaging, 117, 118
   laboratory tests, 118
   MRI studies, 118-119
   puncture biopsy, 120
   radiographic examination, 118-119
   surgical management, 117-126
   technetium nuclear scan, 119

Skeletal tumors (cont)
   see also Musculoskeletal tumors
Sliding nail device for trochanteric fractures, 290
Sodium cellulose phosphate, See Renal stones
Sodium fluoride, 605-612
   calcium-mediated, 606
   dosage and duration, 606
   osteoporosis therapy, 605-612
   serum measurements, 611
   vertebral fractures, 10
   treatment model, 606
   see also Fluoride therapy
Sorbent hemoperfusion in aluminum-related bone disease, 598
Soy formula, phosphorus-deficient, 418-419
SPA (single photon absorptiometry), 153, 154
Spinal osteoporosis, 165-172
   bone loss, 145-147
   bone preservation, 173-179
   calcitonin and diphosphonates, 199-203
   calcium and estrogen, 181-197
   clinical features, 147
   densitometry, 153-163
   future research, 141-143
   heterogeneity of syndromes, 145-152
   perimenopausal treatment, 181-204
   prevention, 191-193
   steroid problem, 211-223
   teenage female, 165-172
   vitamin D metabolites, 205-210
   young adult female, 173-179
Spine, fluoride effect, 294, 299
Sports medicine
   microdamage physiology, 33-34
   see also Orthopedics
Staging
   sarcomas and lesions, 121-124
   skeletal tumors, 117, 120-124
   see also Surgical management
Stem cells
   availability, 111
   bone marrow, 105
Steroid hormones
   assessment and management, 213-215
   bone remodeling, 444
   epidemiology and pathogenesis, 211-213
   metaphyseal bone changes, 222
   osteoporosis, 136, 211-223
   rheumatoid arthritis, 219
Stochastic models
   femoral bone loss, 253-263
   hip fracture risk, 253-263
   Monte Carlo techniques, 253
Strabismus in osteopetrosis, 374
Stress
   fluoride effect, 609, 611
   fractures, 609, 611
   mechanical usage, 20-21
   and strain, 20-21
Strong bones, development and preservation, 165-179
Supracellular organization in bone remodeling, 45
Suppressor gene theory of multiple endocrine neoplasia, 324

Surface-based bone formation, 10-12
Surface-specific bone remodeling, 7-14
   appendicular and axial, 7-8
   biochemistry and histology, 11
   primary hyperparathyroidism, 8-10
Surgery, parathyroid, 353-358
Surgical management
   bone tumors, 92
   hyperparathyroidism, 353-358
   osteosarcoma, 124
   parathyroid hormone function, 353-354
   primary hyperparathyroidism, 353-358
   sarcomas and lesions, 121-124
   serum calcium, 353-354
   skeletal tumors, 117-126
   staging margins, 122-124

T-cell lymphomas and hypercalcemia, 519
Table surface, bone distance from, 243
Technetium
   nuclear bone scan, 119
   see also Scintigraphy
Teeth, See Shell teeth
Tetracycline labeling in transilial biopsy, 60, 73
Therapeutic advances
   aluminum-related bone disease, 597-604
   bisphosphonate treatment, 581-587
   estrogen administration, 613-620
   gallium nitrate and WR-2721, 589-595
   metabolic bone disease, 575-579
   parathyroid peptide therapy, 621-630
   sodium fluoride in osteoporosis, 605-612
Thiazide treatment of renal stones, 547
Thiophosphate, See WR-2721
Thyroid hormone
   receptors, 442
   trabecular remodeling, 74
   see also Parathyroid hormone
Tissue
   defects, 450
   mechanical usage, 30-31
   response modes, 30-31
TNSALP (tissue nonspecific alkaline phosphatase)
   biosynthesis, 388
   ectoenzyme, 390
   genetic defect, 387-388
   hypophosphatasia, 383, 389-390
   leukocyte form, 385
   pediatric and mutant, 383, 384
   physiologic role, 389-390
Tomography, 92
   skeletal tumors, 118-119
   see also Radiocalcium kinetics
Topical steroids in osteoporosis therapy, 211, 214
Total alkaline phosphatase as bone formation marker, 52
Trabecular bone
   architecture, 621
   fluoride effect, 607-608
   osteoporosis, 621
   parathyroid peptide,, 621-623
   proximal femur, 238
Trabecular remodeling, 74
   acromegaly, 83-84

Trabecular remodeling (cont)
  activation frequency, 74
  age-related changes, 61
  anatomic envelope, 73
  bone mass changes, 75
  calcitonin, 74
  connectivity measurements, 60, 71
  endocrine disorders, 78
  estrogen effects, 82-83
  ethnic differences, 71
  histomorphometry, 76-77
  hormonal effects, 73-87
  hyperparathyroidism, 81-82
  hyperthyroidism, 77-79
  hypothyroidism, 79-80
  medullary thyroid carcinoma 83
  mineralization lag time, 62
  morphology and geometry, 61
  osteoporosis, 82-83
  stereology, 73, 76
  tetracycline labeling, 73
Transdermal estrogen, 615-617
Transilial biopsy, tetracycline labeling, 60
TRAP (tartrate-resistant acid phosphate), 45, 51
Trochanteric fractures
  fixed nail device, 290
  Jewett nail, 290
  orthopedic management, 289-290
  see also Femoral neck
Tumor clonality
  bone resorption, 509-510
  DNA analysis, 312
  gene expression, 315
  parathyroid adenomas, 311-316
  phosphate metabolism, 469
Turnover
  bone, 29, 249-251
  cancellous and cortical, 249-250
  iliac crest biopsy, 249-251
  skeletal in thyroid disorders, 73-87
Two-hit theory
  multiple endocrine neoplasia, 324
  retinoblastoma, 553

Uremia, iliac crest biopsy, 251
Urinary calcium
  ethnic differences, 481, 484
  and obesity, 483
  resorption marker, 51
Urinary hydroxyproline
  age factor, 50
  resorption marker, 50-51
  vitamin D metabolites, 206

VDRR (vitamin D resistant hypophosphatemic rickets)
  adult treatment, 426-427
  basic defect, 425-426
  childhood, 425-432
  clinical features, 425
  1,25-dihydroxyvitamin D, 425-427, 430-431
  hyperparathyroidism, 426, 429
  long-term effects, 426
  osteosclerosis, 429
  pathogenesis and treatment, 371, 425-432
  phosphate repletion, 425-426
Vertebral fractures, 145
  cancellous bone remodeling, 10-12
  estrogen-mediated, 613
  fluoride treatment, 10
  vs. hip fractures, 42
  osteopenic, 11-12
  pathogenesis, 10-12
  postmenopausal, 10-12
  risk heterogeneity, 147-148
Vitamin A, See Retinol
Vitamin B6 and hypophosphatasia, 390, 392
Vitamin D
  active forms, 205
  age effects, 273-285
  cellular uptake, 435-436
  deficiency, 283-284, 417-418
  dosage and safety, 206-207, 220
  endocrine system, 439
  estrogen receptor, 444-445
  femoral fractures, 265-271
  infants, 417-419
  malabsorption, 275
  metabolites, 205-210
  nuclear binding, 435-436
  nutrition, 273-285
  older patients, 274-275
  osteitis fibrosa, 553-554
  osteomalacia, 282
  osteoporosis, 138, 205-210, 273-285, 444-445
  premature infants, 417-418
  pseudohypoparathyroidism, 345, 348
  renal function, 206-207
  sources and sites, 273-274
  spinal osteoporosis, 205-210
  theoretical considerations, 273-274
  Williams syndrome, 395, 396
  see also 1,25-Dihydroxyvitamin D
Vitamin D metabolism, 273-285, 435-437
  clinical disorders, 469-474
  diseases, 475-476
  endocrine system, 439, 481-491
  ethnic differences, 481-491
  geography and nutrition, 484, 488
  hereditary resistance, 435, 447-453
  and obesity, 481-491
  phosphorus-modulated, 455-467
  receptor function, 435, 439-446
  renal phosphate transport, 469-473
  sarcoidosis, 475-480
  Williams syndrome, 396
Vitamin D receptors, 444-445
  galactose catabolism, 442-443
  gene regulation, 442
  hinge mechanism, 440, 441
  molecular action, 442-443
  serines and threonines, 443
  structure and function, 439-446
  transcriptional model, 443
Vitamin D2 in osteoporosis, 205
Vitamin D3, See 1,25-Dihydroxyvitamin D

Wall thickness, age-related changes, 61
Ward's triangle region in hip fractures, 155

Water treatment units, aluminum from, 557-558
Whole body retention
    bone-seeking agents, 64
    remodeling measurements, 60
Whooping cough and G proteins, 337
Williams syndrome, 395-401
Wolff's law and bone remodeling, 24-25
Women
    creatinine clearance, 266-267
    fractures and falls, 189, 191, 232
    hip fractures, 234
    primary hyperparathyroidism, 7-14
    radiocalcium absorption, 266-267
    surface-specific bone resorption, 7-14
    see also Osteoporosis
WR-2721
    bone resorption, 592
    hypercalcemia and hyperparathyroidism, 589-595
Wrist fracture, See Colles' fracture

X-chromosomes
    methylation patterns, 313-314
    monoclonal tumors, 312
XLH (X-linked hypophosphatemia)
    animal models, 471-473
    metabolic defect, 426
    renal phosphate transport, 469-470
    vitamin D metabolism, 469-470

Young adult female
    bone preservation, 173-179
    calcium and exercise, 175-176
    menstrual cycle, 174
Young's modulus of elasticity, 21

Zinc
    detoxification, 464
    finger in vitamin D metabolism, 440